AF316749

Contemporary Management of Spinal Cord Injury: From Impact to Rehabilitation

AANS Publications Committee
Charles H. Tator, MD, and
Edward C. Benzel, MD, Editors

Neurosurgical Topics

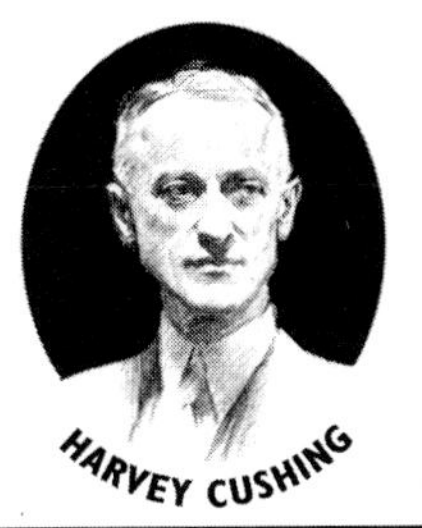

American
Association of
Neurological
Surgeons

Contemporary Management of Spinal Cord Injury: From Impact to Rehabilitation
Charles H. Tator, MD, and Edward C. Benzel, MD, Editors

The CME activity was planned and produced in accordance with the ACCME Essentials.
Released July 2000.

Library of Congress Catalog
ISBN: 1-879284-72-3

Neurosurgical Topics ISBN: 0-9624246-6-8

Warren R. Selman, MD, Chairman
AANS Publications Committee

Gay L. Palazzo, AANS Staff Editor

AANS1M700

Neurosurgical Topics SERIES

FORTHCOMING BOOKS

2000/2001

Neural Prostheses
Edited by Robert J. Maciunas, MD

Neurosurgical Injuries in Sports
Edited by Julian Bailes, MD

Surgical Management of Low Back Pain
Edited by Daniel K. Resnick, MD, and Regis William Haid, Jr., MD

Dedication

We dedicate this book to the individuals
with spinal cord injury
who have taught us so much and
from whom we have much to learn.

CONTENTS

LIST OF CONTRIBUTORS

Sheila M. Alton, MD, FACEP
Department of Emergency Medicine
Liberty Hospital
Liberty, Missouri

Jose Arias, MD
Department of Neurological Surgery
University of Miami
Jackson Memorial Medical Center
Miami, Florida

Nevan G. Baldwin, MD
Division of Neurosurgery
University of New Mexico School of Medicine
Albuquerque, New Mexico

Perry A. Ball, MD
Section of Neurosurgery
Dartmouth-Hitchcock Medical Center
Lebanon, New Hampshire

Edward C. Benzel, MD, FACS
Department of Neurosurgery
The Cleveland Clinic Foundation
Cleveland Ohio

Ronald E. Chicoine, MD
Department of Anesthesiology
Central Maine Medical Center
Lewiston, Maine

William F. Collins, MD
Department of Neurological Surgery
Yale University School of Medicine
New Haven, Connecticut

H. Alan Crockard, FRCS
Department of Surgical Neurology
National Hospital for Neurology and
    Neurosurgery
Queen Square
London, England

John F. Ditunno, Jr., MD
Director
Regional Spinal Cord Injury Center
    of Delaware Valley
Thomas Jefferson University Hospital
Philadelphia, Pennsylvania

Devanand A. Dominique, MD, BCh
Fellow, Spinal Program
Division of Neurosurgery
Toronto Western Hospital
University of Toronto
Toronto, Ontario, Canada

Marc E. Eichler, MD
Division of Neurosurgery
Brigham and Women's Hospital
Boston, Massachusetts

Michael G. Fehlings, MD, PhD, FRCS(C)
Professor of Surgery, Division of Neurosurgery
Robert O. Lawson Chair in
    Neural Repair and Regeneration
Research Director, Division of Neurosurgery
Head, Spinal Program,
    University Health Network
Toronto Western Hospital
University of Toronto
Toronto, Ontario, Canada

Christopher S. Formal, MD
Magee Rehabilitation Hospital
Philadelphia, Pennsylvania

Fred H. Geisler, MD, PhD
Department of Neurosurgery
Chicago Institute of Neurosurgery and
    Neuroresearch
Rush University
Chicago, Illinois

Andrew Gettinger, MD
Department of Anesthesiology
Dartmouth-Hitchcock Medical Center
Lebanon, New Hampshire

Ziya L. Gokaslan, MD
Assistant Professor
Chief, Spine Program
Department of Neurosurgery
Clinical Assistant Professor of Neurosurgery
Baylor College of Medicine
Houston, Texas

Barth A. Green, MD, FACS
Professor and Chair
Department of Neurological Surgery
University of Miami School of Medicine
Miami, Florida

James D. Guest, MD, PhD
Assistant Professor of Neurological Surgery
University of Miami
The Miami Project to Cure Paralysis
The Miami Veterans Administration
Medical Center
Miami, Florida

Sender Herschorn, BSc, MDCM, FRCSC
Professor of Surgery/Urology
University of Toronto
Director of Urodynamics
Sunnybrook and Women's Health Sciences Centre
Toronto, Ontario, Canada

Howard J. Landy, MD, FACS
Associate Professor of Neurological Surgery
University of Miami School of Medicine
Miami, Florida

Peter J. Lennarson, MD
Division of Neurosurgery
University of Iowa Hospitals and Clinics
Iowa City, Iowa

Dennis J. Maiman, MD, PhD
Spinal Cord Injury Center
Milwaukee, Wisconsin

Paul McCormick, MD
Neurosurgical Associates, PC
The Neurological Institute
New York, New York

Arnold H. Menezes, MD
Division of Neurosurgery
University of Iowa Hospitals and Clinics
Iowa City, Iowa

William Mitchell, MD
Department of Neurosurgery
Jefferson Medical College
Thomas Jefferson University
Philadelphia, Pennsylvania

Walter Montanera, MD, FRCP(C)
Associate Professor
Department of Medical Imaging
University of Toronto
Division of Neuroradiology
Toronto Western Hospital
Toronto, Ontario, Canada

Raul C. Ordorica, MD
Assistant Professor
Division of Urology
University of South Florida
James A. Haley Veterans Hospital
Tampa, Florida

David Peterson, BSc, FRCS
Department of Neurosurgery
Charing Cross Hospital
London, England

Gregory J. Przybylski, MD
Assistant Professor
Department of Neurosurgery
Jefferson Medical College
Thomas Jefferson University
Philadelphia, Pennsylvania

Setti S. Rengachary, MD
Wayne State University
Department of Neurosurgery
Detroit, Michigan

Donna J. Rodriguez, MS, RD, CNSD
Independent Consultant, Medical Writer
Albuquerque, New Mexico

Ranjan S. Roy, MD, PhD
Rowan Neurosurgical Associates
Salisbury Professional Center
Salisbury, North Carolina

Lali S. Sekhon, MBBS, PhD, FRACS
Fellow, Division of Neurosurgery
Toronto Western Hospital
University of Toronto
Toronto, Ontario, Canada

Ran Vijai P. Singh, MD
University of Miami
Miami, Florida

Volker K.H. Sonntag, MD
Barrow Neurological Institute
St. Joseph's Hospital and Medical Center
Phoenix, Arizona

Charles B. Stillerman, MD
Clinical Professor
Department of Surgery
University of North Dakota School of Medicine
Director of Neurosurgery
Trinity Medical Center
Minot, North Dakota

Sonia Suys, MD
University of Miami
Miami, Florida

**Charles H. Tator, CM, MD, PhD,
    FRCS(C), FACS**
Professor, Division of Neurosurgery
Department of Surgery
Toronto Western Hospital and
    University of Toronto
Toronto, Ontario, Canada

Cathleen S. Van Buskirk, MD
Alpine Spine Center
Boulder, Colorado

Philip A. Villanueva, MD
Department of Neurosurgery
University of Miami
Miami, Florida

W. Waring III, MD
Spinal Cord Injury Center
Milwaukee, Wisconsin

Jack E. Wilberger, MD
Professor and Acting Chairman
Department of Neurosurgery
Allegheny General Hospital
Medical College of Pennsylvania
    Hahnemann University School of Medicine
Pittsburgh, Pennsylvania

AANS Publications Committee

HOME STUDY EXAMINATION INFORMATION

Contemporary Management of Spinal Cord Injury: From Impact to Rehabilitation
Charles H. Tator, MD, and Edward C. Benzel, MD, Editors
Released July 2000
CME Credits Expiration: July 2003

The American Association of Neurological Surgeons (AANS) is accredited by the Accreditation Council for Continuing Medical Education (ACCME) to sponsor Continuing Medical Education (CME) for physicians. *Neurosurgical Topics* Home Study Examinations were planned and produced in accordance with the ACCME Essentials.

The AANS designates this CME activity for a maximum of 15 hours in category 1 credit toward the AMA Physician's Recognition Award. Each physician should claim only the number of hours that he or she actually spent studying the CME enduring material.

Participants have 3 years from the date of publication shown on this enduring material to complete the Home Study Examination Questions, submit the evaluation form, and request Category 1 credit. The Home Study Examination is presented in the back of this book and in the Education section of the NEUROSURGERY://ON-CALL web site. For more information on CME credits, please refer to the enclosed card or contact the AANS at 888-566-AANS (2267).

The test is to be self-scored. A CME certificate will be mailed upon submission of the evaluation form along with a $30 processing fee.

After reading this book, a physician should be able to:

- diagnose the most common spine fractures
- understand and evaluate today's state-of-the-art concepts regarding the management of spinal cord injury
- apply appropriate surgical techniques
- develop a multidisciplinary approach to the management of the spinal cord injured-patient

PREFACE

This book is born out of mutual interests in spinal cord injury. Although our interests are derived from different orientations and backgrounds, there are more similarities than differences. The similarities have permitted us to add depth to this treatise. Our differences have allowed us to add breadth.

This book is also born out of an earlier publication, *Contemporary Management of Spinal Cord Injury,* published by the AANS Publications Committee. This work harbors some similarities to our previous work. Multiple additions, as well as revisions, have been made. This book has many authors. It is hoped that the multi-authored approach used herein is appropriate from an educational perspective, or at the very least, adds variety and stimulates interest. In this context, repetition is inevitable. We, however, learn best by being repetitively exposed to stimuli. Therefore, "repetition is indeed good" and should be encouraged and not discouraged, as is sometimes done.

We truly hope that this volume provides significant added value to the armamentarium of the neurosurgeon, orthopaedic surgeon, physiatrist, urologist, and others caring for the victims of spinal cord injury. If, in any way, it can contribute to an increased awareness of this devastating problem and its management by educating and provoking thought, it will have been a worthwhile endeavor. Thank you in advance for partaking in the fruits of our labor.

Charles H. Tator, MD
Toronto, Ontario, Canada

Edward C. Benzel, MD
Cleveland, Ohio

June 2000

CHAPTER 1

THE CONTRIBUTIONS OF ALLEN, RIDDOCH, AND GUTTMANN TO THE HISTORY OF SPINAL CORD INJURY

WILLIAM F. COLLINS, MD

The first known written history of a surgical subject is almost by tradition the Egyptian Papyrus, more commonly known as the Edwin Smith Surgical Papyrus.[3] Even though the Papyrus gives a clear description of the findings of sensory and motor loss as well as loss of bladder control after spinal cord injury (SCI) in Cases 31 and 33, the references to the treatment of SCI are brief and state "an ailment not to be treated."

Despite this admonition, many physicians over the next three to four thousand years have attempted to treat patients with SCI. About 400 BC, Hippocrates recommended treatment with large amounts of liquids, preferably milk from a donkey, mixed with honey along with Egyptian white wine. These commonly recommended treatment regimens are used even to this day and imply that doctors do not know what to do. Hippocrates, a wise man, hedged his bets and developed a traction apparatus, described by Aulus Cornelius Celsus and illustrated by Vidus Vidius in the book *Chirurgia è Graeco in Latinum Connersa*[12] (Figure 1). An illustration of the instrument appears in Ludwig Guttmann's book *Spinal Cord Injuries: Comprehensive Management and Research*.[5] The reduction technique and instru-

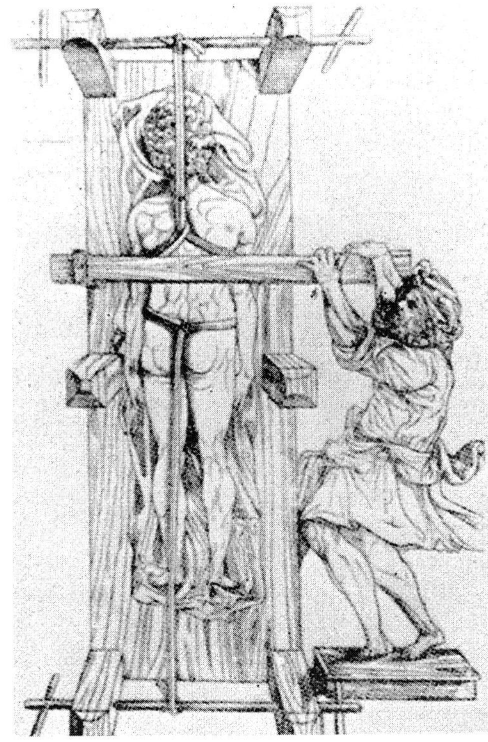

Figure 1: Hippocrates' extension bench, depicted by Oribasius and described in Vidus Vidius' *Chirurgia è Graeco in Latinum Connersa.*

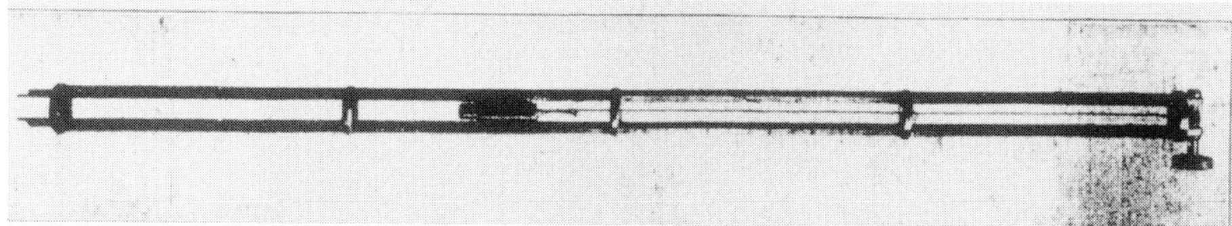

Figure 2: Instrument used by Allen to produce a measured impact on the spinal cord.

mentation were used with various modifications for many centuries. In the 16th century, it was described as the preferred treatment of SCI by the famous French surgeon Paré. In 150 BC, Galen observed the difference between transverse and longitudinal incisions in the spinal cord; the latter did not cause much change in function, whereas the former caused a loss in function.

It is not known who first described the operation of spinal cord decompression by lamina removal, but it is generally attributed to Paulus of Aegina in the 7th century. The operation was used intermittently throughout the centuries with isolated reports of successfully treated cases. Over the years, critics of the forceful and brisk reductions accomplished by the use of Hippocrates' instrument and by decompressive surgery concluded that neither methods appeared to significantly decrease mortality rates and the consensus for SCI therapy returned to "an ailment not to be treated."

This negative notion of care for the SCI patient, particularly the use of surgical decompression, was accepted well into the 19th century. In 1824, Charles Bell could say with conviction, "Laying a patient upon his belly and by incisions laying bare the bones of the spine, breaking up these bones and exposing the spinal marrow itself, exceeds all belief." Even into the turn of the 20th century, few options for effective treatment were available. Experimental studies of the problem by a number of workers, however, began to have some influence on the treatment of SCI. Despite these studies, or perhaps because of them, conflicting treatment positions have continued and even firmed. A dichotomy evolved where one position believed that surgical treatment is advantageous in regaining neurological function after SCI, whereas the opposing view held that it causes an increase in the resulting neurological deficit.

It is not possible to discuss all those who have contributed to the treatment of SCI. Alfred Reginald Allen, George Riddoch, and Ludwig Guttmann, the first two neurologists and the third a neurosurgeon-turned physiatrist, were selected for discussion because their work and influence can be considered a centrum for both the current concepts of treatment and the dichotomy regarding surgery. A brief review of the work and teachings will demonstrate how the modern era of SCI management evolved. It also describes how the work and teachings of these three men facilitated as well as inhibited the development of the treatment of SCI, not an unusual result of differences in opinion in medical care.

ALFRED REGINALD ALLEN

Scientific experimental studies of SCI began during the latter part of the 19th century. In 1890, Schmaus[11] struck boards attached to the backs of rabbits to study the pathological changes in the spinal cord after injury. He noted that, with the passage of time, degeneration and cavitation developed in the area of the blows. Apparent with these studies was that the amount of force, its direction, and the area of delivery were poorly controlled and the neurological outcome could not be predicted. In 1911, Alfred Reginald Allen[2] reported the development of a drop-weight impact experimental model of SCI, where the impact was applied to the dura of the exposed spinal cord in a manner that allowed quantification of the amount of injury and prediction of the neurological outcome (Figure 2). The force was measured by the weight of the object dropped in grams multiplied by the distance dropped in centimeters (gram-centimeters). Histological analysis confirmed that the gray matter of the cord was more sensitive to

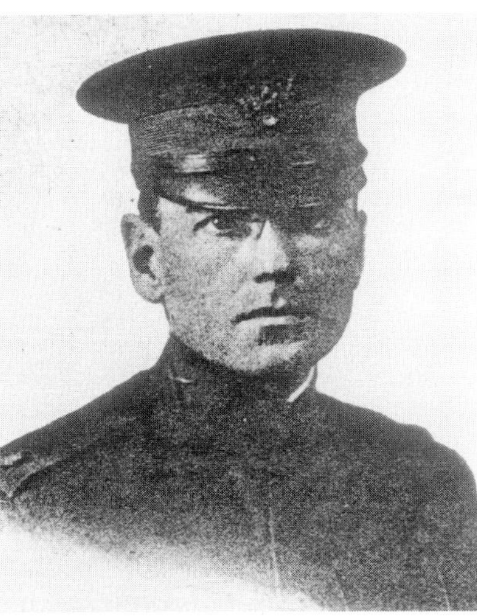

Figure 3: Alfred Reginald Allen. Reproduced courtesy of the University of Pennsylvania Archives, Philadelphia, Pennsylvania.

contusion and that it responded with hemorrhage and what appeared to be necrosis. This progressed to cavitation if the injury caused a severe neurological deficit. These findings led to the hypothesis that a progressive lesion occurred after trauma ("progressive central hemorrhagic necrosis") and that the progression was in part responsible for the resulting neurological deficit. This hypothesis of a secondary injury caused by the response of the nervous system to injury remains the basis for much of the experimental work on SCI, including the recent steroid trials for the acute treatment of SCI. Allen's drop-weight model has remained, with various modifications, the most frequently used model of experimental SCI. The ability to produce a SCI with a predictable outcome has allowed the study of possible therapeutic responses from various treatment regimens. Allen recognized this and used the model to study possible therapeutic approaches to SCI. In a preliminary report in 1911,[2] Allen noted a positive effect, both functionally and histologically, from a longitudinal myelotomy over the area of injury in dogs. In a later report in 1914 entitled "Remarks on the histopathological changes in the spinal cord due to impact: an experimental study,"[1] he expanded this to include the results of myelotomy performed on three patients by Dr. Charles Frazier, the Philadelphia neurosurgeon. These reports by Allen and his presentations at the American Neurological Association considerably influenced American surgeons in the early part of this century (i.e., to use surgery for the acute treatment of SCI).

Allen was born in East Greenwich, Rhode Island, in 1876 (Figure 3). He was descended from a long line of original settlers in New England and Pennsylvania, the Dewolfs, Howes, Pomeroys, and Allens. His preparatory education was at Selwin Hall in Pennsylvania, after which he attended Lehigh University and graduated from the University of Pennsylvania School of Medicine in 1898. A few years later, he joined S. Weir Mitchell for training in neurology. By 1907, he was an instructor in neurology and neuropathology and was appointed assistant neurologist at the University Hospital and chief of the neurology clinic. He also was assistant neurologist at the Pennsylvania Hospital. He attained recognition for his reports on Korsakoff's syndrome, hydrocephalus, and SCI. He was secretary and treasurer of the American Neurological Association from 1907 to 1917 and, because of his interest in the function, anatomy, and response of the spinal cord to injury, was appointed to the faculty of the Department of Experimental Medicine and Surgery and the Department of Neurology at the University of Pennsylvania School of Medicine. He also was a founding member of the Savoy Opera Company of Philadelphia and wrote songs and an opera for the company.

Allen collaborated with Frazier to write *Surgery of the Spine and Spinal Cord*,[4] which was finished in 1917. This was Allen's final written contribution. One might assume that the experimental spark had burned low, but the reason was more tragic. When Germany invaded Belgium, Allen joined the Army Reserve Forces and upon the United States' entry into World War I, he enlisted in the 314th United States Infantry division as an infantry officer, attaining the commission rank of major when his unit was sent to France in July 1918. He was killed at Verdun on September 30, 1918.

A few paragraphs from his 1911 contribution on experimental SCI, in which he demonstrated that longitudinal incisions in the spinal cord did not cause major neurological loss (shades of the work of Galen 2000 years before), demonstrated the pivotal nature of his experimental hypotheses.

Given as the hypothesis that there is a twofold injury factor after impact: 1) the direct injury to axon cylinders from the impact; 2) the outpouring of serum and blood into the substance of the cord; given the condition of the closely investing pia-arachnoid and the inability of drainage; given the comparative absence of symptoms after median longitudinal incision into the spinal cord—the corollary which presented itself was: What effect would a median longitudinal incision into the spinal cord have on subjects submitted to hyperimpact?

The factors suggesting this course were the need for spinal cord drainage thereby accomplishing a spinal cord decompression and the fact the heteromeric neurons in the dog and in man are not of vital importance. In five dogs I have used a hyperimpact of 540 gram-centimeters and then made a medial longitudinal incision from 1 to 1.5 cm. in length directly through the impact level and passing altogether through the spinal cord. These dogs made uneventful recoveries showing only slight spasticity and awkwardness in the hind limbs but not enough to prevent running and jumping. This impact would have led to dire consequences had not the median incision been made.

The final paragraph of this paper stated "The first important step to determine is: How long after injury to the dog's spinal cord can one wait and still obtain the good effect of the drainage from a median longitudinal incision?" The 1914 report answered this query in part but the full answer was not to be completed before Allen joined the army.

Allen's work and his hypothesis of a secondary injury from the response of the nervous system have withstood more than 75 years of studies by other investigators. Many investigators, using variations of his experimental SCI model, continued the format of studying possible physical and pharmacological treatment of SCI by evaluating changes in outcome and supported his hypothesis even though only a few used myelotomy, the technique Allen believed most efficacious.

GEORGE RIDDOCH

Why discuss the work of George Riddoch? Riddoch helped change the playing field for the SCI patient from no hope to one of hope, first

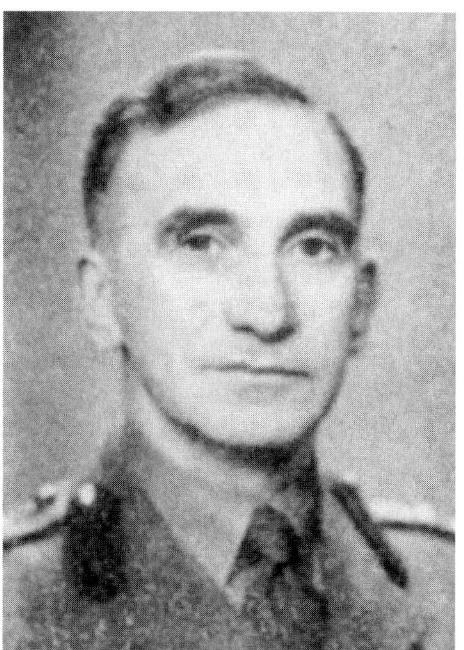

Figure 4: George Riddoch.

through his work with Henry Head and then by appointing Ludwig Guttmann to direct the SCI center at Stoke Mandeville Hospital. George Riddoch (Figure 4) was born in 1888 at Keith Hospital in Banffshire, Scotland, and died in London in 1947. He received his premedical and medical education at Gordon's College in Aberdeen and at Aberdeen University and moved to London just before World War I. In London, he began a career in neurology with Sir Henry Head who assigned him to the development of a unit for the care of nervous system injuries. The level of knowledge in the treatment of SCI at the beginning of World War I is well demonstrated by the report published by Hartwell[8] in 1917 describing the results of 133 cases of SCI admitted to the Massachusetts General Hospital. The series included cases reported by Mixter and Chase, neurosurgeons on the staff of the hospital, treated with decompressive laminectomy. No one with a complete or very severe spinal cord lesion survived either surgical or nonsurgical treatment. Hartwell, who was not a neurosurgeon, believed that the only value of surgery was to lessen the suffering of the operated patients by shortening their lives.

Riddoch and Head established a British Army unit where they developed a system that reversed the survival ratio from less than 10% to almost 90%. Their treatment regimen consisted of special care of the bladder, skin, and nutrition in SCI patients. As more patients with spinal cord injuries were returned to Britain from the warfront, the unit's success became striking. The mortality rates were drastically altered. George Riddoch reported that the human spinal cord, when separated from descending tracts, had all of the spinal reflexes Sherrington had shown in animals. These new findings meant that not only could the incidence of mortality in patients with SCI be markedly reduced by appropriate medical care but, in addition, the isolated spinal cord could and did function so that repair or regeneration of the spinal cord was again a possible dream.[9,10]

The success of this treatment however, was, short-lived because the survivors either did not return to a productive life, were confined to nursing homes, or died from the inevitable breakdown of their treatment in such institutions. This led in the 1930s, 1940s, and 1950s to further attempts at invasive treatments that could possibly regain function. To United States neurosurgeons, this took the form of further attempts at both early and late surgical treatment of the spinal column.

Sir Ludwig Guttmann

In 1943, just as in 1917, the lack of a long survival and the chance for a productive life prepared the way to bring to the fore someone with the belief in and the ability to follow new concepts for the treatment of SCI. As an orderly in Upper Silesia, Sir Ludwig Guttmann, CBE, FRS, FRCP (Figure 5) had witnessed active reduction of the fractured spine followed by casting of the patient. Even in later life he remembered this case and believed that the treatment had caused the patient's increased suffering and death.

Ludwig Guttmann was born in Tost, Upper Silesia, in 1899. His father was an innkeeper who, along with his sister and brother-in-law, was

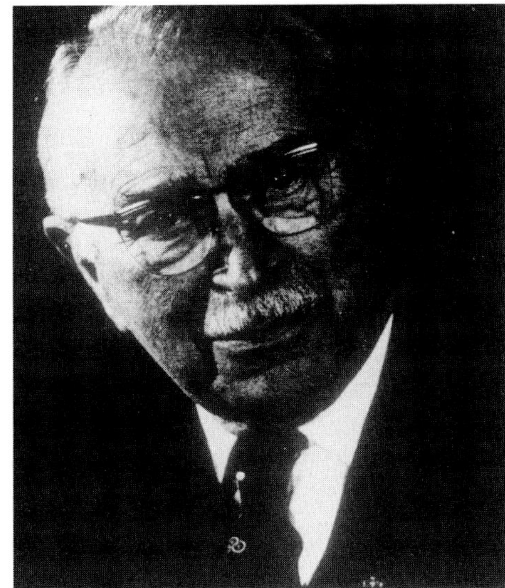

Figure 5: Sir Ludwig Guttmann.

killed at Auschwitz. Guttmann started his medical training in Breslau and completed it with studies in Würzburg and Freiberg, both major centers of surgery at that time. He then worked as an assistant to Otfrid Foerster from 1924 to 1928. In 1928 at the age of 29 years, Guttmann started a neurosurgical unit in Hamburg and had control of the patients and facilities.

In 1929 Foerster asked him to return to Breslau and, because he felt indebted to his teacher, he reluctantly did so, advancing to first associate by 1933. Within a few years, the Nazis forced all Jews to leave Aryan hospitals and Guttmann took over the neurological unit of the Jewish Hospital in Breslau. In 1935, the racial laws took away his right to treat anyone but Jewish patients as well as most of his civilian rights. In 1938 during Krystallnacht, he admitted 64 patients to his service in order to protect them from the Nazi mobs, a fact not overlooked by the Gestapo. This placed him on the Gestapo's list of unreliable citizens and in grave danger. He continued, however, to aid those escaping persecution. In 1939, just before the outbreak of war, he emigrated to England with his family. His emigration was aided by Antonio Salazar, the Dictator of Portugal, who requested that Guttmann see a patient in Lisbon, a request granted because of Germany's desire to maintain Salazar's friendship.

After emigrating to England, Guttmann no longer practiced neurosurgery but instead worked on experimental studies of nerve regeneration with Peter Medawar at Oxford University. In 1941 he wrote a review of rehabilitation after nervous system injuries, which he expanded in 1942;[6,7] this review included his concepts of non-invasive treatment for spinal cord and cauda equina injuries. George Riddoch, a brigadier and consultant to the Emergency Medical Services for treatment of nervous system injuries, recognized that Guttmann had much to offer in the system of special units that he was establishing for care of the large number of wounded soldiers with nervous system injuries. Riddoch offered Guttmann the directorship of a spinal cord unit at Stoke Mandeville Hospital, giving him a reasonably free hand to try to return at least some of the patients to a useful life. The appointment began what was to become the most successful treatment of SCI patients up to that time, and even to this time, with the return of a majority of the patients to a useful and productive life.[5] The results were so striking that his concepts became the accepted treatment of SCI by most European surgeons.

A few lines from a paper Dr. Guttmann presented at a SCI conference in Edinburgh in 1963 portray his concepts very concisely. "Since the National SCI Centre at Stoke Mandeville was opened during the last war, 3000 women and children have been treated at the center, of these, 1963 were paralyzed as a result of injuries to the spinal cord. It is gratifying that during the last 6 years or so the number of patients admitted immediately or within the first few days after injury has greatly increased. This indicates a growing awareness of many surgeons in Great Britain of the value of sending acute cases as quickly as possible to a spinal unit equipped with facilities for immediate as well as late treatment and rehabilitation of these patients.

"The guiding principles in the initial management of the fractured spine resulting in immediate damage to the spinal cord or cauda equina are great gentleness and avoidance of hasty immediate operative procedures such as laminectomy or open reduction as well as forceful conservative procedures by manipulation."

A FINAL HISTORICAL ASSESSMENT

Allen, Riddoch, and Guttmann each played major roles in the conceptual development of the treatment of SCI patients. Unknowingly, they also may have inhibited the development of the field. Allen constricted progress when his patriotism took him from the field of study of SCI where he was arguably the only person at that time who was approaching the problem in a logical manner. He also, possibly because he was leaving to enlist in the Army, pushed treatment before the information was complete and left little room for further objective clinical trials of a treatment that still has, on an experimental basis, great potential.

Riddoch recognized in 1915 and 1916 that the treatment that he and Head developed prevented the multisystem failure that caused the death of spinal cord-injured patients. As a neurologist and a neuroscientist, he also recognized that these results demonstrated that there was no effective treatment of the injured spinal cord. Thus, he stressed the need for protection of the systems of the body as a whole and that invasive management schemes were not indicated because they stressed the patient's general viability.

Later, as an administrator, Riddoch failed to be critical of the substance of the success that Guttmann attained. He neglected to maintain the same standard when he evaluated the results at the Stoke Mandeville Hospital. He allowed Guttmann's results to imply that treatment for the SCI patient resulted in treatment of the injured spinal cord. What Guttmann's results in fact signified was unchanged from his previous work (i.e., that improved patient care resulted in decreased morbidity and mortality, but that there was no effective treatment for the injured spinal cord itself). It should only have been concluded that with protection against further SCI, with care of the vulnerable systems of the body, and with planned rehabilitation, patients with SCI can regain productive lives.

Guttmann was so certain that his regimen was the "only way" an SCI should be treated that he failed to even consider any other treatment. This conclusion from a famous and successful expert led to a lack of incentives to investigate the problem and inhibited other possible approaches to SCI.

CONCLUSION

What deductions can be reached from the work of these men? First, the response of the nervous system to the injury causes a portion of the resulting neurological deficit after SCI. Second, with few exceptions, until there is clinical evidence that an invasive treatment is effective and has a low possibility of causing a second injury, conservative noninvasive treatment of the SCI appears to be the best treatment. Third, even with rehabilitation techniques that allow an injured patient to return to a productive life, one should continue to look at all possibilities of improving neurologic functional outcome. Finally, it appears that the gain from controlling the response of the nervous system to trauma will be small. This makes it imperative, if we are to improve functional outcome, that we continue our efforts to decipher the problems of regeneration of the central nervous system, a dream that Riddoch's work showed could have merit when he demonstrated that the isolated spinal cord retained its local function.

REFERENCES

1. Allen AR: Remarks on the histopathological changes in the spinal cord due to impact: an experimental study. **J Nerv Ment Dis 41:**141-147, 1914
2. Allen AR: Surgery of experimental lesion of spinal cord equivalent to crush injury of fracture dislocation of spinal column. A preliminary report. **JAMA 57:** 878-880, 1911
3. Elsberg CA: The Edwin Smith surgical papyrus and the diagnosis and treatment of injuries to the skull and spine 5000 years ago. **Ann Med Hist 3:**271-279, 1931
4. Frazier CH, Allen AR: **Surgery of the Spine and Spinal Cord.** New York, NY: D Appleton and Co, 1918
5. Guttman L: **Spinal Cord Injuries: Comprehensive Management and Research. 2nd ed.** Oxford, England: Blackwell Scientific, 1976
6. Guttmann L: Rehabilitation after injury to the central nervous system. **Proc R Soc Med 35:**305-308, 1942
7. Guttmann L: **Review on Rehabilitation after Lesions of the Nervous System.** Great Britain: Medical Research Council, 1941
8. Hartwell JB: An analysis of 133 fractures of the spine treated at the Massachusetts General Hospital. **Boston Med Surg J 177:**31-41, 1917
9. Head H, Riddoch G: The automatic bladder, excessive sweating and some other reflex conditions, in gross injuries of the spinal cord. **Brain 40:**188-263, 1917
10. Riddoch G: The practical significance of the mass reflex in the treatment of injuries of the spinal cord. **Lancet 2:**839-841, 1917
11. Schmaus H: Beiträge zur pathologischen anatomie der rückenmarkserschütterung. **Virchows Arch 122:** 470-495, 1890
12. Vidus Vidius: **Chirurgia è Graeco in Latinum Connersa.** Paris, 1544

CHAPTER 2

THE EVOLUTION OF MODERN SPINE SURGERY: AN HISTORICAL PERSPECTIVE

CHARLES H. TATOR, MD, CM, PHD, FRCS(C), FACS, AND
EDWARD C. BENZEL, MD, FACS

The management of spinal cord injury (SCI) is an excellent example of a multidisciplinary endeavor requiring a large number of health care professionals for optimal patient management. Similarly, a large number of disciplines have contributed to the advances in basic research and clinical knowledge of SCI. Within the surgical specialties, both neurosurgery and orthopaedic surgery have contributed a great deal to the clinical advances and fundamental knowledge and both have been affected by a historically conservative (non-operative) influence. This, perhaps, began with the ancient Egyptians. The Egyptian Papyrus, discovered by Edwin Smith in 1862, argues against the treatment of SCI.[36] It is likely that this set the stage for a strong and global non-operative philosophy. In 1814, H.J. Cline, Jr.,[14] had a fatality related to the surgical treatment of a thoracic fracture/dislocation. This adverse event propelled the non-operative "attitude" well into the 20th century. Nevertheless, subsequent surgical interventions by others met with success and eventually led to the establishment of surgery for SCI as a viable option. Pioneers from both neurosurgery and orthopaedic came to the forefront.

NEUROSURGICAL CONTRIBUTIONS

The following account concentrates on the role of neurosurgeons in the development of knowledge regarding the pathophysiology, the clinical manifestations, and the treatment of patients with acute SCI.

Research Contributions

Allen[3,4] in Philadelphia in the early 1900s investigated the role of central hemorrhagic necrosis and central hematomyelia in dogs injured by a novel experimental mechanism of injury produced by dropping a weight onto the exposed spinal cord. He found that evacuation of the necrotic debris produced clinical improvement. In the 1950s, Tarlov[56,57] performed several ingenious experiments to examine the effect of continuing compression of the spinal cord produced by extradural balloon catheters. He demonstrated that early relief of compression was an effective means of improving neurological recovery after acute SCI. In the 1960s, Albin et al[2] conducted a series of experiments on cooling of the injured spinal cord to improve neurological recovery. Although this treatment showed promising results in experimental studies in animals, the clinical results in a small number of patients were disappointing. In outstanding studies reported in 1979 and 1980, Richardson et al[47,48] demonstrated for the first time that peripheral nerve grafts placed in the spinal cord of rats supported the regeneration of central axons and disproved the previously held view that central axons were incapable of regenerating. Recently, Cheng et al[13] combined this strategy with neurotrophic factors to show regeneration of the corticospinal tract.

Biomechanical Studies

The subject of biomechanics of the spine has recently been of major interest to neurosurgeons and, since the 1980s, neurosurgeons have contributed to the knowledge of the biomechanics of the spine. Benzel et al[5,6] examined the effects of spinal bracing on the cervical spine, and Maiman et al[42] elucidated the biomechanics of compression injuries.

Clinical Syndromes and Indications for Surgery

Richard Schneider and his anatomist collaborator, Elizabeth Crosby, helped define some of the clinical syndromes associated with cervicomedullary and incomplete cervical SCI syndromes.[51-53] For example, their anatomical-pathological studies of football players with cervical cord injuries helped explain the central cord syndrome. Schneider was one of the first neurosurgeons to develop guidelines for surgical treatment. It is of interest that he advocated non-operative management for most cases of central cord syndrome, except when a ruptured disc was demonstrated. Harris[30] in Scotland also advocated strict indications for surgical treatment. For many years, Harris served as editor of the journal *Paraplegia* and oversaw its transition into the journal *Spinal Cord*.

Organization of Care

Guttmann[25] in England pioneered specialty hospitals for the management of SCIs, and in North America a similar movement was started by Munro in Boston and Botterell in Toronto along with their colleagues in rehabilitation medicine.[44,58] Neurosurgeons were central players in the movement toward specialized centers for the rehabilitation of SCI patients. In the early 1970s, the Toronto group and others started a trend toward the concentration of acute SCI patients in regionalized centers.[59]

Traction for Reduction of Dislocation

Neurosurgeons were very inventive in developing methods of applying skeletal traction for reducing the dislocated cervical spine. Crutchfield[20] was one of the first to use a tong-like apparatus attached to the skull, although several others, including Gallie[23] and Cone,[15] offered their own versions at about the same time during the 1930s.

Clinical Trials

Collins was instrumental in organizing the first multicenter trials in acute SCI in the 1980s. With his colleague Bracken, Collins organized the National Acute Spinal Cord Injury Study group of investigators.[9-11] This group established the effectiveness of methylprednisolone for acute SCI. They also demonstrated the validity of the concept of secondary injury and that the therapeutic window for methylprednisolone was approximately 8 hours from the time of injury. In Japan, Abe has been a leader in the field of SCI[32] and was involved in the Japanese multicenter trial, which confirmed the effectiveness of methylprednisolone.[46] There have been 10 randomized control trials in the field of acute SCI (see recent review[60]), and neurosurgeons have had a leadership role in most of them.

Studies of Early Management of Cord Compression

Ducker and Saul[21] developed a new paradigm for the clinical management of acute SCI, which involved the performance of an immediate myelogram and early decompression in the presence of persisting cord compression. With a non-randomized study, no definite answer about the role of early decompression was possible. There has been only one randomized prospective controlled trial of early versus late decompression, and this study failed to show a significant difference; however, it should be noted that the "early" group in this trial underwent decompression at a mean of more than 24 hours after injury.[62] In 1993, a group of investigators formed the Surgical Treatment of Acute Spinal Cord Injury Study and conducted multicentered pilot studies. They demonstrated the feasibility of conducting a multicenter randomized control trial of early decompression at a time compatible with the therapeutic window identified in the methylprednisolone drug trial.[45,61] Decompression within 8 hours was believed to be an attainable goal, but to date this trial has not proceeded because of lack of funding.

Innovations in Surgical Management

There have been a large number of neurosurgeons who have made major contributions to the methods of surgical management of patients with acute SCI. Verbiest[63] in The Netherlands explored new ways of approaching the cervical spine and called attention to the importance of vertebral artery injury. Larson et al[40] popularized the lateral extracavitary approach to thoracic and thoracolumbar injuries and established the first neurosurgery spine training program. Sonntag and Dickman[55] improved methods for C1-2 fusion, and Cooper[16] was an early advocate for lateral mass plates for managing unstable cervical fractures. Crockard et al[19] simplified the methods for approaching the cervicomedullary junction anteriorly. Many neurosurgeons have been strong advocates of a variety of anterior approaches in SCI in the cervical, thoracic, or thoracolumbar region.

ORTHOPAEDIC CONTRIBUTIONS

Much of the current "state-of-the-art" of spine surgery developed from work by orthopaedic surgeons. The vast majority of this work applies to SCI.

The Foundations

Early orthopaedic contributions to research regarding spine trauma (particularly biomechanics research), were collected, modified, and eloquently reported by White and Panjabi.[64] The large number of works that emanated from their laboratory culminated in their ultimate treatise *Clinical Biomechanics of the Spine.* This book played a seminal role in the advancement of spine surgery during the last three decades of the 20th century.

The Evolution of Surgical Decompression

It is impossible to give credit to all who have contributed to the advancement of the field of spine surgery. Therefore, the segment that follows provides only an overview. The tragic outcome of Cline's patient was fortunately followed by clinical successes, including the first documented successful decompression for trauma in 1829.[54] This operation was a laminectomy for traumatic paraplegia. The patient not only survived, but also enjoyed neurological recovery. Unfortunately, this phenomenal success went largely unnoticed.

Clinical failures of laminectomy for SCI led to the quest for alternatives. The costotransversectomy by Menard[43] was the first nondorsal alternative to laminectomy. This was followed by a lateral rhachotomy by Capener.[12] Hodgson and Stock[33] developed a true ventral approach to the thoracic and lumbar spine as a treatment for Pott's disease. This surgical strategy, unbeknownst to them at the time, played a major role in the development of surgical strategies for thoracic and lumbar trauma.

The Evolution of Spinal Stabilization Techniques

Sir Frank W. Holdsworth[34] was the first to systematically study internal fixation for spine trauma. Although the surgical strategies were rudimentary by today's standards (i.e., spinous process fixation), Holdsworth developed surgical strategies that were based on biomechanical principles. He ultimately developed a classification scheme for subaxial spine fractures.[35] All other subsequent classification schemes were built upon the foundation created by Holdsworth.

Spinal stabilization surgery nearly always involves a consideration of arthrodesis. Fortunately, spine fusion strategies were well developed prior to their instrumentation counterparts. Albee[1] and Hibbs[31] independently reported the use of spinal fusion in 1911. The advent of the use of autologous iliac crest significantly advanced the field.[8] This, however, did not transpire until later in the century.

Hadra[26] and Lange[39] used a variety of strategies, including wire and rods, to stabilize the spine. Of particular note is that Lange's efforts employed rods without wire, hook, or screw fixation adjuncts. Therefore, their techniques found limited use.

During the two decades that followed World War II, much of the foundation for modern day spinal surgery was laid. This era was opened by two seminal pioneering efforts. The first was the description of the use of interspinous cervical spine wiring in the 1940s by Rogers.[49,50] The second was the introduction of an instrumentation system in the 1960s by Harrington.[27,28] Both advances revolutionized the care of spine trauma patients, in spite of the fact that Harrington's device was initially designed for the management of scoliosis secondary to poliomyelitis. Luque[41] addressed one of the major deficits of the Harrington system by providing a strategy for multilevel fixation of the thoracic and lumbar spine using wires and rods. This strategy was also applied with the Harrington system, allowing both distraction and multisegmental fixation. In 1969, Harrington and Tullos[29] were the first to describe the use of pedicle screw fixation; however, they abandoned this strategy because of difficulties associated with the secure attachment of the screws to rods. Roy-Camille was the first to successfully and routinely utilize this type of fixation; then Steffe significantly refined these strategies and, thus, made major contributions to the advancement of spinal instrumentation.

The first true universal instrumentation system for the thoracic and lumbar spine was developed by Cotrel and Dubousset.[7,18] This system allowed the use of wires, screws, and/or hooks to be used in a multisegmented manner to apply distraction and/or compression to the spine via rods. Many varieties followed. None, however, has differed significantly from the system originally employed by Cotrel and Dubousset.

Ventral thoracic and lumbar instrumentation strategies were pioneered by Dwyer et al,[22] Giehl and Zielke,[24] and, ultimately, Kaneda et al.[38] These strategies ranged from single cables to paired ventral rods. These techniques laid the groundwork for the development of many of the plate systems in current use.

In the cervical spine, the development of the ventral cervical spine fixation plate by Caspar laid the groundwork for subsequent ventral fixation strategies, such as that developed by Morcher.[37] The latter employed a fixed momentum cantilever beam strategy, as opposed to the nonfixed momentum cantilever beam employed by the Caspar technique. Roy-Camille is credited with the application of lateral mass plate fixation of the cervical spine.[17] Recently, this fixation strategy has blossomed. The development of a myriad of related fixation techniques to the cervical spine, skull, and cervicothoracic junction has aided this process.

POSTSCRIPT

Much has changed in the last 150 years. The industrial revolution has left in its wake the foundation for the technical age in which we currently live. Spine surgery most certainly has paralleled these historical events. Although many advances have been made during these years, many more are yet to be made. The disciplines of neurosurgery and orthopaedic surgery can be proud of their contribution to this effort to date. Great things are anticipated in the future.

REFERENCES

1. Albee FH: Transplantation of a portion of the tibia into the spine for Pott's disease. A preliminary report. **JAMA** 57:885-886, 1911
2. Albin MS, White RJ, Locke GE, et al: Spinal cord hypothermia by localized perfusion cooling. **Nature** 210:1059-1060, 1966
3. Allen AR: Remarks on the histopathological changes in the spinal cord due to impact. An experimental

study. **J Nerv Ment Dis** 41:141-147, 1914

4. Allen AR: Surgery of experimental lesion of spinal cord equivalent to crush injury of fracture dislocation of spinal column. A preliminary report. **JAMA 57:** 878-880, 1911

5. Benzel EC: **Biomechanics of Spine Stabilization: Principles and Clinical Practice.** New York, NY: McGraw-Hill, 1994

6. Benzel EC, Hadden TA, Saulsbery CM: A comparison of the Minerva and halo jackets for stabilization of the cervical spine. **J Neurosurg** 70:411-414, 1989

7. Birch JG, Herring JA, Roach JW, et al: Cotrel-Dubousset instrumentation in idiopathic scoliosis. A preliminary report. **Clin Orthop** 227:24-29, 1988

8. Boucher HH: A method of spinal fusion. **J Bone Joint Surg (Br)** 41:248-259, 1959

9. Bracken MB, Collins WF, Freeman DF, et al: Efficacy of methylprednisolone in acute spinal cord injury. **JAMA** 251:45-52, 1984

10. Bracken MB, Shepard MJ, Collins WF, et al: A randomized, controlled trial of methylprednisolone or naloxone in the treatment of acute spinal-cord injury. Results of the second National Acute Spinal Cord Injury Study. **N Engl J Med** 322:1405-1411, 1990

11. Bracken MB, Shepard MJ, Holford TR, et al: Administration of methylprednisolone for 24 or 48 hours of tirilazad mesylate for 48 hours in the treatment of acute spinal cord injury. Results of the third National Acute Spinal Cord Injury Randomized Controlled trial. **JAMA** 277:1597-1604, 1997

12. Capener N: The evolution of lateral rhachotomy. **J Bone Joint Surg (Br)** 36:173-179, 1954

13. Cheng H, Cao Y, Olson L: Spinal cord repair in adult paraplegic rats: partial restoration of hind limb function. **Science** 273:510-513, 1996

14. Cline JH Jr (cited by Hayward G): An account of a case of fracture and dislocation of the spine. **N Engl J Med Surg** 4:13, 1815

15. Cone W, Turner WG: The treatment of fracture-dislocations of the cervical vertebrae by skeletal traction and fusion. **J Bone Joint Surg** 19:584-602, 1937

16. Cooper PR: Stabilization of fractures and subluxations of the lower cervical spine, in Cooper PR (ed): **Management of Posttraumatic Spinal Instability.** Park Ridge, Ill: American Association of Neurological Surgeons, 1990, pp 111-133

17. Cooper PR, Cohen A, Rosiello A, et al: Posterior stabilization of cervical spine fractures and subluxations using plates and screws. **Neurosurgery** 23:300-306, 1988

18. Cotrel Y, Dubousset J, Guillaumat M: New universal instrumentation in spinal surgery. **Clin Orthop** 227: 10-23, 1988

19. Crockard HA, Calder I, Ransford AO: One-stage transoral decompression and posterior fixation in rheumatoid atlanto-axial subluxation. **J Bone Joint Surg (Br)** 72:682-685, 1990

20. Crutchfield WG: Skeletal traction for dislocation of the cervical spine. **South Surg** 2:156-159, 1933

21. Ducker TB, Saul TG: Early myelography in acute cervical cord injury, in Tator CH (ed): **Early Management of Acute Spinal Cord Injury.** New York, NY: Raven Press, 1982, pp 145-151

22. Dwyer AF, Newton NC, Sherwood AA: An anterior approach to scoliosis. A preliminary report. **Clin Orthop** 62:192-202, 1969

23. Gallie WE: Skeletal traction in the treatment of fractures and dislocations of the cervical spine. **Ann Surg** 106:770-776, 1937

24. Giehl JP, Zielke K: Zielke procedures in scoliosis correction, in Birdwell KH, DeWald RL (eds): **The Textbook of Spinal Surgery.** Philadelphia, Pa: JB Lippincott, 1991, pp 163-182

25. Guttmann L: **Spinal Cord Injuries. Comprehensive Management and Research.** 2nd ed. Oxford: Blackwell Scientific, 1976

26. Hadra BE: The classic: wiring of the vertebrae as a means of immobilization in fracture and Pott's disease (reprinted from the original). **Clin Orthop** 112: 4-8, 1988

27. Harrington PR: The history and development of Harrington instrumentation. **Clin Orthop** 93:110-112, 1973

28. Harrington PR: Treatment of scoliosis. Correction and internal fixation by spine instrumentation. **J Bone Joint Surg (Am)** 44:591-610, 1962

29. Harrington PR, Tullos HS: Reduction of severe spondylolisthesis in children. **South Med J** 62:1-7, 1969

30. Harris P: The diagnosis and early treatment of patients with spinal cord injury, in: Proceedings of the 16th Veterans Administration Spinal Cord Injury Conference, 1967, pp 14-18

31. Hibbs RA: An operation for progressive spinal deformities. **NY State Med J** 93:1013-1016, 1911

32. Hida K, Iwasaki Y, Imamura H, et al: Posttraumatic syringomyelia: its characteristic magnetic resonance imaging findings and surgical management. **Neurosurgery** 35:886-891, 1994

33. Hodgson AR, Stock FE: Anterior spinal fusion. A preliminary communication on the radical treatment of Pott's disease and Pott's paraplegia. **Br J Surg** 44: 266-275, 1956

34. Holdsworth FW: Fractures, dislocations, and fracture-dislocations of the spine. **J Bone Joint Surg (Br)** 45: 6-20, 1963

35. Holdsworth FW, Hardy A: Early treatment of paraplegia from fractures of the thoraco-lumbar spine. **J Bone Joint Surg (Br)** 35:540-550, 1953

36. Hughes JT: The Edwin Smith Surgical Papyrus: an analysis of the first case reports of spinal cord injuries. **Paraplegia** 26:71-82, 1988

37. Jonsson H Jr, Cesarini K, Petren-Mallmin M, et al: Locking screw-plate fixation of cervical spine fractures with and without ancillary posterior plating. **Arch Orthop Trauma Surg** 111:1-12, 1991

38. Kaneda K, Abumi K, Fujiya M: Burst fractures with neurologic deficits of the thoracolumbar-lumbar spine. Results of anterior decompression and stabilization with anterior instrumentation. **Spine** 9: 788-795, 1984

39. Lange F: Support for the spondylitic spine by means of buried steel bars, attached to the vertebrae. **Clin Orthop** 203:3-6, 1986

40. Larson SJ, Holst RA, Hemmy DC, et al: Lateral extracavitary approach to traumatic lesions of the thoracic and lumbar spine. **J Neurosurg** 45:628-637, 1976

41. Luque ER: The anatomic basis and development of segmental spinal instrumentation. **Spine** 7:256-259, 1982

42. Maiman DJ, Sances A Jr, Myklebust JB, et al: Compression injuries of the cervical spine: a biomechani-

cal analysis. **Neurosurgery 13:**254-260, 1983

43. Menard V: Causes de la paraplegia dans le mal de Pott. Son traitment chirurgical par l'ouverture direct du foyer tuberculeux des vertebras. **Rev Orthop 5:** 47-64, 1984

44. Munro D: The rehabilitation of patients totally paralyzed below the waist, with special reference to making them ambulatory and capable of earning their own living. V. An end-result study of 445 cases. **N Engl J Med 250:**4-14, 1954

45. Ng WP, Fehlings MG, Cuddy B, et al: Surgical treatment for acute spinal cord injury study pilot study #2: Evaluation of protocol for decompressive surgery within 8 hours of injury. **Neurosurg Focus 2(1):** January 1999

46. Otani K, Abe H, Kadoya S, et al: Beneficial effect of methylprednisolone sodium succinate in the treatment of acute spinal cord injury. **Sekitsui Sekizui J 7:** 633-647, 1994

47. Richardson PM, McGuinness UM, Aguayo AJ: Axons from CNS neurones regenerate into PNS grafts. **Nature 284:**264-265, 1980

48. Richardson PM, McGuinness UM, Aguayo AJ: Regeneration following sciatic nerve grafting to the rat spinal cord. **Can J Neurol Sci 6:**395, 1979

49. Rogers WA: Fractures and dislocations of the cervical spine. An end-result study. **J Bone Joint Surg (Am) 39:**341-376, 1957

50. Rogers WA: Treatment of fracture-dislocation of the cervical spine. **J Bone Joint Surg (Am) 24:**245-258, 1942

51. Schneider RC: A syndrome in acute cervical injuries for which early operation is indicated. **J Neurosurg 8:** 360-367, 1951

52. Schneider RC, Crosby EC, Russo RH, et al: Traumatic spinal cord syndromes and their management. **Clin Neurosurg 20:**424-492, 1973

53. Schneider RC, Thompson JM, Bebin J: The syndromes of the acute central cervical spinal cord injury. **J Neu**rol **Neurosurg Psychiatry 21:**216-227, 1958

54. Smith AG: Account of a case in which portions of three dorsal vertebrae were removed for the relief of paralysis from fracture, with partial success. **North Am Med Surg J 8:**94-97, 1829

55. Sonntag VKH, Dickman CA: Operative management of occipitocervical and atlantoaxial instability. **J Spinal Dis 5:**144-149, 1992

56. Tarlov IM: **Spinal Cord Compression: Mechanisms of Paralysis and Treatment.** Springfield, Ill: Charles C Thomas, 1957

57. Tarlov IM, Klinger H: Spinal cord compression studies. II. Time limits for recovery after acute compression in dogs. **Arch Neurol Psychiatry 71:**271-290, 1954

58. Tator CH: Botterell—contributions in spinal cord injury. **Can J Neurol Sci 26:**239-241, 1999

59. Tator CH, Duncan EG, Edmonds VE, et al: Neurological recovery, mortality and length of stay after acute spinal cord injury associated with changes in management. **Paraplegia 33:**254-262, 1995

60. Tator CH, Fehlings MG: Clinical trials in spinal cord injury, in Biller J, Bogousslavsky J (eds): **Clinical Trials in Neurologic Practice.** Woburn, Mass: Butterworth Heinemann, 2000 (In press)

61. Tator CH, Fehlings MG, Thorpe K, et al: Current use and timing of spinal surgery for management of acute spinal surgery for management of acute spinal cord injury in North America: results of a retrospective multicenter study. **J Neurosurg (Spine) 91:**12-18, 1999

62. Vaccaro AR, Daugherty RJ, Sheehan TP, et al: Neurologic outcome of early versus late surgery for cervical spinal cord injury. **Spine 22:**2609-2613, 1997

63. Verbiest H: Anterolateral operations for fractures or dislocations of the cervical spine due to injuries or previous surgical interventions. **Clin Neurosurg 20:** 334-366, 1973

64. White AA, Panjabi M: **Clinical Biomechanics of the Spine.** Philadelphia, Pa: JB Lippincott, 1990

CHAPTER 3

Epidemiology and General Characteristics of the Spinal Cord-Injured Patient

Charles H. Tator, MD, CM, PhD, FRCS(C), FACS

Effective management of the patient with acute spinal cord injury (SCI) requires an appreciation of how the injuries occur. In addition, knowledge of the epidemiology of an SCI will alert the physician or surgeon to the possible occurrence of such an injury. Recognition of an SCI can be especially difficult in the acute phase, in the context of multiple trauma, or if other conditions are pre-existing such as metastatic disease, congenital anomalies, or spinal arthropathies (including ankylosing spondylitis).

The Incidence of Spinal Cord Injury

Acute SCI is relatively uncommon, affecting about one in 40 patients who present to a major trauma center.[3] Estimates of the annual incidence in developed countries vary from 11.5 to 53.4 per million population.[2,4,12-14,19] Despite the relatively low incidence, these injuries have profound consequences for the patients, their families, and society in general. For example, mortality rates (both immediate and delayed) are high. Kraus et al[13] reported a case fatality rate of 48.3%, with 79% of the fatalities occurring at the scene of the accident or on arrival at the hospital.

For survivors at hospital admission, reported mortality rates range from 4.4% to 16.7%.[12] Morbidity rates among SCI patients are also high, and survivors of acute SCI may require prolonged and/or multiple hospitalization in acute treatment units and rehabilitation centers.[10,27] Frequently associated with these physical injuries is significant damage to the social and psychological well-being of the patients and their families. Finally, the financial burden to the patient, the health care system, and society is great.[27] Added to the expenses for acute and long-term management are indirect costs from lost income and lost productivity. In 1990, Stripling[21] estimated that the cost to the United States of caring for all SCI patients was $4 billion annually.

The causes of frequently seen adult SCI, the level of injury, the type of bony injury, and the severity of neurological injury are described below and listed in Table 1.

Causes of Injury

The epidemiology of SCI varies from one country to another, and within a given country there are variations depending on location, such as urban or rural sites. In addition, the causes

TABLE 1

ETIOLOGY, VERTEBRAL LEVEL, SEVERITY OF
NEUROLOGICAL INJURY AND
TYPE OF BONY INJURY IN ADULT SCI

Cause of Injury	Traffic accidents (motor vehicle, bicycle, pedestrian)	40% – 50%
	Work	10% – 25%
	Sports and recreation	10% – 25%
	Falls (home, elsewhere)	20%
	Violence	10% – 25%
Level of Injury	Cervical (C1 to C7-T1)	55%
	Thoracic (T1-11)	15%
	Thoracolumbar (T11-12 to L1-2)	15%
	Lumbosacral (L2-S5)	15%
Severity of Neurological Injury*	Complete ASIA/IMSOP Grade A	45%
	Incomplete ASIA/IMSOP	
	Grade B	15%
	Grade C	10%
	Grade D	30%
Type of Bony Injury†	Minor fracture (including compression)	10%
	Fracture dislocation	40%
	Dislocation only	5%
	Burst fracture	30%
	SCIWORA	5%
	SCIWORET (including osteoarthritis and cervical spondylosis)	10%

* See Chapter 4 for description of American Spinal Injury Association (ASIA)/International Medical Society of Paraplegia (IMSOP) grades.

† See text for description of SCIWORA and SCIWORET.

and effects of SCI differ among various age groups. Younger victims, with their greater preponderance of injuries in high-velocity, high-impact force activities such as traffic accidents, motorsports, and diving, tend to be subject to higher forces of injury. Younger victims are also subject to different physiological factors that affect the spine such as undeveloped paraspinal musculature and more-elastic ligaments. Older victims, on the other hand, tend to have spines that are more rigid and additional pathological features such as osteoporosis or pre-existing cervical or lumbar spondylosis.

The most common cause of SCI in developed countries is traffic accidents, whereas in many less-developed countries, falls are the most com-

mon cause.[26] Violence is also a variable factor, with gunshot wounds one of the most frequent causes of SCI in urban locations in developed countries.[22] The epidemiology of SCI within a given location will vary with time. For example, in many developed countries, sports and recreational activities have recently become much more frequent causes of SCI as leisure time has increased and the variety of risk-taking recreational activities proliferated.[26]

Worldwide, traffic accidents (motor vehicle, bicycle, and pedestrian) account for the greatest number of SCIs , and in most countries are the cause of approximately one half of all cases. As noted above, sports and recreational causes of injury have increased, and in some countries they have replaced work as the second most frequent cause of injury. The reasons for this shift are multifactorial and include activities in which there is a combination of risk-taking and very high physical forces on the vertebral column such as rock climbing, parachuting, and surfing. In some locations, sports and recreational causes account for up to 25% of SCI. Conversely, work accidents in some countries have diminished as safer practices are promulgated and targeted prevention programs are instituted, especially in the mining, logging, and construction industries. Falls (particularly those occurring in the home) are usually the third most common cause, tending to affect older age groups. Indeed, in individuals aged over 65 years, falls may even exceed traffic accidents as a cause of SCI. Violence (including homicide, suicide, and war) has shown a substantial increase in the past 10 years, especially in some developed countries;[3] in some locations, violence is the most common cause of SCI.[22]

Level of Injury

Overall, approximately 55% of injuries to the spinal cord occur in the cervical spine region from C1 to C7–T1, with approximately 15% of injuries in each of the other three regions as shown in Table 1. However, certain causes produce a significantly different distribution of injuries. For example, diving accidents are almost exclusively cervical injuries, whereas mining and logging tend to produce much higher numbers of thoracic and thoracolumbar injuries.

Type of Vertebral Column Injury

The types of vertebral column injuries encountered in patients with SCI are listed in Table 1. Improved imaging by computed tomography (CT) and magnetic resonance imaging has markedly reduced the relative frequency of patients with SCI without radiological abnormality (SCIWORA) and has increased the incidence of those who have burst fractures with identified intracanalicular space-occupying lesions. In the past, many injuries in this latter group were classified as simple compression fractures. There is still a significant number of patients, especially children, with true SCIWORA. Improved imaging, particularly high-resolution bone window CT, also has improved the ability to diagnose the offending lesion in patients with SCI without radiological evidence of trauma (SCIWORET).[24] The majority of these patients have cervical spondylosis, and the remainder have congenital anomalies.

Severity of Neurological Injury

Since 1969, there has been a marked change in the relative incidence of complete and incomplete SCI, and this change has been reflected in series of cases reported from several countries.[1,6,9,17] Previously, approximately two thirds of SCIs were complete, whereas more recent reports show that approximately 45% are complete.[26] There are many possible reasons for this favorable and substantial change, such as the increasing use of seat belts, air bags, and child-restraint systems, and improved first-aid care and ambulance retrieval. These latter factors include better management of systemic hypotension and hypoxia and a reduced incidence of additional mechanical damage to the injured cord caused by injudicious movement of the injured and unstable spine.

The Effect of Level and Type of Injury on Severity

Thoracic injuries have a higher incidence of complete injuries than do cervical or thoracolumbar cord injuries.[25] Anterior dislocations and fracture dislocations are more likely to be complete cord injuries than compression fractures or

TABLE 2

AGE OF PATIENTS WITH SCI

Age (Years)	
Birth – 10	10%
11 – 20	20%
21 – 30	25%
31 – 40	15%
41 – 50	10%
51 – 60	10%
Over 60	10%
Total	100%

burst fractures. In complete injuries, neurological recovery was greatest in patients with cervical injuries, second in those with thoracic injuries, and lowest in those with thoracolumbar injuries; the likelihood of neurological recovery is approximately the same in patients with cervical and thoracic injuries and considerably less in thoracolumbar injuries.[25] In all three regions, the ability of patients with incomplete injuries to recover is related to the severity of the initial neurological deficit: the greater the deficit at admission, the worse the neurological recovery.

OTHER FACTORS IN SPINAL CORD INJURY

Patient Age and Gender

In almost all series of cases, 80% to 85% of patients with SCI are male and 15% to 20% are female.[26] Young patients comprise the majority of victims, with the usual mean and median ages ranging from the late 20s to the early 30s in series of patients from most countries (Table 2).

Relationship of Spinal Cord Injury to Head Injury

Significant head injuries are five to 10 times more common than SCIs; in several reports, a considerable number of patients have both.[18,20,23] Approximately 5% to 10% of head-injured patients have an associated spinal injury and, 25% to 50% of SCI patients have an associated head injury.

Relationship of Spinal Cord Injury to Multiple Trauma

Management of patients with SCI in the presence of multiple trauma is a great challenge because of the many difficulties and potential pitfalls. For example, an adequate airway establishment may be extremely difficult and hazardous in the presence of a cervical SCI. Hypoxia due to respiratory failure is common in these patients because of diaphragmatic and/or intercostal muscle paralysis. Abdominal distension, ileus, vomiting, and aspiration may add to the hypoxia. Hypotension is often present in SCI with multiple trauma due to spinal neurogenic shock and/or systemic shock. Patients with SCI, especially those with cervical injuries, have a sympathectomy effect[11] with unopposed vagotonia that may cause cardiac arrhythmia or even reflex cardiac arrest. Intra-abdominal hemorrhage or visceral rupture in patients with SCI may be overlooked because of the absence of the typical physical findings associated with those conditions.

Meguro and Tator[15] found that approximately 20% of patients with SCI have significant other major injuries such as cerebral contusion or flail chest. In other reports, the incidence of multiple trauma has varied from 24% to 57%.[5,7,8,16] In a recent study,[3] isolated SCI was present in only 20% of SCI patients. The most common cause of both isolated SCI and SCI associated with multiple trauma in this study was motor-vehicle accidents. Meguro and Tator found reduced neurological recovery and increased mortality in patients with SCI who also had multiple trauma. There was evidence that the reduced neurological recovery in patients with multiple trauma may have been related to systemic hypoxia or hypotension, which were frequent in these patients. In addition, the SCIs in multiple-trauma patients were more severe than in those with isolated SCI.

Alcohol or Other Drugs

In approximately 25% of SCI patients, alcohol consumption was a factor in the mode of injury; other drugs were a factor in a much smaller number.[26]

Associated Spinal Pathological States

The most common pre-existing abnormality of the spinal column in SCI patients is cervical spondylosis. In some series, this condition is present in about 10% of patients with SCI.[26] Less common pathological entities include congenital anomalies such as congenital fusion, metastatic spinal disease with pathological fractures, and spinal arthropathies (e.g., ankylosing spondylitis or rheumatoid arthritis). Trauma may be superimposed on a pre-existing condition such as an acute flexion injury in a patient with a congenital os odontoideum or Down's syndrome and atlantoaxial dislocation. The forces that lead to SCI in these cases are often much less severe than in patients without these associated lesions or anomalies.

REFERENCES

1. Baker SP, O'Neill B, Haddon W Jr, et al: The injury severity score: a method for describing patients with multiple injuries and evaluating emergency care. **J Trauma 14:**187-196, 1974
2. Botterell EH, Jousse AT, Kraus AS, et al: A model for the future care of acute spinal cord injuries. **Can J Neurol Sci 2:**361-380, 1975
3. Burney RE, Maio RF, Maynard F, et al: Incidence, characteristics, and outcome of spinal cord injury at trauma centers in North America. **Arch Surg 128:** 596-599, 1992
4. Gjone R, Nordlie L: Incidence of traumatic paraplegia and tetraplegia in Norway: a statistical survey of the years 1974 and 1975. **Paraplegia 16:**88-93, 1978
5. Guttmann L: History of the National Spinal Injuries Centre, Stoke Mandeville Hospital, Aylesbury. **Paraplegia 5:**115-126, 1967
6. Hachen HJ: Idealized care of the acutely injured spinal cord in Switzerland. **J Trauma 17:**931-936, 1977
7. Harris P. Associated injuries in traumatic paraplegia and tetraplegia. **Paraplegia 5:**215-220, 1968
8. Harris P: **Proceedings of the Third International Congress of Neurological Surgeons, Copenhagen.** Excerpta Medica International Congress Series No. 110. 1965, 347 pp
9. Harris P: Zarmi MZ, McClemont E, et al: The prognosis of patients sustaining severe cervical spine injury (C2-C7 inclusive). **Paraplegia 18:**324-330, 1980
10. Heinemann AW, Yarkony GM, Roth EJ, et al: Functional outcome following spinal cord injury: a comparison of specialized spinal cord injury center vs. general hospital short-term care. **Arch Neurol 46:** 1098-1102, 1989
11. Kiss ZHT, Tator CH: Neurogenic shock, in Geller ER

(ed): **Shock and Resuscitation.** New York, NY: McGraw-Hill, 1993, pp 421-440

12. Kraus JF: Injury to the head and spinal cord: the epidemiological relevance of the medical literature published from 1960 to 1978. **J Neurosurg 53 (Suppl):** S3-S10, 1980

13. Kraus JF, Franti CE, Riggins RS, et al: Incidence of traumatic spinal cord lesions. **J Chron Dis 28:** 471-492, 1975

14. Kurtzke JF: Epidemiology of spinal cord injury. **Exp Neurol 48:**163-236, 1975

15. Meguro K, Tator CH: Effect of multiple trauma on mortality and neurological recovery after spinal cord or cauda equina injury. **Neurol Med Chir 28:**34-41, 1988

16. Meinecke PW: Frequency and distribution of associated injuries in traumatic paraplegia and tetraplegia. **Paraplegia 5:**196-209, 1968

17. Meyer PR, Sullivan DE: Injuries to the spine. **Emerg Med Clin North Am 2:**313-329, 1984

18. Michael DB, Guyot DR, Darmody WR: Coincidence of head and cervical spine injury. **J Neurotrauma 6:** 177-189, 1989

19. Minaire P, Castanier M, Girard R, et al: Epidemiology of spinal cord injury in the Rhône-Alpes region, France, 1970-75. **Paraplegia 16:**76-87, 1978

20. Pagni CA, Massaro F: Concomitant cranio-cerebral and vertebro-medullary injuries: analysis of 121 cases. **Acta Neurochir 111:**1-10, 1991

21. Stripling TE: The cost of economic consequences of traumatic spinal cord injury. **Paraplegia News 8:** 50-54, 1990

22. Sutherland MW: The prevention of violent spinal cord injuries. **Spinal Cord Injury Nurs 10:**91-95, 1993

23. Tator CH: Management of associated spine injuries in head injury patients, in Narayan RK, Wilberger JE Jr, Povlishock JT (eds): **Neurotrauma.** New York, NY: McGraw-Hill, 1996, pp 263-267

24. Tator CH: Spinal cord syndromes with physiologic and anatomic correlations, in Menezes AH, Sonntag VKH (eds): **Principles of Spinal Surgery.** New York, NY: McGraw-Hill, 1996, pp 785-799

25. Tator CH: Spine-spinal cord relationships in spinal cord trauma. **Clin Neurosurg 30:**479-494, 1983

26. Tator CH, Duncan EG, Edmonds VE, et al: Changes in epidemiology of acute spinal cord injury from 1947 to 1981. **Surg Neurol 40:**207-215, 1993

27. Tator CH, Duncan EG, Edmonds VE, et al: Complications and costs of management of acute spinal cord injury. **Paraplegia 31:**700-714, 1993

CHAPTER 4

CLINICAL MANIFESTATIONS OF ACUTE SPINAL CORD INJURY

CHARLES H. TATOR, MD, CM, PHD, FRCS(C), FACS

The effective management of patients with acute spinal cord injury (SCI) depends upon accurate clinical examination and classification of the neurological injury and detailed radiological assessment of the vertebral column injury.[15] The most useful clinical classification is based on the assessment of the functional neurological damage as determined by the clinical examination rather than on other criteria such as the pathological, electrophysiological, or imaging features. Accurate clinical and radiological assessments permit the development of a rational treatment plan and the determination of the likely prognosis. The neurological assessment and classification must be sufficiently reliable to allow accurate comparisons of serial observations by the same or different observers. In the early 1990s, the American Spinal Injury Association (ASIA) convened consensus meetings of representatives from several disciplines involved in the management of patients with acute SCI and from several countries, and in 1992, ASIA along with the International Medical Society of Para-plegia (IMSOP) published the *International Standards for Neurological and Functional Classification of Spinal Cord Injury.*[1] This new ASIA/IMSOP classification is a considerable improvement and should be used by all physicians and surgeons who manage patients with acute SCI, just as the Glasgow Coma Scale is used to assess head injuries.

THE INITIAL CLINIC EXAMINATION

Table 1 shows the "safe assumptions" to make when initially encountering a trauma victim in order to avoid missing the diagnosis or worsening the injury. Since head and spinal injuries can occur together, assume that an unconscious patient also has a spinal injury. To avoid your attention being diverted to the chest or abdomen, assume that, in every case, the multiple-trauma victim has a spinal injury. Since most spinal

TABLE 1

"SAFE ASSUMPTIONS"—
TO AID IN THE DIAGNOSIS OF SCI

- Every patient with a head injury and every unconscious patient has an SCI.
- Every patient with multiple trauma has an SCI.
- Every motor-vehicle accident victim has an SCI.
- Every victim of a sports or recreational accident has an SCI.
- Every severely injured worker has an SCI.
- Every victim of a fall at home has an SCI.
- Every SCI has an unstable spinal column and any movement of the spinal column after trauma will cause further damage to the spinal cord.

injuries result from traffic accidents, work accidents, sports and recreational activities, or from falls at home, assume an SCI in every victim of these accidents. When the spinal cord is injured, always assume that the spinal column is unstable and that any movement can worsen the neurological deficit.

The diagnosis of SCI may be missed because of an inadequate or incomplete history or physical examination or because multiple factors may obscure the diagnosis. For example, inebriated victims of a car accident who were not wearing a seatbelt may have sustained a head injury as well as an SCI. The combination of the head injury and inebriation make it extremely difficult to examine the patient. Also, the presence of multiple trauma may divert the examiner's attention toward more obvious, but often less important, injuries such as limb fractures. Other difficult situations include patients who are psychologically upset by the injury or who are hypoxic and become restless, uncooperative, or agitated. In all of these instances, the practitioner's diagnostic acumen is severely taxed. Indeed, the patient's reactions may be so bizarre that the diagnosis of hysteria may be mistakenly made. This diagnosis is extremely dangerous in situations involving trauma. Thus, in the presence of alcohol, multiple trauma, head injury, or bizarre behavior, one must make the "safe assumption" that there is an accompanying SCI. With major trauma to the abdomen or chest, one should always suspect

that the trauma might have been sufficient to dislocate the spine.

The history provided by the accident victim, a witness, or the ambulance personnel may provide important clues that lead to the diagnosis of the presence and severity of an SCI. At the accident scene, was there leg movement only to have this function disappear later, or were the limbs motionless with subsequent gradual improvement? The former situation would indicate an unstable spine with severe pressure on the cord from progressive dislocation, whereas the latter may indicate a period of spinal shock that is now passing. Symptoms such as the inability to move one or more limbs or a relative lack of movement of one or more limbs are highly suspicious. Complaints of weakness, tingling, or loss of sensation are extremely important. Similarly, post-traumatic urinary retention and incontinence are danger signs.

The physical examination can yield specific indications of the presence of an SCI. These "spinal clues" are obtained from a detailed testing of the vital signs as well as strength, sensation, and reflexes in all four limbs (Table 2). The spine must be palpated in its entirety, paying special attention to tenderness, swelling, step-deformity, or crepitus. It is important to realize that the examiner's hand can be passed safely between the patient and the mattress or stretcher, and the spine palpated from the foramen magnum to the sacrum. This must be done in every instance.

Hypotension, bradycardia, and warm extremities are due to a cervical SCI and not to systemic shock, which usually causes hypotension, tachycardia, and cold extremities. It should be recognized that a cervical injury causes paradoxical respiration in which inspiration causes the chest cage to be drawn in while the abdomen expands due to intercostal muscle paralysis and preserved diaphragmatic contraction. Also, do not misinterpret reflex withdrawal of the limbs in response to "painful" stimulation of the extremities as being due to voluntary movement.

ASIA/IMSOP
IMPAIRMENT SCALE

Table 3 shows the ASIA/IMSOP impairment scale containing five grades of impairment:

TABLE 2

"SPINAL CLUES" — TO AID IN THE DIAGNOSIS OF SCI (ESPECIALLY USEFUL IN IMPAIRED CONSCIOUSNESS OR COOPERATION)

- Hypotension and bradycardia occur in spinal shock
- Paradoxical respiration
- Low body temperature and high skin temperature
- Priapism
- Bilateral paralysis of arms and legs, especially flaccid
- Bilateral paralysis of either arms only or arms more than legs, especially flaccid
- Bilateral paralysis of legs, especially flaccid
- Lack of response to painful stimuli
- Detection of an anatomic level in response to painful stimuli
- Painful stimulation produces only head movement or facial grimacing
- Sweating level
- Horner's syndrome
- Brown-Séquard syndrome

Grade A denotes a complete injury, Grades B, C, and D denote varying levels of incomplete injury, and Grade E denotes a patient with normal motor and sensory spinal cord function. A complete injury (Grade A) is now defined as absence of sensory and motor function in the lowest sacral segment, as originally described by Waters et al.[27] A Grade B patient has sensory preservation only below the level of injury. Grades C and D were originally described by Frankel et al[8] as preserved motor function being "useless" in Grade C and "useful" in Grade D. The new scale defines the function more precisely on the basis of the Medical Research Council muscle grading system:[14] in Grade C the majority of key muscles below the neurological level have a muscle grade of lower than 3, and in Grade D the majority of key muscles below the neurological level have a muscle grade of 3 or greater. The latter modifications are based on the classification of Tator et al.[25]

The new ASIA/IMSOP grading scale improves the ability to distinguish precisely between complete and incomplete injuries. To make this distinction, the clinician must test

TABLE 3

ASIA AND IMSOP ASIA/IMSOP IMPAIRMENT SCALE: SPINAL CORD INJURY BASED ON THE INTERNATIONAL STANDARDS FOR NEUROLOGICAL AND FUNCTIONAL CLASSIFICATION

Grade A	Complete injury	No motor or sensory function is preserved in the sacral segments S4–5.
Grade B	Incomplete injury	Sensory but not motor function is preserved below the neurological level and extends through the sacral segments S4–5.
Grade C	Incomplete injury	Motor function is preserved below the neurological level, and the majority of key muscles below the neurological level have a muscle grade less than 3.
Grade D	Incomplete injury	Motor function is preserved below the neurological level, and the majority of key muscles below the neurological level have a muscle grade 3 or greater.
Grade E	Normal	Motor and sensory function are normal.

both touch and pin prick sensation in the lowest sacral dermatomes perianally at the mucocutaneous junction, as well as deep anal sensation. Also, voluntary motor contraction of the external anal sphincter must be tested by digital examination. The distinction between complete and incomplete injury is crucial in order to plan treatment and to predict outcome.

As noted in Chapter 3, the prognosis for neurological recovery is vastly better in incomplete than in complete injuries at all levels of the spinal cord.[23] However, even complete cord injuries have some potential for recovery. Most large series of acute SCI patients have shown a small percentage of initially complete cases (usually 1% to 2%) with significant recovery of distal cord function.[9] It could be argued that patients who recover from a complete injury represent a misdiagnosis due to the difficulties described above, including inebriation, sedative or other drug effects, spinal shock, uncooperativeness, or a concomitant head injury. The author believes that approximately 1% to 2% of patients with complete SCI recover significant distal cord function, even in the absence of all factors that can interfere with precise, early classification, and that early appropriate treatment can increase this number.

NEUROLOGICAL AND VERTEBRAL LEVELS OF SCI

The new ASIA/IMSOP classification provides precise definitions for the neurological, sensory, and skeletal levels, as well as zone of partial preservation (Figure 1). The neurological level is the most caudal segment of the spinal cord with normal sensory and motor function on both sides of the body. Because normal segments may differ on the two sides and may differ in terms of motor and sensory function, there may be up to four different segments identified in determining the neurological level (i.e., right sensory, left sensory, right motor, and left motor). These levels are determined by neurological examination of a key sensory point in each of 28 right and 28 left dermatomes and a key muscle in each of 10 right and 10 left myotomes. A zone of partial preservation may be present in complete injuries

and is defined as encompassing those dermatomes and myotomes caudal to the neurological level that remain partially innervated (Table 4).

The vertebral level of an injury is defined as the level of greatest vertebral damage on radiological examination. It is clear that the vertebral level and the neurological levels may be similar or may differ by one or more segments.

Recently, there has been an emphasis on determining the effect of SCI on the overall function of the patient. To date, a specific functional measure has not been developed for SCI, but there is evidence that the functional independence measurement (FIM) developed for other neurological disorders[10] is useful for SCI patients as well. For example, in the recently completed third National Acute Spinal Cord Injury study of methylprednisolone versus tirilazad, the FIM result was one of the outcome measures of this clinical trial.[6]

SPINAL SHOCK

Spinal shock is a type of neurogenic shock that occurs in major SCI and can be a source of considerable confusion. Systemic shock, such as a thoracic cord injury with a concomitant aortic injury, also can occur in SCI patients. Spinal shock implies the loss of somatic motor, sensory, and sympathetic autonomic function due to SCI.[12] The more severe the SCI and the higher the level of injury, the greater the severity and duration of spinal shock. Thus, spinal shock is most severe in complete upper cervical cord injuries, less severe in incomplete thoracic injuries, and minimal in lumbar cord injuries.

The somatic motor component of spinal shock consists of paralysis, flaccidity, and areflexia with respect to deep tendon reflexes and cutaneous reflexes, and the sensory component is anesthesia to all modalities. The autonomic component is systemic hypotension, skin hyperemia and warmth, and bradycardia due to loss of sympathetic function but persisting parasympathetic function (unopposed vagotonia). The exact mechanism of spinal shock is unknown but may be due to temporary local effects on impulse conduction in the traumatized spinal cord caused by electrolyte or neurotransmitter changes.

In the first few hours and days after an SCI,

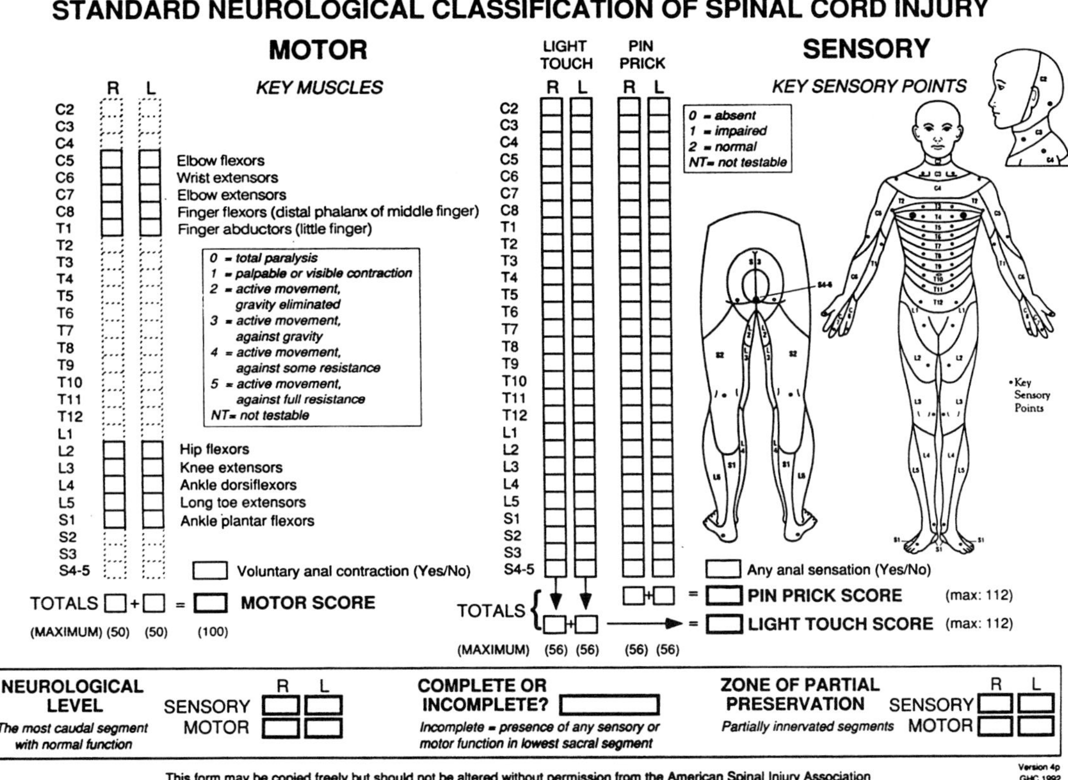

Figure 1: Neurological classification of SCI (ASIA/IMSOP). This diagram contains the principal information about motor, sensory, and sphincter function necessary for accurate classification and scoring of acute SCI. The 10 key muscles to be tested for the motor examination are shown on the left along with the Medical Research Council grading system, and the 28 dermatomes to be tested on each side for the sensory examination are shown on the right. The system for recording the neurological level(s), the completeness of the injury, and the zone of partial preservation (in complete injuries) are shown at the bottom.

there is often a combination of the temporary physiological effects of spinal shock and the more permanent pathological effects of the cord injury. Another problem is the variable duration of spinal shock. The author recommends the following guidelines: 1) the somatic motor and sensory components of spinal shock last only 1 hour or less, and thus have terminated by the time the majority of patients are examined in the initial hospital admission, which in most countries is within 1 to 4 hours of injury; and 2) the reflex and autonomic components of spinal shock may last from days to months, depending on the level and severity of cord injury. In practical terms, these guidelines mean that the motor and sensory deficits detected 1 hour or more after SCI are due to physical SCI rather than to

spinal shock. This is certainly a safe course to follow because it eliminates the possible error of missing a serious SCI because the observed deficits were presumed due to spinal shock.

INCOMPLETE ACUTE SCI SYNDROMES

There are many types of incomplete acute neurological syndromes occurring in an SCI (Table 4). These syndromes are generally named according to the presumed location of the injury in the transverse plane of the spinal cord (Figures 2 to 8).[24] In addition to grading patients according to the ASIA/IMSOP scale, it is helpful for practitioners to categorize the incomplete

TABLE 4

ACUTE SPINAL CORD INJURY SYNDROMES
IN TRAUMA PATIENTS

Complete spinal cord injury
ASIA/IMSOP Grade A
Unilevel: no zone of partial preservation
Multiple level: zone of partial preservation

Incomplete spinal cord injury
ASIA/IMSOP Grades B, C, and D
Cervicomedullary syndrome
Central cord syndrome
Anterior cord syndrome
Posterior cord syndrome
Brown-Séquard syndrome
Conus medullaris syndrome

Complete cauda equina injury
ASIA/IMSOP Grade A

Incomplete cauda equina injury
ASIA/IMSOP Grades B, C, and D

Reversible or transient syndromes
Cord concussion
Burning hands syndrome
Contusio cervicalis
Hysteria

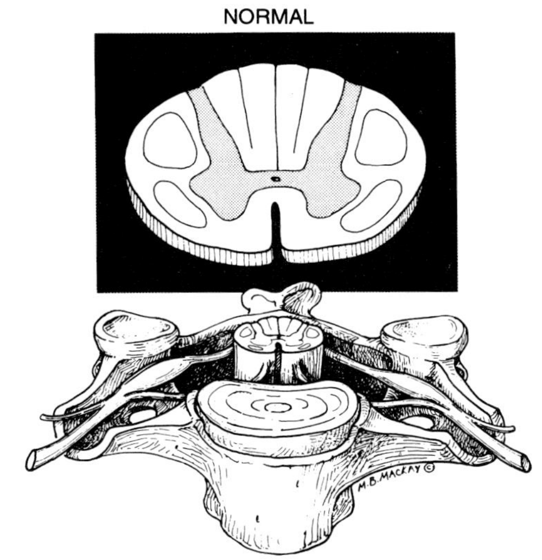

Figure 2: The normal spinal cord and spinal column. The normal relationships between the spinal cord, spinal column, and nerve roots are depicted in the mid-cervical region. The dura has been omitted for clarity. In the upper diagram, the gray matter is finely stippled, and the corticospinal and spinothalamic tracts are outlined. The intervertebral disc is shown. Reprinted with permission from Tator.[23]

patients according to the location of the injury in the spinal cord. First, recognition of the type of incomplete syndrome provides some information about the mechanism of injury, which in turn provides useful information for the selection of treatment. Second, the various categories of incomplete injury have differing prognoses for recovery.

Cervicomedullary Syndrome

A high proportion of injuries to the upper cervical cord will include damage to the medulla as well. These injuries may extend down to C4 or even lower and may extend up to the pons, due either to direct or vascular injury to the vertebral arteries. "Cervicomedullary syndrome" is a useful term to describe the syndromes that involve the upper cervical cord and brainstem, although several other terms have been used, including cruciate paralysis.

The essential features of these include respiratory insufficiency or arrest, hypotension, vary-ing degrees of tetraparesis and hyperesthesia from C1-4, and sensory loss over the face conforming to the onion skin or Déjerine pattern.[19,21] Of course, the higher the lesion, the more severe the manifestations such as those present in patients with atlanto-occipital dislocation. The mechanisms of SCI also include traction injury from severe dislocation as in atlantoaxial dislocation, anterior-posterior compression from burst fracture or odontoid fracture, or ruptured disc. More-prompt and better first-aid account for an increased incidence of these injuries compared with previous experience, due to the larger number of survivors arriving at neurosurgical centers.

It is important to test facial sensation in all patients with cervical SCI, as first urged by Schneider,[19,21] to detect damage to the fibers or cell bodies of the descending spinal tract of the trigeminal nerve or the nucleus of the spinal tract of the trigeminal nerve, respectively, which begin in the pons and medulla and extend downward to at least the C4 cervical segment.

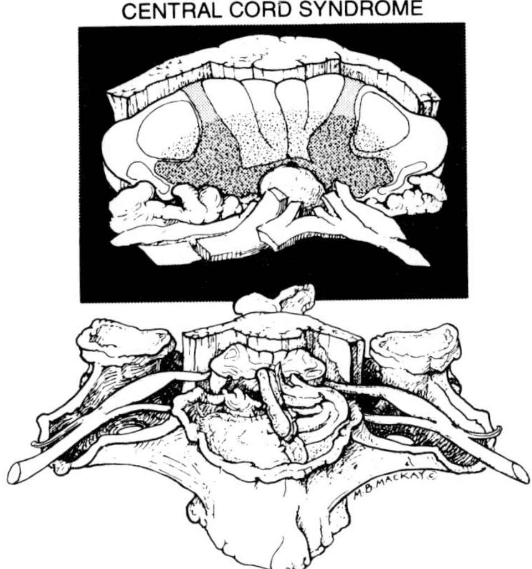

Figure 3: Central cord syndrome. The drawing depicts a case of cervical spondylosis with osteoarthritis of the cervical spine including anterior and posterior osteophytes and hypertrophy of the ligamentum flavum. Superimposed is an acute hyperextension injury that has caused rupture of the intervertebral disc and infolding of the ligamentum flavum. The spinal cord is compressed anteriorly and posteriorly. The central portion of the cord shown in rough stippling sustained the greatest damage. The damaged area includes the medial segments of the corticospinal tracts presumed to subserve arm function. Reprinted with permission from Tator.[23]

Due to the onion-skin or Déjerine pattern of topographic representation, a perioral distribution of sensory loss denotes a lesion in the lower medulla and upper cervical cord, whereas a more peripheral facial distribution of sensory loss involving the forehead, ear, and chin denotes a lesion in the cord at C3-4. Cervicomedullary injuries often mimic the central cord syndrome because of a greater weakness in the arm than the leg.

Acute Central Cord Syndrome

Schneider[21,22] described the acute central cervical cord injury syndrome characterized by a disproportionally greater loss of motor power in the upper extremities than the lower extremities with varying degrees of sensory loss. He hypothesized that acute compression was an etiological factor in many cases such as cord compression between bony bars or spurs anteriorly and infolded ligamenta flava posteriorly (Figure 3). Table 5 shows the similarities and differences between the central cord syndrome and the syndrome of cruciate paralysis. Clinically, it may be very difficult to make this distinction. Fortunately, the combination of plain films, computed

TABLE 5

CENTRAL CORD SYNDROME VS. CRUCIATE PARALYSIS WITH ARMS WEAKER THAN LEGS

	Central Cord Syndrome	Syndrome of Cruciate Paralysis
Site of Lesions	Mid to lower Anterior horn cells Lateral corticospinal tract (medial part)	Lower medulla and upper cervical cord, anterior aspect Corticospinal decussation caudal to the pyramids
Clinical Manifestations	Arms weaker than legs Flaccid arms acutely Legs normal or variably weak Lower motor neuron deficits in upper limbs persist	Arms weaker than legs Flaccid arms acutely Legs normal or variably weak Upper motor neuron deficits in upper limbs develop ± Trigeminal sensory deficit (onion skin, spinal tract of 5th cranial nerve) ± Cranial nerve dysfunction (9th, 10th, or 11th cranial nerve)
Prognosis for Neurological Recovery	Variable	Usually good

tomography (CT), and magnetic resonance imaging (MRI) can usually accurately localize the lesion to either the mid to lower cervical spine in the central cord syndrome or to the cervicomedullary junction in the syndrome of cruciate paralysis.[7]

There is recent evidence that syndromes characterized by greater weakness of the arm than leg are not based on previously enunciated mechanisms such as the presumed differing locations of the arm and leg fibers in the corticospinal tract.[13] In contrast, the new explanation is derived from careful clinical-pathological-MRI correlations[17] and of cases of SCI. The new understanding is based on the finding that the corticospinal tract subserves mainly distal limb musculature and, thus, the functional deficit would be more pronounced in the hands when the tract is the primary site of damage.

It is of interest that Schneider initially admonished against operating on individuals with central cord syndrome because of their good prognosis for spontaneous recovery. Indeed, in some instances, his patients showed very rapid spontaneous clinical recovery. Furthermore, Schneider reported deterioration following laminectomy in some patients. Although it is true that a considerable number of patients with central cord syndrome make a substantial recovery without surgery, many remain with significant deficits,[3] especially with serious impairment of the hands due to a combination of severe weakness and severe proprioceptive loss. When there is persistent compression, instability, or neurological deterioration, a patient with central cord syndrome should be considered a surgical candidate.

Anterior Cord Syndrome

Anterior cord syndrome was originally described in the setting of acute cervical trauma by Schneider,[20] who presented two patients with "immediate complete paralysis with hyperesthesia at the level of the lesion and an associated sparing of touch and some vibration sense." Both patients, one of which was a young football player, had a ruptured disc (the football player also had bone fragments in the canal), and both made a substantial recovery following surgical removal of the intracanalicular space-occupying lesions (Figure 4). This syndrome, in Schneider's

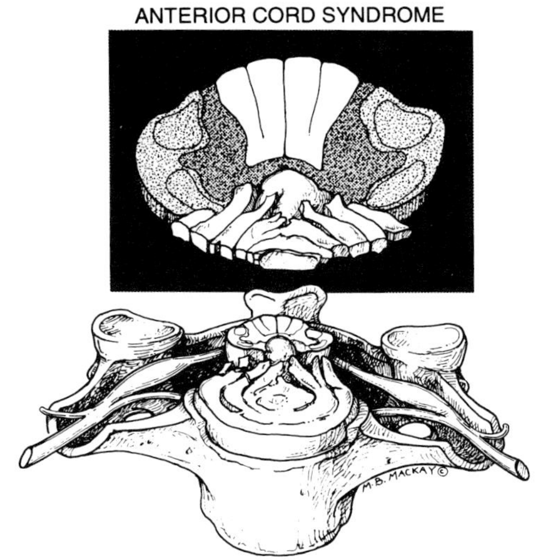

Figure 4: Anterior cord syndrome. A large disc herniation is shown compressing the anterior aspect of the cord and resulting in damage (rough stippling) to the anterior and lateral white matter tracts and to the grey matter. The posterior columns remain intact. Reprinted with permission from Tator.[23]

view, was "a syndrome for which early operative intervention is indicated." The anterior aspect of the cord is damaged and, in severe cases, there may only be sparing of the posterior columns (Figure 4). In less severe cases, there may be some retention of motor function due to sparing of some fibers in the lateral corticospinal tracts.

Posterior Cord Syndrome

Posterior cord syndrome is a rarely seen type of incomplete SCI syndrome. Many researchers, including the author, have doubted its existence. It supposedly occurs after major destruction of the posterior aspect of the cord but with some residual functioning spinal cord tissue anteriorly (Figure 5). Thus, clinically, the patient has retained spinothalamic function but lost movement and proprioception due to damage to the posterior half of the cord, including the corticospinal tracts and posterior columns.

Brown-Séquard Syndrome

The Brown-Séquard syndrome is caused by a lesion of the lateral half of the spinal cord (Fig-

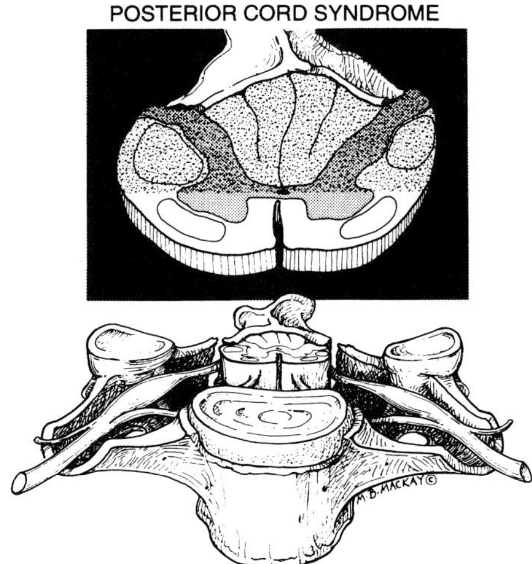

Figure 5: Posterior cord syndrome. A laminar fracture is depicted with anterior displacement of the fractured bone and compression of the posterior aspect of the spinal cord. The damaged area of the cord (roughly stippled in the upper diagram) includes the posterior columns and the posterior half of the lateral columns including the corticospinal tracts. Reprinted with permission from Tator.[23]

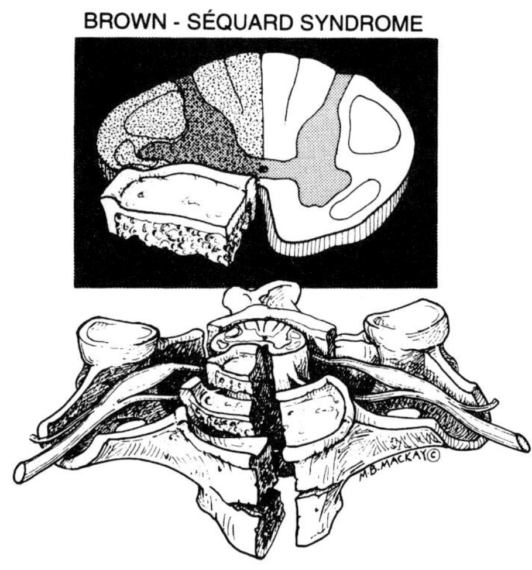

Figure 6: Brown-Séquard syndrome. A burst fracture is depicted, with posterior displacement of bone fragments and disc, resulting in unilateral compression and damage (rough stippling) to one-half of the spinal cord. Reprinted with permission from Tator.[23]

ure 6) and is characterized by ipsilateral motor and proprioceptive loss and contralateral pain and body temperature loss. The syndrome can be associated with a variety of mechanisms of injury, but in the series of Braakman and Penning[4] was most often observed with hyperextension injuries; also reported were cases with flexion injuries, locked facets, and compression fractures.

The Brown-Séquard syndrome may be present at the onset of injury in some patients; in others, it may become apparent only several days after injury as a gradual evolution from a bilateral incomplete injury. Hybrid combinations of Brown-Séquard and other incomplete syndromes may occur. For example, the author has seen examples of central cord injuries that are quite asymmetric, with the more severely damaged side of the cord showing features of a Brown-Séquard syndrome. The Brown-Séquard syndrome occurs most often following cervical injuries and less frequently in the thoracic cord and conus medullaris. In milder cases, there may be no sphincter deficit.

Conus Medullaris Syndrome

Almost all of the lumbar cord segments are opposite the T12 vertebral body, and almost all of the sacral cord segments are opposite the L1 vertebral body with the cord ending opposite the L1-2 disc space (Figure 7). Because injuries at T11-12 and T12-L1 are relatively common due to the mobility of these segments compared with the relatively immobile thoracic segments, injuries to the conus medullaris are frequent. These injuries usually produce a combination of lower motor neuron deficits with initial flaccid paralysis of the legs and anal sphincter. This is followed in the chronic phase by a combination of some degree of muscle atrophy and spasticity or reflex hyperactivity with, possibly, an extensor plantar response. The sensory picture may be variable, and in some cases the only evidence of incompleteness is retention of some perianal sensation, which is an example of sacral sparing. In the more severe conus lesions, bowel and bladder deficits may be profound with the ultimate development of a low-pressure, high-capacity neurogenic bladder.

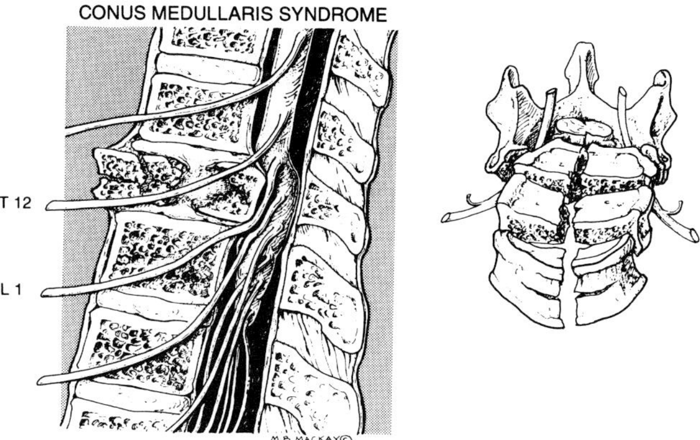

Figure 7: Conus medullaris syndrome. A burst fracture of T12 is depicted with posterior dislocation of bone fragments from the vertebral body into the spinal canal resulting in compression of the conus medullaris. Almost all the lumbar cord segments are opposite the T12 vertebral body, so that a severe compression injury at this level could affect all lumbar and sacral segments of the cord. Reprinted with permission from Tator.[23]

CAUDA EQUINA INJURIES

With the spinal cord normally terminating opposite the L1-2 disc space (Figure 7), injuries at this level or below involve the roots of the cauda equina, although injuries one or two levels above also involve the origins of some of the roots comprising the cauda equina. Clinically, these injuries may be complete (Grade A on the new ASIA/IMSOP scale), whereas incomplete injuries vary in severity and range from Grades B to D. Similar to SCI, the motor fibers tend to be more susceptible to trauma so that incomplete cases always have sensory preservation with or without some motor preservation. Cases with only motor preservation are extremely rare. The degree of bowel and bladder deficits parallels those found with cord injury. It is believed that cauda equina injuries have a much better prognosis for neurological recovery compared with SCI because the lower motor neuron inherently has more resilience to trauma, with fewer secondary injury mechanisms and greater regenerative capacity than the upper motor neuron and its tracts.

One interesting and dangerous cauda equina syndrome is associated with acute central disc herniation at L4-5 or L5-S1 and results in major damage to the sacral roots that lie centrally within the dural sac (Figure 8). Partial or complete sparing of the lumbar roots and often the

S1 roots may be present as well. Thus, these patients may have total preservation of leg strength but complete bowel and bladder paralysis as well as perineal anesthesia. The sacral roots are very delicate and sometimes may not recover, even when decompressed reasonably expeditiously.

REVERSIBLE OR TRANSIENT SYNDROMES

There are a number of complete or incomplete SCI syndromes that are reversible or transient (Table 4). One of the most interesting is the "burning-hands syndrome," which frequently occurs in athletes.[28] The syndrome is characterized by transient paresthesiae and dysesthesiae in the upper limbs, especially the hands. It may exist with or without long-tract signs, which, if present, are usually evanescent. Biemond[2] found pathological changes in the posterior horn of one case and termed the condition "contusio cervicalis posterior." Braakman and Penning[5] found that hyperextension was the most frequent mechanism of injury. Intramedullary lesions may be demonstrable by MRI.[28] Torg et al[26] described a transient incomplete spinal cord syndrome with sensory and motor deficits that lasted up to 48 hours in football players and used the inappropriate term "neurapraxia." They found that all of the patients had radiological

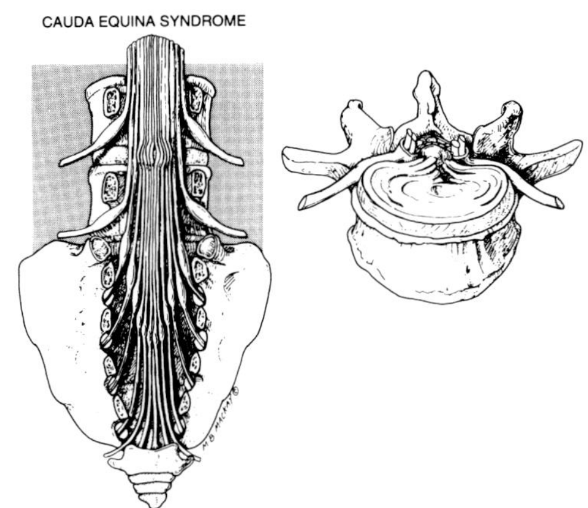

Figure 8: Cauda equina syndrome. The drawing shows an acute central disc herniation of L4-5 with major compression of the central aspect of the cauda equina. The medially placed sacral roots from S2 downward sustain the maximal compression, whereas the more laterally located L5 and S1 roots are completely or partially spared. Reprinted with permission from Tator.[23]

spinal abnormalities such as ligamentous instability, disc disease, or spinal stenosis. These transient cord injury syndromes are usually bilateral, which distinguishes them from the other syndrome of "stingers" or "burners" in athletes due to unilateral nerve root or brachial plexus lesions (especially traction injury), most of which are also transient.[28]

Spinal cord concussion is a transient loss of motor or sensory function of the spinal cord, with recovery of function usually within minutes but always within hours. In most instances, the patient reports that the symptoms are rapidly diminishing and a normal neurological examination is found. The exact pathophysiology of spinal cord concussion is unknown, but most likely is caused by a biochemical abnormality in the cord such as leakage of potassium from the intracellular to the extracellular space due either to direct mechanical injury or secondary to a vascular mechanism. The latter possibility was suggested by Schneider et al.[21]

Acute Spinal Cord Syndrome without Radiological Evidence of Trauma

The syndrome of SCI without radiological abnormality (SCIWORA) is more common in children than in adults and represents a significant percentage of pediatric SCIs.[16] Children with SCIWORA tend to be less severely injured than those with definite evidence of bony injury, although complete injuries have been described. By definition, the negative radiological examination includes only plain films and tomography, either conventional or CT. If a negative MRI was included in the definition, the number of cases would diminish dramatically, because of the extreme sensitivity of MRI in detecting mild cord injury and spinal column injuries such as torn ligaments and ruptured discs. Children are more susceptible to these injuries, presumably because of the laxity of their spinal ligaments and the weakness of their paraspinal muscles.

True SCIWORA can also occur in adults, but is much less frequent than the syndrome of SCI without radiological evidence of trauma (SCIWORET). In patients with SCIWORET, radiological examinations are abnormal but x-rays show no evidence of trauma. Prior to the use of CT in spinal trauma, the incidence of SCIWORET in adults was approximately 14%.[24] The addition of CT has reduced the reported incidence of SCIWORET to about 5%. There has been a recent analysis of the incidence of SCIWORET in a Japanese study of acute SCI[18] which shows that many of these patients have demonstrable compression by myelography or MRI and should be considered for early surgical decompression. It is likely that very few SCIs will remain undetected by MRI, because of its high sensitivity for detecting mild SCI and nonbony spinal column lesions. Cervical spondylosis is the most common associated condition in adults with SCIWORET, but other arthropathies (e.g., spinal stenosis, ankylosing spondylitis, and disc herniation) may on rare occasion be associated with SCI and not show radiological evidence of trauma.

Trauma Patients with an Acute Spinal Cord Syndrome but Without Direct Trauma to the Spine

In some trauma patients, there is an acute spinal cord syndrome but no direct trauma to the spine. This relatively rare syndrome differs from SCIWORET and SCIWORA in that these patients sustain a lesion of the spinal cord that manifests as an acute spinal cord syndrome and is associated with trauma although the trauma is not to the spine. The syndrome can occur in both children and adults and produces the clinical findings known as the "anterior spinal artery syndrome." Keith[11] described several cases in children with major abdominal, thoracic, or limb trauma and concluded that many had sustained an aortic injury that caused occlusion of intercostal or lumbar arteries with subsequent occlusion of medullary arteries and spinal cord infarction. Rarely, penetrating injuries such as gunshot wounds can interrupt major arterial feeders to the cord without direct trauma to the spine. Severe hypotension and systemic shock in trauma patients can also result in spinal cord ischemia and infarction, even without causing concomitant cerebral ischemia.

REFERENCES

1. American Spinal Injury Association, International Medical Society of Paraplegia: **International Standards for Neurological and Functional Classification of Spinal Cord Injury. Revised 1992.** Chicago, Ill: ASIA/IMSOP, 1992
2. Biemond A: Contusio cervicalis posterior. **Nederl T Geneesk 108:**1333-1335, 1964
3. Bosch A, Stauffer S, Nickel VL: Incomplete traumatic quadriplegia: a ten year review. **JAMA 216:**473-478, 1971
4. Braakman R, Penning L: Injuries of the cervical spine. **Excerpta Medica.** Amsterdam, 1971
5. Braakman R, Penning L: Injuries of the cervical spine, in Vinken PJ, Bruyn GW (eds): **Handbook of Clinical Neurology. Vol 25.** New York, NY: American Elsevier, 1976, pp 227-380
6. Brackman MB, Shepard MJ, Holford TR, et al: Administration of methylprednisolone for 24 or 48 hours of tirilazad mesylate for 48 hours in the treatment of acute spinal cord injury. Results of the Third National Acute Spinal Cord Injury Randomized Controlled Trial. **JAMA 277:**1597-1604, 1997
7. Dickman CA, Hadley MN, Pappas CTE, et al: Cruciate paralysis: a clinical and radiographic analysis of injuries to the cervicomedullary junction. **J Neurosurg 73:**850-858, 1990
8. Frankel HL, Hancock DO, Hyslop G, et al: The value of postural reduction in the initial management of closed injuries of the spine with paraplegia and tetraplegia. **Paraplegia 7:**179-192, 1969
9. Hansebout RR: A comprehensive review of methods of improving cord recovery after acute spinal cord injury, in Tator CH (ed): **Early Management of Acute Spinal Cord Injury.** New York, NY: Raven Press, 1982, pp 181-196
10. Keith RA, Granger CV, Hamilton BB, et al: The functional independence measure: a new tool for rehabilitation. **Adv Clin Rehab 1:**6-18, 1987
11. Keith WS: Traumatic infarction of the spinal cord. **Can J Neurol Sci 1:**124-126, 1974
12. Kiss ZHT, Tator CH: Neurogenic shock, in Geller ER (ed): **Shock and Resuscitation.** New York, NY: McGraw-Hill, 1993, pp 421-440
13. Levi ADO, Tator CH, Bunge RP: Clinical syndromes associated with disproportionate weakness of the upper versus the lower extremities after cervical spinal cord injury. **Neurosurgery 38:**179-185, 1996
14. Medical Research Council: **Aids to Investigation of Peripheral Nerve Injuries: Medical Research Council War Memorandum.** 2nd ed. London: HM Stationery Office, 1943
15. Michaelis LS, Braakman R: Current terminology and classification of injuries of spine and spinal cord, in Vinken PJ, Bruyn GW (eds): **Handbook of Clinical Neurology. Vol 25.** New York, NY: American Elsevier, 1976, pp 145-153
16. Pang D, Wilberger JE Jr: Spinal cord injury without radiographic abnormalities in children. **J Neurosurg 57:**114-129, 1982
17. Quencer RM, Bunge RP, Egnor M, et al: Acute traumatic central cord syndrome: MRI—pathological correlations. **Neuroradiology 34:**85-94, 1992
18. Saruhashi Y, Hukuda S, Katsuura A, et al: Clinical outcomes of cervical spinal cord injuries without radiographic evidence of trauma. **Spinal Cord 36:** 567-573, 1998
19. Schneider RC: Concomitant craniocerebral and spinal trauma, with special reference to the cervicomedullary region. **Clin Neurosurg 17:**266-309, 1970
20. Schneider RC: A syndrome in acute cervical injuries for which early operation is indicated. **J Neurosurg 8:** 360-367, 1951
21. Schneider RC, Cherry G, Pantek H: The syndrome of acute central cervical spinal cord injury. **J Neurosurg 11:**546-577, 1954
22. Schneider RC, Crosby EC, Russo EH, et al: Traumatic spinal cord syndromes and their management. **Clin Neurosurg 20:**424-492, 1973
23. Tator CH: Classification of spinal cord injury based on neurological presentation, in Narayan RK, Wilberger JE Jr, Povlishock JT (eds): **Neurotrauma.** New York, NY: McGraw-Hill, 1996, pp 1053-1073
24. Tator CH: Spine-spinal cord relationships in spinal cord trauma. **Clin Neurosurg 30:**479-494, 1983
25. Tator CH, Rowed DW, Schwartz ML: Sunnybrook cord injury scales for assessing neurological injury and neurological recovery, in Tator CH (ed): **Early Management of Acute Spinal Cord Injury.** New York, NY: Raven Press, 1982, Vol 2, pp 7-24
26. Torg JS, Pavlov H, Genuario SC, et al: Neurapraxia of the cervical spinal cord with transient quadriplegia. **J Bone Joint Surg (Am) 68:**1354-1370, 1986
27. Waters RL, Adkins RH, Yakura JS: Definition of complete spinal cord injury. **Paraplegia 29:**573-581, 1991
28. Wilberger JE Jr, Maroon JC: Cervical spine injuries in athletes. **Physician Sports Med(March)18:**57-70, 1990

CHAPTER 5

CELLULAR, IONIC, AND BIOMOLECULAR MECHANISMS OF THE INJURY PROCESS

MICHAEL G. FEHLINGS, MD, PHD, FRCSC, AND
LALI H.S. SEKHON, MBBS, PHD, FRACS

Spinal cord injury (SCI) occurs in various countries throughout the world with an annual incidence of 15-40 cases per million population. The causes of these injuries range from motor-vehicle accidents and community violence to recreational activities and workplace-related injuries.[176] Of the estimated 12,000 paraplegic and quadriplegic injuries that occur in the U.S. each year, 4000 die before reaching hospital and 1000 die during their hospitalization.[5,40,120,157] Although there has been much work done, the only treatment known to date to ameliorate neurological dysfunction that occurs at or below the level of neurological injury has been methylprednisolone.[31-38] Despite this, a great deal of research over the past 30-40 years has focused on SCI, with the complex pathophysiological processes slowly being unraveled. Given the enormous expense of SCI to the community,[7] only by a full understanding of the pathophysiological changes that occur at cellular and subcellular levels can the hopes of reversal or augmentation of recovery be realized.

THE CONCEPTS OF PRIMARY AND SECONDARY MECHANISMS

It is now generally accepted that acute SCI is a two-step process involving primary and secondary mechanisms. The primary mechanism involves the initial mechanical injury due to local deformation and energy transformation, while the secondary mechanisms encompass a cascade of biochemical and cellular processes that are initiated by the primary process and that may cause ongoing cellular damage and even cell death (Table 1).[43,88,158,178] The concept of a secondary mechanism to acute SCI was first postulated in 1911, when Allen noted an improvement in neurological function after the removal of post-traumatic hematomyelia in dogs who underwent experimental acute SCI.[7] Three years later, Allen[6] speculated that there was a putative "biochemical factor" present in the hemorrhagic necrosis material that may be instigating ongoing damage. Since that time, the concept of primary and secondary mechanisms and their duality in acute

TABLE 1

PRIMARY AND SECONDARY MECHANISMS OF
ACUTE SPINAL CORD INJURY

Primary Injury Mechanism
  Acute compression
  Impact
  Missile
  Distraction
  Laceration
  Shear

Secondary Injury Mechanisms
Systemic effects
  Heart rate—brief increase, then prolonged
    bradycardia
  Blood pressure—brief hypertension,
    then prolonged hypotension
  Decreased peripheral resistance
  Decreased cardiac output
  Increased catecholamines, then decreased
  Hypoxia
  Hyperthermia
  Injudicious movement of the unstable spine
    leading to worsening compression
Local vascular changes
  Loss of autoregulation
  Systemic hypotension (neurogenic shock)
  Hemorrhage (especially gray matter)
  Loss of microcirculation
  Reduction in blood flow: Vasospasm;
    Thrombosis
Electrolyte changes
  Increased intracellular calcium
  Increased intracellular sodium
  Increased sodium permeability
  Increased intracellular potassium
Biochemical changes
  Neurotransmitter accumulation
  Catecholamines (e.g., norepinephrine and
    dopamine)
  Excitotoxic amino acids (e.g., glutamate)
  Arachidonic acid release
  Free radical production
  Eicosanoid production: Prostaglandins
  Lipid peroxidation
  Endogenous opioids
  Cytokines
Edema
Loss of energy metabolism: Decreased adenosine
  triphosphate production
Apoptosis
Loss of neurotrophic factor support

SCI has also been embraced in the understanding of the pathophysiology of subarachnoid hemorrhage (SAH), cerebral and spinal ischemia, and head trauma.

MODELING SPINAL CORD INJURY

Although much of the understanding of the pathophysiology of SCI has come from analysis of clinical cases, most of the more detailed knowledge has come from the laboratory, particularly from looking at experimental models of SCI. In the majority of human SCIs, the mechanism of primary injury is acute compression or laceration of the spinal cord due to displacement of bone or disc into the spinal cord during fracture or dislocation of the vertebral column.[175] In an attempt to replicate this injury in the laboratory, several experimental models were developed that simulated the compressive type of acute SCI.[70] The was first described by Allen in 1911,[7] where he employed a weight-dropping technique in dogs. A variety of modifications to the Allen model have been developed, including the NYU impactor model,[82] to enhance the precision and reproducibility of experimental SCI. Compressive models are either static or kinetic, depending on the biomechanics of the forces that are applied. Kinetic models typically involve rapid compression of the spinal cord in less than 1 second or, more usually, less than 100 msec. The applied load compresses the spinal cord with increasing velocity (acceleration >0) to the point of maximal compression. Static compression models used forces that slowly compress the cord at an approximately constant velocity. Of the many kinetic compression models available, the extradural balloon compression method,[174] the aneurysmal clip compression model,[55,112] and recent modifications of the Allen technique (e.g., the NYU impactor model) most closely simulate human acute SCI. Kinetic models more closely represent the human clinical scenario than static compression models. The reader is referred to Fehlings and Tator[69] for a more detailed review of these models.

Aside from compression, distraction injuries have been simulated in animal models.[56] Models utilizing spinal cord transection have also been described; however, this scenario is rarely encountered in the clinical situation.[76,106] Utilization of these models has allowed for the isolation of putative factors and pathways believed to play a key role in acute SCI. In order to fully understand the cellular and biochemical processes involved in acute SCI, the primary and particularly the secondary mechanisms, gleaned from the research done with these models, need to be evaluated.

Primary Mechanisms of Spinal Cord Injury

Primary SCI is most commonly a combination of the initial impact as well as subsequent persisting compression. This will typically occur with fracture dislocation, burst fractures, missile injuries, and acutely ruptured discs. Clinical scenarios where impact alone occurs without ongoing compression may include severe ligamentous injuries where the spinal column dislocates and then spontaneously reduces. Similarly, spinal cord laceration from sharp bone fragments or missile injuries can produce a mixture of spinal cord laceration, contusion and compression, or concussion.[176]

Secondary Mechanisms of Spinal Cord Injury

The various theories of secondary mechanisms of SCI have undergone a process of maturation in the past three decades. In the 1970s, the free radical hypothesis, as advocated by Demopoulos et al,[51] was believed to be crucial to the injury process. Ten years later, the focus shifted to the role of calcium, opiate receptors, and lipid peroxidation. As we enter the new millennium, modern research is implicating apoptosis, intracellular protein synthesis inhibition, and glutaminergic mechanisms among a myriad of pathophysiological pathways that mediate secondary injury mechanisms. The complexity and interrelationship of these secondary mechanisms are now being embraced. The following secondary mechanisms of SCI are discussed below: ischemia; free radical-mediated cell injury;

ionic mechanisms; receptor-mediated cell injury; inflammatory-mediated cell injury; and apoptosis.

Ischemia

Changes in spinal cord blood flow (SCBF) and the perturbations that follow are an important part of the changes induced by acute SCI. The changes that occur in SCBF after an acute injury can be divided into systemic and local. Immediately after an SCI, a major reduction in local blood flow occurs (Figure 1).[29,80,114,161,178] If left untreated, the ischemia becomes progressively worse over the first few hours.[71] Experimentally, ischemia may persist for at least 24 hours after major SCI in rats[155] or monkeys.[158] The precise mechanisms behind this are unclear. Vasospasm secondary to mechanical damage or a vasoactive amine may be partially responsible.[178] Endothelial swelling or damage may be occurring.[53] Hemorrhages may promote ischemia[183] or thrombosis may occur via platelet aggregation.[48,140] Finally, excitatory amino acids (EAAs), particularly glutamate, may be involved. Ischemia may play a role in the formation of local cord edema, although whether edema formation is injurious in itself or is an epiphenomenon is still unclear.

Because of differences in relative vascularity, the central gray matter, along with adjacent white matter, is more severely affected by acute SCI than peripheral white matter.[188] In the normal situation, gray matter to white matter blood flow is maintained at a 3:1 ratio.[96] Studies on *in vivo* SCBF have confirmed this dichotomy between central gray matter and surrounding white matter.[20,67] White matter perfusion typically decreases within 5 minutes of an acute SCI and begins to return to normal within 15 minutes. Thereafter, it remains near normal preinjury values during the first 24 hours. In contradistinction, in central gray matter, numerous hemorrhages typically occur as early as 5 minutes after an acute SCI. Perfusion is relatively absent 1 hour after an injury, and this state remains so for at least the first 24 hours. It has been suggested that the peripheral changes seen in SCBF are due to initial vasospasm, but it seems unlikely that this alone causes the central

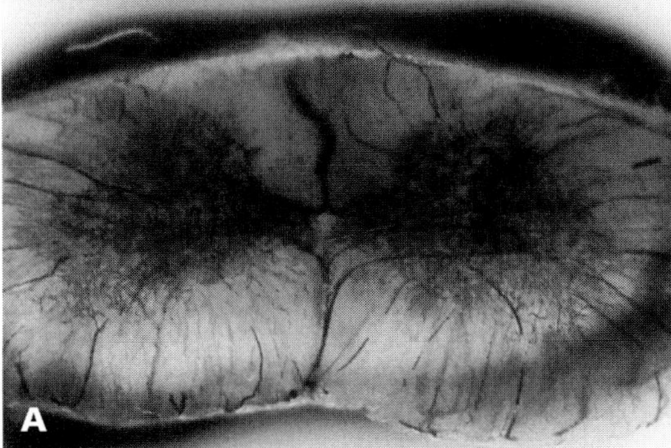
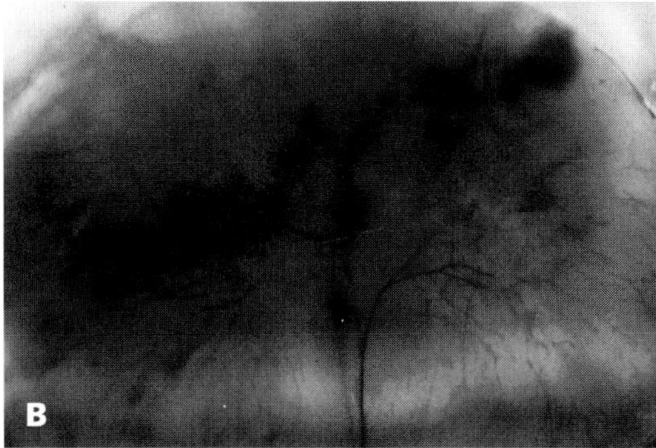

Figure 1: A) Spinal angiogram demonstrating a normal cord. Note the extensive, well-organized microcirculation, concentrated in the gray matter. The prominent anterior spinal artery and anterior sulcal arteries are well defined. **B)** Spinal angiogram after acute SCI demonstrating cord ischemia. Extensive disruption has occurred at the point of impact, with local hemorrhage. Surrounding this immediate zone of hematoma formation, relative ischemia in the microcirculation is apparent. In this example, the anterior sulcal artery is patent.

phenomenon. This vascular standstill has been confirmed using microangiography,[74,178] fluorescent tracer studies,[54] and the operating microscope;[14] it plays a major role in the devastating outcomes following acute SCI.

The contribution of vascular mechanisms in the pathophysiology of human SCI was meticulously reviewed by Tator and Koyanagi.[179] Using silicon rubber microangiography, the authors shed light on the role of the sulcal arterial system and pial arteries in the spinal cord. The centrifugal sulcal arterial system supplies the anterior gray matter, the anterior half of the posterior gray matter, the inner half of the anterior and lateral white columns, and the anterior half of the posterior white columns. Traumatized spinal cords show severe hemorrhages predominantly in gray matter, and it may be obstruction of these anterior sulcal arteries that leads to the hemorrhagic necrosis and subsequent central myelomalacia seen at the site of injury.

Alterations in endothelial cell function causing an increase in vascular permeability and edema formation have been well documented.[81,102,168] Endothelial damage occurs early, with the formation of craters, adherence of noncellular debris, over-riding of endothelial cell junctions, and microglobular formations occurring 1-2 hours after acute SCI.[52]

Histopathologically, progressive hemorrhages develop early in the central region of the spinal cord (especially in the gray matter). It is very likely that these occur because of the forces imparted by the primary injury, with direct mechanical disruption of the capillaries and venules occurring.[53] Angiographic studies both experimentally and in the human scenario confirm that the large arteries remain patent, but a major change occurs in the local microcirculation (mainly capillaries and venules) in the vicinity of the injury, spreading peripherally for a considerable distance.[117,118] The anterior spinal artery is rarely thrombosed.[188]

Autoregulation is also impaired after acute SCI.[115,162,193] Systemic hypotension can cause further decreases in SCBF with induced hypertension not necessarily reversing the ischemia, but rather causing marked hyperemia at adjacent sites.[84,178] Experimentally, it has been shown in animal studies that autoregulation is intact during the initial 60 to 90 minutes after SCI, but is then lost coincident with the onset of ischemia. It has been suggested that the ischemic response to SCI is mediated both by the loss of autoregulation and by relative constriction of the resistance vessels.[162]

Disturbances of venous drainage may play a role in the secondary damage that occurs after acute SCI, particularly in terms of exacerbating ischemia of the posterior columns.[118,119,163] This hypothesis gains credibility from studies that show that venous occlusion in various pathological conditions causes white matter lesions.[113, 142,150] It may be that peculiarities of venous drainage of the spinal cord make it more susceptible to damage.[119]

Following an acute SCI, an immediate but transient increase in mean arterial blood pressure may occur followed by profound hypotension.[58,63,93,172,186,195] The reason for this transient hypertension is unknown, but may be mediated by both the thoracic sympathetic ganglia and the adrenal glands.[194] Acute SCI is one of the causes of neurogenic shock,[15] typically being related to the magnitude and severity of the cord injury. Decreased sympathetic tone, unopposed cardiac vagal tone, and other cardiac changes are all contributory.[83] At its extreme, systemic effects including hypotension and bradycardia may be profound. These changes may persist for an extended period, sometimes months. In concert with these changes, total peripheral resistance and cardiac output may remain depressed for a prolonged period.

Of all purported mechanisms of secondary injury, the vascular hypothesis has considerable weight, with biochemical, angiographic, histopathological, and clinical support for its key role in damage following acute SCI. Proven effects include loss of the microcirculation, direct disruption of small vessels and hemorrhage, failure of autoregulation, and glutamate-mediated excitotoxicity. Ischemia has a direct linear dose-response relationship with the severity of the injury, becoming progressively worse a few hours after the injury and persisting for 24 hours or more.[178] Like so many secondary mechanisms of acute SCI, the precise mechanisms are still unclear.

Free Radical-Mediated Cell Injury

Free radicals are highly reactive molecules that posses an extra electron in the outer orbit. There is ample evidence for the early occurrence and pathophysiological importance of oxygen free radical formation with cell membrane lipid peroxidation in central nervous system (CNS) injury.[49] Free radicals most commonly form from molecular oxygen. Superoxide (O_2) is formed by incomplete electron transport in mitochondria. Superoxide is converted to H_2O_2

by superoxide dismutase and this in turn H_2O and O_2 by catalase. In the presence of free iron released from hemoglobin, transferrin, or ferritin by either lowered pH or oxygen radicals, H_2O_2 forms highly reactive hydroxyl radicals (HO). If unchecked, these can cause geometrically progressive lipid peroxidation, spreading over the cellular surface and causing impairment of phospholipid-dependent enzymes, disruption of ionic gradients, and, if severe enough, membrane lysis. This process also forms additional lipid peroxides and, consequently, additional free radicals.[90]

Much work has been done on the role of free radicals in SCI. After experimental contusive or compressive injuries, there is an increase in polyunsaturated fatty acid oxidation products such as malonyldialdehyde,[89,121,137] with a decrease in tissue cholesterol and the appearance of cholesterol oxidation products,[9,50] radical and lipid peroxidase-sensitive activation of guanylate cyclase, and a consequent increase in cyclic guanosine monophosphate,[89] early inhibition of the Na^+/K^+ ATPase which is lipid peroxidase-sensitive, and a decrease in tissue antioxidant levels (e.g., α-tocopherol).[148,159] These are all markers of early oxygen radical reactions. Lipid peroxidation may also play a role in posttraumatic hypoperfusion after SCI.[92]

High-dose steroids may improve SCBF and microvascular perfusion[8,93,195] as well as clinical neurological recovery after experimental SCI.[9] They may also provide some cytoprotection through the inhibition of lipid peroxidation and may facilitate spinal cord impulse generation and the inhibition of prostaglandin-induced vasoconstriction.[91] Because lipid peroxidation begins within the first 5 minutes after an acute SCI, the administration of high-dose steroids should occur as close to the time of injury as possible for maximal efficacy. In the clinical situation, high-dose methylprednisolone improves neurological function if given within 8 hours of an acute SCI;[34,37] however, the improvements noted have been modest and there have been some methodological problems with the study. Nevertheless, the clinical crossover of methylprednisolone therapy from the laboratory to the bedside demonstrates that therapeutic interventions are possible with a clearer understanding of secondary mechanisms.

Ionic Mechanisms

Sodium

The role of sodium in the secondary mechanisms of SCI has recently been delineated. Spinal cord axons possess voltage-gated Na^+ channels as well as a variety of ion exchanges, including the Na^+-H^+ and Na^+-Ca^{2+} exchangers.[138,153,170] With the reduction in blood flow that occurs after SCI leading to a depletion of adenosine 5'-diphosphate stores, a loss of ionic homeostasis occurs.[109] This leads to a depolarization of the cell membrane causing voltage-dependent Na^+ channels to open, with an influx of sodium ions. The rise in sodium concentration can be damaging to the cell via several mechanisms. It may lead to the formation of cytotoxic edema.[152] It may stimulate intracellular phospholipase activity.[85] It may promote intracellular acidosis via gating of the Na^+-H^+ exchanger.[87,153] Finally, sodium influx may increase intracellular Ca^{2+} by reversing operation of the Na^+-Ca^{2+} exchanger.[87,169,170] Following traumatic SCI in the dorsal column of the rat, it has been shown that axons depend to a large extent on a persistent membrane Na^+ conductance that allows Na^+ to rise sufficiently to promote operation of the Na^+-H^+ exchanger.[1,2,68] Agrawal and Fehlings[1] demonstrated further in the rat spinal cord that the administration of QX-314, a potent Na^+ channel blocker, provided partial neuroprotection after SCI. This has been shown to be the case in other CNS tissue, including hippocampus[30] and the optic nerve,[169] and with other Na^+ channel blockers, such as tetrodotoxin.[180] Agrawal and Fehlings[1] have also shown that, in the rat, pharmacological inhibition of the Na^+-Ca^{2+} exchanger with benzamil or bepridil did not improve outcome after compression injury to the dorsal column segment. They postulated that reverse operation of the Na^+-Ca^{2+} exchanger did not explain the mechanisms of Na^+-induced neurotoxicity that are seen in acute SCI.

Recently, Li et al[123] demonstrated that in isolated spinal dorsal columns endogenous glutamate is released by reversal of Na^+-dependent glutamate transport. They also showed that the myelin sheath is the target for glutamate-mediated excitotoxicity through the activation of L-amino-3-hydroxy-5-methyl isoxazole-4-proprionic acid (AMPA) receptors. This explains why either sodium channel blockade or AMPA antagonism is neuroprotective in SCI.

Sodium influx can also be harmful through other mechanisms. Glutamate and gamma-aminobutyric acid uptake, as well as many other cellular processes, are dependent on the maintenance of transmembrane gradients of sodium ions.[116] Consequently, a reduction in sodium fluxes associated with SCI may preserve these vital processes and maintain homeostasis, with less subsequent secondary injury.[156]

Calcium

Calcium is a ubiquitous ion that plays a role in numerous critical cellular pathways.[181] Calcium regulation in normal cellular function is tightly regulated. The role of Ca^{2+} in CNS dysfunction has been intensively explored in the past decade, with its role in cerebral ischemia and SAH more clearly delineated. Pharmacological intervention in those clinical scenarios is now possible. The magnitude and importance of calcium in the pathogenesis of SCI, however, are still being defined. Experimental SCI can produce a significant accumulation of Ca^{2+} axons,[21,22] possibly because of white matter ischemia.[181] Although elevated intracellular Ca^{2+} is linked to cell death, the precise mechanisms remain unclear. The mechanisms by which Ca^{2+} leads to neurotoxicity can be classified into one of two stages. Either the pathological mechanisms trigger and sustain an excess of intracellular Ca^{2+} (Figure 2) or secondary phenomena are precipitated by the sustained excess of intracellular Ca^{2+} (Figure 3). The concept of a two-stage mechanism may play a role in determining pharmacological inputs, although the use of Ca^{2+} antagonists in an attempt to ameliorate the effects of acute SCI have so far shown no efficacy.[147,177]

The rise in intracellular calcium is believed to act as a nonphysiological stimulus to phospholipases, proteases, plasmalogenases, calpains, nitric oxide synthetase, guanylate cyclase, calcineurins, and endonucleases which, at the endpoint, alter the functions of receptors, membrane channels, and ion translocases by phosphorylation and lead to the formation of free radicals, as well as potentially lethal changes in the cellular genetic characteristics. The proteases cause a breakdown of cytoskeletal components and parts of the plasma membrane, resulting in an acute cell in-

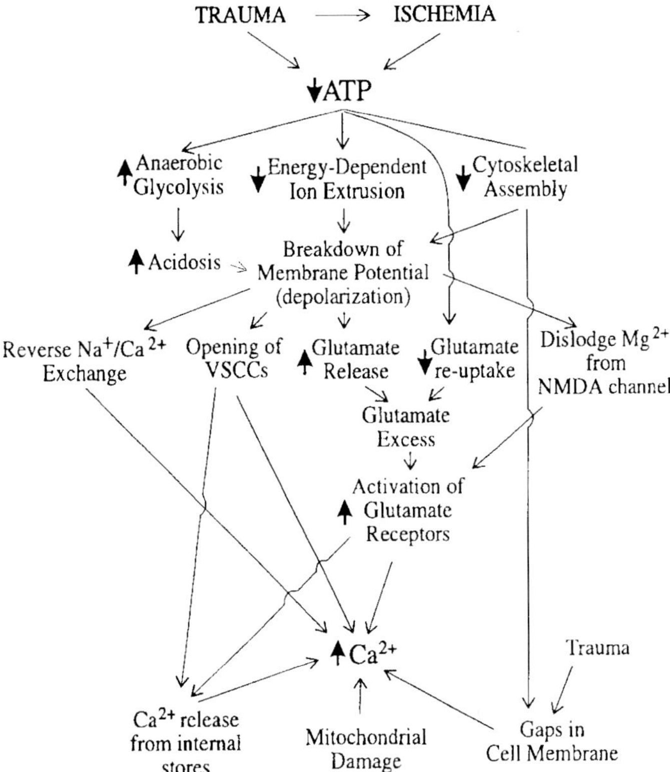

Figure 2: Algorithm showing mechanisms by which trauma and ischemia produce intracellular Ca²⁺ elevations. VSCC = voltage-gated Ca²⁺ channel. (Reprinted with permission from Tymianski and Tator[181])

jury (see below). The precise cascades affected remain controversial. The reader is referred to an excellent review of calcium and its role in CNS pathology by Tymianski and Tator.[181] The role of calcium through its glutaminergic mechanisms is also discussed below under "Glutaminergic Mechanisms."

Recent work has suggested that the rise in intracellular calcium after ischemic insults is driven by an increase in intracellular sodium concentration and is mediated by "reverse mode" of Na⁺-Ca²⁺ exchange.[169] This is discussed in this chapter, but in the spinal cord this does not appear to be the case[87] (see "Sodium").

Calcium ions play a role in axonal degeneration after acute SCI. The proteolytic degradation of neurofilament proteins is a critical step in the secondary mechanisms associated with acute SCI.[23] This degradation may be mediated by calpain, an intracellular Ca²⁺-activated neutral cysteine protease. Calpain very likely plays a regulatory rather than a degradative physiological role, with limited proteolysis by calpain of its substrates under normal conditions. The role of the Ca²⁺-activated protease calpain in causing the breakdown of cytoskeletal proteins in the pathophysiology of acute SCI has been recently examined.[151,160] Schumacher et al[151,160] examined a rat SCI model and showed that the level of calpain I (mu-calpain)-mediated spectrin breakdown products are increased at 15 minutes post-injury, with peak levels reached by 2 hours post-injury. Over that same time period, the dephosphorylated form of the neurofilament protein NF200 is substantially lost. NF200 is a cytoskeletal calpain substrate, and the study by Schumacher et al demonstrated a temporal and spatial relationship between calpain I-mediated spectrin breakdown within NF200-positive neuronal processes post-injury (Figure 4). Similar

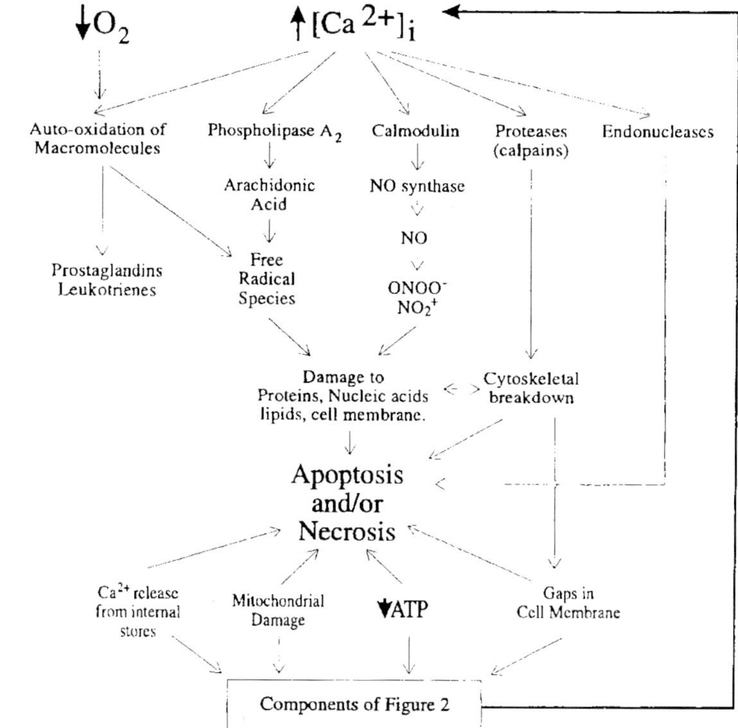

Figure 3: Algorithm showing mechanisms by which intracellular Ca²⁺ elevations trigger secondary Ca²⁺-dependent phenomena, which result in neurotoxicity. (Reprinted with permission from Tymianski and Tator[181])

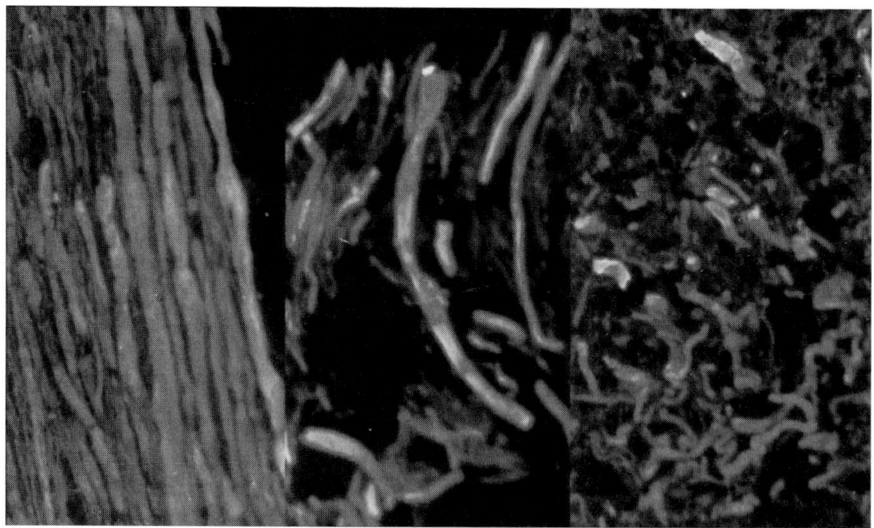

Figure 4: Progressive axonal degeneration after SCI. Immunohistochemical fluorescein labeling of spinal cord sections with anti-NF200 antibody. The normal spinal cord *(left)* shows progression 8 hours after injury *(center)* with a substantial reduction in immunoreactivity and the presence of a few swollen axons. At 24 hours *(right)*, the immunoreactivity is further reduced, with decreased axonal density and marked disorganization present.

effects of calpain I on microtubule-associated protein 2 (MAP2) have been demonstrated, with a loss of dendritic MAP2 in concert with a rise in calpain I after acute SCI. Calpain may also play a role in acute reactive gliosis following acute SCI.[57] Experimentally, the treatment of animals with riluzole, an inhibitor of glutamate release, before the acute SCI has been shown to ameliorate this reduction in MAP2 levels, 24 hours after the injury.[166] The issue of calpain-mediated proteolysis and its implications for pathology and therapy was reviewed by Kampfl et al.[108]

The use of calcium antagonists experimentally does not ameliorate the changes seen following SCI.[64] The failure of numerous clinical trials to demonstrate the efficacy of calcium antagonists in clinical scenarios outside SAH testifies to the complexity of the interactions being studied. The precise role of Ca^{2+} in SCI is still being defined.

Receptor-Mediated Cell Injury

Glutaminergic Mechanisms

The role of excitatory amino acid (EAA) neurotransmitters has generated much interest in many spheres of study in CNS disease. The earliest reports of their effects, where monosodium glutamate was reported to have caused neuronal and retinal death,[132,143,144] raised much controversy. Van Harreveld[182] in 1959 noted that glutamate and aspartate were capable of causing prolonged depolarization in the cortical neurons of rabbits and suggested, in reference to glutamate, that "it is likely that it also plays a major part in the asphyxial cortical changes which have a striking resemblance to this phenomenon." Since then, several subtypes of glutamate and aspartate receptors have been identified, based upon differential sensitivities to specific agonists, and the possible pathogenesis of glutamate-mediated excitotoxicity has been delineated.[165,185] These receptors are the high- and low-affinity kainate (KA), quisqualate, amino-3-hydroxy-5-methyl-4-isoazole propionic acid (AMPA), N-methyl-D-aspartate (NMDA), and the "metabotropic receptor."[128] All of these have been shown to be capable of mediating excitotoxicity, although the NMDA receptor has been the most extensively studied. The NMDA receptor has several features that distinguish it from the other receptor subtypes. The receptor is linked to an Na^+/Ca^{2+} ion channel that has much greater Ca^{2+} conductance than the ion channels associated with the other EAA receptor subtypes,[133] and the NMDA ion channel is subject to voltage-dependent Mg^{2+} blockade.[135] Acting at a site separate to the NMDA, Zn^{2+} ion channel is an inhibitory modulator of channel function.[187] Finally, the NMDA receptor is closely associated with recognition sites through which glycine[104] and certain polyamines[39] facilitate the opening of the NMDA ion channel and, with phencyclidine receptors[127] (which are positioned within this channel), permitting phencyclidine agonists to perform an open-channel block.[110] The NMDA receptors are quite different to the non-NMDA receptors. The former are highly Ca^{2+} permeable, whereas the KA and AMPA receptors are impermeable to Ca^{2+} but are permeable to monovalent ions such as Na^+ and K^+.[13] Also, NMDA receptors, unlike AMPA and KA receptors, are not found on axons or glia, and so may play a doubtful role in acute SCI.[3]

The precise mechanisms by which EAAs exert their neurotoxicity are unclear. Presynaptic depolarization, due to the successive activation of Na^+ channels, results in voltage-sensitive calcium channels (VSCCs) opening, which allow the influx of Ca^{2+} and the release of EAAs, predominantly in the region of the dendrites and soma.[79] The released glutamate acts on the AMPA and the NMDA receptors. The AMPA receptors allow an Na^+ influx, causing membrane depolarization. This membrane depolarization relieves the Mg^{2+} blockade of the NMDA receptor, allowing a postsynaptic influx of monovalent cations and calcium. The marked rise in intracellular calcium then acts via a secondary messenger system, possibly nitric oxide,[47] to initiate cell damage. The concept that non-NMDA receptors cause Ca^{2+} influx only indirectly by Na^+-dependent depolarization with subsequent opening of VSCC is now being qualified. Several types of AMPA and KA receptors can be important sources of Ca^{2+} influx in neurons[101,103] and astrocytes.[77] Cloning studies of non-NMDA receptor subtype cell lines support this hypothesis.[100]

The mechanisms of cation-dependent axonal injury after spinal cord trauma have not been fully elucidated. While initial interest has concentrated on the NMDA receptor, non-NMDA-

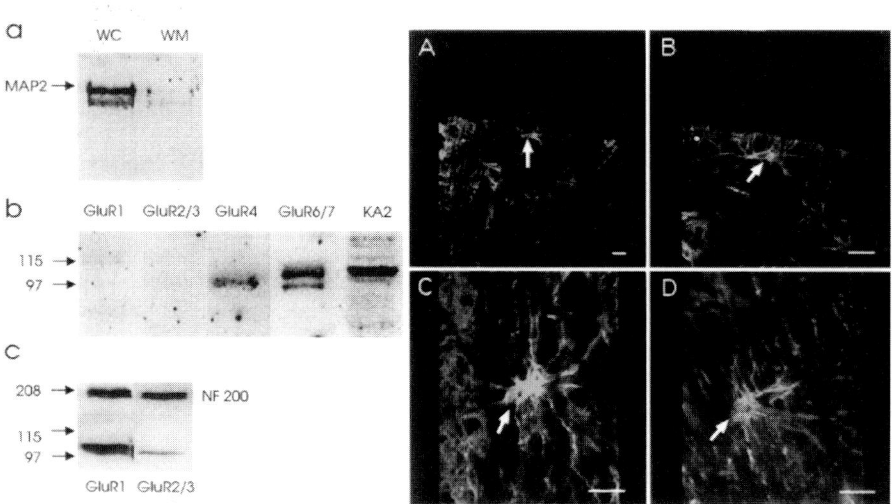

Figure 5: Expression of AMPA/KA glutamate receptors in spinal cord white matter. *Left:* **a)** Western blot illustrating MAP2 presence in whole spinal cord (WC) and exclusion in an isolated dorsal column white matter preparation (WM). **b)** Spinal cord white matter (dorsal column) homogenates (10 mg protein) were subjected to SDS-PAGE and immunoblotted with antibodies to GluR1, GluR2/3, GluR4, GluR6/7, and KA2. As illustrated, GluR4, GluR6/7, and KA2 were detected in spinal cord white matter. **c)** These immunoblots show equal amounts of protein loading with NF200 and positive controls for GluR1 and GluR2/3 using olfactory bulb. (Reprinted with permission from Agrawal and Fehlings.[2]) *Right:* The presence of GluR4 (**A** and **B**), GluR6/7 **(C)**, and KA2 **(D)** immunoreactivity (FITC labeling shown) in 10-mm sections of thoracic spinal cord dorsal column. Double labeling with GFAP (Texas Red) confirmed these immunopositive cells to be astrocytes *(arrows)*. Scale bars = 50 mm. (Reprinted with permission from Agrawal and Fehlings[3])

type glutamate receptors gated by AMPA or KA play a greater role in the pathophysiology of acute SCI.[189,190] The blockade of the AMPA or KA receptors, but not NMDA receptors, improves the recovery of dorsal column compound action potentials recorded in the rat after acute SCI.[2] Conversely, from the same study, the infusion of AMPA or KA worsened post-injury axonal function. The failure of NMDA receptor antagonists to ameliorate injury after SCI has been repeatedly demonstrated[66,78] and, interestingly, in contradistinction to the findings in cerebral ischemia, it appears that the non-NMDA receptors play a greater pathophysiological role than the NMDA receptors. These non-NMDA receptors seem restricted predominantly to astrocytes in the CNS white matter. Immunohistochemistry and Western blot analyses have shown that the AMPA and KA receptors are found on the periaxonal astrocytes,[2] lending further support to their role in glutamate-mediated SCI (Figure 5).

Metabotropic glutamate receptors (mGluRs) may also play a role in the pathogenesis of acute SCI. The mGluRs are not associated with an ion channel but mediate their actions through gua-nosine triphosphate-binding protein-dependent mechanisms to elicit phosphoinositide hydrolysis, the formation of 1,4,5-triphosphate, and diacylglycerol with mobilization of Ca^{2+} stores.[181] These receptors are split into three groups of a total of eight subtypes based on amino acid sequences, pharmacology, and signal transduction. The Group I mGluRs include mGluRa, mGluR5, and their variants, with activation of this group stimulating phospholipase C. Stimulation of phospholipase C leads to phosphatidylinositol hydrolysis and subsequent activation of the intracellular Ca^{2+} signal transduction pathway. Using Western blot techniques and immunohistochemistry, it has been shown that the pathophysiology of acute SCI involves the activation of Group I mGluRs, which are coupled to phospholipase C, with the mGluRa receptors found on astrocytes in spinal cord white matter (Figure 5).[4]

Opiate Receptors

Faden et al[62] first reported in 1980 that improvement from the effects of experimental SCI could be initiated by the use of naloxone. Naloxone is a potent blocker of the mu-subtype of opiate receptors. Faden's work has since been confirmed by others, in the experimental setting.[12,27,73,86] SCI releases dynorphin in the region of injury,[10,65] a compound known to induce cellular injury experimentally.[19] This substance activates kappa receptors, with no obvious adverse affects, yet those opiate receptors believed to play a role in SCI are not activated by dynorphin.[129] Opiate receptors also play a role in regulating CNS monoamine and serotonergic neurotransmitter levels,[171] as well as interacting with descending adrenergic systems[124] and EEAs.[61] The role of opiates in SCI is complex and still not delineated. The only clinical trial to date, using thyrotropin-releasing hormone as an endogenous opioid antagonist, demonstrated no significant recovery between treated and placebo groups after acute SCI.[149]

Inflammatory-Mediated Cell Injury

Inflammatory mediators can cause progressive damage in CNS tissue. In the acutely injured spinal cord, there is an accumulation of many mediators, including bradykinin, prostaglandins, leukotrienes, serotonin, and platelet-activating factor.[192] Neutrophils act as phagocytes of red blood cells and necrotic tissue, but may also play a role in the pathogenesis and extension of SCI, which currently has only been demonstrated in the rat.[94,173,191] Neutrophils can release proteases and reactive oxygen species,[95] and activated neutrophils have been found to be associated with ischemia.[98] Neutrophil invasion increases the oxidative stress on neurons and, similarly, oxidative stress encourages neutrophil invasion. Secondary injury after acute SCI may be minimized by limiting oxidative stress via: 1) maintaining reduced-glutathione levels through the administration of cysteine precursors such as N-acetylcysteine, and 2) limiting neutrophil invasion by administering platelet-activating factor antagonists.[105]

The migration of neutrophils is controlled by specific adhesion proteins on both endothelial cells and neutrophils. Within the CNS, ICAM-1 and VCAM-1 facilitate cell-to-cell interactions between astrocytes, microglia and endothelial cells, and the peripheral blood macrophages, lymphocytes, and neutrophils. It has been shown experimentally that antibodies for specific cell adhesion molecules reduce the level of ischemic injury to the CNS when administered *in vivo*, as the influx of neutrophils that release cytokines, prostaglandins, and the like are modulated.[125]

Inflammatory responses may be mediated and/or enhanced by induced gene expression. A major regulator of inflammatory gene expression is the nuclear factor-κB (NF-κB) family of transcription factors (cRel, RelA/p65, RelB, p50, and p52).[16-18] Transcriptionally, NF-κB transcription factors regulate gene expression in inflammatory responses in the CNS and may be key determinants in cell death and disease in the CNS.[16-18,107] NF-κB activates the genes encoding prostaglandin synthase-2,[141] cytokines,[136] cell adhesion molecules (CAM),[107] and inducible nitric oxide synthase.[145] It has been found in degenerating as opposed to non-degenerating neurons.[41] NF-κB may play a role in apoptosis[17] as well as in normal neural transduction.[145] Bethea et al,[28] using immunohistochemical and Western blot analyses in a contusion model in the rat, recently demonstrated that NF-κB is activated after SCI. This is the first time that NF-κB activation has been shown to occur following trauma. Bethel et al provide an excellent review of the current state of play of inflammation in SCI. In the future, strategies aimed at blocking this activation may play a role in inducing neuroprotection from the secondary mechanisms that occur after SCI.

The cytokines play an important role in the inflammatory response after SCI. Their production is regulated primarily at the transcription level. NF-κB has a role in this regulation.[18,145] Tumor necrosis factor-α (TNF-α), interleukin-1, and interleukin-6 are all prototypical inflammatory cytokines that are produced following a CNS insult.[136] TNF-α has been detected after an SCI in the rat[184] and, again, NF-κB plays a key role in regulating the responses of TNF-α at the transcription level.[18,145] Studies *in vivo* and *in vitro* confirm that TNF-α plays a key role in secondary damage after SCI via potent activation of the inflammatory system, as well as possibly activating NF-κB. TNF-α also potentiates microgliosis, astrogliosis, and cell death.[72] The effect of TNF-α and the other cytokines illustrates the net downstream amplificatory cascade induced by NF-κB activation in acute SCI with inflammation and possible cell death occurring, a process leading to exacerbation of the primary injury.

Apoptosis

Cell death occurs via either necrosis or apoptosis. Apoptosis is a form of programmed cell death that occurs in a wide variety of disease states in eukaryotic cells. Unlike necrosis, apoptosis is an active process that is characterized by cell shrinkage, chromatin aggregation, and nuclear pyknosis.[99] The cells die and are engulfed by phagocytes without initiating an inflammatory response or without discharging their cellular contents into the extracellular environment. This is initiated by physiological stimuli, either internal or external.[130] Apoptosis is a tightly regulated process with a sequence of activation steps that requires energy and specific macromolecular synthesis as *de novo* gene transcription.[111]

Necrosis, on the other hand, is characterized by a more passive cellular swelling, with mitochondrial damage and disruption of internal homeostasis, leading to membrane lysis, release of intracellular contents, and provocation of an intense inflammatory response.[42,134] It arises from nonphysiological disturbances.[130] Necrosis has no energy requirements because there is no *de novo* gene transcription and, thus, no new protein or nucleic acid synthesis occurs.[24,44]

Apoptosis is recognized as occurring *in utero* as a form of neuronal cell death during embryonic development[97] and is also now believed to play a role in many postdevelopmental disorders of the CNS, including ischemia, trauma, inflammation, and neurodegenerative states.[11,26,139,146,154] A family of cysteine proteins, the caspases, are believed to play an important role in apoptosis. Caspase-3 cleaves several essential downstream substrates involved in the apoptosis pathway, including PAK2, fodrin, and gelsolin. Caspase-3 activation *in vitro* can be triggered by upstream events, leading to the release of cytochrome c from the mitochondria and the subsequent transactivation of procaspase-9 by Apaf-1. These upstream and downstream components of the caspase-3 apoptotic pathway are activated after traumatic SCI in rats and may occur early in neurons in the injury site and hours to days later in oligodendroglia adjacent to and distant

from the injury site.[167] In the spinal cord, apoptosis was identified first in 1995 as occurring in rats[46] and, more recently, in the human spinal cord.[60] It is believed that oligodendrocytes are the major cell type in compressive SCI that undergoes apoptosis[45,122] and are seen in areas of Wallerian degeneration and are detectable between 24 hours and 3 weeks postinjury[45,46] (Figure 6). The mechanism behind this is unclear, but it may occur due either to adverse changes in the cellular environment resulting in axonal demyelination or to Wallerian degeneration, or by a combination of both processes.[25,59]

It has also been suggested that the death of oligodendrocytes may be a consequence of microglial activation and peaks at 8 days postinjury.[164] This hypothesis has been suggested by Shuman et al[164] following their observations of activated microglia in the same regions undergoing apoptosis, with apparent contact between some of the microglial processes and apoptotic oligodendrocytes. Apoptosis occurs around the lesion epicenter as well as within areas of Wallerian degeneration in both ascending and descending white matter tracts.[60] In time, it may be that targeting the upstream events of the caspase cascade to protect neurons and oligodendrocytes from undergoing apoptotic death has therapeutic potential in the treatment of acute SCI. Already, agents such as the oncogene Bcl-2 have been shown to limit the degree of histological injury in acute experimental SCI in rats, possibly by regulating an antioxidant pathway that limits free radical generation.[131] Similarly, cycloheximide treatment can improve outcome after contusion trauma in the spinal cords of rats.[126]

CONCLUSION

The cellular and ionic processes that take place following an acute SCI are a complex cascade of interrelated events that occur within minutes, hours, days, and weeks of the event. As our knowledge of cellular physiology grows, the intricate interrelationship of these processes is slowly being unraveled and the enormous complexity begins to be appreciated. Whereas lipid peroxidation and vascular disruptions were initially believed to be key mediators, the increasing contribution of glutaminergic pathways, sodium,

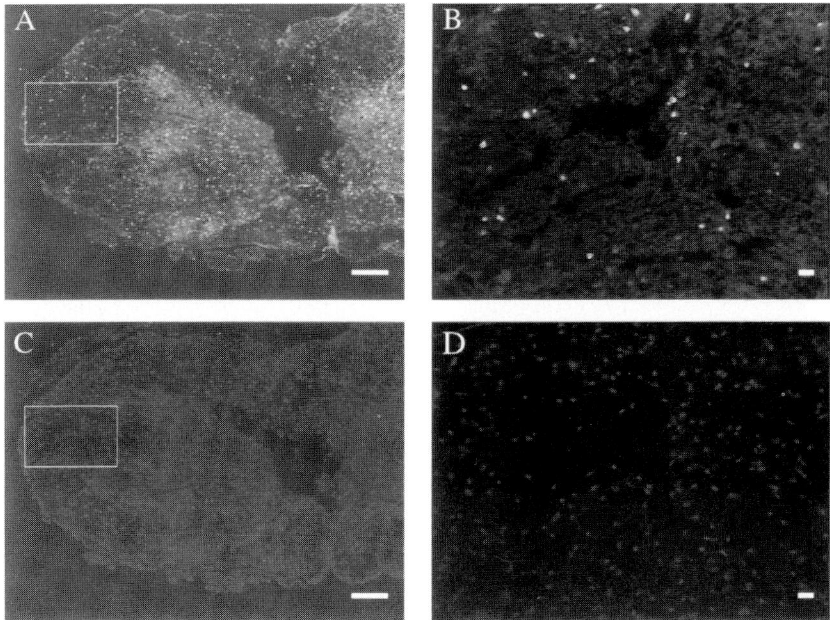

Figure 6: Apoptosis after SCI. Spinal cord sections stained using the TUNEL technique[75] and double labeled with propidium iodide (nuclear marker) to demonstrate DNA fragmentation, the hallmark of apoptosis (scale bar = 1 mm).

and calcium-mediated mechanisms as well as programmed cell death, are also now known to play a part. Despite our burgeoning knowledge, acute intervention for acute SCI is still limited, and our ability to ameliorate or temporize these secondary mechanisms is similar to that which we possessed decades previously. With time and a greater appreciation of the complex cellular and subcellular pathways, it is hoped that the terrible consequences of acute SCI will one day be able to be slowed and, perhaps, even reversed.

REFERENCES

1. Agrawal SK, Fehlings MG: The effect of the sodium channel blocker QX-314 on recovery after acute spinal cord injury. **J Neurotrauma 14:**81-88, 1997
2. Agrawal SK, Fehlings MG: Mechanisms of secondary injury to spinal cord axons in vitro: role of Na^+, $Na^{(+)}$-$K^{(+)}$-ATPase, the $Na^{(+)}$-H^+ exchanger, and the $Na^{(+)}$-Ca^{2+} exchanger. **J Neurosci 16:**545-552, 1996
3. Agrawal SK, Fehlings MG: Role of NMDA and non-NMDA inotropic glutamate receptors in traumatic spinal cord axonal injury. **J Neurosci 17:**1055-1063, 1997
4. Agrawal SK, Theriault E, Fehlings MG: Role of group I metabotropic glutamate receptors in traumatic spinal cord white matter injury. **J Neurotrauma 15:** 929-941, 1998
5. Albin MS, White RJ: Epidemiology, physiopathology, and experimental therapeutics of acute spinal cord injury. **Crit Care Clin 3:**441-452, 1987
6. Allen AR: Remarks on the histopathological changes in the spinal cord due to impact. An experimental study. **J Nerv Ment Dis 41:**141-147, 1914
7. Allen AR: Surgery for experimental lesions of spinal cord equivalent to crush injury of fracture dislocation of spinal column. A preliminary report. **JAMA 57:** 878-880, 1911
8. Anderson DK, Means ED, Waters TR, et al: Microvascular perfusion and metabolism in injured spinal cord after methylprednisolone treatment. **J Neurosurg 56:**106-113, 1982
9. Anderson DK, Saunders RD, Demediuk P, et al: Lipid hydrolysis and peroxidation in injured spinal cord: partial protection with methylprednisolone or vitamin E and selenium. **Cent Nerv Syst Trauma 2:** 257-267, 1985
10. Andrew J, Sweetnam DR, Williams RA, et al: Separate dens with subluxation and paraplegia treated by occipitocervical fusion. **Proc R Soc Med 62:**581-583, 1969
11. Arends MJ, Wyllie AH: Apoptosis: mechanisms and role in pathology. **Int Rev Exp Pathol 32:**223-254, 1991
12. Arias MJ: Effect of naloxone on functional recovery after experimental spinal cord injury in the rat. **Surg Neurol 23:**440-442, 1985
13. Ascher P, Nowak L: Quisqualate- and kainate-activated channels in mouse central neurones in culture. **J Physiol (Lond) 399:**227-245, 1988

14. Assenmacher DR, Ducker TB: Experimental traumatic paraplegia. The vascular and pathological changes seen in reversible and irreversible spinal-cord lesions. **J Bone Joint Surg (Am) 53:**671-680, 1971
15. Atkinson PP, Atkinson JL: Spinal shock. **Mayo Clin Proc 71:**384-389, 1996
16. Baeuerle PA: The inducible transcription activator NF-êB: regulation by distinct protein subunits. **Biochim Biophys Acta 1072:**63-80, 1991
17. Baeuerle PA, Baltimore D: NF-κB: ten years after. **Cell 87:**13-20, 1996
18. Baeuerle PA, Henkel T: Function and activation of NF-êB in the immune system. **Annu Rev Immunol 12:**141-179, 1994
19. Bakshi R, Newman AH, Faden AI: Dynorphin A-(1-17) induces alterations in free fatty acids, excitatory amino acids, and motor function through an opiate-receptor-mediated mechanism. **J Neurosci 10:** 3793-3800, 1990
20. Balentine JD: Pathology of experimental spinal cord trauma. II. Ultrastructure of axons and myelin. **Lab Invest 39:**254-266, 1978
21. Balentine JD, Dean DL Jr: Calcium-induced spongiform and necrotizing myelopathy. **Lab Invest 47:** 286-295, 1982
22. Balentine JD, Greene WB: Ultrastructural pathology of nerve fibers in calcium-induced myelopathy. **J Neuropathol Exp Neurol 43:**500-510, 1984
23. Banik NL, Hogan EL, Powers JM, et al: Degradation of cytoskeletal proteins in experimental spinal cord injury. **Neurochem Res 7:**1465-1475, 1982
24. Bargmann CI: Death from natural and unnatural causes. Elegant studies of the nematode are providing answers to the question of how programmed cell death and neurodegeneration are regulated. **Curr Biol 1:**388-390, 1991
25. Barres BA, Jacobson MD, Schmid R: Does oligodendrocyte survival depend on axons? **Curr Biol 3:** 489-497, 1993
26. Bauer J, Wekerle H, Lassman H: Apoptosis in brain-specific autoimmune disease. **Curr Opin Immunol 7:** 839-843, 1995
27. Benzel EC, Lancon JA, Bairnsfather S, et al: Effect of dosage and timing of administration of naloxone on outcome in the rat ventral compression model of spinal cord injury. **Neurosurgery 27:**597-601, 1990
28. Bethea JR, Castro M, Keane RW, et al: Traumatic spinal cord injury induces nuclear factor-κB activation. **J Neurosci 18:**3251-3260, 1998
29. Bingham WG, Goldman H, Friedman SJ, et al: Blood flow in normal and injured monkey spinal cord. **J Neurosurg 43:**162-171, 1975
30. Boening JA, Kass IS, Cottrell JE, et al: The effect of blocking sodium influx on anoxic damage in the rat hippocampal slice. **Neuroscience 33:**263-268, 1989
31. Bracken MB: Treatment of acute spinal cord injury with methylprednisolone: results of a multicenter, randomized clinical trial. **J Neurotrauma 8 (Suppl 1):** S47-S52, 1991
32. Bracken MB, Collins WF, Freeman DF, et al: Efficacy of methylprednisolone in acute spinal cord injury. **JAMA 251:**45-52, 1984
33. Bracken MB, Holford TR: Effects of timing of methylprednisolone or naloxone administration on recovery of segmental and long-tract neurological function in NASCIS 2. **J Neurosurg 79:**500-507, 1993
34. Bracken MB, Shepard MJ, Collins WF, et al: A randomized, controlled trial of methylprednisolone or naloxone in the treatment of acute spinal-cord injury. Results of the second National Acute Spinal Cord Injury Study. **N Engl J Med 322:**1405-1411, 1990
35. Bracken MB, Shepard MJ, Collins WF Jr, et al: Methylprednisolone or naloxone treatment after acute spinal cord injury: 1-year follow-up data. Results of the second National Acute Spinal Cord Injury Study. **J Neurosurg 76:**23-31, 1992
36. Bracken MB, Shepard MJ, Hellenbrand KG, et al: Methylprednisolone and neurological function 1 year after spinal cord injury. Results of the National Acute Spinal Cord Injury Study. **J Neurosurg 63:**704-713, 1985
37. Bracken MB, Shepard MJ, Holford TR, et al: Administration of methylprednisolone for 24 or 48 hours or tirilazad mesylate for 48 hours in the treatment of acute spinal cord injury. Results of the third National Acute Spinal Cord Injury Randomized Controlled Trial. **JAMA 277:**1597-1604, 1997
38. Bracken MB, Shepard MJ, Holford TR, et al: Methylprednisolone or tirilazad mesylate administration after acute spinal cord injury: 1-year follow up. Results of the third National Acute Spinal Cord Injury randomized controlled trial. **J Neurosurg 89:**699-706, 1998
39. Carter C, Benavides J, Legendre P: Ifenprodil and SL 82.0715 as cerebral anti-ischemic agents. II. Evidence for N-methyl-D-aspartate receptor antagonist properties. **J Pharmacol Exp Ther 247:**1222-1232, 1988
40. Carter RE Jr: Etiology of traumatic spinal cord injury: statistics of more than 1,100 cases. **Tex Med 73:**61-65, 1977
41. Clemens JA, Stephenson DT, Smalstig EB, et al: Global ischemia activates nuclear factor-κB in forebrain neurons of rats. **Stroke 28:**1073-1081, 1997
42. Cohen JJ: Apoptosis. **Immunol Today 14:**126-130, 1993
43. Collins WF: A review and update of experiment and clinical studies of spinal cord injury. **Paraplegia 21:** 204-219, 1983
44. Collins WF, Piepmeier J, Ogle E: The spinal cord injury problem-a review. **Cent Nerv Syst Trauma 3:** 317-331, 1986
45. Crowe MJ, Bresnahan JC, Shuman SL, et al: Apoptosis and delayed degeneration after spinal cord injury in rats and monkeys. **Nat Med 3:**73-76, 1997
46. Crowe MJ, Shuman SL, Masters JN, et al: Morphological evidence suggesting apoptotic nuclei in spinal cord injury. **Soc Neurosci Abstr 21:**232, 1995 (Abstract)
47. Dawson VL, Dawson TM, London ED, et al: Nitric oxide mediates glutamate neurotoxicity in primary cortical cultures. **Proc Natl Acad Sci USA 88:** 6368-6371, 1991
48. de la Torre JC: Spinal cord injury. Review of basic and applied research. **Spine 6:**315-335, 1981
49. Demopoulos HB, Flamm ES, Pietronigro DD, et al: The free radical pathology and the microcirculation in the major central nervous system disorders. **Acta Physiol Scand Suppl 492:**91-119, 1980
50. Demopoulos HB, Flamm ES, Seligman ML, et al: Further studies on free-radical pathology in the

major central nervous system disorders: effect of very high doses of methylprednisolone on the functional outcome, morphology, and chemistry of experimental spinal cord impact injury. **Can J Physiol Pharmacol 60:**1415-1424, 1982

51. Demopoulos HB, Flamm ES, Seligman ML, et al: Membrane perturbations in central nervous system injury: theoretical basis for free radical damage and a review of the experimental data, in Popp AJ, et al (eds) **Neural Trauma.** New York, NY: Raven Press, 1979, pp 63-78

52. Demopoulos HB, Yoder M, Gutman EG, et al: The fine structure of endothelial surfaces in the microcirculation of experimentally injured feline spinal cords, in Becker RP, Johari O (eds): **Scanning Electron Microscopy II AMF.** O'Hare, Ill: Scanning Electron Microscopy, Inc, 1978, pp 677-682

53. Dohrmann GJ, Allen WE III: Microcirculation of traumatized spinal cord. A correlation of microangiography and blood flow patterns in transitory and permanent paraplegia. **J Trauma 15:**1003-1013, 1975

54. Dohrmann GJ, Wick KM: Intramedullary blood flow patterns in transitory traumatic paraplegia. **Surg Neurol 1:**209-215, 1973

55. Dolan EJ, Tator CH, Endrenyi L: The value of decompression for acute experimental spinal cord compression injury. **J Neurosurg 53:**749-755, 1980

56. Dolan EJ, Transfeldt EE, Tator CH, et al: The effect of spinal distraction on regional spinal cord blood flow in cats. **J Neurosurg 53:**756-764, 1980

57. Du S, Rubin A, Klepper S, et al: Calcium influx and activation of calpain I mediate acute reactive gliosis in injured spinal cord. **Exp Neurol 157:**96-105, 1999

58. Ducati A, Schieppati M, Giovanelli MA: Effects of deep barbiturate coma on acute spinal cord injury in the cat. **Surg Neurol 21:**405-413, 1984

59. Dusart I, Schwab ME: Secondary cell death and the inflammatory reaction after dorsal hemisection of the rat spinal cord. **Eur J Neurosci 6:**712-724, 1994

60. Emery E, Aldana P, Bunge MB, et al: Apoptosis after traumatic human spinal cord injury. **J Neurosurg 89:** 911-920, 1998

61. Faden AI: Dynorphin increases extracellular levels of excitatory amino acids in the brain through a non-opioid mechanism. **J Neurosci 12:**425-429, 1992

62. Faden AI, Jacobs TP, Holaday JW: Endorphin-parasympathetic interactions in spinal shock. **J Autonomic Nerv Syst 2:**295-304, 1980

63. Faden AI, Jacobs TP, Holaday JW: Thyrotropin-releasing hormone improves neurologic recovery after spinal trauma in cats. **N Engl J Med 305:** 1063-1067, 1981

64. Faden AI, Jacobs TP, Smith MT: Evaluation of calcium channel antagonist nimodipine in experimental spinal cord ischemia. **J Neurosurg 60:**796-799, 1984

65. Faden AI, Molineaux CJ, Rosenberger JG, et al: Endogenous opioid immunoreactivity in rat spinal cord following traumatic injury. **Ann Neurol 17:**386-390, 1985

66. Faden AI, Simon RP: A potential role for excitotoxins in the pathophysiology of spinal cord injury. **Ann Neurol 23:**623-626, 1988

67. Fairholm D, Turnbull I: Microangiographic study of experimental spinal injuries in dogs and rabbits. **Surg Forum 21:**453-5:453-455, 1970

68. Fehlings MG, Agrawal S: Role of sodium in the pathophysiology of secondary spinal cord injury. **Spine 20:** 2187-2191, 1995

69. Fehlings MG, Tator CH: An evidence-based review of decompressive surgery in acute spinal cord injury: rationale, indications, and timing based on experimental and clinical studies. **J Neurosurg 91 (Spine 1):** 1-11, 1999

70. Fehlings MG, Tator CH: A review of models of acute experimental spinal cord injury, in Illis LS (ed): **Spinal Cord Dysfunction: Assessment.** New York, NY: Oxford University Press, 1988, pp 3-33

71. Fehlings MG, Tator CH, Linden RD: The effect of nimodipine and dextran on axonal function and blood flow following experimental spinal cord injury. **J Neurosurg 71:**403-416, 1989

72. Feuerstein GZ, Liu T, Barone FC: Cytokines, inflammation, and brain injury: role of tumor necrosis factor-α. **Cerebrovasc Brain Metab Rev 6:**341-360, 1994

73. Flamm ES, Young W, Collins WF, et al: A phase I trial of naloxone treatment in acute spinal cord injury. **J Neurosurg 63:**390-397, 1985

74. Fried LC, Goodkin R: Microangiographic observations of the experimentally traumatized spinal cord. **J Neurosurg 35:**709-714, 1971

75. Gavrieli Y, Sherman Y, Ben-Sasson SA: Identification of programmed cell death in situ via specific labeling of nuclear DNA fragmentation. **J Cell Biol 119:** 493-501, 1992

76. Geisler FH, Dorsey FC, Coleman WP: Recovery of motor function after spinal-cord injury—a randomized, placebo-controlled trial with GM-1 ganglioside. **N Engl J Med 324:**1829-1838, 1991

77. Glaum SR, Holzwarth JA, Miller·RJ: Glutamate receptors activate Ca^{2+} mobilization and Ca^{2+} influx into astrocytes. **Proc Natl Acad Sci USA 87:** 3454-3458, 1990

78. Gómez-Pinilla F, Tram H, Cotman CW, et al: Neuroprotective effect of MK-801 and U-50488H after contusive spinal cord injury. **Exp Neurol 104:** 118-124, 1989

79. Greenberg DA: Calcium channels and calcium channel antagonists. **Ann Neurol 21:**317-330, 1987

80. Griffiths IR: Spinal cord blood flow after acute experimental cord injury in dogs. **J Neurol Sci 27:** 247-259, 1976

81. Griffiths IR, Miller R: Vascular permeability to protein and vasogenic oedema in experimental concussive injuries to the canine spinal cord. **J Neurol Sci 22:**291-304, 1974

82. Gruner JA: A monitored contusion model of spinal cord injury in the rat. **J Neurotrauma 9:**123-128, 1992

83. Guha A, Tator CH: Acute cardiovascular effects of experimental spinal cord injury. **J Trauma 28:** 481-490, 1988

84. Guha A, Tator CH, Rochon J: Spinal cord blood flow and systemic blood pressure after experimental spinal cord injury in rats. **Stroke 20:**372-377, 1989

85. Gusovsky F, Hollingsworth EB, Daly JW: Regulation of phosphatidylinositol turnover in brain synaptosomes: stimulatory effects of agents that enhance influx of sodium ions. **Proc Natl Acad Sci USA 83:** 3003-3007, 1986

86. Haghighi SS, Chehrazi B: Effect of naloxone in experimental acute spinal cord injury. **Neurosurgery 20:** 385-388, 1987

87. Haigney MCP, Lakatta EG, Stern MD, et al: Sodium channel blockade reduces hypoxic sodium loading and sodium-dependent calcium loading. **Circulation** 90:391-399, 1994

88. Hall ED: Pathophysiology of spinal cord injury. Current and future therapies. **Minerva Anesthesiol 55:** 63-66, 1989

89. Hall ED, Braughler JM: Effects of intravenous methylprednisolone on spinal cord lipid peroxidation and Na$^+$ + K$^+$)-ATPase activity. Dose-response analysis during 1st hour after contusion injury in the cat. **J Neurosurg** 57:247-253, 1982

90. Hall ED, Braughler JM: Free radicals in CNS injury. **Res Publ Assoc Res Nerv Ment Dis** 71:81-105, 1993

91. Hall ED, Braughler JM: Glucocorticoid mechanisms in acute spinal cord injury: a review and therapeutic rationale. **Surg Neurol 18:**320-327, 1982

92. Hall ED, Wolf DL: Post-traumatic spinal cord ischemia: relationship to injury severity and physiological parameters. **Cent Nerv Syst Trauma 4:**15-25, 1987

93. Hall ED, Wolf DL, Braughler JM: Effects of a single large dose of methylprednisolone sodium succinate on experimental posttraumatic spinal cord ischemia. Dose-response and time-action analysis. **J Neurosurg** 61:124-130, 1984

94. Hamada Y, Ikata T, Katoh S, et al: Involvement of an intercellular adhesion molecule 1-dependent pathway in the pathogenesis of secondary changes after spinal cord injury in rats. **J Neurochem** 66:1525-1531, 1996

95. Harlan JM: Consequences of leukocytes-vessel wall interactions in inflammatory and immune reactions. **Semin Thromb Hemost 13:**425-433, 1987

96. Hayashi N, Green BA, Gonzalez-Carvajal M, et al: Local blood flow, oxygen tension, and oxygen consumption in the rat spinal cord. Part 1: Oxygen metabolism and neuronal function. **J Neurosurg 58:** 516-525, 1983

97. Henderson CE: Programmed cell death in the developing nervous system. **Neuron** 17:579-585, 1997

98. Hernandez LA, Grisham MB, Twohig B, et al: Role of neutrophils in ischemia-reperfusion-induced microvascular injury. **Am J Physiol** 253:H699-H703, 1987

99. Hockenberry D: Defining apoptosis. **Am J Pathol** 146:16-19, 1995

100. Hollman M, Hartley M, Heinemann S: Ca^{2+} permeability of KA-AMPA-gated glutamate receptor channels depends on subunit composition. **Science** 252:851-854, 1991

101. Holopainen I, Enkvist MOK, Akerman KEO: Glutamate receptor agonists increase intracellular Ca^{2+} independently of voltage-gated Ca^{2+} channels in rat cerebellar granule cells. **Neurosci Lett** 98:57-62, 1989

102. Hsu CY, Hogan EL, Gadsden RH Sr, et al: Vascular permeability in experimental spinal cord injury. **J Neurol Sci 70:**275-282, 1985

103. Iino M, Owaza S, Tsuzuki K: Permeation of calcium through excitatory amino acid receptor channels in cultured rat hippocampal neurones. **J Physiol (Lond)** 424:151-165, 1990

104. Johnson JW, Ascher P: Glycine potentiates the NMDA response in cultured mouse brain neurons. **Nature** 325:529-531, 1987

105. Juurlink BH, Paterson PG: Review of oxidative stress in brain and spinal cord injury: suggestions for pharmacological and nutritional management strategies. **J Spinal Cord Med 21:**309-334, 1998

106. Kakulas BA: Pathology of spinal injuries. **Cent Nerv Syst Trauma** 1:117-129, 1984

107. Kaltschmidt B, Baeuerle PA, Kaltschmidt C: Potential involvement of the transcription factor NF-κB in neurological disorders. **Mol Aspects Med 14:**171-190, 1993

108. Kampfl A, Posmantur RM, Zhao X, et al: Mechanisms of calpain proteolysis following traumatic brain injury: implications for pathology and therapy: a review and update. **J Neurotrauma 14:**121-134, 1997

109. Kass IS, Abramowicz AE, Cottrell JE, et al: The barbiturate thiopental reduces ATP levels during anoxia but improves electrophysiological recovery and ionic homeostasis in the rat hippocampal slice. **Neuroscience** 49:537-543, 1992

110. Kemp JA, Foster AC, Wong EHF: Non-competitive antagonists of excitatory amino acid receptors. **Trends Neurosci** 10:294-299, 1987

111. Kerr JFR, Wyllie AH, Currie AR: Apoptosis: a basic biological phenomenon with wide-ranging implications in tissue kinetics. **Br J Cancer** 26:239-257, 1972

112. Khan M, Griebel R: Acute spinal cord injury in the rat: comparison of three experimental techniques. **Can J Neurol Sci** 10:161-165, 1983

113. Kim RC, Smith HR, Henbest ML, et al: Nonhemorrhagic venous infarction of the spinal cord. **Ann Neurol** 15:379-385, 1984

114. Kobrine AI, Doyle TF, Martins AN: Local spinal cord blood flow in experimental traumatic myelopathy. **J Neurosurg** 42:144-149, 1975

115. Kobrine AI, Doyle TF, Rizzoli HV: Spinal cord blood flow as affected by changes in systemic arterial blood pressure. **J Neurosurg** 44:12-15, 1976

116. Koch RA, Barish ME: Pertubation of intracellular calcium and hydrogen ion regulation in cultured mouse hippocampal neurons by reduction of the sodium ion concentration gradient. **J Neurosci** 14:2585-2593, 1994

117. Koyanagi I, Tator CH, Lea PJ: Three-dimensional analysis of the vascular system in the rat spinal cord with scanning electron microscopy of vascular corrosion casts. Part 1: Normal spinal cord. **Neurosurgery** 33:277-284, 1993

118. Koyanagi I, Tator CH, Lea PJ: Three-dimensional analysis of the vascular system in the rat spinal cord with scanning electron microscopy of vascular corrosion casts. Part 2: Acute spinal cord injury. **Neurosurgery** 33:285-292, 1993

119. Koyanagi I, Tator CH, Theriault E: Silicone rubber microangiography of acute spinal cord injury in the rat. **Neurosurgery** 32:260-268, 1993

120. Kraus JF: Epidemiologic features of head and spinal cord injury. **Adv Neurol** 19:261-279, 1978

121. Kurihara M: Role of monoamines in experimental spinal cord injury in rats. Relationship between Na$^+$-K$^+$-ATPase and lipid peroxidation. **J Neurosurg 62:** 743-749, 1985

122. Li GL, Brodin G, Farooque M, et al: Apoptosis and expression of Bcl-2 after compression trauma to rat spinal cord. **J Neuropathol Exp Neurol** 55:280-289, 1996

123. Li S, Mealing GAR, Morley P, et al: Novel injury mechanism in anoxia and trauma of spinal cord white matter: glutamate release via reverse Na$^+$-

dependent glutamate transport. **J Neurosci 19:**1-9, 1999

124. Li YJ, Xie YF, Qiao JT: Effects of intrathecal monoamine antagonists and naloxone on the descending inhibition of the spinal transmission of noxious input in rats: study with a new experimental model. **Brain Res 568:**131-137, 1991

125. Lindsberg PJ, Sirén AL, Feuerstein GZ, et al: Antagonism of neutrophil adherence in the deteriorating stroke model in rabbits. **J Neurosurg 82:**269-277, 1995

126. Liu XZ, Xu XM, Hu R, et al: Neuronal and glial apoptosis after traumatic spinal cord injury. **J Neurosci 17:** 5395-5406, 1997

127. Lodge D, Anis NA: Effects of phencyclidine on excitatory amino acid activation of spinal interneurons in the cat. **Eur J Pharmacol 77:**203-204, 1982

128. Lodge D, Collingridge G: Les agents provocateurs: a series on the pharmacology of excitatory amino acids. **Trends Pharmacol Sci 11:**22-24, 1990

129. Long JB, Martinez-Arizala A, Petras JM, et al: Endogenous opioids in spinal cord injury: a critical evaluation. **Cent Nerv Syst Trauma 3:**295-315, 1986

130. Lou J, Lenke LG, Ludwig FJ, et al: Apoptosis as a mechanism of neuronal cell death following acute experimental spinal cord injury. **Spinal Cord 36:** 683-690, 1998

131. Lou J, Lenke LG, Xu F, et al: *In vivo Bcl*-2 oncogene neuronal expression in the rat spinal cord. **Spine 23:** 517-523, 1998

132. Lucas DR, Newhouse JP: The toxic effect of sodium L-glutamate on the inner layers of the retina. **Arch Ophthalmol 58:**193-210, 1957

133. Macdermott AB, Mayer ML, Westbrook GL, et al: NMDA-receptor activation increases cytoplasmic calcium concentration in cultured spinal cord neurones. **Nature 321:**519-522, 1986

134. Majno G, Joris I: Apoptosis, oncosis, and necrosis. An overview of cell death. **Am J Pathol 146:**3-15, 1995

135. Mayer ML, Westbrook GL, Guthrie PB: Voltage-dependent block by Mg^{2+} of NMDA responses in spinal cord neurones. **Nature 309:**261-263, 1984

136. Merrill JE, Benveniste EN: Cytokines in inflammatory brain lesions: helpful and harmful. **Trends Neurosci 19:**331-338, 1996

137. Milvy P, Kakari S, Campbell JB, et al: Paramagnetic species and radical products in cat spinal cord. **Ann N Y Acad Sci 222:**1102-1111, 1973

138. Mullins LJ, Requena J, Whittembury J: Ca^{2+} entry in squid axons during voltage-clamp pulses is mainly Na^+/Ca^{2+} exchange. **Proc Natl Acad Sci USA 82:** 1847-1851, 1985

139. Namura S, Zhu J, Fink K, et al: Activation and cleavage of caspase-3 in apoptosis induced by experimental cerebral ischemia. **J Neurosci 18:**3659-3668, 1998

140. Nemecek S: Morphological evidence of microcirculatory disturbances in experimental spinal cord trauma. **Adv Neurol 20:**395-405, 1978

141. Nogawa S, Zhang F, Ross ME, et al: Cyclo-oxygenase-2 gene expression in neurons contributes to ischemic brain damage. **J Neurosci 17:**2746-2755, 1997

142. Ohshio I, Hatayama A, Kaneda K, et al: Correlation between histopathologic features and magnetic resonance images of spinal cord lesions. **Spine 18:** 1140-1149, 1993

143. Olney JW: Brain lesions, obesity and other disturbances in mice treated with monosodium glutamate. **Science 164:**719-721, 1969

144. Olney JW: Glutamate-induced retinal degeneration in neonatal mice. Electron microscopy of the acutely evolving lesion. **J Neuropathol Exp Neurol 28:** 455-474, 1969

145. O'Neill LAJ, Kaltschmidt C: NF-κB: a crucial transcription factor for glial and neuronal cell function. **Trends Neurosci 20:**252-258, 1997

146. Pender MP, Nguyen KB, McCombe PA, et al: Apoptosis in the nervous system in experimental allergic encephalomyelitis. **J Neurol Sci 104:**81-87, 1991

147. Petitjean ME, Pointillard V, Daverat P, et al: Administration of methylprednisolone or nimodipine or both versus placebo at the acute phase of spinal cord injury. **J Neurotrauma 14:**456, 1995 (Abstract)

148. Pietronigro DD, Hovsepian M, Demopoulos HB, et al: Loss of ascorbic acid from injured feline spinal cord. **J Neurochem 41:**1072-1076, 1983

149. Pitts LH, Ross A, Chase GA, et al: Treatment with thyrotropin-releasing hormone (TRH) in patients with traumatic spinal cord injuries. **J Neurotrauma 12:**235-243, 1995

150. Rao KR, Donnenfeld H, Chusid JG, et al: Acute myelopathy secondary to spinal venous thrombosis. **J Neurol 56:**107-113, 1982

151. Ray SK, Shields DC, Saido TC, et al: Calpain activity and translational expression increased in spinal cord injury. **Brain Res 816:**375-380, 1999

152. Regan RF, Choi DW: Glutamate neurotoxicity in spinal cord cell culture. **Neuroscience 43:**585-591, 1991

153. Reithmeier RAF: Mammalian exchangers and cotransporters. **Curr Opin Cell Biol 6:**583-594, 1994

154. Rink A, Fung KM, Trojanowski JQ, et al: Evidence of apoptotic cell death after experimental traumatic brain injury in the rat. **Am J Pathol 147:**1575-1583, 1995

155. Rivlin AS, Tator CH: Regional spinal cord blood flow in rats after severe cord trauma. **J Neurosurg 49:** 844-853, 1978

156. Rosenberg LJ, Teng YD, Wrathall JR: Effects of the sodium channel blocker tetrodotoxin on acute white matter pathology after experimental contusive spinal cord injury. **J Neurosci 19:**6122-6133, 1999

157. Sances A Jr, Myklebust JB, Maiman DJ, et al: The biomechanics of spinal injuries. **Crit Rev Biomed Eng 11:**1-76, 1984

158. Sandler AN, Tator CH: Effect of acute spinal cord compression injury on regional spinal cord blood flow in primates. **J Neurosurg 45:**660-676, 1976

159. Saunders RD, Dugan LL, Demediuk P, et al: Effects of methylprednisolone and the combination of α-tocopherol and selenium on arachidonic acid metabolism and lipid peroxidation in traumatized spinal cord tissue. **J Neurochem 49:**24-31, 1987

160. Schumacher PA, Eubanks JH, Fehlings MG: Increased calpain I-mediated proteolysis, and preferential loss of dephosphorylated NF200, following traumatic spinal cord injury. **Neuroscience 91:** 733-744, 1999

161. Senter HJ, Venes JL: Altered blood flow and secondary injury in experimental spinal cord trauma. **J Neurosurg 49:**569-578, 1978

162. Senter HJ, Venes JL: Loss of autoregulation and posttraumatic ischemia following experimental spinal

cord trauma. J Neurosurg 50:198-206, 1979

163. Shingu H, Kimura I, Nasu Y, et al: Microangiographic study of spinal cord injury and myelopathy. Paraplegia 27:182-189, 1989

164. Shuman SL, Bresnahan JC, Beattie MS: Apoptosis of microglia and oligodendrocytes after spinal cord contusion in rats. J Neurosci Res 50:798-808, 1997

165. Siesjö BK: Pathophysiology and treatment of focal cerebral ischemia. Part I: Pathophysiology. J Neurosurg 77:169-184, 1992

166. Springer JE, Azbill RD, Kennedy SE, et al: Rapid calpain I activation and cytoskeletal protein degradation following traumatic spinal cord injury: attenuation with riluzole pretreatment. J Neurochem 69: 1592-1600, 1997

167. Springer JE, Azbill RD, Knapp PE: Activation of the caspase-3 apoptotic cascade in traumatic spinal cord injury. Nat Med 5:943-946, 1999

168. Stewart WB, Wagner FC: Vascular permeability changes in the contused feline spinal cord. Brain Res 169:163-167, 1979

169. Stys PK, Waxman SG, Ransom BR: Ionic mechanism of anoxic injury in mammalian CNS white matter: role of Na+ channels and the Na^+- Ca^{2+} exchanger. J Neurosci 12:430-439, 1992

170. Stys PK, Waxman SG, Ransom BR: Na^+-Ca^{2+} exchanger mediates Ca^{2+} influx during anoxia in mammalian central nervous system white matter. Ann Neurol 30:375-380, 1991

171. Sufka KJ, Hoganson DA, Hughes RA: Central monoaminergic changes induced by morphine in hypoalgesic and hyperalgesic strains of domestic fowl. Pharmacol Biochem Behav 42:781-785, 1992

172. Taoka Y, Naruo M, Koyanagi E, et al: Superoxide radicals play important roles in the pathogenesis of spinal cord injury. Paraplegia 33:450-453, 1995

173. Taoka Y, Okajima K, Uchiba M, et al: Role of neutrophils in spinal cord injury in the rat. Neuroscience 79:1177-1182, 1997

174. Tarlov IM, Klinger H, Vitale S: Spinal cord compression studies. I. Experimental techniques to produce acute and gradual compression. Arch Neurol Psychiatry 70:813-819, 1953

175. Tator CH: Spine-spinal cord relationships in spinal cord trauma. Clin Neurosurg 30:479-494, 1983

176. Tator CH: Update on the pathophysiology and pathology of acute spinal cord injury. Brain Pathol 5:407-413, 1995

177. Tator CH, Fehlings MG: Review of clinical trials of neuroprotection in acute spinal cord injury. Neurosurg Focus 6(1):Article 8, 1999

178. Tator CH, Fehlings MG: Review of the secondary injury theory of acute spinal cord trauma with emphasis on vascular mechanisms. J Neurosurg 75: 15-26, 1991

179. Tator CH, Koyanagi I: Vascular mechanisms in the pathophysiology of human spinal cord injury. J Neurosurg 86:483-492, 1997

180. Teng YD, Wrathall JR: Local blockade of sodium channels by tetrodotoxin ameliorates tissue loss and long-term functional deficits resulting from experimental spinal cord injury. J Neurosci 17:4359-4366, 1997

181. Tymianski M, Tator CH: Normal and abnormal calcium homeostasis in neurons: a basis for the pathophysiology of traumatic and ischemic central nervous system injury. Neurosurgery 38:1176-1195, 1996

182. Van Harreveld A: Compounds in brain extracts causing spreading depression of cerebral cortical activity and contraction of crustacean muscle. J Neurochem 3:300-315, 1959

183. Wallace MC, Tator CH, Frazee P: Relationship between posttraumatic ischemia and hemorrhage in the injured rat spinal cord as shown by colloidal carbon angiography. Neurosurgery 18:433-439, 1986

184. Wang CX, Nuttin B, Heremans H, et al: Production of tumor necrosis factor in spinal cord following traumatic injury in rats. J Neuroimmunol 69: 151-156, 1996

185. Watkins JC: Excitatory amino acids, in McGreer E, Olney JW, McGreer P (eds): Kainic Acid as a Tool in Neurobiology. New York, NY: Raven Press, 1978, pp 37-69

186. Wells JD, Hansebout RR: Local hypothermia in experimental spinal cord trauma. Surg Neurol 10: 200-204, 1978

187. Westbrook GL, Mayer ML: Micromolar concentrations of Zn^{2+} antagonize NMDA and GABA responses of hippocampal neurons. Nature 328: 640-643, 1987

188. Wolman L: The disturbance of circulation in traumatic paraplegia in acute and late stages: a pathological study. Paraplegia 2:213-216, 1965

189. Wrathall JR, Choiniere D, Teng YD: Dose-dependent reduction of tissue loss and functional impairment after spinal cord trauma with the AMPA/kainate antagonist NBQX. J Neurosci 14:6598-6607, 1994

190. Wrathall JR, Teng YD, Choiniere D: Amelioration of functional deficits from spinal cord trauma with systemically administered NBQX, an antagonist of non-N-methyl-D- aspartate receptors. Exp Neurol 137: 119-126, 1996

191. Xu JA, Hsu CY, Liu TH, et al: Leukotriene B_4 release and polymorphonuclear cell infiltration in spinal cord injury. J Neurochem 55:907-912, 1990

192. Young W: Secondary injury mechanisms in acute spinal cord injury. J Emerg Med 11 (Suppl 1):13-22, 1993

193. Young W, Decrescito V, Tomasula JJ: Effect of sympathectomy on spinal blood flow autoregulation and posttraumatic ischemia. J Neurosurg 56:706-710, 1982

194. Young W, Decrescito V, Tomasula JJ, et al: The role of the sympathetic nervous system in pressor responses induced by spinal injury. J Neurosurg 52:473-481, 1980

195. Young W, Flamm ES: Effect of high-dose corticosteroid therapy on blood flow, evoked potentials, and extracellular calcium in experimental spinal injury. J Neurosurg 57:667-673, 1982

CHAPTER 6

THE APPLICATION OF BIOMECHANICS TO THE SPINE AND SPINAL CORD

WILLIAM MITCHELL, MD, AND GREGORY J. PRZYBYLSKI, MD

The application of biomechanical principles to spinal anatomy and physiology over the past three decades has substantially enhanced our understanding of the mechanisms of spine and spinal cord injury (SCI). Since the spine represents multisegmented scaffolding supporting the body to allow upright posture and motion, the evaluation of normal spine kinematics has led to an appreciation of the contributions of structures in the spine to the normal physiological range of motion. Similarly, the study of kinematics in SCI models has facilitated both a framework for describing the mechanism of injury and a guide for defining the best treatment. The application of biomechanics to SCI is less understood, but may be equally important in refining recommendations for medical and surgical treatments of patients sustaining SCIs.

TERMINOLOGY

In order to apply a biomechanical analysis of the spine and spinal cord to the clinical management of these injuries, one must first understand basic biomechanical terminology and related anatomy. Motion of spinal components is described in terms of displacement. This vector quantity (measured in meters) defines both the distance from the original to the final positions as well as the direction between them. Velocity represents the displacement over time (m/sec), whereas acceleration represents the rate at which the velocity changes (m/sec^2). Force (or load) is determined by the product of an object's mass and its acceleration (measured in newtons with units of kg-m/sec^2). For example, weight measures an object's mass subjected to gravitational acceleration. A bending moment (or torque) is the product of an applied load at a given point and the distance from that point to a constrained point on that object (Nm or kg-m^2/sec^2).

Forces and moments applied to an object can cause not only deformation but also motion of that object. The direction of displacements (vector) within a three-dimensional space can be simplified into individual translational or rotational components in three orthogonal (perpendicular) planes. This system has been applied to the human body and can be helpful in understanding movements of the spine. The three orthogonal planes with three perpendicular axes consist of the sagittal, coronal, and transverse planes (Figure 1). Since motion can occur either along or about an axis, there are a total of six degrees of freedom within this system. For example, movement of the spine in the sagittal plane consisting of rotation about the x-axis perpendicular to this plane results in flexion or extension. Likewise, rotation about the z-axis perpendicular to the coronal plane results in lateral bending, whereas rotation about the y-axis in the transverse plane results in axial rotation.

The structural and material properties of objects help define the predicted effects of forces placed on these objects. The structural proper-

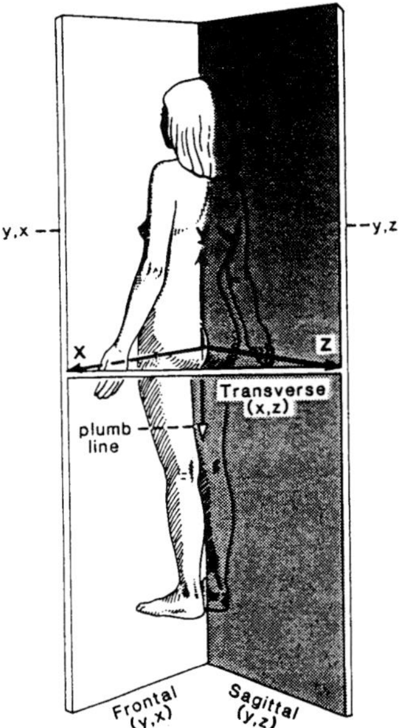

Figure 1: Representation of the three orthogonal planes of motion (reprinted with permission).

ties of an object are easier to measure and involve determination of the relationship between force and displacement. Tension describes the application of forces away from the object, whereas compression describes the application of forces toward the object. Material testing machines typically apply a given force and measure the resultant displacement or apply a given placement. The rate of change along a measured load-displacement curve is termed "stiffness" (N/m). For a linear relationship between force and displacement, an elastic constant is identified. For example, the force to stretch a simple spring is proportional to the displacement attained. Consequently, a structure with large elasticity requires larger forces to achieve deformation.

However, testing of many biological tissues identifies a nonlinear relationship between force and displacement. Although a nonlinear relationship can be modeled by a dashpot, this inadequately describes the behavior of biological tissues such as ligaments. Instead, these structures are viscoelastic. This term refers to the behaviors observed, such as creep and stress relaxation. Creep describes the phenomenon of smaller progressive displacements over time after a single force is applied and maintained on an object. In contrast,

stress relaxation describes the progressively smaller degrees of force required to maintain a viscoelastic object at a given length. These time-dependent properties demonstrate the importance of dynamic tests in examining the properties of human tissues.

An ultrastructural examination of an object allows the measurement of material properties, such as stress and strain. Stress describes the force applied to a given area of a surface (N/m^2), whereas strain (a unitless quantity) measures the ratio of the change in length of a material and its original length. The property of elasticity allows an object to return to its original shape after being deformed. However, when an object is deformed beyond its elastic limit, plastic deformation occurs with only incomplete recovery of the object's original shape after removal of the applied force. Finally, after deformation exceeds an object's plastic limit, failure occurs.

Structural Biomechanics and Kinematics

The application of biomechanical principles to the spine and spinal cord requires some understanding of their structural components. The simplest basic subset of the spine is termed the functional spinal unit. This consists of two adjacent vertebrae with their intervening discoligamentous structures. Bone is comprised predominantly of calcium salts, which impart strength. Tensile forces are applied to the vertebrae by attached muscles and ligaments. Although the tensile strength of bone is greatest along its axis,[15] most forces applied to the vertebrae are typically in compression. Consequently, vertebrae are strongest in compression. Moreover, the stiffness of vertebrae is related to the rate of loading, with increased strength and energy absorption at higher rates of loading. This tissue behavior correlates with the increasing height of each caudal vertebral body.[79] The vertebrae typically fail in flexion-compression, as partial flexion eliminates the spinal curvature to attain maximal stiffness in axial compression.[1,52,56,83,84]

The kinematics of the vertebrae are influenced by the orientation of the facet joints, which can limit motion depending upon their alignment. For example, the coronal orientation of cervical facet joints facilitates axial rotation while allowing sagittal plane bending. In contrast, the sagittal orientation of lumbar facet joints facilitates sagittal plane bending at the expense of limited axial rotation. Consequently, more diverse mobility is observed in the cervical spine, whereas prominent resistance to axial rotation occurs in the lumbar spine.[79] Finally, the direct contact of adjacent facet joints limits the allowable range of motion, with extension and lateral bending resisted in the cervical spine and axial rotation and lateral bending resisted in the lumbar spine.

The other major structural component of the functional spinal unit is the intervertebral disc. This joint is composed of circumferential layers of annular ligaments oriented at a 30° angle to the plane of the end plate and in opposite directions in alternating layers. The central viscoelastic nucleus pulposus contained by the annulus fibrosis helps distribute axial loads by causing compression of the cartilaginous end plate and tension within the annular ligaments. The aging process reduces the ability of the nucleus to distribute axial forces.

The kinematic effects of annular ligaments are observed in tension. In axial rotation, alternating annular layers are placed in tension to resist excess rotation. In contrast, bending in either the sagittal or coronal planes places ligaments on the convex side of the bend in tension.[45,59] Finally, some internal displacement of the nucleus is observed toward the convex side.[10,38]

Although usually considered independently from the annular ligaments, the other spinal ligaments are similarly composed of collagen, elastin, and reticulin fibers. While these ligaments are designed to resist tensile forces, their behavior is dependent on the ratio of the component fiber types. For example, the flaval ligament is composed of the greatest proportion of elastin fibers of all the body ligaments, thereby allowing less resistance to tension. The strength of ligaments varies by the ligament type as well as by the spinal segment of attachment.[14,47,48,50,53,54,70,79]

The spinal ligaments stabilize joints when placed in tension. Since the instantaneous axis of rotation is typically located within the posterior third of the intervertebral disc, the distance between the ligament and the axis of rotation will also contribute to the ability of a ligament to resist a given displacement.[49] Moreover, tension will lengthen the ligaments on the convex side of

a bend and shorten or buckle ligaments on the opposite side of the bend. For example, the anterior longitudinal ligament and anterior annulus resist extension,[62,79] whereas the posterior annular, posterior longitudinal, capsular, flaval, and interspinous ligaments all resist flexion.[6,79] In addition, capsular and annular ligaments resist lateral bending.[40] However, there is some evidence suggesting that certain ligaments may not be placed in tension within the physiological range of motion of the functional spinal unit.[55,60]

One of the least understood components of the spine is the musculature. Although muscles provide both motion and stability to the spine, the complicated neurophysiological behavior of muscles has limited the understanding of their contribution to spinal stabilization. By location of the muscular attachments, one can infer that the erector spinae provide extension and lateral bending, whereas the longus colli, iliopsoas, and rectus abdominus muscles produce flexion. In addition, muscle activity may provide spinal stability while reducing ligamentous tension within the physiological range of motion.[81]

Likewise, the biomechanical behavior of the spinal cord has not been well elucidated. The spinal cord is a viscoelastic material, with a semifluid parenchyma supported structurally by the fibroelastic pia. The arachnoid is composed of a fine fibroelastic membrane with traversing strands from the dura to the pia, which thickens at the level of the ventral and dorsal roots to form the supporting dentate ligaments in the cervicothoracic spinal cord. These act as stabilizers of the spinal cord, providing axial forces to balance axial tension of the spinal cord and transverse forces which provide stability in the axial plane.

As the spinal cord lengthens from its original length,[9] the initial longitudinal displacement of the spinal cord occurs with small forces. Subsequently, the second phase of lengthening requires larger forces to cause incrementally smaller deformations. With axial compression, the spinal cord initially folds and buckles, whereas, in extension, this folding is eliminated. The nonlinear behavior initially reflects the structural properties of the "accordion-like" spinal cord, followed by the viscoelastic material properties of the spinal cord.[35,36]

Finally, the integration of these components into the entire spine must also be considered to predict their interaction after spinal injuries. The spine is curved in the sagittal plane, with a concave cervical and lumbar "lordosis" and convex thoracic "kyphosis." The center of gravity of the body is located anterior to the thoracic spine, which places a flexion bending moment upon the thoracic region. The interrelationship of the spinal cord with the protective vertebral column relates to these curvatures. In flexion, the ventral spinal cord tissue becomes compressed, whereas the dorsal cord is placed in tension. Nearly 75% of the capacity of the spinal cord to lengthen is related to unfolding.[9] External compression of the spinal cord, as may occur in trauma, imparts a variety of forces upon the spinal cord, including compression, tension, and a bending moment. The compressive stress decreases with progressively larger distances from the point of impingement. Tensile forces are present across the transverse plane of the spinal cord. The bending of the spinal cord across a compressive mass results in a moment, causing tensile stress on the convex side and compressive stress on the concave side. Stresses are greatest peripherally and least in the central neutral axis of the cord.

Determining Spinal Stability

Although describing spinal instability has been the topic of many publications, a consensus agreement among spinal surgeons and scientists remains elusive. While displacement beyond the normal boundaries of motion may be sufficient to indicate instability in acute injury, the absence of such excess displacement on a static radiograph should not imply maintenance of stability. White and Panjabi[79] proposed that spinal instability represents the "loss of the ability of the spine under physiologic loads to maintain relationships between vertebrae in such a way that there is neither damage nor subsequent irritation to the spinal cord or nerve roots, and, in addition, there is no development of incapacitating deformity or pain due to structural changes." Rather than suggesting an absolute limit, White and Panjabi describe a continuum of spinal stability in which an accumulation of deficiencies within the normal properties of the spine leads to progressive instability. A simpler definition of stability describes an ability of the spine to resist

displacement and resume its resting position.[25]

In order to understand the effects of partial injury to the spine on its stability, the structure of the spine has been divided into components termed columns. The two-column model separates the vertebral bodies and supporting ligaments from the elements dorsal to the posterior longitudinal ligament. Instability occurs after all of the elements of one column and any additional element of the second column are disrupted.[36] In contrast, the three-column model separates the ventral column into an anterior and middle column based on the elements in the anterior two-thirds of the vertebra and the elements in the posterior third. Instability occurs after the elements of two columns are disrupted.[16] These theories provide a framework to assist the spine specialist in translating the imaging findings of injured spinal elements to an estimation of the instability of the spine. This method is applicable to any segment of the spine.

Furthermore, a mechanistic classification was devised for the subaxial cervical spine, which can also be applied to the entire spinal axis.[1] The scheme is based upon compression or distraction occurring with the spinal segment in one of three positions (neutral, flexion, or extension). Compression in the neutral position with forces transmitted along the vertebral body axis results in a "burst" fracture, with displacement of the body outward in the coronal plane. Compression in flexion with forces transmitted anterior to the axis of rotation results in a wedge-shaped fracture. Progressively greater forces can additionally cause dorsal retropulsion and/or posterior ligamentous and facet damage. Compression in extension with forces transmitted posterior to the axis of rotation results in posterior fractures. Progressively greater forces can additionally cause ventral ligamentous injury. Distraction in flexion results in dorsal ligamentous rupture, resulting in various degrees of facet subluxation to dislocation. Distraction in extension produces widening of the disc space anteriorly as the anterior longitudinal and annular ligaments fail. Progressively greater forces can additionally cause posterior ligamentous rupture.

Although these methods analyze the bony structure of the spine, assessment of the remaining spinal components is likewise essential in estimating instability. Neurological injury secondary to trauma implies instability. Bony displacements beyond the normal range imply ligamentous disruption. Modern imaging techniques can reveal ligamentous, muscular, and intervertebral disc injuries.[17,27,51] Although there is no definitive algorithm for every spinal injury, one can synthesize an understanding of the normal anatomy, physiological range of motion, column theory, and mechanism of injury to estimate spinal stability as well as direct appropriate treatment.

SPINAL BIOMECHANICS

Cervical

The upper cervical spine primarily allows rotation in the axial and sagittal planes. The normal axial rotation of the atlanto-occipital and atlantoaxial joints are 8° and 56°, respectively, whereas the normal flexion-extension range is 25° for both joints.[22,80] The tectorial membrane and alar ligaments provide the majority of the ligamentous stability of the craniovertebral junction.[11,23,77] Atlanto-occipital dislocation is a hyperextension injury in which disruption of the craniovertebral ligaments, particularly the tectorial and alar ligaments, results in atlanto-occipital instability. This injury typically occurs in children, perhaps related to the flatter articulation plane of the superior facet joints of the atlas with the immature occipital condyles.[74] Approximately half of the patients sustaining this injury have substantial neurological injuries involving the cervicomedullary tissues as well as the lower cranial nerves. Since ligaments typically do not heal well, this ligamentous injury requires reduction and internal fixation. In contrast, occipital condyle fractures result from axial compression. These are typically stable injuries unless avulsion of the alar ligaments and tectorial membrane also occurs from off-axis loading. Neurological injuries are uncommon. Although fractures alone can be managed with external immobilization, significant disruption of the supporting ligaments may require surgical stabilization.[4]

The transverse ligament provides much of the resistance of sagittal translation of the atlas upon the axis. Atlas fractures result from axial loading of the occipital condyles upon the lateral masses of C1, displacing the lateral masses centripetally. This fracture is not usually associated with neurological injury and may be treated with external immobilization. However, lateral displacement of the lateral masses beyond 7 mm, as measured on an open-mouth radiograph,[64] or an atlantodental interval greater than 3 mm on a lateral radiograph[26] imply injury to the transverse ligament, which may require surgical stabilization. Odontoid fractures are classified into three types based upon the scheme proposed in 1974 by Anderson and D'Alonzo.[2] These fractures are also not typically associated with neurological injuries. An avulsion of the tip of the dens (Type 1) is unusual, and is typically treated with rigid collar immobilization. The more common fracture at the base of the dens (Type 2) typically occurs from lateral bending.[44] Advanced patient age and increased subluxation have been associated with frequent nonunion from external immobilization.[5,28] Whereas some patients can be successfully treated with external immobilization, others at increased risk for nonunion may benefit from surgical fusion. In contrast, fractures extending into the vertebral body and facet (Type 3) occur from flexion and usually achieve satisfactory union with external immobilization.[44] Finally, traumatic C2 spondylolisthesis (hangman's fracture) typically occurs following hyperextension,[61] resulting in bilateral axis fractures near the articular facets. These fractures are classified based on displacement and angulation.[24] Neurological injuries are likewise uncommon. Unless substantial displacement from ligamentous injury occurs with facet dislocation (Type 3), these bony injuries can often be treated with external immobilization.

In the subaxial spine, the parameters measured on plain radiographs that suggest potential instability include sagittal plane angulation beyond 11° on static or 20° on dynamic lateral radiographs, or sagittal translation beyond 3.5 mm on lateral radiographs.[78] Normal segmental ranges of motion include 5°-10° of axial rotation, 6°-10° of flexion-extension, and 6°-10° in lateral bending.[33,40] All four common mechanisms of injury can cause cervical injuries.[73] The more common compression or flexion-compression injuries may cause neurological injury if bony intrusion into the spinal canal occurs. Increased susceptibility of neurological injury may be related to a pre-existing narrowing of the canal diameter.[71,72] Flexion-distraction injuries with an axis of rotation ventral to the anterior

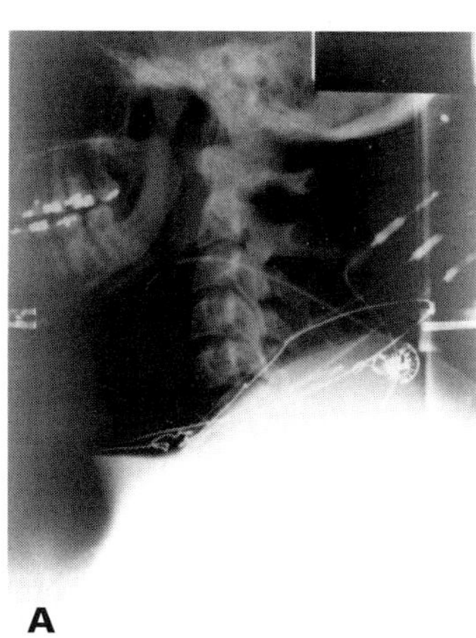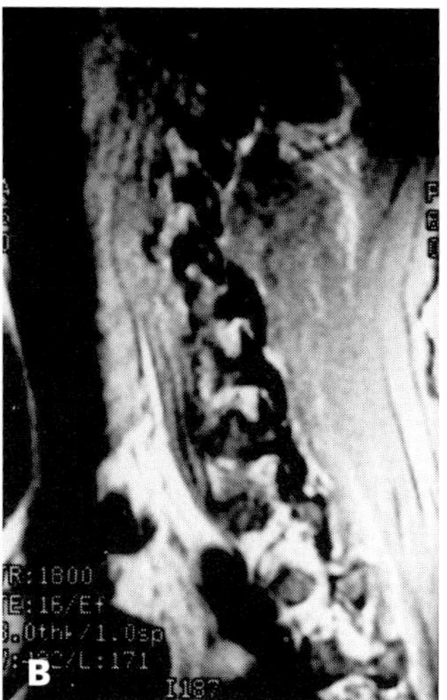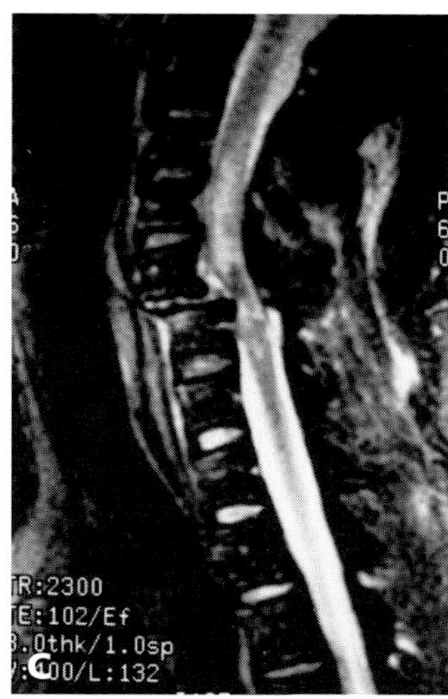

Figure 2: A 27-year-old man sustained a C5 ASIA A SCI, using the American Spinal Injury Association (ASIA) grading classification, from a flexion-distraction mechanism upon sliding into first base while playing softball. A lateral cervical radiograph **(A)** demonstrated facet dislocation at C5-6. Parasagittal magnetic resonance imaging (MRI) **(B)** confirmed a right facet dislocation. Midsagittal T2-weighted MRI **(C)** demonstrated extensive parenchymal edema.

longitudinal ligament can cause facet dislocations (Figure 2). These are often associated with significant neurological injuries. Extension injuries may be difficult to diagnose on plain radiographs alone (Figure 3). Both latter injury types are often treated with surgical fusion.

Thoracic

The thoracic region of the spine has several unique characteristics, including a kyphotic curvature as well as increased stiffness, imparted by the large moment inertia of the chest. The attachment of the ribs between the costovertebral and costosternal joints provides substantial stability to this region. Although injuries in this area are less common, the significant forces required to damage the thoracic spine often results in significant neurological impairment. Sagittal angulation exceeding 5° or translation exceeding 2.5 mm indicates instability.[29] Since the center of gravity lies anterior to the thoracic spine, flexion-compression injuries are common (Figure 4). Reduction of the dorsal vertebral body height by half or canal compromise greater than half suggests posterior ligamentous instability that will be inadequately treated with external immobilization.[12,31,32] Fracture-dislocation, shear injuries, and rotation can be observed on radiographs and signify instability requiring operative treatment.[31,32]

Thoracolumbar Junction

The thoracolumbar junction region of the spine is particularly vulnerable to injury as the spinal curvature changes from kyphosis to lordosis. The loss of costosternal joints reduces the stiffness imparted by the chest, whereas the smaller vertebral size and sparse muscular attachments provides less integrity than that observed in the lumbar spine. The normal parameters of motion are intermediate between those observed in the thoracic and lumbar areas. In addition to compression and flexion-compression injuries, this is a common area to observe shear injuries. The "Chance" fracture represents a transverse disruption of the spinal column, either through the vertebral body, pedicles, and posterior bony elements or through the discoligamentous structures without apparent bony injury. Reducible osseous Chance fractures will often heal with secure external immobilization.[13,63] Many injuries occurring after distractive, shear, or rotational forces are treated surgically.

Lumbar

The lumbar region of the spine contains the largest components since the entire loads of the torso are transmitted through the lumbar spine. Additional stiffness is imparted by the sagittal

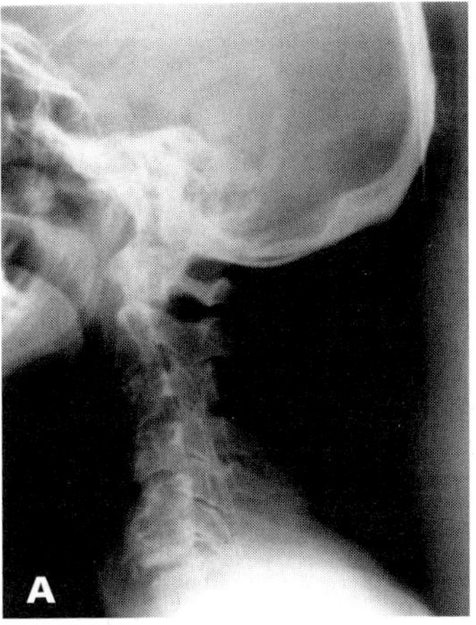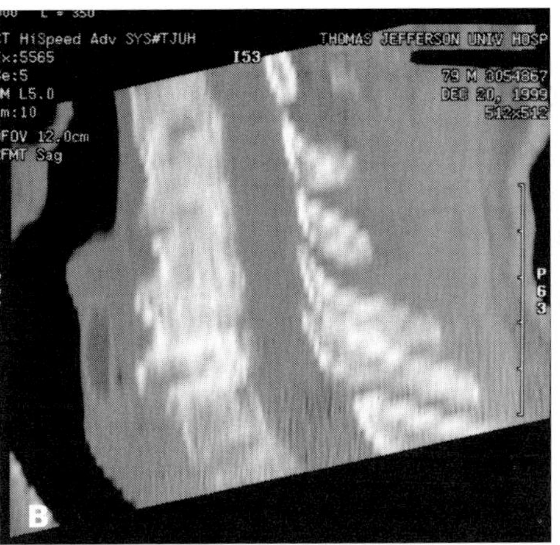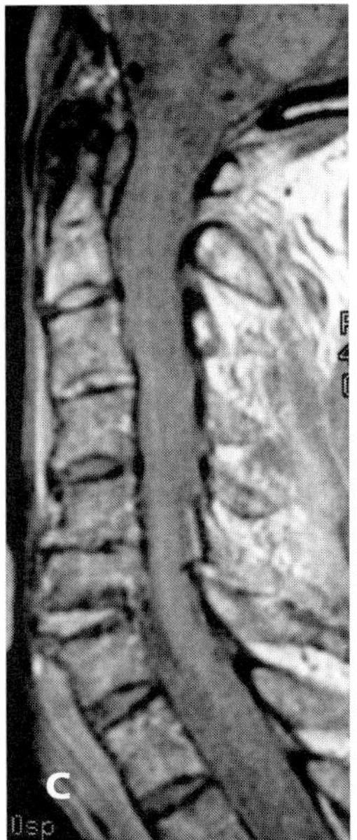

Figure 3: A 79-year-old man with no neurological injury sustained a C6-7 extension injury during a motor-vehicle accident. A lateral cervical radiograph **(A)** revealed spontaneous fusion of the C5-6 interspace and slight anterior widening of the C6-7 interspace, which was confirmed on midsagittal computed tomography (CT) reconstruction **(B)**. Midsagittal MRI **(C)** showed increased signal within the C6-7 interspace. Complete disruption of the disc was identified intraoperatively.

orientation of the facet joints, which limit axial rotation and lateral bending. Sagittal rotation beyond 22° or translation beyond 3 mm suggests instability.[8,53] Flexion-compression injuries are most common. Unless the conus extends below the thoracolumbar junction (Figure 5), many of these injuries are not accompanied by neurological impairment. If vertebral body height is maintained without angulation or rotation, external immobilization is usually sufficient. Substantial burst fractures or evidence of rotational or distraction injuries may imply sufficient ligamentous injury to warrant surgical stabilization. If the force is ventral to the anterior longitudinal ligament, a transverse injury to the osseous body and/or ligaments may result. This may be treated with external immobilization, if reduction can be achieved and maintained.[13,63]

BIOMECHANICS OF SCI

Traumatic compression of the spinal cord causes early parenchymal changes from vascular impairment.[19] Venous channels distend within 5 minutes followed by extravasation of erythrocytes within the first 30 minutes. Hemorrhages then occur within the hour, followed by chromatolysis and vacuolization of neurons within 4 hours. Edema develops in the white matter and reaches its maximum after 5 days.[19,82] However, diminished blood flow occurs immediately after injury and extends a considerable distance.[58] In experimental models, animals attaining complete recovery had increased blood flow after injury. This ischemic mechanism of injury is consistent with the irreversibility after two hours.

In addition, the degree of mechanical compression contributes to the extent of recoverability after deformation of the spinal cord. For example, a 1.0-cc balloon inflated within the spinal canal for only 5 minutes caused irreversible injury, whereas recovery was observed if compression by an 0.8-cc balloon is discontinued within 2 hours of compression.[67] In addition, tensile forces can also contribute to SCI.[20,41,42]

Moreover, gradually applied compressive forces can be reversed within a longer time interval.[18,66] Improved recovery has been demonstrated after decompression of the spinal cord in experimentally injured animals.[18,65-68] A linear relationship between the log of compression time and clinical performance in rats after acute spinal cord compression has been observed.[57] Although rapid decompression has been investigated in the management of human SCI, studies have failed to demonstrate a benefit with early decompressive surgery. In fact, surgical timing may not influence recovery from complete or

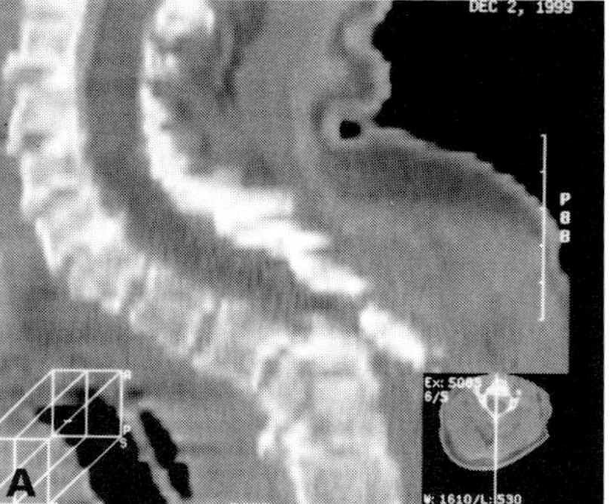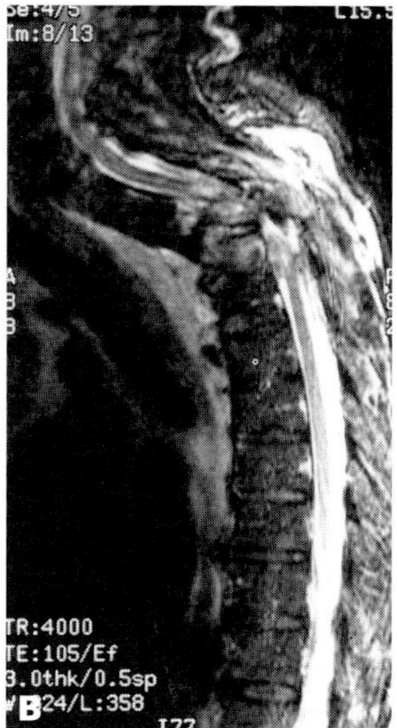

Figure 4: A 65-year-old man sustained a T4 ASIA A SCI, using the ASIA grading classification, from a flexion-compression mechanism following a fall. Midsagittal CT reconstruction **(A)** demonstrated kyphotic deformity with compression fractures of T3 and T4 accompanied by retropulsion of bone into the spinal canal. Midsagittal T2-weighted MRI **(B)** demonstrated the significant signal change observed in the thoracic spinal cord.

incomplete injuries.[7,21,30,39,43,46,69,75] Although the second National Acute Spinal Cord Injury Study revealed a significant difference in outcome at 6 weeks favoring surgery beyond 5 days, compared to surgery within 24 hours, this difference was not significant at 1 year.[21] However, studies examining the effects of early decompression may be limited by the excessive time elapse until decompression, given the rapid ultrastructural changes observed from ischemia in animal studies. Although most patients with complete SCIs do not recover long tract function, many will achieve some nerve root recovery either with ventral decompression[3,34,39,76] or without decompression.[76]

CONCLUSION

The application of biomechanical principles can assist the spinal surgeon in assessing the extent of bony and ligamentous injury. An analysis of the stability of the traumatized spine is essential to guide appropriate treatment. Investigations into the evolution of irreversible experimental SCI have identified the potential benefit of rapid decompression in facilitating the likelihood of reversing spinal cord ischemia. Current efforts are underway to prospectively study the feasibility of early decompression within a shorter time interval.

REFERENCES

1. Allen BL Jr, Ferguson RL, Lehmann TR, et al: A mechanistic classification of closed, indirect fractures and dislocations of the lower cervical spine. Spine 7:1-27, 1982
2. Anderson LD, D'Alonzo RT: Fractures of the odontoid process of the axis. J Bone Joint Surg (Am) 56: 1663-1674, 1974
3. Anderson PA, Bohlman HH: Anterior decompression and arthrodesis of the cervical spine: Long-term motor improvement. Part II: Improvement in complete tramatic quadriplegia. J Bone Joint Surg (Am) 74: 683-692, 1992
4. Anderson PA, Montesano PX: Morphology and treatment of occipital condyle fractures. Spine 13:731-736, 1988
5. Apuzzo MLF, Heiden JS, Weiss MH, et al: Acute fractures of the odontoid process. An analysis of 45 cases. J Neurosurg 48:85-91, 1978
6. Bailey RW: Fractures and dislocations of the cervical spine. Postgrad Med 35:588-599, 1964
7. Benzel EC, Larson SJ: Functional recovery after decompressive spine operation for cervical spine fractures. Neurosurgery 20:742-746, 1987
8. Bernhardt M, Bridwell KH: Segmental analysis of the sagittal plane alignment of the normal thoracic and lumbar spines and thoracolumbar junction. Spine 14: 717-721, 1989
9. Brieg A: **Biomechanics of the Central Nervous System: Some Basic Normal and Pathological Phenomena.** Stockholm: Almquist and Wiksell, 1960
10. Broberg KB: On the mechanical behaviour of intervertebral discs. Spine 8:151-165, 1983
11. Bucholz RW, Burkhead WZ: The pathological anatomy of fatal atlanto-occipital dislocations. J Bone Joint Surg (Am) 61:248-250, 1979
12. Capen DA, Gordon ML, Zigler DE, et al: Nonoperative treatment of upper thoracic spine fractures. Orthop Rev 23:818-821, 1994
13. Chance GQ: Note on a type of flexion fracture of the spine. Br J Radiol 21:452-453, 1948
14. Chazal J, Tanguy A, Bourges M, et al: Biomechanical properties of spinal ligaments and a histological study of the supraspinal ligament in traction. J Biomech 18: 167-176, 1985
15. Cowin SC: The mechanical and stress adaptive properties of bone. Ann Biomed Eng 11:263-295, 1983
16. Denis F: The three-column spine and its significance in the classification of acute thoracolumbar spinal injuries. Spine 8:817-831, 1983
17. Dickman CA, Mamourian A, Sonntag VKH: Magnetic resonance imaging of the transverse atlantal

Figure 5: A 38-year-old man sustained a conus medullaris injury from an L1 burst fracture due to a compression mechanism following a fall. Lateral lumbar radiograph **(A)** demonstrated the fracture with loss of superior vertebral body height. Midsagittal T2-weighted MRI **(B)** revealed increased signal in the spinal cord at the level of the retropulsed bone. Postoperative T2-weighted MRI **(C)** 7 months after anterior column spinal reconstruction revealed residual hyperintensity at the conus.

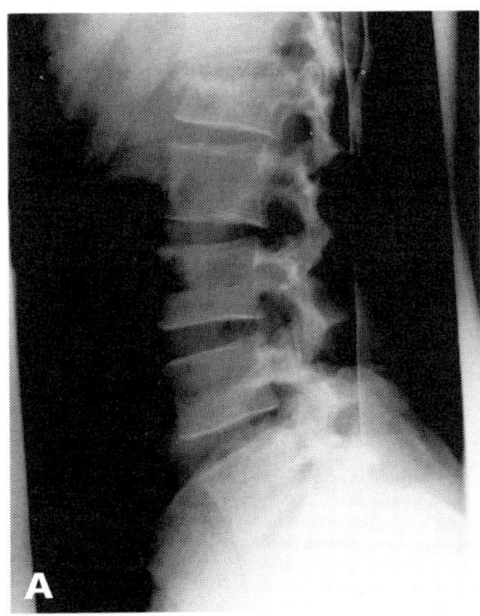
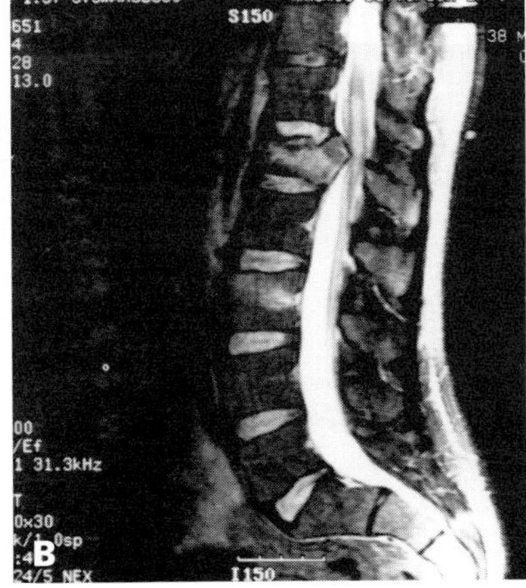
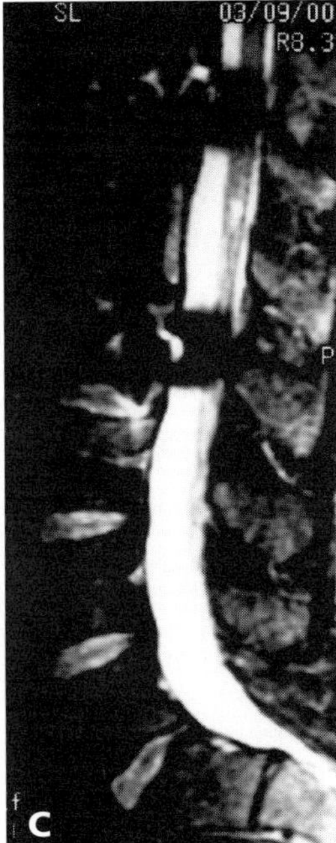

ligament for the evaluation of atlanto-axial instability. **J Neurosurg** 75:221-227, 1991

18. Dolan EJ, Tator CH, Endrenyi L: The value of decompression for acute experimental spinal cord compression injury. **J Neurosurg** 53:749-755, 1980

19. Ducker TB: Experimental injury of the spinal cord, in Vinken PJ, Bruyn GW (eds): **Handbook of Clinical Neurology,** V 25, Amsterdam: N Holland, 1976, pp 9-26

20. Ducker TB, Salcman M, Daniell HB: Experimental spinal cord trauma, III: Therapeutic effect of immobilization and pharmacologic agents. **Surg Neurol 10:** 71-76, 1978

21. Duh MS, Shephard MJ, Wilberger JE, et al: The effectiveness of surgery on the treatment of acute spinal cord injury and its relation to the pharmacological treatment. **Neurosurgery** 35:240-249, 1994

22. Dvorak J, Hayek J, Zehnder R: CT-functional diagnostics of the rotatory instability of the upper cervical spine Part 2. **Spine** 12:726-731, 1987

23. Dvorak J, Schneider E, Saldinger P, et al: Biomechanics of the craniocervical region: The alar and transverse ligaments. **J Orthop Res** 6:452-461, 1988

24. Effendi B, Roy D, Cornish B: Fractures of the ring of the axis: a classification based on the analysis of 131 cases. **J Bone Joint Surg (Br)** 63:319-327, 1981

25. Farfan HF, Gracovetsky S: The nature of instability. **Spine** 9:714-719, 1984

26. Fielding JW, Cochran GV, Lawsing JF: Tears of the transverse ligament of the atlas. **J Bone Joint Surg (Am)** 56:1683-1691, 1974

27. Greene KA, Dickman CA, Marciano FF, et al: Transverse atlantal ligament disruption associated with odontoid fractures. **Spine** 19:2307-2314, 1994

28. Hadley MN, Browner C, Sonntag VKH: Axis fractures: a comprehensive review of management and treatment in 107 cases. **Neurosurgery** 17:281-289, 1985

29. Hausfield JN: A Biomechanical Analysis of Clinical Stability in the Thoracic and Thoracolumbar Spine. Thesis, Yale University School of Medicine, 1977

30. Heiden JS, Weiss MH, Rosenberg AW, et al: Management of cervical spinal cord injury trauma in Southern California. **J Neurosurg** 43:732-736, 1975

31. Holdsworth FW: Fractures, dislocations, and fracture-dislocations of the spine. **J Bone Joint Surg (Br) 45:** 6-20, 1963

32. Holdsworth FW: Fractures, dislocations, and fracture-dislocations of the spine. **J Bone Joint Surg (Am) 52:** 1534-1551, 1970

33. Holmes A, Wang C, Han ZH, et al: The range and nature of flexion-extension motion in the cervical spine. **Spine** 19:2505-2510, 1994

34. Horsey WJ, Tucker WS, Hudson AR, et al: Experience with early anterior operation in acute injuries of the cervical spine. **Paraplegia** 15:110-122, 1977

35. Hung TK, Chang GL: Biomechanical and neurological response of the spinal cord of a puppy to uniaxial tension. **J Biomech Eng** 103:43- 47, 1981

36. Hung TK, Chang GL, Chang JL, et al: Stress-strain relationship and neurological sequelae of uniaxial elongation of the spinal cord of cats. **Surg Neurol** 15:471-476, 1981

37. Kelly RP, Whitesides TE Jr: Treatment of lumbodorsal fracture-dislocations. **Ann Surg** 167:705-717, 1968

38. Krag MK, Seroussi RE, Wilder DG, et al: Internal displacement distribution from in vitro loading of human thoracic and lumbar spinal motion segments: Experimental results and theoretical predictions. **Spine** 12:1001-1007, 1987

39. Levi, L, Wolf A, Rigamonti D, et al: Anterior decompression in cervical spine trauma: Does timing of surgery affect the outcome? **Neurosurgery** 29:216-222, 1991

40. Lysell E: Motion in the cervical spine. **Acta Orthop Scand Suppl** 123:1-61, 1969

41. Maiman DJ, Coats J, Myklebust JB: Cord/spine motion

in experimental spinal cord injury. **J Spinal Disord 2:** 14-19, 1989

42. Maiman DJ, Myklebust JB, Ho KC, et al: Experimental spinal cord injury produced by axial tension. **J Spinal Disord 2:**6-13, 1989

43. Maynard FM, Reynolds GG, Fountain S, et al: Neurological prognosis after traumatic quadriplegia. Three-year experience of California Regional Spinal Cord Injury Care System. **J Neurosurg 50:**611-616, 1979

44. Mouradian WH, Fietti VG Jr, Cochran GVB: Fractures of the odontoid: a laboratory and clinical study of mechanisms. **Orthop Clin N Am 9:**985-1001, 1978

45. Munro D. The factors that govern the stability of the spine. **Paraplegia 3:**219-228, 1965

46. Murphy KP, Opitz JL, Cabanela ME, et al: Cervical fractures and spinal cord injury: Outcome of surgical and nonsurgical management. **Mayo Clin Proc 65:** 949-959, 1990

47. Myklebust JB, Pintar F, Yoganandan N, et al: Tensile strength of spinal ligaments. **Spine 13:**526-531, 1988

48. Nachemson A, Evans J. Some mechanical properties of the third lumbar inter-laminar ligament. **J Biomech 1:** 211-217, 1968

49. Panjabi MM, Greenstein G, Duranceau J, et al: Three-dimensional quantitative morphology of lumbar spinal segments. **J Spinal Disord 4:**54-62, 1991

50. Panjabi MM, Hausfield JN, White AA: A biomechanical study of the ligamentous stability of the thoracic spine. **Acta Orthop Scand 52:**315-326, 1981

51. Pathria MN, Petersilge CA: Spinal trauma. **Radiol Clin North Am 29:**847-865, 1991

52. Pintar FA, Yoganandan N, Droese K, et al: Biomechanics of cervical spine column injury. **Proceedings of the Fourth Annual Injury Prevention through Biomechanics Symposium, Vol 4.** 1995, pp 117-126

53. Posner I, White AA III, Edwards WT, et al: A biomechanical analysis of the clinical stability of the lumbar and lumbosacral spine. **Spine 7:**374-389, 1982

54. Przybylski GJ, Carlin GJ, Patel PR, et al: Human anterior and posterior cervical longitudinal ligaments possess similar tensile properties. **J Orthop Res 14:** 1005-1008, 1996

55. Przybylski GJ, Patel PR, Carlin GJ, et al: Quantitative anthropometry of the subatlantal cervical longitudinal ligaments. **Spine 23:**893-898, 1998

56. Roaf R: A study of the mechanics of spinal injuries. **J Bone Joint Surg (Br) 42:**810-823, 1960

57. Rivlin AS, Tator CH: Effect of duration of acute spinal cord compression in a new acute injury model in the rat. **Surg Neurol 10:**39-43, 1978

58. Rivlin AS, Tator CH: Regional spinal cord blood flow in rats after severe cord trauma. **J Neurosurg 49:** 844-853, 1978

59. Sances A Jr, Weber, RC, Larson SJ, et al: Bioengineering analysis of head and spine injuries. **Crit Rev Bioeng 5:** 79-122, 1981

60. Schendel MJ, Wood KB, Buttermann GR, et al: Experimental measurement of ligament force, facet force, and segment motion in the human lumbar spine. **J Biomech 26:**427-438, 1993

61. Schneider RC, Livingston KE, Cave AJE, et al: "Hangman's fracture" of the cervical spine. **J Neurosurg 22:** 141-154, 1965

62. Shea M, Wittenberg RH, Edwards WT, et al: In vitro hyperextension injuries in the human cadaveric cervical spine. **J Orthop Res 10:**911-916, 1992

63. Smith WS, Kaufer H: Patterns and mechanisms of lumbar injuries associated with lap seat belts. **J Bone Joint Surg (Am) 51:**239-254, 1969

64. Spence K Jr, Decker S, Sell KW: Bursting atlantal fracture associated with rupture of the transverse ligament. **J Bone Joint Surg (Am) 52:**543-549, 1970

65. Tarlov IM: Acute spinal cord compression paralysis. **J Neurosurg 36:**10-20, 1972

66. Tarlov IM: Spinal cord compression studies. III. Time limits for recovery after gradual compression in dogs. **Arch Neurol Psychiatry 71:**588-597, 1954

67. Tarlov IM, Klinger H: Spinal cord compression studies. II. Time limits for recovery after acute compression in dogs. **Arch Neurol Psychiatry 71:**271-290, 1954

68. Tarlov IM, Klinger H, Vitale S: Spinal cord compression studies. I. Experimental techniques to produce acute and gradual compression. **Arch Neurol Psychiatry 70:**813-819, 1953

69. Tator CH, Duncan EG, Edmonds VE, et al: Comparison of surgical and conservative management in 208 patients with acute spinal cord injury. **Can J Neurol Sci 14:**60-69, 1987

70. Tkaczuk H: Tensile properties of human lumbar longitudinal ligaments. **Acta Orthop Scand 115 (Suppl):** 1-69, 1968

71. Torg JS: Pavlov's ratio: determining cervical spinal stenosis on routine lateral roentgenograms. **Contemp Orthop 18:**153-160, 1989

72. Torg JS, Pavlov H, Genuario SE, et al: Neuropraxia of the cervical spinal cord with transient quadriplegia. **J Bone Joint Surg (Am) 68:**1354-1370, 1986

73. Torg JS, Thibault L, Sennett B, et al: The Nicholas Andry Award. The pathomechanics and pathophysiology of cervical spinal cord injury. **Clin Orthop 321:** 259-269, 1995

74. Traynelis VC, Marano GD, Dunker RO, et al: Traumatic atlanto-occipital dislocation: case report. **J Neurosurg 65:**863-870, 1986

75. Wagner FC Jr, Chehrazi B: Early decompression and neurological outcome in acute cervical spinal cord injuries. **J Neurosurg 56:**699-705, 1982

76. Weinshel SS, Maiman DJ, Baek P, et al: Neurologic recovery in quadriplegia following operative treatment. **J Spinal Disord 3:**244-249, 1990

77. Werne S: Studies in spontaneous atlas dislocation. **Acta Scand (Suppl) 23:**1-150, 1957

78. White AA, Johnson RM, Panjabi MM: Biomechanical analysis of clinical stability in the cervical spine. **Clin Orthop 109:**85-96, 1975

79. White AA, Panjabi M: **Clinical Biomechanics of the Spine, 2nd ed.** Philadelphia: JB Lippincott, 1990

80. White AA, Panjabi MM: The clinical biomechanics of the occipitoatlantoaxial complex. **Orthop Clin N Am 9:**867-878, 1978

81. Wilke HJ, Wolf S, Claes LE, et al: Stability increase of the lumbar spine with different muscle groups: A biomechanical in vitro study. **Spine 20:**192-198, 1995

82. Yashon D, Bingham WG Jr, Faddoul EM, et al: Edema of the spinal cord following experimental impact trauma. **J Neurosurg 38:**693-697, 1973

83. Yoganandan N, Pintar FA, Sances A Jr, et al: Strength and kinematic response of dynamic cervical spine injuries. **Spine 16 (Suppl):**S511-S517, 1991

84. Yoganandan N, Sances A Jr, Pintar FA, et al: Injury biomechanics of the human cervical column. **Spine 15:**1031-1039, 1990

CHAPTER 7

RESUSCITATION AND EARLY MEDICAL MANAGEMENT OF THE SPINAL CORD INJURY PATIENT

SETTI S. RENGACHARY, MD, AND SHEILA M. ALTON, MD, FACEP

PRE-HOSPITAL CARE

Motor-vehicle accidents account for 36% of spinal cord injuries (SCIs) reported. Other contributors include acts of violence (particularly gunshot wounds), falls, and recreational sporting activities.[27] All victims of major trauma should therefore be treated presumptively by pre-hospital personnel as having an SCI until proven otherwise. The force involved in producing other injuries often has the potential for damaging the spinal cord. Care must be taken not to further any damage during transport to the hospital or during the early course of treatment in the emergency department.

Immobilization of the Spine at the Scene of the Accident

When the patient is found lying on the ground at the scene of an accident (Figure 1A), initial manual in-line immobilization of the neck should be obtained. This is accomplished by gently grasping the head and moving it into a neutral in-line, or "eyes forward," position[17] (Figure 1B).

This should not be forced, however, and the maneuver should be abandoned if pain increases, the airway becomes compromised, or if neurological symptoms develop. If such effects are noted, the neck should be immobilized in the deformed position found. It has been the authors' experience that this rarely occurs and most individuals can be turned to the "eyes forward" position. Once a neutral position is obtained, an appropriately sized hard cervical collar is applied by a second individual while manual in-line immobilization is maintained by the first (Figure 1C).

The same principles are used in securing the neck for victims of motor-vehicle collisions. One individual maintains the patient in manual in-line immobilization, while a second individual applies a hard cervical collar (Figure 2A and B). Full spine immobilization is then accomplished with patient's torso and extremities secured onto a long spine board (Figure 2C). The cervical collar alone does not adequately immobilize the cervical spine as it allows for rotational movement. The head must be secured to the spine board with tape across the forehead (Figure 2D).[19] In the past, sandbags had been used for further immobilization of the head but their use

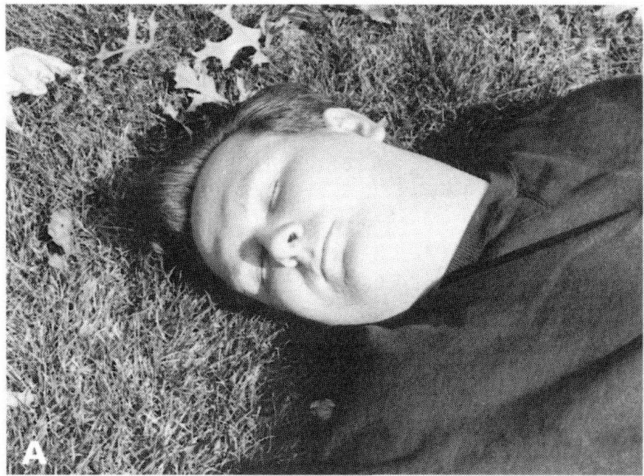
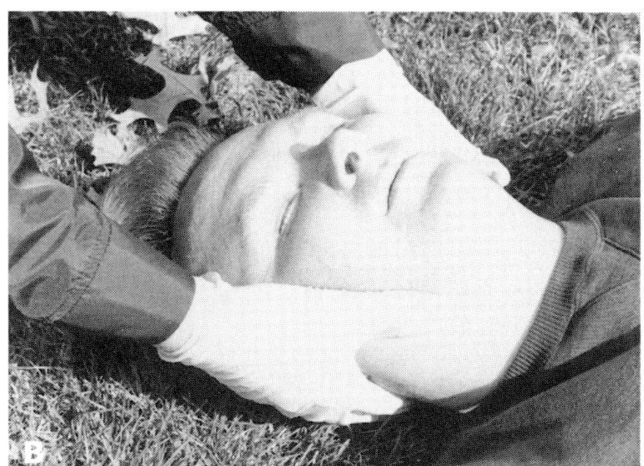
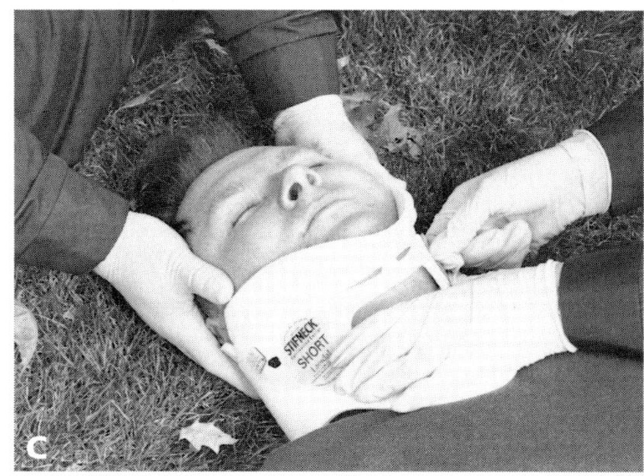

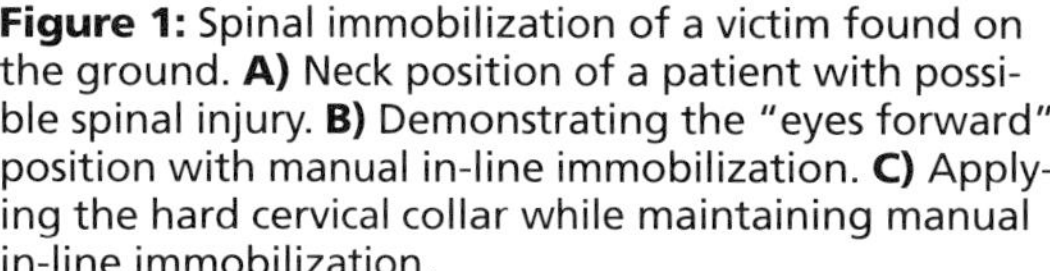

Figure 1: Spinal immobilization of a victim found on the ground. **A)** Neck position of a patient with possible spinal injury. **B)** Demonstrating the "eyes forward" position with manual in-line immobilization. **C)** Applying the hard cervical collar while maintaining manual in-line immobilization.

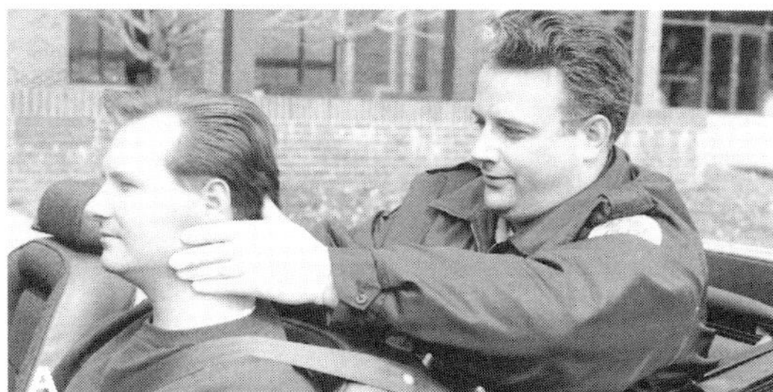
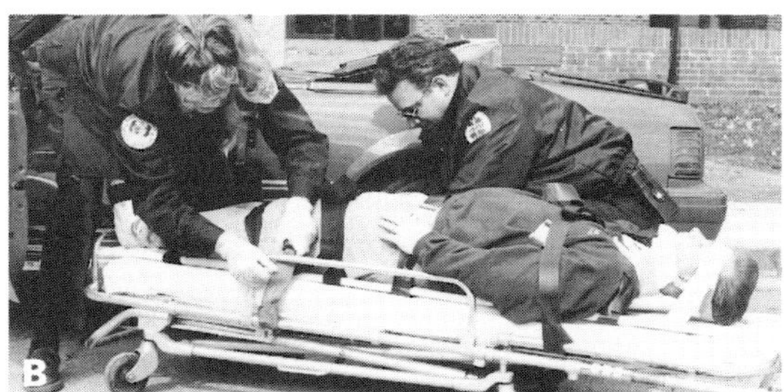
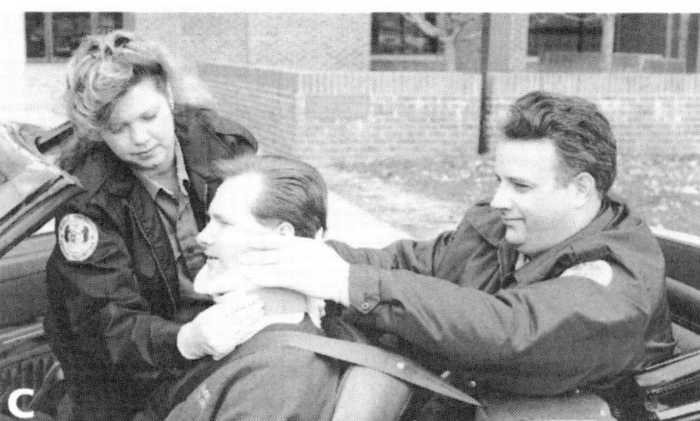
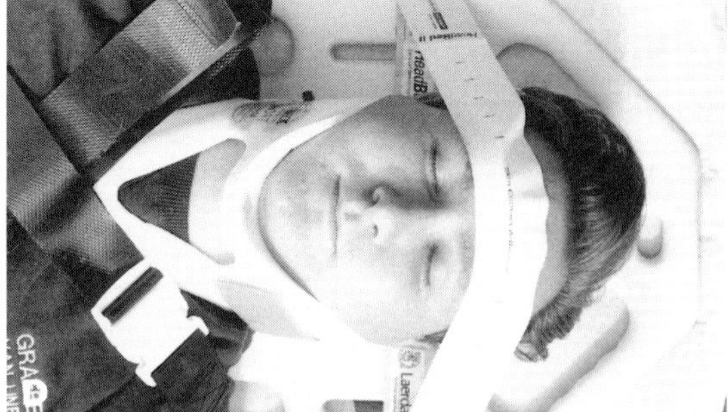

Figure 2: Spinal immobilization of a victim of a motor-vehicle accident. **A)** Manual in-line immobilization is maintained while in the vehicle by the first rescuer. **B)** The second rescuer applying the hard cervical collar. **C)** Full spinal immobilization on a long spine board (spine board has been placed on a stretcher). **D)** The victim's head is immobilized to the spine board by tape.

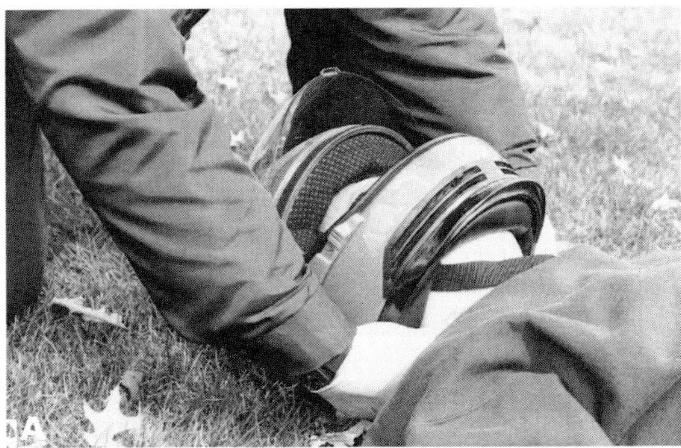

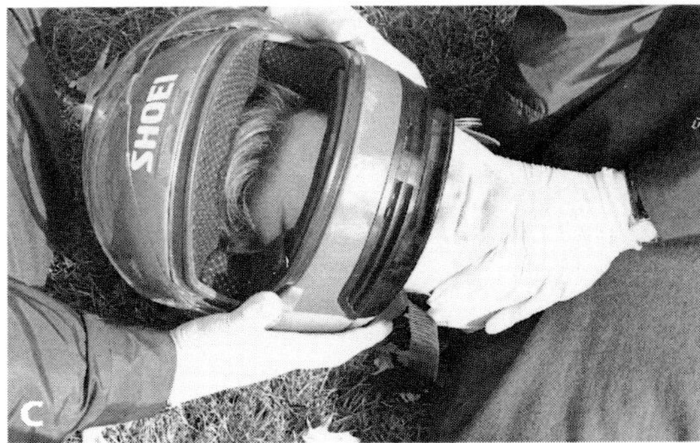

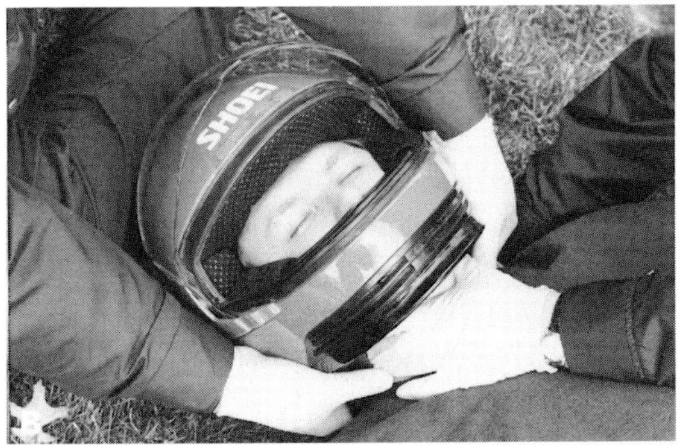

Figure 3: Two-rescuer helmet removal.
A) Position of the first rescuer during helmet removal.
B) Position of the second rescuer during helmet removal.
C) Removal of the helmet by the first rescuer.

is discouraged in contemporary practice. The concern is the potential risk of infection from the inability to clean the sandbags of blood and other body fluids. There are many disposable foam products that can be used in place of the sandbags.

If the patient is or becomes unconscious, the board should be tilted onto the left side, supporting the patient's torso with pillows, to avoid aspiration of secretions.

Removal of Helmet

If the accident victim is wearing a helmet at the time of injury, the patient may be brought to the emergency department with the helmet still on, although the pre-hospital care personnel are trained in their removal. The helmet does not necessarily need to be removed in the pre-hospital setting unless it is interfering with the patient's airway, concealing life-threatening hemorrhage, too large (causing extreme flexion of the neck), or too loose to provide adequate immobilization.[17] To remove the helmet, two individuals are needed. One person (situated at the patient's head) places a hand on either side of the mandible, supporting the head in the neutral

position (Figure 3A). The second person (situated at the patient's side) loosens the chin strap and then places one hand on the mandible supporting the chin with the second hand under the neck (Figure 3B). The first person then removes the helmet, expanding the sides to clear the ears. The second person then moves a hand from the neck up to support the occiput (Figure 3C). After the helmet is removed, the first person maintains the head with in-line immobilization while the second individual (Figure 1C) applies the hard cervical collar. Full spinal immobilization on a long spine board is then performed (Figure 2C and D).

Special consideration is given, however, to the removal of a football helmet. Investigations have discovered that removal of either the shoulder pads or the helmet individually increases the risk of furthering SCI.[10,35] When shoulder pads are in place, the neck is extended further with helmet removal.[35] It is recommended that the pads and helmet be removed in the controlled setting of the emergency department with the assistance of at least three, and preferably four, individuals.[10] Initially, the chin strap and cheek pads are removed. The head is supported by the occiput and the helmet is removed as described in Figure 3. The only difference is that the head is maintained in line with the spine, which is elevated by the shoulder pads. The shoulder pads are removed and a collar is applied. The patient should then be fully immobilized on a long spine board with foam blocks and tape. The helmet may also be removed by cutting with heavy shears, if necessary.

Underwater Rescue of Spine-Injured Patients

Diving accidents are a frequent cause of SCI. The injury results when a person plunges head-first, striking the head on the ground or on a protruding rock. Any drowning victim has a presumed SCI until proven otherwise. The first maneuver is to position the patient on his/her back with a rescuer placing one arm along the patient's spine and the other arm under the chest. The rescuer then slowly backs away while rotating the patient into a supine position. One hand is kept under the thoracic spine with the head supported on the upper arm. The other hand is used to stabilize the victim's head while mouth-to-mouth ventilation is performed, if needed. Two rescuers may be needed to rotate the body safely, with the head and trunk maintained as one unit.

A second rescuer floats the backboard out into the water and slides the backboard under the victim. The head and trunk are then secured to the backboard, and the victim is removed from the water. The first rescuer continues mouth-to-mouth or mouth-to-mask artificial respirations during the immobilization. The patient's head is then immobilized between two blanket rolls, a hard cervical collar is placed, and full spinal immobilization is achieved with strapping of the patient's torso and legs onto the board.[9] Once the victim is removed from the water and properly immobilized, circulation is assessed. If indicated, cardiopulmonary resuscitation is initiated. Ventilation can then be maintained with the use of a bag-valve-mask apparatus utilizing 100% oxygen. If the patient is unconscious, transport should be with the patient on his/her left side. This can be accomplished when the patient is fitted secure to the board and buttressed with pillows.

These principles of manual in-line immobilization need to be practiced throughout the patient's initial care, especially while the patient is being moved and examined in the emergency department. All involved hospital personnel should be aware of and versed in proper spine immobilization to prevent initiating or worsening SCI.

Resuscitation

All SCI patients should be managed initially using a standardized protocol. The approach described in this section closely follows the guidelines established by the American College of Surgeons.[1]

The initial management of all trauma patients begins with addressing the ABC's (*a*irway, *b*reathing, *c*irculation). Although this chapter is concerned primarily with SCIs, life-threatening injuries need to be addressed first. An initial "primary survey" should be rapidly performed addressing *a*irway maintenance with cervical spine immobilization; *b*reathing; *c*irculation with hemorrhage control; *d*isability (i.e., addressing the neurological status), and *e*xposure. This can be remembered by the mnemonic "ABCDE."

Establishment of the Airway

The airway may be maintained initially with the chin lift. This maneuver aids in releasing the obstruction of the posterior pharynx caused by the tongue. In a patient with a suspected cervical spine injury, the jaw-thrust maneuver should be performed rather than the chin lift. The jaw thrust displaces the mandible forward and is performed by grasping the angles of the mandible bilaterally and gently lifting in an upward motion. This is the same motion that is used when utilizing the bag-valve-mask. The jaw-thrust method is preferable over the chin-lift maneuver, as the former releases the obstruction of the posterior pharynx caused by the soft tissues but produces less neck extension.

If this is not successful, an oral or nasopharyngeal airway may be placed to aid in maintaining the airway. If still unsuccessful or the patient's mental status is such that protection of the airway is at risk, endotracheal intubation is required. Airway management is further discussed in Chapter 10, but it is the authors' bias that nonsurgical methods should be attempted first (i.e., oral or nasal endotracheal intubation).

In patients with suspected cervical spine injuries, it has been commonly taught that nasotracheal intubation or surgical airway is preferred over orotracheal intubation. Orotracheal intubation has not been shown to worsen cervical spine injuries if manual in-line immobilization is maintained.[18,25,30] Advanced Trauma Life Support guidelines emphasize the importance of experience rather than technique. Nasotracheal intubation requires that the patient have spontaneous respirations. It is a "blind" procedure and is technically difficult for the inexperienced; in addition, it increases the risk of bleeding and subsequent loss of airway. If the patient is apneic, orotracheal intubation with manual in-line immobilization is the procedure of choice. Fiberoptic intubation should also be considered if experienced personnel are available. It produces little or no cervical movement but requires the full cooperation of the patient or full anesthesia. Excessive secretions may also complicate the procedure.[31]

Axial traction, which was previously used to maintain cervical spine immobilization, has been shown to produce distraction and may aggravate pre-existing injuries.[2,4] It is currently recommended that manual cervical in-line immobilization such as shown in Figure 1B be performed during any intervention with potential for neck movement.[1,36,38] The rigid collar has been shown to significantly impede mouth opening and further complicate attempts at orotracheal intubation. It is permissible to open the front of the cervical collar as long as strict in-line immobilization is maintained.[16]

Surgical airways should be reserved for those instances where extensive central facial or upper airway injury occurs, or following the failure of initial attempts at oral or nasal intubation of the airway.[1,36] Complications associated with emergent surgical airways, particularly with cricothyroidotomy,[5,11,25,26,37] include hemorrhage and unsuccessful or incorrect placement. These complications occur most often when there is a lack of clinician familiarity with the procedure.

Percutaneous transtracheal ventilation (needle cricothyroidotomy) is an alternative method that is associated with less risk of hemorrhage than the open cricothyroidotomy. The potential complications include barotrauma, aspiration, and inadequate ventilation.[20,36] This technique requires the use of specialized equipment and a familiarity with the anatomy, technique, and use of equipment.

Another concern when using surgical airways is that of the potential for infection. This may delay attempts at surgical cervical spine stabilization, as the needle or surgical cricothyroidotomy was performed in the planned surgical field. It is imperative that the surgeon uses the method that he/she is most comfortable with because the establishment of the airway is of prime importance.

Ventilation

Breathing, or ventilation, is addressed after the airway is established. The respiratory rate must be observed for possible ventilatory compromise. Four traumatic conditions that may compromise ventilation include flail chest, tension pneumothorax, open pneumothorax, and paralysis of the diaphragm and respiratory accessory muscles from SCI.

Flail chest occurs with multiple rib fractures resulting in a free-floating chest wall segment. Disruption of normal chest movement is seen with paradoxical inward movement of the flail segment during inspiration and outward movement during expiration. There is usually an associated underlying pulmonary contusion that can be severe enough to require intubation and mechanical ventilation.

Tension pneumothorax develops when air enters into the pleural cavity with no means of escape. The involved lung collapses and the resulting pressure forces the mediastinum and trachea to the opposite side, interfering with venous return to the heart. Tension pneumothorax is manifested by absent or decreased breath sounds on the involved side, tracheal deviation away from the involved side, distended neck veins from obstruction of venous flow, hypoxia from collapsed lung and further compression of the opposite lung, and eventually shock. The diagnosis is based on clinical rather than radiographic criteria. Immediate needle decompression should be performed in the second intercostal space at the midclavicular line, allowing a rush of air through the catheter. Definitive treatment entails the subsequent placement of a chest tube.

Open pneumothorax occurs as a result of a

defect in the chest wall opening into the pleural space. Ventilation may be impaired if the opening approaches two thirds the diameter of the trachea, causing preferential movement of air through the chest wound rather than the trachea. The defect should be closed using a sterile occlusive dressing, taped on three sides to allow a flutter-type valve. If completely occluded, an open pneumothorax may rapidly progress to a tension pneumothorax. Definitive treatment requires thoracostomy placement in a clean site away from the open wound, and surgical closure if the defect is large enough. If the patient is to be transferred via air or is undergoing general anesthesia, a chest tube must be placed to prevent conversion to a tension pneumothorax.

Paralysis of the diaphragm and respiratory accessory muscles. In SCI patients, ventilation may be impaired without any of the above traumatic causes. Branches from the C3-5 nerve roots innervate the diaphragm. In a high cervical lesion where these might be disrupted, paradoxical breathing may be observed. The abdominal wall is sucked in secondary to a negative-pressure gradient created by accessory muscle contractions raising the diaphragm. In lower cervical spine injuries, although the diaphragmatic function may be intact, respiratory compromise may occur because of the lack of the stabilizing effects of the intercostal muscles. Paradoxical inward motion of the upper and midthoracic cage occurs on inspiration due to unopposed diaphragm contraction with loss of the intercostal muscle function. Ventilatory failure may occur insidiously in the SCI patient because some muscle function is maintained. If, however, the patient is observed to be tiring, elective intubation may be required to prevent further hypoxic spinal cord damage. It is recommended that intubation be performed if the PaO_2 is <70 mm Hg or the $PaCO_2$ is >45 mm Hg on room air. The determination, however, should be based on considerations of the entire clinical picture.[22] It is important that hypoxia is presumed to play a major role in furthering SCI. Therefore, all efforts should be made to maintain adequate oxygenation and ventilation.

Management of Hemodynamic Status

The patient's hemodynamic status requires rapid assessment after the airway and breathing are secured. Hypovolemic shock is the most common cause of circulatory failure in the trauma patient. Assessment should include evaluating the patient's vital signs, capillary refill, and level of consciousness. All trauma patients in shock should initially be presumed to be hypovolemic until proven otherwise.

Two large-bore intravenous catheters should be placed and the initial fluid resuscitation performed with a balanced salt solution. Although some advocate the use of colloid solutions initially, crystalloid solutions are more readily available and minimize infection risk. Ringer's lactate solution should be used because hyperchloremic acidosis may be produced when using normal saline. The initial fluid bolus is given as rapidly as possible, with the usual dosage of 1 to 2 liters in the adult and 20 cc/kg in the child. If the patient does not respond after 2 to 3 liters are instilled and there is an obvious source of bleeding, blood is infused. Fully cross-matched blood is preferable; however, unmatched type-specific blood can be used if severe hemorrhage dictates emergent transfusion. If type-specific blood is unavailable, type O packed cells can be used, preferably Rh-negative for women of childbearing age.

Other causes of shock in a trauma patient include cardiogenic, neurogenic, and less likely, septic etiologies. Cardiogenic shock may occur from tension pneumothorax, cardiac tamponade, myocardial contusion, air embolus, or myocardial infarction. Cardiac tamponade should be suspected when there is penetrating trauma to the thorax and is manifested by muffled heart sounds, distended neck veins, tachycardia, and persistent hypotension despite volume replacement. This condition is treated by pericardiocentesis using the subxiphoid approach.

Neurogenic shock presents with the classic picture of hypotension without tachycardia. Sympathetic outflow of the autonomic nervous system arises from spinal segments T1 through L2. This innervation is normally responsible for increases in heart rate, increases in contractility of the heart, and peripheral vasoconstriction. The opposing parasympathetic outflow is transmitted through the vagus nerve, which slows the heart and slightly reduces cardiac contractility. Injuries to the spinal cord involving levels T1-L2 will result in interruption of the sympathetic outflow, controlling the vasopressor and cardiac reflexes to one degree or another. Unopposed parasympathetic influence will then prevail.

The patient in neurogenic shock exhibits hypotension with bradycardia, warm extremities from vasodilatation, and good urine output. This is in contrast to the classic picture of hypotension with tachycardia, cool extremities from vasoconstriction, and markedly decreased urine output that occurs from hypovolemia. The systolic blood pressure will usually be <70 mm Hg, with a pulse rate <60 beats.[24] The hypotension is a result of a lowered systemic vascular resistance with pooling of blood in the extremities. Inadequate central blood return occurs, causing an inability to maintain sufficient cardiac preload. Cardiac dysfunction occurs as well, secondary to unopposed vagal stimulation. Dysrhythmias are common. They include atrioventricular blocks, supraventricular tachycardias, and cardiac arrest.

The initial management of the patient in neurogenic shock includes patient placement in the Trendelenburg position to decrease the pooling of blood in the lower extremities. Atropine may be used to treat cardiac rhythm disturbances, although it may be only a temporary measure. Hypotension associated with neurogenic shock is best treated with vasopressors (dopamine). A Swan-Ganz catheter should be placed to determine accurate fluid status and to gauge further management because neurogenic shock is a distributive rather than a hypovolemic phenomenon. Care must be taken to avoid overhydration.

Neurological and Physical Assessment

The neurological status should be assessed briefly during the initial survey. A rapid neurological examination should be performed to determine the patient's level of consciousness, pupillary size, and reactivity, using either the "AVPU" scale (*a*lert, responds to *v*oice, responds to *p*ain, and *u*nresponsive) or, more commonly, the detailed Glasgow Coma Scale. Finally, the patient should be fully exposed, removing all pieces of clothing.

A detailed neurological examination should be performed after the initial stabilization. One should look for signs of SCI, which can include weakness or paralysis of trunk and/or extremities, absence of sensation in the trunk and/or

extremities, and loss of bowel or bladder control. During the rectal examination, it is important to note the absence of rectal tone as well as any sparing of perianal sensation. Intact motor and/or sensory function of the rectum indicates an incomplete lesion, which potentially alters prognosis.

After the initial life-threatening injuries are addressed, a more detailed head-to-toe examination should be performed. It is during this survey that stomach and bladder decompression is accomplished. A nasogastric tube is inserted unless evidence of a cribriform plate fracture exists. An orogastric tube should then be used to avoid the potential risk of insertion of the nasogastric tube into the intracranial cavity. A Foley catheter is placed if there is no evidence of urethral trauma, manifested by blood at the urinary meatus, blood in the scrotum, or a high-riding prostate palpated on rectal examination. If any of these findings are present, a Foley catheter should not be inserted until further radiological studies rule out urethral injury.

A diagnostic peritoneal lavage or computed tomography (CT) scan of the abdomen may be needed to rule out occult abdominal injury in a patient with altered mental status or SCI.

Radiographic Assessment

Initial radiographic films are obtained at this time and should always include a cross-table lateral cervical spine, chest, and pelvis. The lateral cervical spine should include C7-T1 articulation. Maneuvers that assist this assessment include bilateral arm traction to depress the shoulders or placement of the patient in a swimmer's position (with one arm extended above the head and the other pulled down). If neither maneuver is successful, limited CT or cervical magnetic resonance imaging of this region is recommended.

Approximately 10% of patients with a cervical spine fracture have a second noncontiguous vertebral column fracture. A complete radiographic screening of the spine is therefore mandatory in patients with a cervical spine fracture and should be considered in the comatose patient.[1]

Spinal Shock

Spinal shock is a transient phenomenon in which the spinal cord temporarily loses function below the level of the injury. Motor and sensory functions, spinal reflexes, and autonomic control are absent below the level of the lesion. This is temporary and usually resolves within 24 hours of injury. Resolution is heralded with the return of the anal-cutaneous and the bulbocavernosus reflexes. The anal-cutaneous reflex is performed by scratching the perianal skin with production of an involuntary anal contraction, the "anal wink." The bulbocavernosus reflex is performed by rapidly squeezing the glans penis, tapping the clitoris, or tugging on the Foley catheter; contraction of the anal sphincter results. For the same degree of SCI, the presence of spinal shock implies a more rapid evolution of injury and a worse prognosis.[3]

Pharmacotherapy of Spinal Cord Injuries

Improvement in outcome after SCI using pharmacological agents is a relatively new concept. Research on SCI has provided an improved understanding of the pathophysiology of neural injury and established the potential for pharmacological intervention. Only recently, however, has pharmacological therapy been used in the clinical setting. Two fundamental theories have been postulated with regard to the cellular mechanism of the primary injury: the neuronal theory (distortion of the neuronal membrane by trauma), and the vascular theory (which proposes that reduced or interrupted blood flow is responsible for the damage).[34] Complete anatomic transection rarely occurs at the initial impact; a contusion commonly exists that initiates a cascade of events (secondary injury). These events include edema, ischemia, microhemorrhages, and eventually neuronal death. Pharmacological therapy is designed to protect the spinal cord from progression of this cascade. Based on these theories, agents believed to be beneficial include corticosteroids, naloxone, thyroid-releasing hormone, dimethyl sulfoxide, vitamin E, nimodipine, gangliosides, Lazaroids, and superoxide dismutase. The broad classes of drugs include antioxidants, opiate receptor antagonists, neurotransmitter receptor blockers, and anti-inflammatory agents. Methylprednisolone, tirilazad (a Lazaroid), and gangliosides (specifically GM-1) have under-

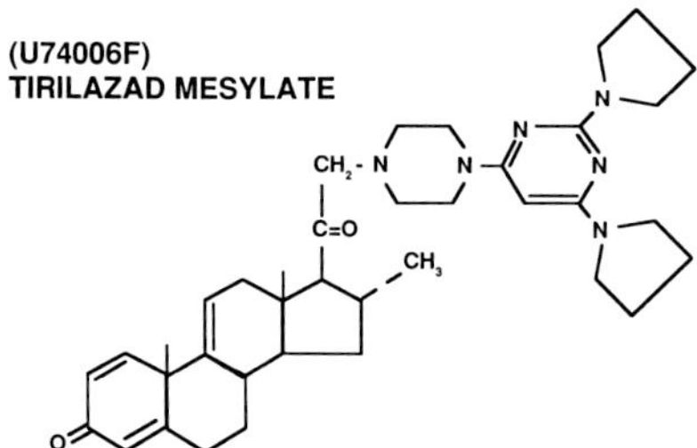

Figure 4: Molecular structure of tirilazad mesylate (U74006F), a Lazaroid.

gone, or are currently undergoing, randomized clinical trials.

Methylprednisolone has been shown in animal studies to increase blood flow to the injured spinal cord and to decrease the accumulation of water and sodium at the lesion site, with almost complete elimination of potassium loss.[29] It has also been shown to protect the injured cord from lipid peroxidation.[15] The National Acute Spinal Cord Injury Study (NASCIS) 2 showed that methylprednisolone, given within 8 hours of injury, significantly improved recovery in patients with SCI without altering morbidity or mortality rates.[6] Based on these results, it was recommended that an initial loading dose of 30 mg/kg of methylprednisolone be given within 8 hours of injury, followed by a continuous infusion of 5.4 mg/kg/hour for the next 23 hours. NASCIS 3 evaluated whether a 48-hour maintenance dose of methylprednisolone would provide greater recovery than the 24-hour methylprednisolone protocol.[7] Results confirmed that patients in whom methylprednisolone treatment was initiated within 3 hours of injury should be maintained on the previous treatment regimen. Patients in whom treatment was initiated 3 to 8 hours after injury should have their maintenance dose extended for 48 hours.

Lazaroids, or 21-aminosteroids, are a class of synthetically derived nonglucocorticoid steroids and have been found to provide even greater antioxidant activity than methylprednisolone. Tirilazad mesylate (U74006F) has been selected for clinical study (Figure 4). Tirilazad appears to offer three protective effects: it has been found to scavenge lipid peroxyl radicals and superoxide radicals; it appears to behave as membrane-lo-

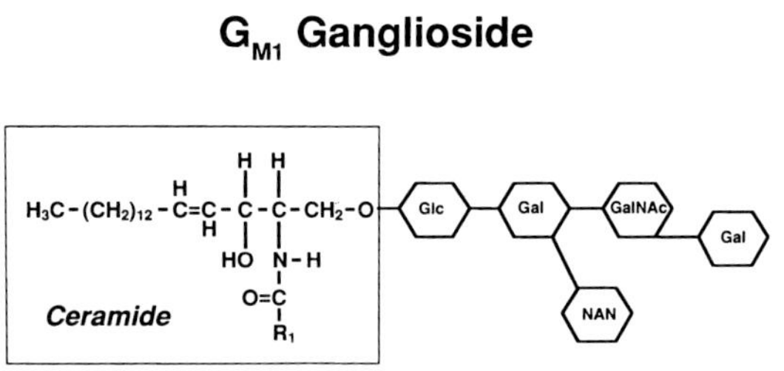

G_{M1} Ganglioside

Figure 5: Molecular structure of GM-1 ganglioside.

calized iron chelator that potently inhibits iron-dependent lipid peroxidation; and it provides membrane-stabilizing effects by limiting lipid hydrolysis.[15] *In vivo* studies have also shown that tirilazad acts to preserve tissue levels of vitamin E in injured central nervous system tissue.[15] Tirilazad does not possess the potential deleterious effects of methylprednisolone such as immunosuppression or hyperglycemia. NASCIS 3 compared the 24-hour administration of methylprednisolone with the 48-hour administration of either methylprednisolone or tirilazad.[7] Patients treated with tirilazad for 48 hours (2.5 mg/kg every 6 hours) showed motor recovery rates equivalent to those who received methylprednisolone for 24 hours. Tirilazad was given after a bolus of 30 mg/kg of methylprednisolone, and the study design did not distinguish the effect of the bolus from the maintenance dose. The 1-year follow-up study showed that the neurological recovery rate for patients treated with tirilazad fell between that seen in the two methylprednisolone regimens.[8]

Chemical variants have been synthesized using the parent U74006F molecule, replacing the steroid with the antioxidant ring structure (chromanol) of alpha tocopherol (vitamin E). These compounds, called 2-methylamino-chromans, appear to have even greater antioxidant effects than Lazaroids.[15]

Gangliosides, or acidic glycolipids, are a major component of the cell's outer lipid bilayer of the plasma membrane.[13] They are derived from sphingosine, an amino alcohol that contains a long, unsaturated hydrocarbon chain. The basic glycolipid is the cerebroside that contains a simple sugar unit (glucose or galactose). The gangliosides are more complex, containing up to seven sugar residues, with at least one acidic sugar. GM-1 ganglioside (Figure 5) has been most commonly used in clinical application. Exogenous gangliosides are assumed to insert into the lipid bilayer and mimic endogenous gangliosides.

Gangliosides have been found to augment neuronal growth *in vitro* and induce regeneration and restoration of neuronal function *in vivo.* Animal models have shown these compounds to stimulate the growth of nerve cells in damaged tissue.[13] Other possible functions may include enhancing neuronal survival in white matter tracts and limiting the neurotoxic effect of excitatory amino acid-induced cell death.[33] The excitatory amino acids glutamate and aspartate exert neurotoxic effects by opening calcium channels, causing a rapid influx of calcium into the cell and triggering lipid peroxidation. Gangliosides limit this neurotoxicity, but not the physiological excitatory amino acid-mediated effect on the calcium channel ("receptor abuse-dependent antagonism").[33]

A clinical trial was undertaken by Geisler et al[14] in 1991 to study whether neurological recovery in SCI could be improved by gangliosides, specifically GM-1. SCI patients were given l00 mg/day of GM-1 sodium salt or placebo intravenously within the first 72 hours after injury (mean initial dose 48 hours after injury) and continued for 18 to 32 doses (mean 26 days). All subjects received the NASCIS 1 steroid bolus. Compared with placebo, the study found significant improvement in the GM-1-treated patients and in those assessed using the ASIA (American Spinal Injury Association) motor score and Frankel grades from baseline to the 1-year follow-up. An analysis of individual muscle recoveries indicated that the increased recovery in the GM-1-treated group was attributable to regained motor strength in the initially paralyzed muscles rather than to the strengthening of paretic muscles. The Sygen (GM-1) Acute Spinal Cord Injury Study sponsored by Fidia Pharmaceutical Corporation contained three parallel groups (placebo, low-dose GM-1, and high-dose GM-1). Those in the low-dose GM-1 group were given a loading dose of 300 mg followed by 100 mg/day for 56 days, and those in the high-dose group were given a loading dose of 600 mg followed by 200 mg/day for 56 days. Chapter 26 offers details on this study.[12] Adverse effects of GM-1 are noted to be rare; however the use of gangliosides has been associated with reported cases of Guillain-Barré syndrome.[28,32]

ACUTE PULMONARY MANAGEMENT

Aggressive pulmonary care should be undertaken early when managing the SCI patient, as the most frequent causes of death in the acute phase are pulmonary failure and shock. Management begins early with a high index of suspicion for impending ventilatory failure and a low threshold for intubation and mechanical ventilation. SCI patients often require mobilization of secretions, adequate maintenance of lung volumes, and the avoidance of a ventilation-perfusion mismatch.[24] Indications for mechanical ventilation include apnea, the presence of dyspnea, hypoxia, and hypercarbia. Specific physiological parameters that correlate with these indications include vital capacity <20 ml/kg, inspiratory force below –30 cm H_2O, and spontaneous minute ventilation (product of the respiratory rate and the tidal volume) >10 L/min.[21]

Positive-pressure ventilation is used in SCI patients. This reverses the normal process of inspiration by inflating lungs via forced pressure on the chest cavity. The two types of positive-pressure ventilation are pressure-limited and volume-limited. Pressure-limited ventilation has a predetermined pressure with a variable volume of gas delivered and cannot compensate for changes in compliance or resistance. Therefore, the tidal volume needs close monitoring. Volume-limited ventilation delivers a preset volume via a variable pressure. This allows for changes in compliance and resistance while continuing to deliver the preset volume until high pressures are reached. Volume-limited ventilation is preferable because SCI patients frequently have poor pulmonary compliance secondary to mucus plugging and the development of adult respiratory distress syndrome.

Regardless of whether pressure- or volume-limited ventilation is used, there are a variety of inspiratory modes to choose.[24] The *assist mode* requires that the patient's negative airway pressure initiate the ventilatory cycle, which then augments the patient tidal volume. The *control mode* cycles at a preset rate regardless of the patient's effort. The *assist/control mode* assists the patient when the breath is initiated and provides breath when there is no effort, delivering a preset tidal volume. *Intermittent mandatory ventilation* (IMV) allows the patient to breathe at his/her own rate and tidal volume but delivers a set volume at preset intervals. This prevents the patient from receiving a full-tidal volume with every breath taken, as would be the case with the assist/control mode. *Synchronized IMV* delivers a preset volume in synchrony with the patient's respiratory effort by waiting for a preset negative inspiratory force before delivering the volume. If a predetermined required number of breaths are not taken, the ventilator originates a cycle to assure that the preset minute ventilation is met.

Positive end-expiratory pressure (PEEP) may be needed when managing respiratory failure. This is a technique that increases airway pressure and therefore improves oxygenation. PEEP is added to the expiratory phase and maintains a certain pressure (generally to a maximum of 20 mm Hg), allowing the alveoli to remain open. In part, PEEP acts by increasing the functional residual capacity that, in turn, maintains adequate lung expansion. This technique is clinically indicated when persistent hypoxia occurs, as in adult respiratory distress syndrome.

Mobilizing secretions is extremely important as well. This entails frequent suctioning as well as adequate hydration to prevent inspissation of mucus and subsequent plugging. This can be accomplished in part by the delivery of warm humidified air. Bronchodilator therapy is also effective not only in mobilizing secretions by dilating the airways but by improving ciliary action.

Aggressive pulmonary care, if maintained, will minimize the often-inevitable respiratory complications that occur in the SCI patient.

REFERENCES

1. American College of Surgeons: **Advanced Trauma Life Support Course Manual. 6th ed.** Chicago: American College of Surgeons, 1997
2. Aprahamian C, Thompson BM, Finger WA, et al: Experimental cervical spine injury model: evaluation

of airway management and splinting techniques. **Ann Emerg Med** 13:584-587, 1984

3. Atkinson PP, Atkinson JL: Spinal shock. **Mayo Clin Proc** 71:384-389, 1996

4. Bivins HG, Ford S, Bezmalinovic Z, et al: The effect of axial traction during orotracheal intubation of the trauma victim with an unstable cervical spine. **Ann Emerg Med** 17:25-29, 1988

5. Bjoraker DG, Kumar NB, Brown ACD: Evaluation of an emergency cricothyrotomy instrument. **Crit Care Med** 15:157-160, 1987

6. Bracken MB, Shepard MJ, Collins WF, et al: A randomized, controlled trial of methylprednisolone or naloxone in the treatment of acute spinal-cord injury. Results of the second National Acute Spinal Cord Injury Study. **N Engl J Med** 322:1405-1411, 1990

7. Bracken MB, Shepard MJ, Holford TR, et al: Administration of methylprednisolone for 24 or 48 hours or tirilazad mesylate for 48 hours in the treatment of acute spinal cord injury. Results of the third National Acute Spinal Cord Injury Randomized Controlled Trial. **JAMA** 277:1597-1604, 1997

8. Bracken MB, Shepard MJ, Holford TR, et al: Methylprednisolone or tirilazad mesylate administration after acute spinal cord injury: 1-year follow up. Results of the third National Acute Spinal Cord Injury Randomized Controlled Trial. **J Neurosurg** 89: 699-706, 1998

9. Caroline NL: **Emergency Medical Treatments. 3rd ed.** Boston: Little, Brown & Co, 1991

10. Donaldson WF III, Lauerman WC, Heil B, et al: Helmet and shoulder pad removal from a player with suspected cervical spine injury. A cadaveric model. **Spine** 23:1729-1733, 1998

11. Erlandson MJ, Clinton JE, Ruiz E, et al: Cricothyrotomy in the emergency department revisited. **J Emerg Med** 7:115-118, 1989

12. Geisler FH: Clinical trials of pharmacotherapy for spinal cord injury. **Ann NY Acad Sci** 845:374-381, 1998

13. Geisler FH, Dorsey FC, Coleman WP: GM-1 ganglioside in human spinal cord injury. **J Neurotrauma 9** (Suppl 1):S517-S530, 1992

14. Geisler FH, Dorsey FC, Coleman WP: Recovery of motor function after spinal-cord injury—a randomized placebo-controlled trial with GM-1 ganglioside. **N Engl J Med** 324:1829-1838, 1991

15. Hall ED, Braughler JM, McCall JM: Antioxidant effects in brain and spinal cord injury. **J Neurotrauma 9 (Suppl 1):**S165-S172, 1992

16. Heath KJ: The effect on laryngoscopy of different cervical spine immobilization techniques. **Anaesthesia** 49:843-845, 1994

17. Heckman JD: **Emergency Care and Transportation of the Sick and Injured. 5th ed.** Park Ridge, Ill: American Academy of Orthopaedic Surgeons, 1992

18. Holley J, Jorden R: Airway management in patients with unstable cervical spine fractures. **Ann Emerg Med** 18:1237-1239, 1989

19. Ivy ME, Cohn SM: Addressing the myths of cervical spine injury management. **Am J Emerg Med** 15: 591-595, 1997

20. Jorden RC: Percutaneous transtracheal ventilation. **Emerg Med Clin North Am** 6:745-752, 1988

21. Kennedy SK: Airway management and respiratory support, in Ropper AH, Kennedy SF (eds): **Neurological and Neurosurgical Intensive Care. 2nd ed.** Rockville, Md: Aspen, 1988, pp 57-84

22. LaSala PA, Frost EA: Intensive care management of spinal cord injury, in Alderson JD, Frost EA (eds): **Spinal Cord Injuries: Anaesthetic and Associated Care.** London: Butterworth, 1990, pp 72-86

23. Majernick TG, Bieniek R, Houston JB, et al: Cervical spine movement during orotracheal intubation. **Ann Emerg Med** 15:417-420, 1986

24. Marshall SB, Marshall LF, Vos HR, et al: **Neuroscience Critical Care: Pathophysiology and Patient Management.** Philadelphia, Pa: WB Saunders, 1990

25. McGill J, Clinton JE, Ruiz E: Cricothyrotomy in the emergency department. **Ann Emerg Med** 11:361-364, 1982

26. Miklus RM, Elliott C, Snow N: Surgical cricothyrotomy in the field: experience of a helicopter transport team. **J Trauma** 29:506-508, 1989

27. National Spinal Cord Injury Statistical Center (NSDISC): **Spinal Cord Injury, Facts and Figures at a Glance.** Birmingham, Alabama. January 1998

28. Nobile-Orazio E, Carpo M, Scarlato G: Gangliosides. Their role in clinical neurology. **Drugs** 47:576-585, 1994

29. Nockels R, Young W: Pharmacologic strategies in the treatment of experimental spinal cord injury. **J Neurotrauma 9 (Suppl 1):**S211-S217, 1992

30. Rhee KJ, Green W, Holcroft JW, et al: Oral intubation in the multiply injured patient: the risk of exacerbating spinal cord damage. **Ann Emerg Med** 19:511-514, 1990

31. Sawin PD, Todd MM, Traynelis VC, et al: Cervical spine motion with direct laryngoscopy and orotracheal intubation. An *in vivo* cinefluoroscopic study of subjects without cervical abnormality. **Anesthesiology** 85:26-36, 1996

32. Schonhofer PS. GM-1 ganglioside for spinal cord injury. **N Engl J Med** 326:493-494, 1992 (Letter)

33. Skaper SD, Leon A: Monosialogangliosides, neuroprotection, and neuronal repair processes. **J Neurotrauma 9 (Suppl 2):**S507-S516, 1992

34. Sonntag VK, Douglas RA: Management of cervical spinal cord trauma. **J Neurotrauma 9 (Suppl 1):** S385-S396, 1992

35. Swenson TM, Lauerman WC, Blanc RO, et al: Cervical spine alignment in the immobilized football player. Radiographic analysis before and after helmet removal. **Am J Sports Med** 25:226-260, 1997

36. Walls RM: Airway management. **Emerg Med Clin North Am** 11:53-60, 1993

37. Walls RM: Cricothyroidotomy. **Emerg Med Clin North Am** 6:725-736, 1988

38. Walls RM: Management of the difficult airway in the trauma patient. **Emerg Med Clin North Am** 16:45-61, 1998

CHAPTER 8

IMAGING OF SPINAL CORD INJURY

DEVANAND A. DOMINIQUE, MB, BCH, WALTER MONTANERA, MD, FRCP(C), AND MICHAEL G. FEHLINGS, MD, PHD, FRCS(C)

Adequate imaging of the spinal column is of paramount importance to determine the level and extent of injury, to classify and categorize the nature of the spinal injury, to detect clinically occult spine injuries, to determine spinal stability, and to plan potential reconstructive and stabilizing measures. The contemporary management of spinal cord and spinal column trauma has been revolutionized since the introduction of computerized multiplanar radiographic techniques such as computed tomography (CT) and magnetic resonance imaging (MRI). Traditionally, spinal trauma has been categorized according to the nature of the forces that produced the injury (flexion, extension, compression, rotation, shearing, and distraction).

The rapid diagnosis of the full extent of a spinal cord injury (SCI) optimizes the potential for patient recovery. The appropriate and complete radiographic evaluation of spinal injuries is not only cost-efficient, but also expedites patient care. The correct interpretation of the studies ordered should ensure appropriate patient management. To completely investigate patients with acute SCI requires a dedicated and experienced multidisciplinary team for monitoring and safe transport.

IMAGING MODALITIES

Plain Films

Although CT and MRI have dramatically improved our delineation of traumatic spinal pathology, plain film radiographs remain indispensable in the initial assessment of acute SCI.[2,3,5,20,31,40,45] When properly obtained, plain radiographs detect the majority of spine fractures and provide an excellent examination of vertebral alignment. Because they are portable, quick, and inexpensive, plain radiographs are ideal in the setting of trauma. Plain films poorly visualize soft-tissue structures. Abnormalities of the intervertebral discs, supporting ligaments, epidural and subdural spaces, and the spinal cord parenchyma cannot be detected.[3] Plain films do not clearly delineate fine bony anatomy and structural relationships as clearly as plain tomograms and CT. Soft tissues and the neural elements are best imaged by MRI. Various parts of the spine are frequently visualized suboptimally due to poor x-ray penetration through surrounding soft-tissue and bony structures, such as the ribs. In spite of the many limitations outlined, plain radiographs of the spine continue to be the initial investigation of choice in all acute spinal injuries.

Conventional Tomography

Conventional tomography has been largely supplanted since the introduction of CT. This modality remains, however, an excellent means by which to define the spatial arrangement of bone fragments and bony alignment.[40] In spite of sagittal and coronal reconstructed CT scans, conventional tomography is superior in detecting horizontally oriented fractures.[36,40] Plain tomograms are technically difficult to perform, require an experienced radiographer, have a higher overall radiation dose, and take longer to perform than CT. For these reasons, CT has replaced conventional tomograms in the setting of spinal trauma.

Computed Tomography

Digitized cross-sectional imaging, first introduced with CT, has significantly improved the classification, diagnosis, and management of spinal trauma. CT is the optimal method for viewing the bony central spinal canal and any encroachment by osseous fragments. It is the most sensitive and specific imaging method for the detection of vertebral fractures, particularly the evaluation of the integrity and alignment of the posterior elements.[27,36,37,40,42,59] CT is the gold standard for the examination of facet joint integrity. Typically, CT is performed with thin (cervical 1.0 to 3.0 mm, thoracolumbar 3.0 to 5.0 mm) contiguous or overlapping axial slices and requires minimum manipulation of the patient. The CT examination should be tailored by the use of preliminary plain radiographs and clinical symptomatology. For visualizing vertically oriented fractures and bony displacement in the axial plane, CT is the best imaging modality. Horizontally oriented fractures (e.g., Type II odontoid fractures and flexion-distraction injuries of the thoracolumbar spine) could be inadequately imaged or may be undetected by axial CT scans. Sagittal, coronal, and three-dimensional reconstructions allow assessment of gross bony displacement in all planes of orientation,[58] but the resolution is poor, and small min-

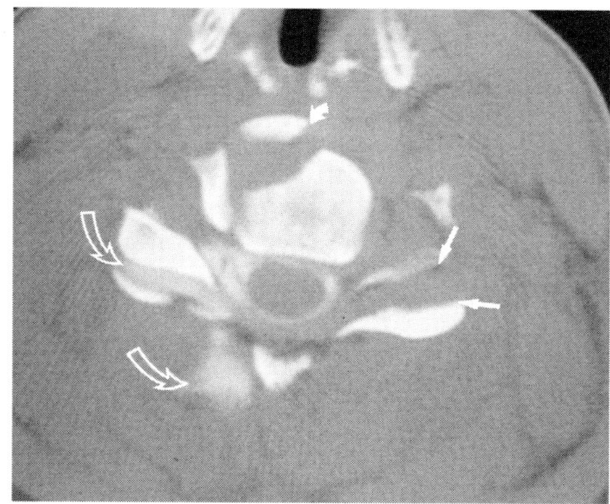

Figure 1: Axial postmyelography CT through the C5-6 disc demonstrating a fracture-dislocation of the cervical spine with dural tear. Fractures of the vertebral body *(solid curved arrow)* and widening of the facet joint space *(straight arrows)* can be seen. Leakage of myelographic contrast into the right C5-6 facet joint space and leakage into the posterior paraspinal soft tissues indicate a dural tear *(open curved arrows)*.

imally displaced fractures may remain radiographically occult.

CT is limited in its ability to evaluate the thecal sac and intraspinal soft tissues. For reliable demonstration of traumatic disc herniation or intraspinal hematoma causing cord compression, CT must be used in conjunction with myelography (Figure 1). To evaluate traumatic dural lacerations, CT myelography remains the technique of choice. In the assessment of the surface and substance of the spinal cord, MRI has replaced CT and CT myelography. Myelography and CT myelography are now largely reserved for when MRI is unavailable, non-diagnostic, or when the patient cannot properly fit into the magnetic resonance scanner.

Magnetic Resonance Imaging

MRI is the only imaging modality capable of directly imaging spinal cord parenchyma. Since its introduction into clinical practice, MRI has substantially improved the ability to assess acute SCI.[16,17,24,36,40] MRI removes bony artifact, provides excellent anatomic definition of soft-tissue structures of the spinal column, allows multiplanar examination of the spine, and is sensitive and specific for the identification of edema and hemorrhage within and around the spinal cord.

To obtain an MRI, the patient must be hidden from direct observation. Attending personnel must therefore ensure adequate patient monitoring capabilities prior to the scan. Coordinated care is crucial. The team must ensure adequate analgesia and sedation and continuously monitor pulse rate, blood pressure, respiratory rate, blood oxygen saturation, and the level of consciousness when applicable. Extra caution is necessary when investigating patients with penetrating injuries in which there may be retained ferromagnetic fragments (e.g., gunshot wounds). Metallic fragments create severe distortion artifacts and may heat up or torque during the procedure. MRI should be obtained after rigid spinal immobilization but prior to the application of traction or surgical intervention.[34,54]

Imaging with surface coils in a high-field strength magnetic resonance scanner is ideal because it produces higher quality images in a shorter period of time and with greater sensitivity to hemorrhage. MRI is most commonly performed in sagittal and axial planes using spin-echo sequences with 3- to 4-mm slice thickness. Sagittal images give excellent visualization of listhesis and any site of ongoing cord compression.[17] Axial images aid in lateralizing abnormalities and determining canal cross-section. Coronal images often prove useful in the evaluation of scoliotic curves. T1-weighted images generally give the best anatomic detail for defining spinal canal diameter, canal compromise, and cord compression.[17] T2- and proton density-weighted images are best suited for detection and delineation of soft-tissue injury and hematoma within and around the spinal cord. Edema in acute SCI is seen as a bright signal on T2-weighted sequences.

Blood may vary in its appearance, depending upon the concentration of hemoglobin metabolites within the clot. The T2-weighted signal is most sensitive for detection of a blood clot. Most commonly, the hematoma appears as a dark signal that represents the degradation of blood into a deoxyhemoglobin metabolite. After approximately 3 to 5 days, the clot appears bright on both T1- and T2-weighted images because of further degradation of blood into methemoglo-

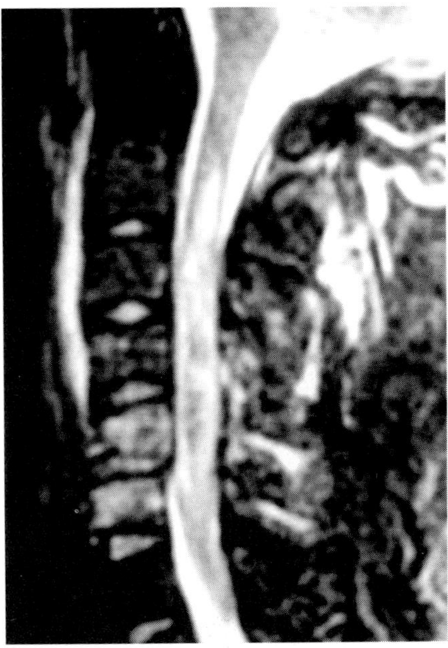

Figure 2: Sagittal long TR/long TE (T2-weighted) MRI demonstrating a Type I (hemorrhagic) cervical SCI. Fracture of the C5 vertebral body with posterior extrusion of a bone fragment into the cervical canal is visualized. Cord enlargement and edema extend from C2 to C6. A large area of decreased signal intensity (dark) opposite C4 and C5 represents hemorrhage within the cord.

bin.[17,36,40] An MRI obtained extremely early in the evolution of an SCI may reveal a "hyperacute" hemorrhage, which will also appear bright on T2-weighted imaging because of oxyhemoglobin.

The pattern of cord edema and hemorrhage as demonstrated on T2-weighted MRI correlates with the degree of initial neurological deficit and the ultimate neurological outcome.[51] These injuries have been described in detail by Schaefer et al[48] according to their T2-weighted imaging characteristics:

- Type I: hypointense (dark)—focal intramedullary hematoma, the most severe initial neurological deficit with poor potential for recovery of motor function (Figure 2).
- Type II: hyperintense (bright)—representing edema without focal hematoma extending over a long segment of the cord (>1 vertebral segment); motor recovery potential is moderate (Figure 3).
- Type III: hyperintense (bright)—intramedul-

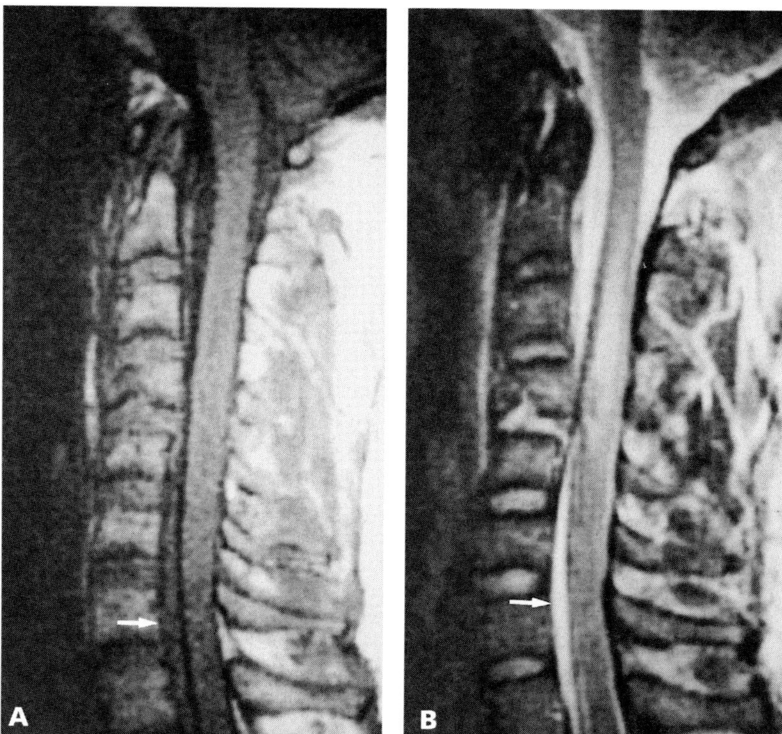

Figure 3: Sagittal short TR/short TE (T1-weighted) **(A)** and sagittal long TR/long TE (T2-weighted) **(B)** spin-echo MRIs demonstrating a Type II cervical SCI. Compression fracture of the C4 vertebral body is accompanied by posterior extrusion of bone into the cervical spinal canal. The T1-weighted sequence shows the cord to be diffusely increased in size. The T2-weighted sequence shows increased signal (brightness) within the cervical spinal cord extending from C2 to C5. This represents increased water within the cord secondary to edema and contusion. There is also a small anterior epidural hematoma *(arrows)* seen below the C5 level. The high-signal intensity of this hematoma on T2-weighted sequence is likely due to hyperacute (oxyhemoglobin) components.

lary focus of edema extending over a short segment of the cord (<1 vertebral segment), with best initial neurological function; best potential for recovery of motor function.

Cerebrospinal fluid (CSF) appears as a bright signal on T2-weighted images. T2-weighted images are particularly useful in assessing cord compression or effacement by bone, disc herniation, or hematoma (Figure 4). A swollen edematous cord will also efface the thecal sac. Both gradient echo and T2-weighted sequences are helpful in assessing the integrity of the anterior and posterior longitudinal ligaments. The MRI appearance of an epidural hematoma will vary depending upon the age of the clot and its biochemical composition (Figure 5).[47]

MRI has demonstrated that disc herniation is an extremely common sequela of spine fracture and ligamentous injury.[36,46] The presence of disc disruption can significantly impact the surgical management of a patient with an SCI. Acute disc herniation occurs as frequently as 54% of the time in acute SCI. Signs of disc injury on MRI include: 1) loss of disc height and widening of the disc space; 2) relative hyperintensity of one disc on a T2-weighted sequence; 3) outer annular fiber or longitudinal ligament disruption; 4) posterior protrusion of disc material into the epidural space; and 5) posterior deviation of the posterior longitudinal ligament (PLL).[46-48,50]

In spite of rapidly improving technology, MRI has yet to replace plain radiographs or CT for the investigation of spinal trauma. Poor resolution of cortical bone impairs the diagnosis of minimally displaced cortical fractures; facet

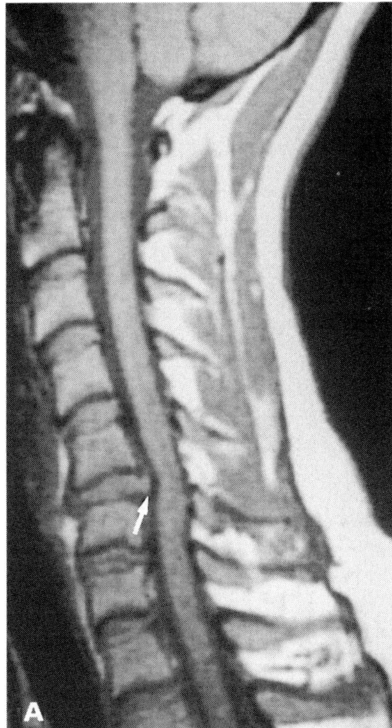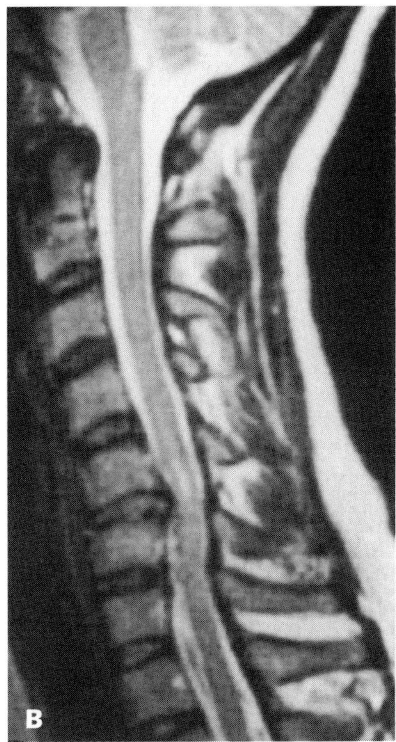

Figure 4: Sagittal short TR/short TE (T1-weighted) **(A)** and sagittal long TR/long TE (T2-weighted) **(B)** spin-echo MRIs demonstrating traumatic cervical disc herniation. Posterior extrusion of disc material causing compression of the cervical spinal cord *(arrow)* can be seen. The T2-weighted sequence also demonstrates increased signal within the cervical cord indicating cervical cord contusion. There is effacement of the CSF space both anterior and posterior to the cord.

fractures or fractures of the posterior elements are also poorly delineated by MRI.[7,36] MRI underestimates ossification of the PLL. CT remains the most reliable technique for examination of the bony spine. MRI is superior to CT for identification of pathological marrow changes (edema and hemorrhage) that occur from fracture (Figure 6). In patients with cervical SCI, the midsagittal T1- and T2-weighted MRI provides an objective, quantifiable, and reliable assessment of spinal cord compression superior to that afforded by CT.[15,44] Posterior ligament and paraspinal soft-tissue injury, evident only on MRI, serves as indicators of ligamentous injury and, therefore, posterior instability (Figure 7).

MRI is the imaging technique of choice in the diagnosis and follow-up of the long-term sequelae of SCI such as syringomyelia, myelomalacia, and cord atrophy.

Injuries of the Spine

A spine injury should be suspected in all trauma patients. In an alert, reliable, and stable trauma patient, with no history of change in level of consciousness, a spine radiograph may not always be required. A cross-table lateral x-ray, in order to be adequate, must clearly image all of the cervical vertebrae to the top of T1.[9,21] In an obese or uncooperative patient, this may prove too difficult and a "swimmer's view" may be necessary to completely examine the cervical spine. A systematic and thoughtful approach to interpreting these films is required to avoid missing pathology.

Atlanto-Occipital Dislocation

The craniovertebral junction is a common site of injury in patients who die following head and

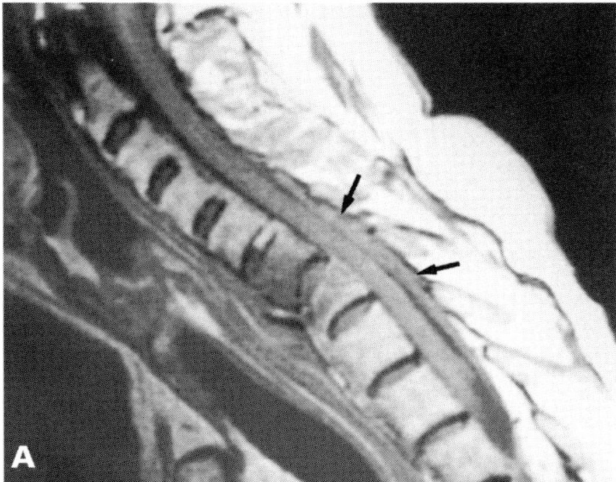
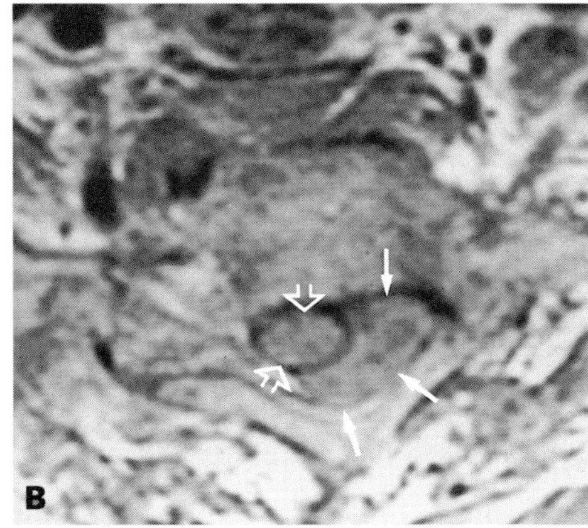
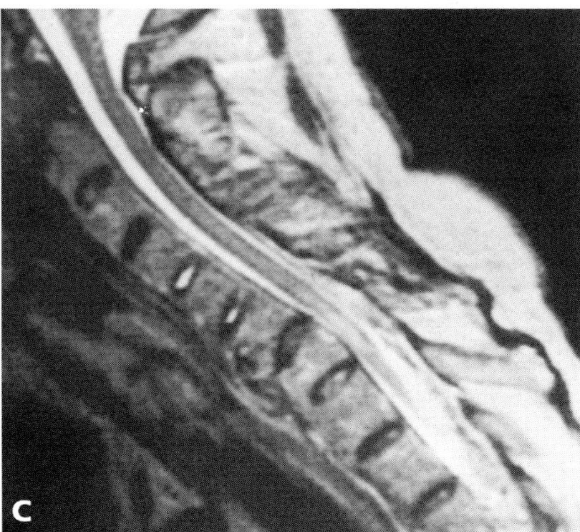

Figure 5: Sagittal **(A)** and axial **(B)** short TR/short TE (T1-weighted) and sagittal long TR/long TE (T2-weighted) **(C)** spin-echo MRIs of the cervical spine demonstrating epidural hematoma. A 61-year-old patient with underlying ankylosing spondylitis presented with a C6-7 cervical injury and symptoms and myelopathy. MRI examination demonstrated an extradural collection on the dorsal and left lateral surface of the cervical thecal sac spanning several vertebral segments (C5-T2) *(arrows)*. The cervical cord *(open arrows)* is compressed and deviated to the right, representing an epidural hematoma. Acute epidural hematomas are usually isointense (gray) on the T1-weighted sequence with variable intensity (dark or bright) on the T2-weighted sequence depending on the clot's composition (oxy-, deoxy-, or methemoglobin). The T2-weighted series also demonstrates increased signal (brightness) indicating edema and contusion within the cord at the site of maximum compression by the epidural hematoma and fracture.

neck trauma. Between 6% and 8% of persons fatally injured following trauma have sustained an atlanto-occipital dislocation. Hyperextension and distraction of the head lead to transection of the spinomedullary junction.[40] Atlanto-occipital dislocation is a radiographic diagnosis and is often difficult to appreciate on plain films. Retropharyngeal hematoma and emphysema are frequently present due to a laceration of the posterior pharyngeal wall. A multitude of lines, measurements, and ratios has been devised to assist in the detection and diagnosis of this condition. Perhaps the easiest way to determine whether an atlanto-occipital dislocation has occurred is to calculate Power's ratio. This ratio accounts for the relationship between the occiput and the atlas. The Power's ratio is obtained by dividing the distance between the basion to the posterior arch of

the atlas by the distance from the opisthion to the anterior arch of the atlas. If the ratio is ≥ 1, atlanto-occipital dislocation has occurred; if it is <0.9, the atlanto-occipital relationship can be considered normal.[43]

Traumatic craniovertebral dislocation requires ligamentous disruption. MRI is the modality of choice when evaluating ligamentous injury and is therefore essential when evaluating patients with suspected atlanto-occipital dislocation.[28] Ordinarily, the anterior foramen magnum and the dens are invested in a fat pad. The signal characteristics will change from high intensity with normal fat to intermediate or low intensity on spin-echo sequences because of hemorrhage and edema. These signal changes imply a ligamentous injury. Hemorrhage and/or edema along the occipital condyles and/or the lateral

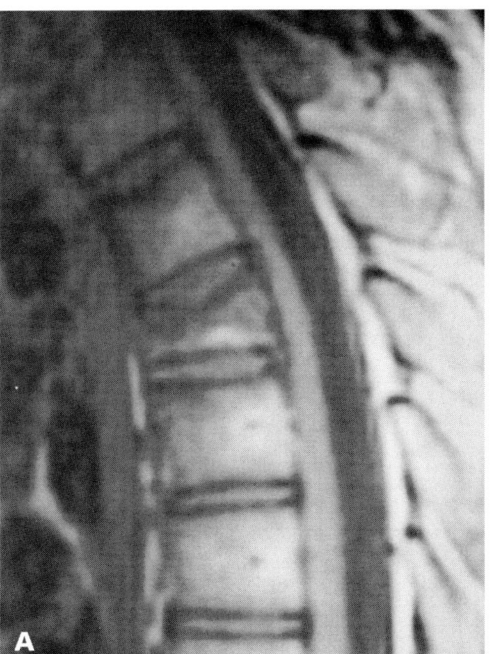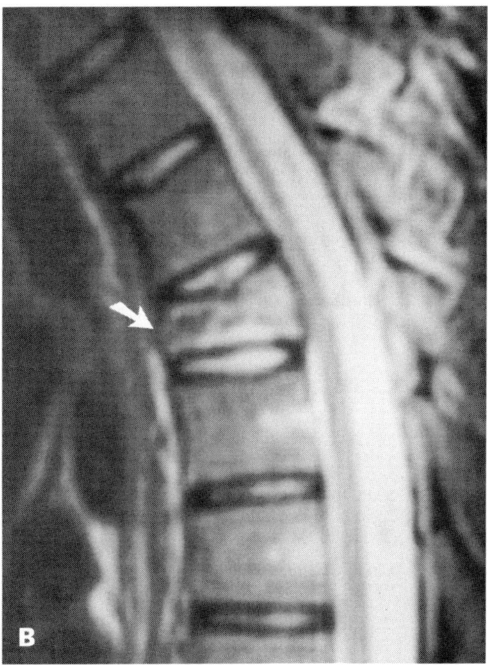

Figure 6: Short TR/short TE (T1-weighted) **(A)** and long TR/long TE (T2-weighted) **(B)** spin-echo MRIs through the upper thoracic spine demonstrating signal alterations in vertebral marrow due to acute fracture. A compression fracture of the T5 body *(arrow)* also includes mild buckling of the posterior vertebral body cortex. The marrow signal is decreased (dark) on the T1-weighted image and increased (bright) on the T2-weighted image due to replacement of normal vertebral marrow fat by edema and hemorrhage.

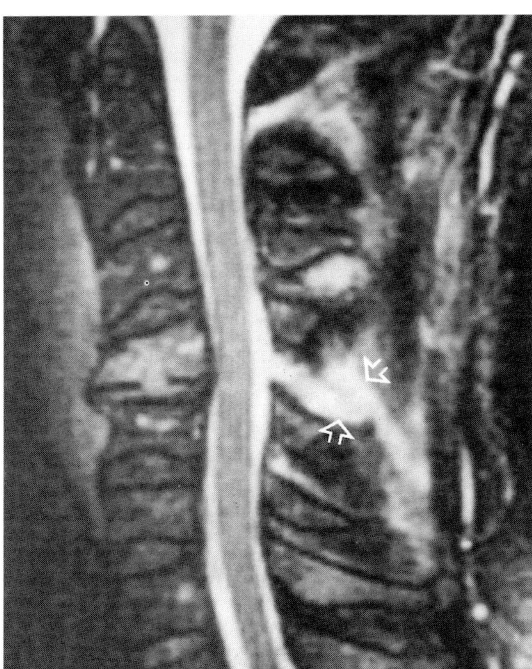

Figure 7: Sagittal long TR/long TE (T2-weighted) MRI of the cervical spine demonstrating vertebral fracture and posterior ligamentous injury. Increased signal (brightness) involving the interspinous ligaments of C4 and C5 *(arrows)* indicates posterior ligamentous disruption. There is a compression fracture of the C4 vertebral body with a vertically oriented fracture as well as discontinuity of its inferior end plate.

masses of C1 may represent disruption of articular capsular ligaments. MRI is also useful for the detection of vertebral artery injury.[29]

Atlanto-occipital dislocation has been classified into three types. Type I atlanto-occipital dislocation consists of an anterior displacement of the occiput in relation to C1. Type III refers to a posterior displacement of the occiput in relation to C1. Types I and III are both amenable to reduction by traction.[13,38,39,43,56] Traction, when employed, may serve to reduce the dislocation and thereby decompress the impinged neural elements. Type II atlanto-occipital dislocation refers to a longitudinal distraction of the skull from the vertebral column. In this circumstance, traction is absolutely contraindicated.[12,43]

Occipital Condyle Fractures

Occipital condyle fractures (OCF) are extremely rarely encountered in clinical practice. They are often associated with severe head injury and, therefore, may remain undetected. This presents a diagnostic challenge. Plain radiographs of the skull base and upper cervical spine poorly visualize the anatomic details of the occipital condyles. CT scanning, however, provides excellent resolution of the occipital condyles, and is the appropriate test for the diagnosis of OCF. A classification system for the management of OCF was presented by Anderson and Montesano[1] based on CT findings. A system of classification utilizing both CT and MRI data has recently been developed by Tuli and coworkers.[57] Their system unifies OCF with craniocervical injuries as a spectrum of pathologies.

The preponderance of patients with OCF has been involved in motor-vehicle accidents. A triad of neck pain, cranial nerve deficits, and normal cervical radiographs has been described as indicative of OCF. Plain cervical radiographs fail to demonstrate these injuries. There is an association between OCF and occipital cervical dislocations, and this is often evident on plain radiographs of the cervical spine. Fractures of the occipital condyle are best imaged by CT. Sequential axial slices obtained at 0 to 30 degrees positive to the canthomeatal line are ideal for optimum fracture definition. Three-dimensional reconstruction protocols are often useful to visualize

normal surrounding structures in their relationship to fracture segments. MRI is helpful to understand the degree and extent of ligamentous injury and to evaluate brain stem injury and SCI. MR angiography or conventional angiography can be helpful when diagnosing or excluding vascular injury.[6]

Using the classification system for managing OCF as proposed by Tuli et al,[57] Type I is a nondisplaced and stable fracture; Type 2A is a displaced but stable fracture; and in Type 2B the fracture is both unstable and displaced. Unstable OCF are defined as >8 degrees of axial rotation, >1 mm occiput to C1 translation, >7 mm overhang of C1 on C2, >45 degrees of axial rotation of C1-2, >4 mm C1-2 translation, <13 mm between the posterior body of C2 to the posterior ring of C1, and an avulsed transverse ligament with MRI evidence of ligamentous disruption.[57]

Jefferson's Fracture

Jefferson's fracture is a burst fracture involving the ring of the atlas. Axial compression of the lateral masses of C1 by the occipital condyles results in either uni- or bilateral fractures of the anterior and posterior arches.[9,36,40] These fractures are best visualized with the "open-mouth" anterior-posterior (AP) technique. The fracture and lateral displacement of the lateral masses are usually clearly evident on plain x-rays. On the lateral view, the only indication of the injury may be pre-vertebral soft-tissue swelling (>5 mm). The normal retropharyngeal soft-tissue shadow at the level of C1-2 is usually less than 5 mm. If the sum of the distances between the lateral masses and the odontoid on each side is greater than 7 mm, the transverse ligament is likely to be torn.[53] The atlanto-dental interval (ADI) is an important radiographic feature of the lateral view. It is a fixed distance, ordinarily not exceeding 3 mm (5 mm in children). An increase in the ADI is often indicative of an anterior fracture. The lateral view is useful for the diagnosis of posterior ring fractures.[36,41]

Fracture morphology is best defined by CT; 1.0- to 1.5-mm cuts with coronal and sagittal reconstructions help delineate the spatial arrangement of fracture segments to normal anatomy. Often, CT may uncover other vertebral and skull base fractures. MRI directly visualizes the transverse atlantal ligament. The integrity of this structure is crucial in determining the management of this injury. Atlas fractures associated with disruption of the transverse atlantal ligament are unstable and do not heal.[18]

Axis Fractures

The axis is the most commonly fractured vertebra in the cervical spine. Approximately 20% of cervical spine fractures involve the axis.[22] Up to 55% of axis fractures are odontoid fractures; they are the most commonly encountered axis fractures. Odontoid fractures were categorized by Anderson and D'Alonzo[2] into three subtypes. The type I odontoid fracture accounts for 5% of odontoid fractures and is an oblique fracture through the dens and an avulsion of the tip of the dens. These fractures are associated with avulsion of the alar ligament from the apex of the dens. A type II odontoid fracture is a horizontal fracture through the base of the dens, at its junction with the C2 body (Figure 8). This is the most commonly encountered axis fracture and accounts for between 40% to 80% of all odontoid fractures. A type III odontoid fracture is a fracture through the body of C2. This type of fracture has been reclassified by Benzel and colleagues and represent 20% to 40% of odontoid fractures.[4]

The *type I odontoid fracture* is relatively rare. It is, however, associated with atlanto-occipital dislocation. These fractures in isolation are generally considered to be stable and have a good prognosis for healing. Ligamentous injury in association with type I odontoid fractures may require surgical fusion.[52] The *type II odontoid fracture* is associated with a high rate of non-union. A precarious blood supply and difficulty in adequate immobilization of fracture segments are commonly ascribed reasons for non-union. Dens displacement of >6 mm is associated with >65% non-union. Conservative therapy for these fractures can vary from minimal (e.g., Philadelphia collar) to halo vest immobilization.[55] At many centers, this is the mainstay of therapy. Surgical remedies include both anterior and posterior approaches. Each technique and approach has its own set of attendant risks, benefits, and alternatives.

Isolated *type III odontoid fractures* have a high

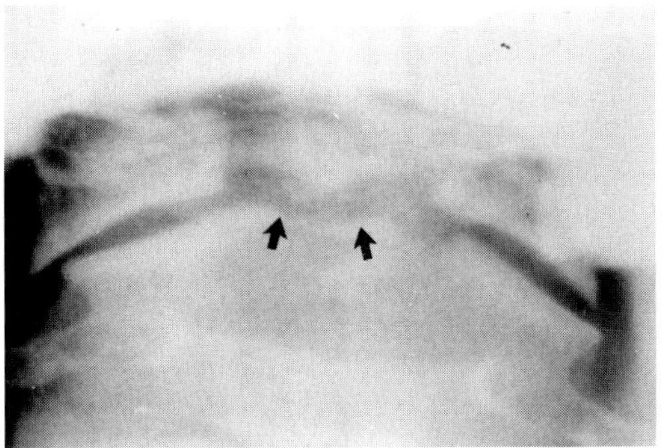

Figure 8: "Open-mouth" AP view of the odontoid process demonstrating a Type II odontoid fracture. There is a transverse fracture of the base of the odontoid process *(arrows)*.

rate of fusion with external orthotic immobilization. The rate of fusion in patients treated with a hard collar for 2 to 3 months has been reported to achieve almost 100%.[8] Type III fractures associated with ligamentous instability are, however, more difficult to treat non-operatively. Often, these require surgical fusion. C1-2 posterior sublaminar wiring and fusion with or without C1-2 transarticular screw fixation are frequently employed to treat type III odontoid fractures with associated ligamentous instability.[8,22]

A *hangman's fracture* is an axis fracture through the pars interarticularis, one of the weakest portions of the entire spine fractures.[30] These fatal fracture-dislocations of the axis are associated with the application of a submental knot, as employed in judicial hangings. As originally described, the hangman's fracture is caused by severe distraction and hyperextension of the cervical spine. The modern-day hangman's fracture differs significantly from its antiquated counterpart.[49] Most commonly, it results from vehicular accidents or a hyperextension and axial compression injury; neurological injury is infrequent. Hangman's fractures were renamed as traumatic spondylolisthesis of the axis by Garber[19] in 1964. A classification system was initially proposed by Effendi et al.[14] This was later modified to a classification system with four subtypes by Levine and Rhyne.[30]

The system developed by Levine and Rhyne accounts for both angulation and translation of

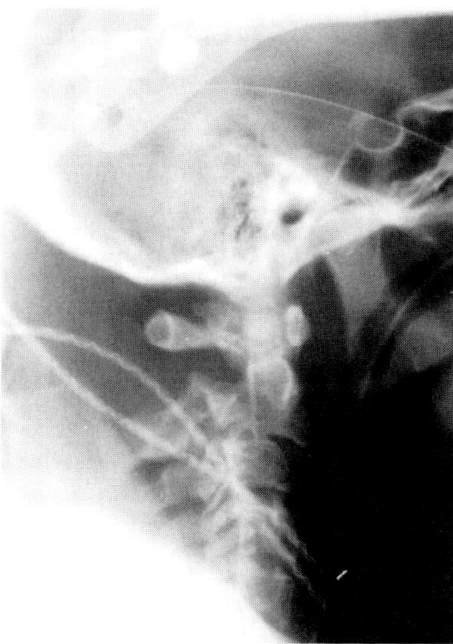

Figure 9: Lateral radiograph of the cervical spine demonstrating fracture of the axis (type 2 hangman's fracture). An oblique fracture of the C2 vertebral body is accompanied by anterior subluxation (>3 mm) of C2 on C3 with no angulation.

C2 on C3. A type 1 hangman's fracture involves the pars with no more than 3 mm of translation, and there is no angulation. Most commonly, the type 1 fracture results from a hyperextension and axial loading injury. These fractures are not associated with significant disc disruption or ligamentous injury (anterior or posterior longitudinal ligament). The type 2 hangman's fracture is similar to a type 1 fracture but has greater than 3 mm of translation and no angulation (Figure 9). The type 2A hangman's fracture has severe angulation, an oblique fracture line through the pars, and no translation. Type 1 and 2 fractures are both secondary to an initial hyperextension and compression injury, but the type 2 fracture results from a secondary flexion injury that disrupts the PLL. High-speed motor-vehicle accidents commonly cause this triad of hyperextension, axial compression, and rebound flexion. Angulation and translation are created by disruption of the disc and ligamentous structures. Commonly, the type 2 fracture is associated with anterior compression of the C3 body. The type 2A fracture is the sequela of a flexion-distraction injury. The anterior longitudinal ligament (ALL) remains intact, but the disc and the PLL are torn. The application of traction for the reduction of

this injury carries significant risk. The majority of type 1 and 2 fractures may be reduced with longitudinal traction. The type 3 hangman's fracture includes facet fracture with a fracture through the pars interarticularis. The mechanism for the type 3 fracture has been postulated to be a combination of flexion and distraction, causing the facet injury and hyperextension fracturing of the neural arch.[22,23,30]

Complex fractures through the body of C2 that also extend into the posterior elements account for up to 20% of axis fractures. They have been classified by Benzel and coworkers. There are three types of C2 body fractures, according to the Benzel system of nomenclature. The type I C2 body fracture consists of a coronally oriented fracture; the type II fracture is sagittally oriented; and the type III fracture is identical to the type III odontoid fracture as described and classified by Anderson and D'Alonzo.[2]

The advent of CT and MRI has revolutionized the understanding and practical management of axis fractures. A complete radiographic evaluation of these fractures includes plain films, CT, and MRI. All modalities must be employed to correctly classify and thereby treat these complex fractures. The lateral radiograph clearly demonstrates alignment and loss of disc height. Plain radiographs often reveal other vertebral fractures and associated soft-tissue swelling. The axial CT scan, augmented with sagittal, coronal, and 3-D reconstructions, clearly defines fractures and their spatial arrangement to normal and vital structures. MRI is also mandatory to evaluate SCI and identify the presence of epidural or parenchymal hematoma, ligamentous integrity, and the condition of intervertebral discs. Strong consideration must be given to magnetic resonance angiography or conventional angiography to diagnose associated vascular injury and/or thrombosis.

Hyperflexion Injuries of the Lower Cervical Spine

In considering fractures of the lower cervical spine, it is often easier to think in terms of the mechanism of injury. Hyperflexion injuries result in the disruption of the posterior elements of the spine. These include the interspinous ligaments, the interfacet ligaments, the articular fa-

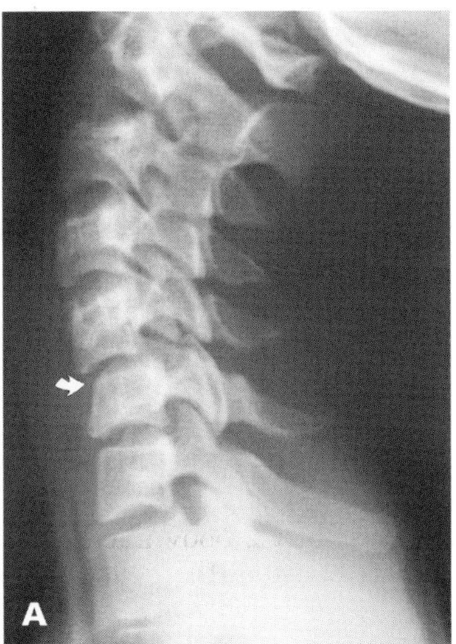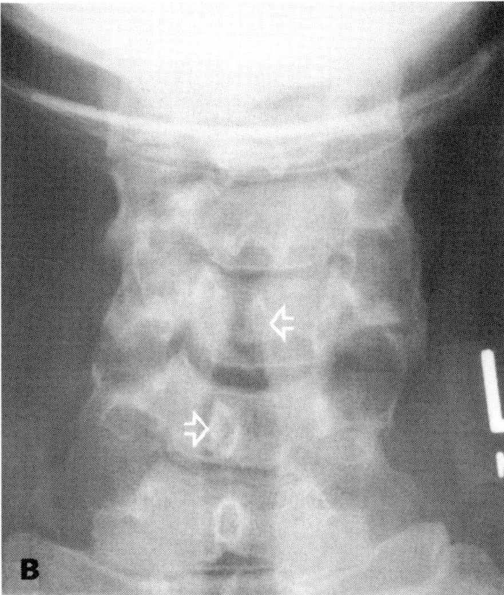

Figure 10: Lateral **(A)** and AP **(B)** radiographs of the cervical spine demonstrating unilateral cervical facet dislocation. There is mild (<25%) anterolisthesis of C5 on C6 *(curved arrow)* and focal malalignment of the cervical facet joints at the C5-6 level ("bow-tie" sign). The AP radiograph shows focal malalignment of the spinous processes *(open arrows)*.

cets and their joint capsules, the ligamentum flavum, and the PLL.[27] Common injuries believed to result primarily from hyperflexion include hyperflexion sprain, wedge fracture, facet dislocation, the flexion teardrop fracture, and the spinous process fracture (including the "clay shoveler's" fracture).[27,36,40]

Hyperflexion Sprain and Wedge Fractures

The hyperflexion sprain is a primary ligamentous injury, and plain films may show an increase in the interspinous and interlaminar distances, as well as subluxation (but not dislocation) of the facet joints.[25] Patients with hyperflexion sprain occasionally present with normal radiographs.[40] Wedge fractures caused by hyperflexion share the same radiographic features as seen in the hyperflexion sprain with the addition of anterior vertebral body compression. The presence of this fracture is confirmed when the height of the anterior vertebral body is at least 3 mm shorter than the height of the posterior part of the body. If compression is greater than 25%, instability may be present.[36]

Facet Dislocation

Facet dislocation may be unilateral or bilateral. Unilateral facet dislocation is caused by a flexion rotation mechanism and most often occurs between the C4 and C6 levels.[36] Cross-table lateral views of this injury show the dislocated facet locked anteriorly with the loss of superimposition of the articular pillars above the level of the injury. This appearance is described as the "bow-tie" sign and is characteristic of the fractures (Figure 10).[36] In addition, lateral radiographs of these injuries often reveal anterior subluxation of the vertebral body. This subluxation will not exceed 50% if the injury is unilateral. AP projections of these injuries show malalignment of the spinous processes with deviation to the side of the dislocation from the level of the injury and above.[36] Bilateral facet dislocation, which is associated with the highest incidence of SCI of all cervical fractures, occurs with hyperflexion. There is disruption of the posterior ligaments (e.g., the ligamentum flavum and interspinous ligaments), the ALL and PLL, the intervertebral disc, and the articular facet joints. Radiographically, this injury is associated with a 50% or greater anterior subluxation at the involved level,

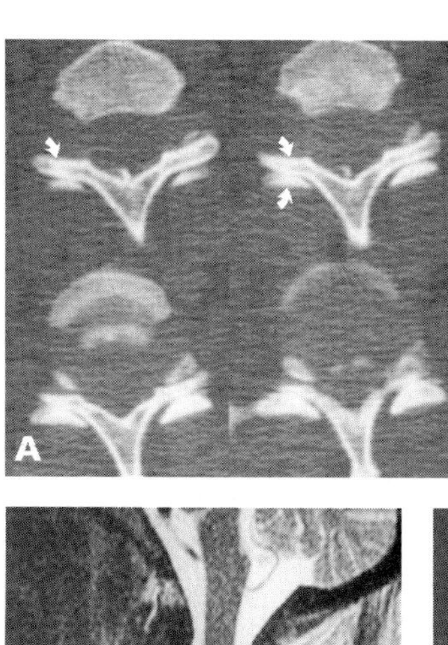
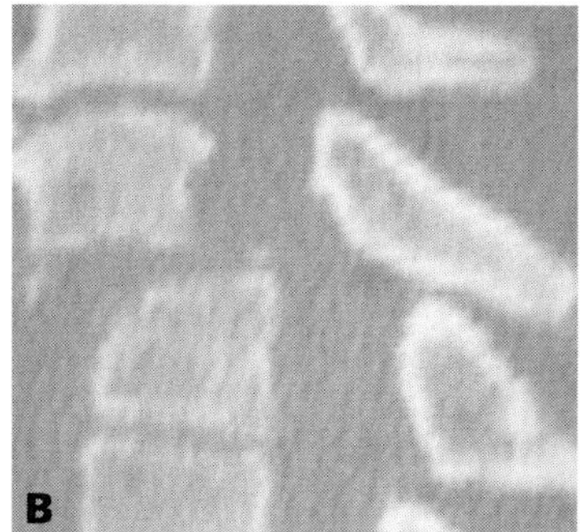
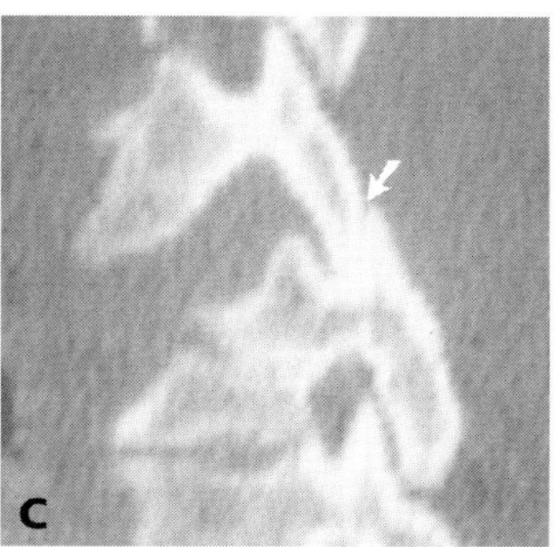
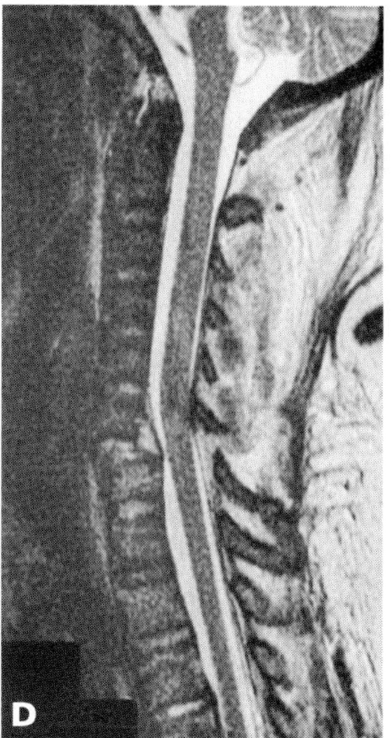
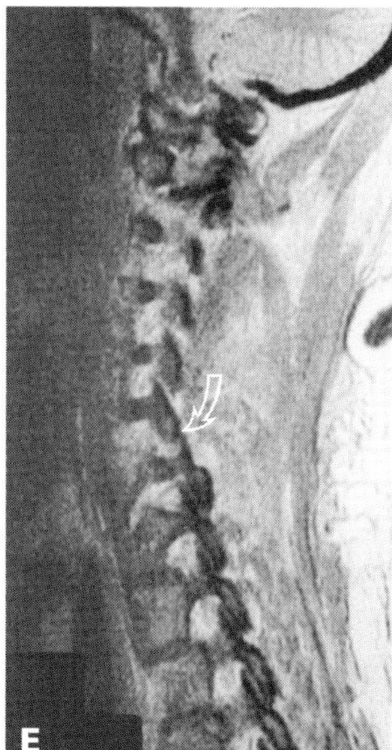

Figure 11: Bilateral C6-7 facet dislocation with the "naked facet" sign. Overlapping axial CT slices through the C6-7 disc space **(A)**. Midsagittal **(B)** and parasagittal **(C)** reformatted CTs at the C6-7 level. Midsagittal **(D)** and parasagittal **(E)** long TR/long TE (T2-weighted) spin-echo MRIs. Preliminary plain radiographs did not show the lower cervical spine. Axial CT at the C6-7 disc level demonstrated "naked facets" *(curved arrows)* indicating bilateral facet fracture-dislocation. This is confirmed on the sagittally reformatted images performed through the plane of the facet joints *(arrow)*. Anterolisthesis and facet dislocation are easily recognized on the parasagittal image.

as well as dislocation of the articular facets and disc space narrowing (Figure 11).[27] The AP view reveals widening of the interspinous distance, which occurs as a result of the posterior ligamentous injury. CT reveals abnormal facet articulation ("naked facets"), and reformatted images may be required for full appreciation of the degree of listhesis. MRI is a crucial diagnostic tool to assess disc space integrity, to detect the presence of hematoma, and to visualize the affected ligaments.

Flexion Teardrop Fracture

The flexion teardrop fracture is believed to occur as a result of combined flexion and axial loading. In this injury, as in bilateral facet dislocation, there is disruption to all anterior and posterior ligamentous structures, including the intervertebral discs and the facet joint capsule. Plain radiographs of the cervical spine show a small "teardrop fragment" that originates from the antero-inferior aspect of the vertebral body. There is posterior displacement of the larger posterior fragment of the vertebral body relative to the body below (Figure 12). Other radiographic findings in patient with this fracture include posterior disc space narrowing, fractures of the lamina, and focal kyphosis.[40]

Avulsion Fractures of the Spinous Process

Avulsion fractures of the spinous process are also known as "clay shoveler's" fractures. These fractures are most commonly encountered at

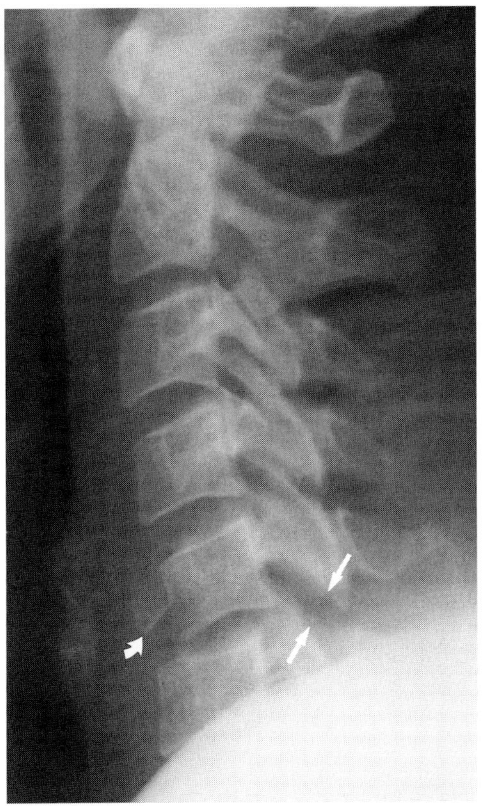

Figure 12: "Shoot through" (trauma) lateral radiograph of the cervical spine demonstrating a flexion teardrop fracture of C5-6. There is malalignment (retrolisthesis) of the C5 vertebral body on C6 with a displaced fracture fragment *(curved arrow)* at the antero-inferior aspect of the C5 vertebral body. Widening of the C5-6 facet joints *(arrows)* and interspinous distance can also be seen.

C6, C7, and T1.[36] They were first described among workers building the German Autobahn, occurring when the head and cervical spine are in flexion and there is rotation against the opposing interspinous ligaments.[27] These fractures are best imaged with cross-table lateral films. Although considered stable, care must be used when examining the lamina, as they may also be involved, in which case the management may differ.[36]

Hyperextension Injuries of the Lower Cervical Spine

Hyperextension injuries of the lower cervical

spine result in distractive anterior forces and compressive posterior forces. Injuries associated with hyperextension include hyperextension sprain, pillar fractures, hyperextension fracture-dislocation, and isolated laminar fractures.[27]

Hyperextension Sprain

In a hyperextension sprain, the force of hyperextension of the neck results in disruption of the ALL, rupture of the intervertebral disc, and stripping of the PLL from below. In addition, there is inward buckling of the ligamentum flavum, which may contribute to the spinal cord compression seen with these injuries.[27,36] Radiographic features include prevertebral soft-tissue swelling, which may be the only abnormality on plain film. Additional features may include avulsion fractures from the antero-inferior aspect of the affected vertebral segment and widening of the disc space anteriorly. The alignment is most commonly normal, as the subluxation reduces spontaneously. Clinically, these patients sustain a central cord syndrome, particularly if they have premorbid cervical stenosis.[36]

Pillar Fractures

Pillar fractures occur as a result of combined hyperextension and rotation and most commonly involve the C6 or C7 segment. They may be difficult to detect on plain films, which may show disruption of the lateral cortical margin on the AP view. Oblique views are best for this type of injury because they display asymmetric foraminal stenosis, which may result in acute radiculopathy in these patients.[36,40]

Hyperextension Fracture-dislocation

Injuries occurring as a result of a combination of hyperextension, compression, and rotational forces are hyperextension fracture-dislocation injuries. This injury produces unilateral articular pillar, lamina, pedicle, and spinous process fractures, as well as subluxation of the contralateral facets and disruption of the ALL and intervertebral disc. Radiographically, the pillar fracture appears on the AP film as described above. Lateral plain films reveal mild anterolisthesis (3-6 mm), narrowing of the disc space, and disruption of the facet joints.[27,40]

Laminar Fractures

Laminar fractures are caused by hyperextension and usually occur in the lower cervical spine between C5 and C7. They result from compression of adjacent lamina that can occur in hyperextension. This type of injury is often seen in elderly patients, and underlying degenerative changes may make it difficult to see the fractures on plain films. They are best seen on the lateral view of plain radiographs.[27,36]

Thoracic and Thoracolumbar Spine Fractures

Fractures that involve the thoracic spine are less common than cervical spine fractures. The thoracic spine has enhanced stability due to the bony thorax, large overlapping facets, and a limited range of movement.[35,40] A considerable force is required to produce a thoracic spine fracture or dislocation, and there is a strong association with neurological injury. Vertebral body integrity and alignment are best determined by AP and lateral screening x-rays. The upper four vertebral segments are often difficult to assess because of overlying soft tissues at the level of the shoulders. Plain radiography offers clues to the presence of a thoracic spine injury, including paraspinal soft tissue swelling and apical pleural capping. CT is best for evaluating the full extent of vertebral fracture and canal encroachment.

The thoracolumbar junction of the spine is a relatively frequent site of vertebral injury due to the relative lack of adjacent supporting structures, high mobility, and changing orientation of the facet joints.[11,36,40] The forces leading to injuries of the thoracolumbar spine and spinal cord usually consist of flexion and/or compression. The initial radiographic evaluation of these injuries requires frontal and lateral x-rays supplemented by CT for better assessment of the spinal canal and posterior elements. These injuries have been classified clinically and radiographically according to the three-column model originated by Denis[11] and the two-column model described by Holdsworth.[26]

To determine the severity of thoracic and thoracolumbar injuries, trauma to the bones and soft tissues must be identified. The ideal classification system would include information regarding the severity of the injury, the number of columns involved, and the planes of disruption. The classification system proposed by Magerl et al and updated by Gertzbein addresses the majority of these requirements.[32,33] This classification is simple and includes a relationship between fracture morphology and neurological injury. The characteristics of the injury categories are best determined by plain, AP, and lateral x-rays and CT scans. The main categories of this system of classification are:

- Type A: compression injuries primarily involving the vertebral bodies;
- Type B: distraction injuries affecting the anterior and posterior elements; and
- Type C: multidirectional injuries with translation also affecting the anterior and posterior elements of the spine.

Type A compression injuries are caused by an axial load onto the vertebral bodies, with or without an element of flexion. There is an associated loss of vertebral body height. Posterior arch fractures do not substantially affect stability. There is no disruption of posterior soft-tissue structures and no translation. Type A injuries are further divided into three groups: Group 1: impaction, with wedge-compression fractures; Group 2: split fractures, with a sagittal or coronal split in the vertebral body; and Group 3: burst fractures, with varying degrees of comminution and displacement.

Type B injuries involve both the anterior and posterior elements with distraction. The distractive forces involved result in a transverse injury. Again, there are three groups of Type B injuries: Group 1: transverse disruption through the posterior soft tissues; Group 2: transverse disruption through the bony arch; and Group 3: transverse disruption anteriorly through the disc space. Group 3 injuries occur with distraction anteriorly and are usually associated with extension forces. The injury may pass through the disc space and may fracture the arch (extension spondylosis) or create a posterior subluxation because of soft-tissue disruption.

Type C injuries also affect the anterior and posterior spinal elements with a significant translational component. These are the most unstable spinal injuries: Group 1: AP translation; Group 2: lateral translation; and Group 3: rotational translation.

This classification system is ordered in a graded fashion of soft tissue and bony injury. The injuries are more unstable as one progresses through the classification, and the neurological deficit increases from Types A to C. The planes of disruption and mechanisms of injury can be used as a guideline for management.[32]

Wedge-Compression Injuries

Wedge-compression injuries involve flexion and compression of the anterior aspect of the vertebral body. The fulcrum is at the posterior aspect of the vertebral body (middle column) and the posterior elements may experience mild distraction. Plain radiographs characteristically show loss of anterior vertebral body height. The posterior vertebral body margin and vertebral body height are preserved. CT demonstrates fragmentation of the anterior aspect of the vertebral body with an intact posterior vertebral body margin.

Burst Fracture

Burst fractures are due to an axial load with injury to both the anterior and middle portions of the spinal column. They are commonly associated with a retropulsed bony fragment originating from the posterior vertebral body encroaching upon the central spinal canal. Plain radiographs reveal a widened interpediculate distance and loss of vertebral body height involving both the anterior and posterior vertebral margins. Discontinuity or obliteration of the posterior vertebral body margin with a posteriorly displaced or rotated fragment may also be seen. CT is most valuable in assessing the degree and site of central spinal canal compromise as well as associated fractures of the laminae or splaying of the pedicles.

Flexion-Distraction Injury

A flexion-distraction injury is caused by extreme flexion with tensile forces applied to the middle and posterior portions of the spinal columns. The anterior vertebral body and ALL

act as a fulcrum or hinge. The anterior portion of the vertebral body may show mild fragmentation under compressive forces, but the anterior column is functionally intact. Plain radiographs are very important in assessing the degree of posterior element injury. There may be "fanning" of the spinous processes or distraction of facet joints. Fractures may extend through the pedicles or pars interarticularis. The transverse orientation of these fractures makes them difficult to appreciate on axial CT scans (Figure 13). Conventional tomography or reformatted CT images in the sagittal or coronal plane are often required.

Fracture-Dislocation Injuries

In fracture-dislocation injuries, there is total failure of all three vertebral columns, frequently, this is the result of a combination of compression, distraction, rotation, and shearing. These patients commonly present with severe neurological deficits. The radiographic hallmark is subluxation or rotational malalignment of the vertebral bodies as well as fracture and splaying of the posterior elements (Figure 14).

Radiological Assessment of Stability

Instability following spinal trauma exists when there is potential for progressive skeletal deformity (under normal physiological loading), pain, or risk of further neurological deficit. Five radiological signs have been described that correlate with potential spinal instability:[10]

1. vertebral displacement (listhesis) greater than 2 to 3.5 mm;[36]
2. focal widening of the interlaminar or interspinous distances (interspinous and ligamentum flavum disruption);
3. focal widening of the facet joints (ligamentous and joint capsule disruption);
4. disruption of the posterior vertebral body line (middle column disruption); and
5. focal widening of the interpediculate distance.

To this list, one may add focal angulation of greater than 11 degrees and vertebral body com-

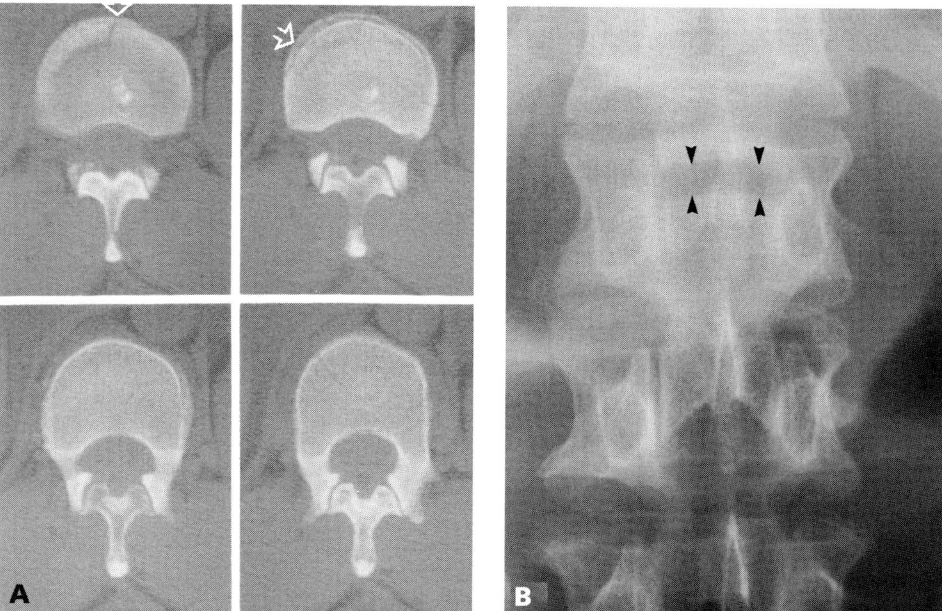

Figure 13: Axial CT **(A)** and AP radiograph **(B)** of the thoracolumbar spine demonstrating flexion-distraction fracture of thoracolumbar spine. A transverse fracture of the lamina and spinous process of T12 is visualized on the AP radiograph *(arrowheads)*. The accompanying CT shows comminution of the superior endplate of L1 *(open arrows)*. However, the fracture of the lamina is not demonstrated due to its transverse orientation.

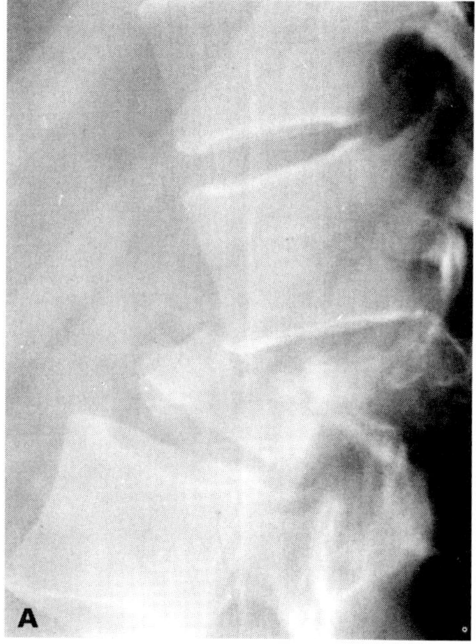

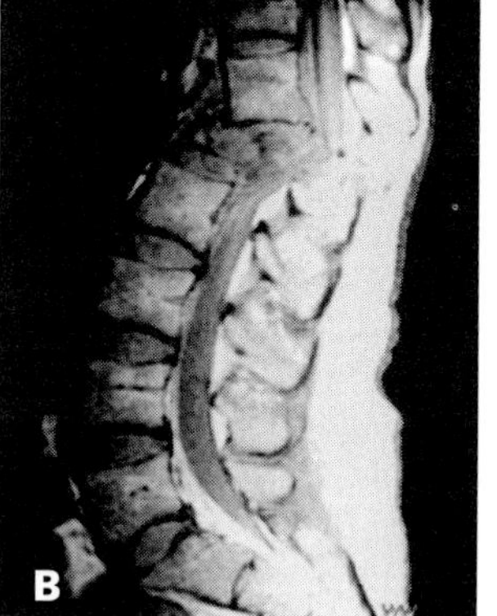

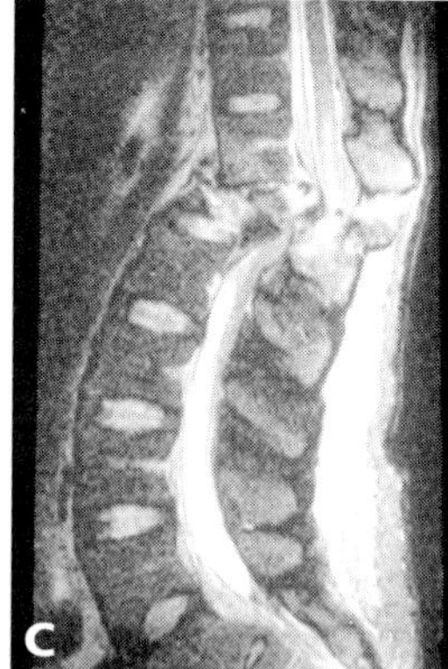

Figure 14: Lateral radiograph of the thoracolumbar spine **(A)** and midsagittal short TR/short TE (T1-weighted) and long TR/long TE (T2-weighted) MRIs **(B and C)** of the thoracolumbar spine demonstrating fracture-dislocation at the T12 and L1 vertebral levels using the Gertzbein classification system. The L1 vertebral is severely fragmented and compressed. There is subluxation as well as disruption of the posterior elements. Posteriorly extruded bone fragments have resulted in compression of the conus medullaris and adjacent cord edema.

pression (25% (cervical) and >50% (thoraco-lumbar)).[36]

Flexion-extension radiographs may be considered for an alert patient when there is clinical concern about possible ligamentous injury without an associated fracture. These should be performed cautiously, with only the patient moving the neck. The initial studies may be falsely negative due to muscle spasm and may warrant repetition after pain and spasm subside.

CONCLUSION

The timely availability and correct interpretation of spine imaging procedures are pivotal to the proper management of patients with spinal trauma. The plain radiograph remains the initial screening procedure of choice. The radiographic pattern of fracture and malalignment aid in the initial classification and in understanding its mechanism. Clinical and plain radiographic assessment are then used to direct further imaging aimed at fully evaluating the extent of bony and soft-tissue injury. A thorough analysis and understanding of these imaging procedures are essential to the goals of preventing further skeletal deformity, relieving ongoing cord compression, and preventing further neurological compromise.

REFERENCES

1. Andersen PA, Montesano PX: Morphology and treatment of occipital condyle fractures. **Spine** 13:731-736, 1988
2. Anderson LD, D'Alonzo RT: Fractures of the odontoid process of the axis. **J Bone Joint Surg (Am)** 56:1663-1674, 1974
3. Bates D, Ruggieri P: Imaging modalities for evaluation of the spine. **Radiol Clin North Am** 29:675-690, 1991
4. Benzel EC, Hart BL, Ball PA, et al: Fractures of the C-2 vertebral body. **J Neurosurg** 81:206-221, 1994
5. Bondurant FJ, Cotler HB, Kulkarni MV, et al: Acute spinal cord injury. A study using physical examination and magnetic resonance imaging. **Spine** 15:161-168, 1990
6. Bridgman SA, McNab W: Traumatic occipital condyle fracture, multiple cranial nerve palsies, and torticollis: a case report and review of the literature. **Surg Neurol** 38:152-156, 1992
7. Brightman RP, Miller CA, Rea GL, et al: Magnetic resonance imaging of trauma to the thoracic and lumbar spine. The importance of the posterior longitudinal ligament. **Spine** 17:541-550, 1992
8. Clark CT, Apuzzo MLJ: The evaluation and management of trauma to the odontoid process, in Cooper PR (ed): **Management of Posttraumatic Spinal Instability.** Park Ridge, Ill: American Association of Neurological Surgeons, 1990, pp 77-97
9. Cook PL: Radiology of spine and spinal cord injury, in Illis LS (ed): **Spinal Cord Dysfunction: Assessment.** Oxford, Engl: Oxford University Press, 1988, pp 41-103
10. Daffner RH, Deeb ZL, Goldberg AL: The radiologic assessment of posttraumatic vertebral stability. **Skeletal Radiol** 19:103-108, 1990
11. Denis F: The three column spine and its significance in the classification of acute thoracolumbar spinal injuries. **Spine** 8:817-831, 1983
12. Dickman CA, Papadopoulos SM, Sonntag VKH, et al: Traumatic occipitoatlantic dislocations. **J Spinal Disord** 6:300-313, 1993
13. Dublin AB, Marks WM, Weinstock D, et al: Traumatic dislocation of the atlanto-occipital articulation (AOA) with short-term survival. With a radiographic method of measuring the AOA. **J Neurosurg** 52:541-546, 1980
14. Effendi B, Roy D, Cornish B, et al: Fractures of the ring of the axis. A classification based on the analysis of 131 cases. **J Bone Joint Surg (Br)** 63:319-327, 1981
15. Fehlings MG, Rao SC, Tator CH, et al: The optimal radiologic method for assessing spinal canal compromise and cord compression in patients with cervical spinal cord injury. Part II: Results of a multicenter study. **Spine** 24:605-613, 1999
16. Flanders AE, Schaefer DM, Doan HT, et al: Acute cervical spine trauma: correlation of MR imaging findings with degree of neurologic deficit. **Radiology** 177:25-33, 1990
17. Flanders AE, Tartaglino LM, Friedman DP, et al: Magnetic resonance imaging in acute spinal injury. **Semin Roentgenol** 27:271-298, 1992
18. Fowler JL, Sandhu A, Fraser RD: A review of fractures of the atlas vertebra. **J Spinal Disord** 3:19-24, 1990
19. Garber JN: Abnormalities of the atlas and axis vertebrae—congenital and traumatic. **J Bone Joint Surg (Am)** 46:1782-1791, 1964
20. Gerlock AJ Jr, Mirfakhraee M, Benzel EC: Computed tomography of traumatic atlantooccipital dislocation. **Neurosurgery** 13:316-319, 1983
21. Goldberg AL, Rothfus WE, Deeb ZL, et al: The impact of magnetic resonance on the diagnostic evaluation of acute cervicothoracic spinal trauma. **Skeletal Radiol** 17:89-95, 1988
22. Hadley MN, Browner C, Sonntag VKH: Axis fractures: a comprehensive review of management and treatment in 107 cases. **Neurosurgery** 17:281-290, 1985
23. Hadley MN, Sonntag VK, Grahm TW, et al: Axis fractures resulting from motor vehicle accidents. The need for occupant restraints. **Spine** 11:861-864, 1986
24. Hall AJ, Wagle VG, Raycroft J: Magnetic resonance imaging in cervical spine trauma. **J Trauma** 34:21-26, 1993
25. Harris JH, Edeiken-Monroe B: **The Radiology of Acute Cervical Spine Trauma.** Baltimore, Md: Williams & Wilkins, 1987
26. Holdsworth FW: Neurological diagnosis and the indications for treatment of paraplegia and tetraplegia, associated with fractures of the spine. **Manitoba Med Rev** 48:16-18, 1968
27. Hudgins PA, Hudgins RJ: Radiology of cervical spine trauma. **Clin Neurosurg** 37:571-595, 1991

28. Lee C, Woodring JH, Goldstein SJ, et al: Evaluation of traumatic atlantooccipital dislocations. **AJNR 8**:19-26, 1987

29. Lee C, Woodring JH, Walsh JW: Carotid and vertebral artery injury in survivors of atlanto-occipital dislocation: case reports and literature review. **J Trauma 31**:401-407, 1991

30. Levine AM, Rhyne AL: Traumatic spondylolisthesis of the axis. **Semin Spine Surg 3**:47-60, 1991

31. MacDonald RL, Schwartz ML, Mirich D, et al: Diagnosis of cervical spine injury in motor vehicle crash victims: how many x-rays are enough? **J Trauma 30**:392-397, 1990

32. Magerl F, Aebi M, Gertzbein SD, et al: A comprehensive classification of thoracic and lumbar injuries. **Eur Spine J 3**:184-201, 1994

33. Magerl F, Harms J, Gertzbein SD: A new classification system of spinal fractures. Presented at the Societe Internationale Orthipedie et Traumatologie Meeting, Montreal, Canada, Sept 9, 1990

34. Masaryk TJ: Spinal trauma, in Modic MT, Masaryk TJ, Ross JS (eds): **Magnetic Resonance Imaging of the Spine.** Chicago: Year Book Medical, 1989, pp 214-239

35. Meyer S: Thoracic spine trauma. **Semin Roentgenol 27**:855-872, 1992

36. Murphey MD, Batnitzky S, Bramble JM: Diagnostic imaging of spinal trauma. **Radiol Clin North Am 27**:855-872, 1989

37. Naidich JB, Naidich TP, Garfein C, et al: The widened interspinous distance: a useful sign of anterior cervical dislocation in the supine frontal projection. **Radiology 123**:113-116, 1977

38. Pang D, Wilberger JE Jr: Traumatic atlanto-occipital dislocation with survival: case report and review. **Neurosurgery 7**:503-508, 1980

39. Papadopoulos SM, Dickman CA, Sonntag VKH, et al: Traumatic atlantooccipital dislocation with survival. **Neurosurgery 28**:574-579, 1991

40. Pathria MN, Petersilge CA: Spinal trauma. **Radiol Clin North Am 29**:847-865, 1991

41. Penning L: Prevertebral hematoma in cervical spine injury: incidence and etiologic significance. **AJR 13**:553-561, 1981

42. Post MJ, Green BA: The use of computed tomography in spinal trauma. **Radiol Clin North Am 21**:327-375, 1983

43. Powers B, Miller MD, Kramer RS, et al: Traumatic anterior atlantooccipital dislocation. **Neurosurgery 4**:12-17, 1979

44. Rao SC, Fehlings MG: The optimal radiologic method for assessing spinal canal compromise and cord compression in patients with cervical spinal cord injury. Part I: An evidence-based analysis of the published literature. **Spine 24**:598-604, 1999

45. Reines HD, Harris RC: Pulmonary complications of acute spinal cord injuries. **Neurosurgery 21**:193-196, 1987

46. Rizzolo SJ, Piazza MR, Cotler JM, et al: Intervertebral disc injury complicating cervical spine trauma. **Spine 16(Suppl)**:S187-S189, 1991

47. Schaefer DM, Flanders A, Northrup BE, et al: Magnetic resonance imaging of acute cervical spine trauma. Correlation with severity of neurologic injury. **Spine 14**:1090-1095, 1989

48. Schaefer DM, Flanders AE, Osterholm JL, et al: Prognostic significance of magnetic resonance imaging in the acute phase of cervical spine injury. **J Neurosurg 76**:218-223, 1992

49. Schneider RC, Livingston KE, Cave AJE: "Hangman's fracture" of the cervical spine. **J Neurosurg 22**:141-154, 1965

50. Silberstein M, McLean K: Fast magnetic resonance imaging in spinal trauma. **Australas Radiol 39**:118-123, 1995

51. Silberstein M, Tress BM, Hennessy O: Prediction of neurologic outcome in acute spinal cord injury: the role of CT and MR. **AJNR 13**:1597-1608, 1992

52. Sonntag VKH, Dickman C: Treatment of upper cervical spine injuries, in Rea GL, Miller CA (eds): **Spinal Trauma: Current Evaluation and Management.** Park Ridge, Ill: American Association of Neurological Surgeons, 1993, pp 25-74

53. Spence KF Jr, Decker S, Sell KW: Bursting atlantal fracture associated with rupture of the transverse ligament. **J Bone Joint Surg (Am) 52**:543-549, 1970

54. Teitelbaum GP, Yee CA, Van Horn DD, et al: Metallic ballistic fragments: MRI imaging safety and artifacts. **Radiology 175**:855-859, 1990

55. Tippets RH, Alvis JM: Treatment of axis fractures, in Menezes A, Benzel EC, Cahill DW, et al (eds): **Principles of Spinal Surgery.** New York: McGraw-Hill, 1996, pp 871-884

56. Traynelis VC, Marano GD, Dunker RO, et al: Traumatic atlanto-occipital dislocation. Case report. **J Neurosurg 65**:863-870, 1986

57. Tuli S, Tator CH, Fehlings MG, et al: Occipital condyle fractures. **Neurosurgery 41**:368-377, 1997

58. Wojcik WG, Edeiken-Monroe B, Harris JH: Three-dimensional computer tomography in acute cervical spine trauma: a preliminary report. **Skeletal Radiol 16**:261-269, 1987

59. Woodring JH, Lee C: Limitations of cervical radiography in the evaluation of acute cervical trauma. **J Trauma 34**:32-39, 1993

CHAPTER 9

IMMOBILIZATION AND TRACTION

JACK E. WILBERGER, MD

The treatment of acute spinal cord injury (SCI) has three primary goals: 1) to maximize neurological recovery; 2) to stabilize the spine; and 3) to mobilize and rehabilitate the patient. Achieving these goals begins at the scene of the injury with a logical management schema. After the traumatized patient is resuscitated and stabilized, spinal immobilization and realignment assumes primary importance. A number of craniospinal traction devices have been used for this purpose. In addition, an appropriate bed is needed to manage the patient with acute SCI.

Opinions vary on the means, methods, and timing of spinal realignment. This chapter focuses on the techniques of closed cervical reduction and its place in the overall management of patients with acute SCI.

CLOSED CERVICAL REDUCTION

Historically, once the radiographic diagnosis of the bony injury has been established, neurosurgical treatment is directed toward acute spinal stabilization and, if appropriate, spinal realignment. The rationale was that spinal stabilization to prevent further injury to the spinal cord and/or the nerve roots is well founded. The degree and extent to which realignment is at-

tempted, especially in the setting of an initially complete SCI, have been subject to debate. Intuitively and anecdotally, it appears reasonable to realign the spine and thereby decompress the spinal canal in an effort to ameliorate the neurological injury. For the most part, however, it has not been possible to determine whether the subsequent degree of neurological recovery is due to the treatment or to the extent of primary injury to the spinal cord.

A recent survey of the current treatment of acute SCI found that traction was applied in only 47% of patients with cervical injuries.[34] It cannot be determined as to whether such a low rate of utilization is related to the lack of significant spinal deformity or to the recent tendency for aggressive surgical treatment of patients with ongoing compression from an unstable spinal injury.

CRANIOSPINAL IMMOBILIZATION

Initial immobilization and attempted realignment have been traditionally accomplished by craniospinal traction.[3-5] In 1933, Crutchfield[14] first reported the use of cranial tongs for this purpose. The Crutchfield tongs or a modification continued in widespread clinical use for five decades.[25,36]

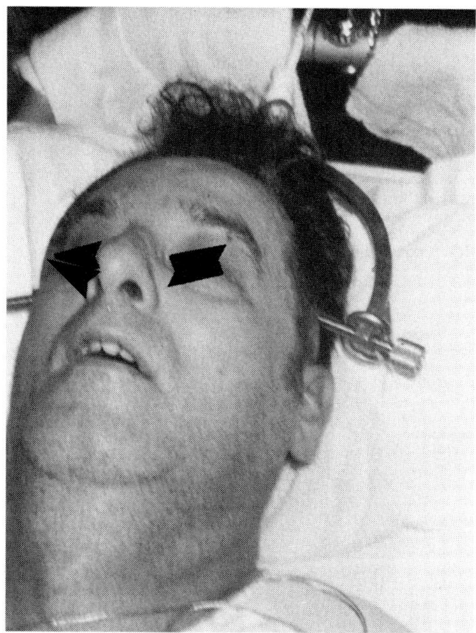

Figure 1: Gardner-Wells tongs are used in a patient for closed cervical reduction.

In 1973, Gardner[18] introduced the spring-loaded tong. The Gardner-Wells (G-W) tongs can be applied readily under local anesthesia and they have rapidly supplanted earlier devices. The G-W tongs are easy to apply in emergency situations. Typically, after antiseptically prepping and anesthetizing the skin, pins are typically introduced in line with the external auditory canals, just below the temporal line. One pin is spring loaded to indicate the amount of compressive force exerted on the outer table of the skull. When the indicator on the spring-loaded pin protrudes 1 mm beyond the hub, approximately 30 pounds of force are being applied and further tightening might cause penetration of the skull. After the tongs have been in place for 24 hours, however, it is important to retighten the tongs until the pin is flush with the hub (Figure 1). The exact location of pin attachment will determine the effects of any traction applied. That is, if the pins are slightly anterior to the external auditory canal, the cervical spine will extend as traction is applied; if the pins are posteriorly placed, flexion will occur. Generally, the G-W tongs will tolerate up to 65 pounds of traction without pulling out.

However, in clinical practice, much higher levels of traction have been tolerated on a short-term basis without adverse consequences.

Gardner reported the use of tongs for up to 8 weeks without evident problems. Likewise, Grundy,[22] in a comprehensive review of complications related to skull traction, found no significant problems in the use of G-W tongs. Currently, there is a graphite version of the G-W tongs available for potential use in the setting of magnetic resonance imaging (MRI) after acute SCI.

The halo device was first introduced in the 1960s.[12,27,32,38,39] With the recent renewed interest in early patient mobilization, its use is being increasingly advocated for the management of patients with acute SCI. The halo device application is somewhat more involved than the G-W tongs.[26,28,31] However, it can be readily used in the acute setting and may have several advantages over the G-W tongs. All halos are currently compatible with both computed tomography scanning and MRI. The halo is considered by many to be the primary method of treatment in a significant number of cervical spine injuries. Placement of the halo requires four skull pins, and careful attention must be paid to the localization of pin placement and how tightly each pin is applied to the skull.

Halo rings are available in a number of sizes and should be fitted to allow 1 cm of clearance between the scalp and the ring around the entire circumference of the head (Figure 2). To prevent migration of the device, the rings should be placed no more than 1 cm above the eyebrows or the top of the ears. Usually, the frontal pins are placed just lateral to the supraorbital notch to avoid the supraorbital and supratrochlear nerves and the frontal sinus. Patients should be instructed to close their eyes tightly while the frontal pins are being applied to avoid the inadvertent retraction of the forehead skin, which subsequently may make it difficult to completely close the eyelids. The occipital pins are usually placed several centimeters behind the ears.

Before pin placement, the scalp and periosteum should be fully anesthetized; otherwise, pin tightening may be extremely uncomfortable. In addition, intravenous sedation with short-acting agents such as midazolam or fentanyl may be appropriate. Once the pins are placed, opposite pins are hand tightened and then tightened

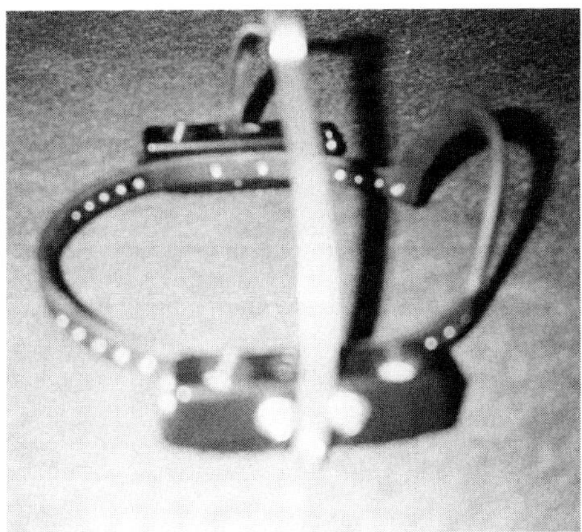

Figure 2: Modification of the halo device to allow for cervical traction during closed cervical reduction.

with a torque wrench to 6-8 pounds. Within 48 hours, the pins should be rechecked and the torque corrected to 6-8 pounds.

The most significant problems associated with acute halo use are pin loosening and pin infection, which occur in up to 25% of cases.[19] Such problems usually are heralded by complaints of pain and discomfort and generally are minimized by careful daily pin-site cleansing and care. There have been rare reports of skull penetration by a halo pin, with subsequent cerebrospinal fluid and/or infection. Patients and/or their caretakers should be fully instructed in local pin care before discharge and should be cautioned to report any unusual appearance or discharge.

TRACTION

Once craniospinal traction devices are applied, attention is turned to maintaining and/or achieving spinal realignment. This usually is accomplished via the use of traction; however, there continue to be advocates of cervical manipulation. Crutchfield advocated slow, controlled attempts at reduction through traction, fearing that the rapid increase in large amounts of weight might further injure the spine and jeopardize the spinal cord. One of Crutchfield's tenets was that no more than 5 pounds of trac-

tion per cervical level should be applied. This recommendation continues to serve as a guideline. However, many have taken issue with Crutchfield's ideas concerning timing and rapid realignment, especially in the presence of an incomplete SCI.

Before cervical traction application, it is very important to understand clearly the nature of the bony and/or ligamentous injury. In certain severe ligamentous injuries, such as atlanto-occipital dislocation, any traction is contraindicated. It has been shown clearly that spondylotic spines are predisposed to overdistraction, even with minimal corrective traction.[17,40] Jackson[24] used cineradiographic studies to demonstrate that 20 pounds of traction can produce visible disc distraction and widening of the intervertebral foramina. Voluntary cervical muscle contraction can, however, overcome the effects of up to 30 pounds of traction.[2,24] Within the past decade, there has been increasing concern over the use of traction in the setting of bilateral locked facets, particularly in the presence of an incomplete SCI. The rates of associated acute disc herniation in conjunction with bilateral locked facets have been reported to be as high as 15%. Realistically, however, the rate appears to be in the 3%-5% range. Concern over applying traction and acutely realigning these patients lies in the fact that the acute disc herniation might cause significant compression once realignment has occurred. Although not universally agreed upon, many are recommending MRI before the application of cervical traction.

If the spine is already aligned, the amount of traction necessary to maintain stabilization is not more than 5-10 pounds. Traditionally, it has been recommended that not more than 5 pounds per level of injury be applied if realignment is attempted (e.g., a C5-6 dislocation will require a maximum of 30 pounds of traction). Nevertheless, on a practical clinical basis, it is often necessary to use 10 pounds or more per level to achieve reduction. It has been suggested that 60-80 pounds may be a reasonable absolute limit.

It is important to monitor clinical signs and radiographic results closely during the application of traction. Attention must be paid to the patient's complaints, such as increased pain and new or worsened neurological symptoms. In a recent review of current use of cervical traction, an 8.1% incidence of neurological worsening was described.[34] Thus, after each new application of weight, the neurological examination should be repeated. Radiographic monitoring is aimed at preventing significant overdistraction before it produces clinical problems. Although there are no absolute radiographic guidelines defining overdistraction, it has been suggested that, as the height of any part of the intervertebral disc space exceeds 5 mm, extreme caution should be exercised while adding weights.[17]

Currently, it is a generally accepted procedure to add cervical traction in increments of 5 to 10 lb every 10 to 15 minutes until one of the following: reduction is achieved; there is clinical or radiographic evidence of overdistraction; or a maximum weight has been achieved. Constant or intermittent fluoroscopic monitoring is a useful adjunct in this process. When large amounts of weights are necessary, elevating the head of the patient's bed may help to provide counter-traction. Given the ability of the cervical muscles to overcome the effects of traction (especially when in spasm), muscle relaxants and analgesics are commonly administered. Such medications, however, should be used with caution as they may interfere with the necessary neurological monitoring. In addition, the precipitous loss of muscle tone may allow for overdistraction at relatively low weights.

If reduction is not achieved with these techniques, slight flexion or extension of the neck, depending on the mechanism of injury may aid in realignment (e.g., flexion for facet dislocations and extension for C2 hangman's fracture with subluxation).

It is also important to insure that traction is actually being applied. Occasionally, the weights may come in contact with the floor, or the knot on the rope connecting the weights to the patient may retract into the pulley system. Both of these events effectively negate the traction.

Manual Manipulation

If closed reduction cannot be accomplished within a predetermined time, operative intervention for open reduction will be indicated. Some, however, continue to support manual manipulation as an adjunct or as a primary means

of closed reduction.

The first report of manipulation to treat cervical dislocation was provided by Walton[37] in 1893. There have been a number of subsequent proponents and opponents of this method of treatment.[9,13,15,16,35] Although popular in Europe and Australia, manipulation has never been widely accepted in the United States or Canada. The U.S. Air Force and Army Technical Bulletin entitled "Care of Patients with Injury to the Spinal Cord" states: "under no circumstances must a grave error be made of trying to reduce any cervical dislocation by closed manipulation."

Nevertheless, Burke and Berryman[11] reported using closed manipulation on 41 patients with flexion facet injuries. The patients were placed under general anesthesia with Pentothal. If no "click" (indicating reduction) was heard with endotracheal intubation, manual traction was applied, followed by lateral flexion and rotation in the direction of the facet injury. This maneuver was repeated in the opposite direction for bilateral facet injuries (manipulation was not successful in achieving reduction in only four of the 41 patients). In addition, no patient became "permanently worse," even though two died shortly after the procedure of "acute respiratory failure."[11]

The only absolute guidelines provided by Burke and Berryman were that manipulations should not be attempted for injuries at the C7-T1 level. They did, however, provide a number of qualifiers that should be considered before closed manipulation is attempted (e.g., the patient's general condition and neurological status, age, and the presence of shock or associated injuries).

Timing

The time allotted to traction for achieving reduction is controversial. Yashon et al[40] in 1975 was one of the first to call for "rapid reduction: within 1-2 hours of injury." This approach was based on the belief that the ultimate neurological dysfunction after SCI was dependent on the time between injury and spinal cord decompression. Yashon et al described the use of this approach in "over 50 patients" but did not provide supporting data on neurological outcome.

Brunette and Rockswold[10] in 1987 reported a single case of "impressive neurological recovery" after a complete C4 SCI secondary to a C3-4 fracture dislocation. Reduction with traction was accomplished within 90 minutes of injury and a neurological examination 14 days later was nearly normal.

While there have been a number of reports on the effect of cervical traction on neurological improvement over the past several decades, few have addressed the issue of the timing of reduction by traction. Dall in 1972 reported on 75 patients and found that, regardless of the timing of anatomical reduction by traction, there was no effect on neurological recovery. Aebi et al[1] in 1986 reported that, of 100 patients, 75% were able to be reduced within 6 hours of injury. In those patients who underwent reduction within 6 hours of injury, 31% manifested significant neurological recovery.

Recently, some evidence has suggested that decompression of the spinal canal by realignment and its timing have an important impact on neurological recovery. In a study of 37 patients with facet fracture dislocations, Hadley et al[23] found that the most important factor with respect to prognosis for neurological recovery was the time from injury to decompression realignment of the spinal canal. In the small number of cases in which there was significant neurological improvement, realignment was achieved within 8 hours of injury. Similarly, in a series of 210 patients, Lee and others noted in 1994 that, with utilization of up to 150 lb of traction, rapid realignment resulted in improved outcomes.[34]

NEUROLOGICAL SEQUELAE

The use of traction or halo immobilization, although possibly providing neurological benefits, may also be a source of neurological deterioration. As mentioned previously, recent review indicated neurological deterioration in 8.1% of patients following the institution of cervical traction.[34] Although reported only rarely, it probably occurs at a rate somewhat lower than what has been recently documented.

Marshall et al,[29] in a comprehensive study of SCI in southern California, documented a 4.9%

incidence of neurological deterioration which, in almost all cases, was due to an identifiable therapeutical intervention. The application of skeletal traction was believed to be responsible in 21% of patients with neurological deterioration and halo application accounted for another 14%. Marshall et al believed that these figures represented acceptable minimal levels, which occurred as a result of necessary and appropriate treatment. Braackman and Penning[6] described three SCI cases that they believed were caused by improperly applied cervical traction. Yashon et al[40] reported no cases in their extensive experience in which large amounts of weight were used.

A special caution should be made when applying traction to elderly patients with severe spondylosis—especially in the setting of ankylosing spondylitis. Fried[17] reported two such patients who had marked disc space distraction with traction and neurological deterioration ultimately leading to death. Marshall et al[29] also noted this concern in their study.

IMMOBILIZATION BEDS

The management of the SCI patient in an appropriate bed is an integral component of spine immobilization and traction. The bed should be able to maintain spinal stability and alignment while enabling easier nursing access and frequent patient repositioning to lessen the complications of immobilization. The two most commonly used specialized beds are the Wedge Turning Frame (Stryker Frame, Stryker Corp., Kalamazoo, MI) and the Kinetic Treatment Table (Roto Rest Kinetic Treatment Table, Kinetic Concepts, Inc., San Antonio, TX) (Figure 3).

The importance of "mobilizing" the patient in spinal traction cannot be overemphasized. In general, SCI patients are susceptible to many systemic complications, regardless of the treatment that is undertaken (Figure 4). The techniques of immobilization, and prolonged immobilization itself, may further increase the complication rate. The National Acute Spinal Cord Injury Study (NASCIS)[7] provides the most current information with regard to the risk of such complications.

Although the Stryker frame has been widely used for many decades, its potential inadequacies

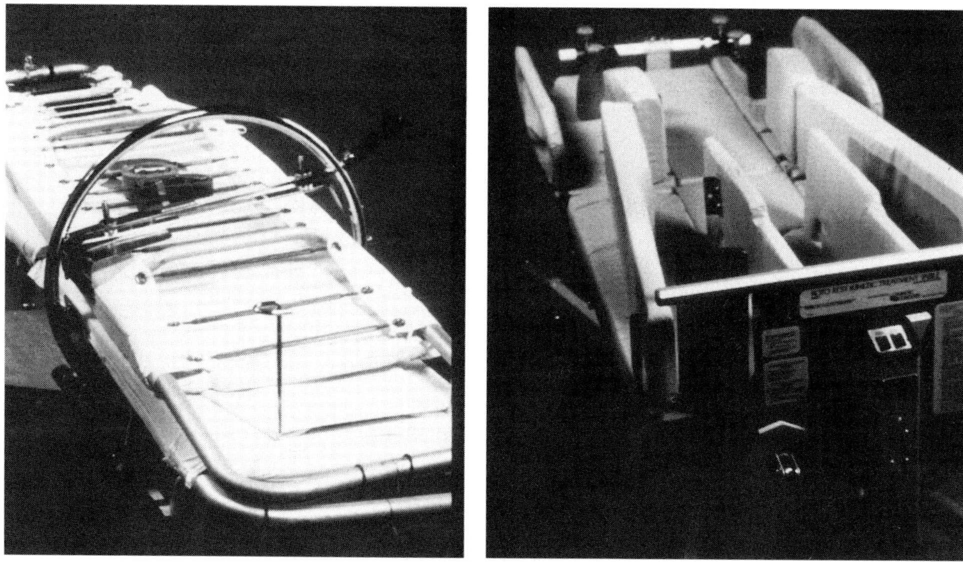

Figure 3: Commonly used specialized immobilization beds: the Wedge Turning Frame *(left)* and the Roto Rest Kinetic Treatment Table *(right)*.

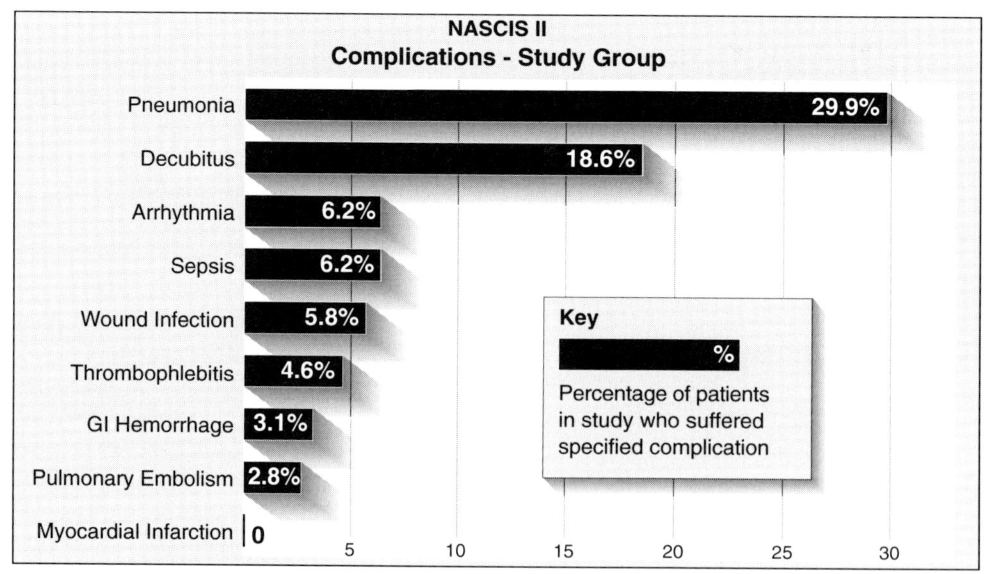

Figure 4: Complications occurring in NASCIS 2 study. GI = gastrointestinal.

in immobilizing a cervical spine were first pointed out by Slabaugh and Nickel[33] in 1978. The frame is a narrow canvas-covered structure that is lightweight and simple to operate. Advocates recommend that the patient be turned from the supine to the prone position every 2 hours while on this frame. During turning, the patient is wedged between the two pieces of the frame as protection against loss of spine immobilization. Slabaugh and Nickel pointed out three specific concerns with the Stryker Frame: 1) loss of immobilization with turning; 2) diminished pulmonary vital capacity; and 3) the development of decubiti in unusual locations. They presented a case of alignment loss of a C5-6 subluxation on turning from the supine to the prone position. Additionally, they found 13%-16% decrements in vital capacity going from the supine to the prone position using the Frame. Finally, they encountered a number of patients with occipital decubitus ulcers.

The Roto Rest Kinetic Treatment Table is a bulky apparatus. It automatically and continually rotates the patient in a cradle-like fashion through an arc of 125 degrees. Added supports maintain the arms, legs, and trunk in proper position and can be easily removed for nursing or other therapeutic interventions. In addition, there are supports for the side of the head to prevent head rotation when the bed is in motion.

The benefits of therapy using the Kinetic bed have been described in a number of reports.[8,20,21,30] Green et al[20,21] reported a series of 105 acute SCI cases treated on a Kinetic bed with only a 1.9% incidence of significant pulmonary complications. Brackett and Condon[8] compared complications in patients treated on either a Stryker Frame or a Kinetic bed. Of 14 patients with complete SCI immobilized on a Stryker Frame, 46% had severe pulmonary problems and, of those, almost one third went on to respiratory failure and death. However, of 17 patients managed using a Kinetic bed, none had severe pulmonary problems and no deaths were reported. The total number of days spent in the intensive care unit was 45% greater for those treated on a Stryker Frame compared to those on a Kinetic bed.

Recently, McGuire et al[30] examined the efficacy of immobilization of the spine, comparing the two beds. Using a cadaver model, unstable injuries were produced in the cervical and lumbar regions of the spine. The spines were then rotated on the beds in a manner typical in clinical management. In spines with unstable lumbar injuries immobilized using the Stryker Frame, significant anteroposterior displacement, angular movement, and distraction were seen at the injury site on turning from the supine to the prone position; similar movements were not identifiable with the spines using a Kinetic bed. Similarly, with an unstable cervical spine injury, turning from the supine to the prone position using the Stryker Frame resulted in considerable change in the extent of distraction and angular movement. No such changes were observed with the spines using a Kinetic bed.

Based on the above, it does not appear that the Stryker Frame is suitable for patients with severely unstable complicated spine injuries or for those with pre-existing pulmonary problems. Additionally, there should be concerns about its use with obese patients or with patients who have marked agitation and restlessness. While the frame is in use, the patient should be carefully checked after each turn for any new complaints or neurological findings. Arterial blood gases or oximetry should be continually monitored for arterial desaturation with turning from one position to another. At least once, a lateral spine radiograph should be obtained with the patient in both the supine and the prone position, to insure that clinically unsuspected significant spine movement is not occurring.

The Kinetic bed automatically rotates the patient through a 125-degree arc every 4-5 minutes and can be stopped in any position to aid nursing care access. The patient's back can be assessed through one of several hatches on the underside of the bed to minimize patient movement. The side supports are easily removed to provide for arrangement of the extremities. The Kinetic bed is not without potential problems, however. A study by Marshall et al[29] reported one patient who deteriorated neurologically during the course of rotation on a Roto Rest bed. Of final note, spine surgery is possible with the patient positioned using the Kinetic bed.

REFERENCES

1. Aebi M, Mohler J, Zach GA, et al: Indication, surgical

technique, and results of 100 surgically-treated fractures and fracture-dislocations of the cervical spine. **Clin Orthop** 203:244-257, 1986

2. Bard G, Jones MD: Cineradiographic recording of traction of the cervical spine. **Arch Phys Med 45:** 403-406, 1964

3. Barton LG: The reduction of fracture dislocations of the cervical vertebrae by skeletal traction. **Surg Gynecol Obstet 67:**94-96, 1938

4. Beatson TR: Fractures and dislocations of the cervical spine. **J Bone Joint Surg (Br)** 45:21-35, 1963

5. Blackburn JAD: A new skull-traction appliance. **South Surg 7:**16-18, 1938

6. Braakman R, Penning L: **Injuries to the Cervical Spine.** Amsterdam: Excerpta Medica Foundation, 1971

7. Bracken MB, Shepard MJ, Holford TR, et al: Methylprednisolone or tirilazad mesylate administration after acute spinal cord injury: 1-year follow-up. Results of the third National Acute Spinal Cord Injury randomized controlled trial. **J Neurosurg 89:**699-706, 1998

8. Brackett TO, Condon N: Comparison of the Wedge Turning Frame and Kinetic Treatment Table in the acute care of spinal cord injury patients. **Surg Neurol 22:**53-56, 1984

9. Brookes TP: Dislocations of the cervical spine. Their complications and treatment. **Surg Gynecol Obstet 57:**772-778, 1933

10. Brunette DD, Rockswold GL: Neurologic recovery following rapid spinal realignment for complete cervical spinal cord injury. **J Trauma 27:**445-447, 1987

11. Burke DC, Berryman D: The place of closed manipulation in the management of flexion rotation dislocations of the cervical spine. **J Bone Joint Surg (Br) 53:** 165-182, 1971

12. Cooper PR, Maravilla KR, Sklar FH, et al: Halo immobilization of cervical spine fractures. Indications and results. **J Neurosurg 50:**603-610, 1979

13. Crooks F, Birkett AN: Fractures and dislocations of the cervical spine. **Br J Surg 31:**252-255, 1944

14. Crutchfield WG: Skeletal traction for dislocation of the cervical spine: report of a case. **South Surg 2:** 156-159, 1933

15. Ellis VH: Injuries of the cervical vertebrae. **Proc R Soc Med 40:**19-25, 1946

16. Evans DK: Reduction of cervical dislocations. **J Bone Joint Surg (Br)** 43:552-555, 1961

17. Fried LC: Cervical spinal cord injury during skeletal traction. **JAMA 229:**181-183, 1974

18. Gardner WJ: The principle of spring-loaded points for cervical traction. Technical note. **J Neurosurg 39:**543-544, 1973

19. Garfin SR. Botte MJ, Waters RL, et al: Complications in the use of the halo fixation device. **J Bone Joint Surg (Am) 68:**320-325, 1986

20. Green BA, Green KL, Klose KJ: Kinetic nursing for acute spinal cord injury patients. **Paraplegia 18:** 181-186, 1980

21. Green BA, Green KL, Klose KJ: Kinetic therapy for spinal cord injury. **Spine 8:**722-728, 1983

22. Grundy DJ: Skull traction and its complications. **Injury 15:**173-177, 1983

23. Hadley MN, Fitzpatrick BC, Sonntag VK, et al: Facet fracture-dislocation injuries of the cervical spine. **Neurosurgery 30:**661-666, 1992

24. Jackson R: **The Cervical Syndrome.** Springfield, Ill: Charles C Thomas, 1956

25. Johnson RM, Hart DL, Simmons EF, et al: Cervical orthoses. A study comparing their effectiveness in restricting cervical motion in normal subjects. **J Bone Joint Surg (Am) 59:**332-339, 1977

26. Koch RA, Nickel VL: The halo vest: an evaluation of motion and forces across the neck. **Spine 3:**103-107, 1978

27. Lind B, Shilbom H, Nordwall A: Halo-vest treatment of unstable traumatic cervical spine injuries. **Spine 13:** 425-432, 1988

28. Maiman DJ, Barolat G, Larson SJ: Management of bilateral locked facets of the cervical spine. **Neurosurgery 18:**542-547, 1986

29. Marshall LF, Knowlton S, Garfin SR, et al: Deterioration following spinal cord injury. A multicenter study. **J Neurosurg 66:**400-404, 1987

30. McGuire RA, Green BA, Eismont FJ, et al: Comparison of stability provided to the unstable spine by the Kinetic therapy table and the Stryker Frame. **Neurosurgery 22:**842-845, 1988

31. Perry J, Nickel VL: Total cervical spine fusion for neck paralysis. **J Bone Joint Surg (Am) 41:**37-60, 1959

32. Sears W, Fazl M: Prediction of stability of cervical spine fracture managed in the halo vest and indications for surgical intervention. **J Neurosurg 72:** 426-432, 1990

33. Slabaugh PB, Nickel VL: Complications with use of the Stryker frame. **J Bone Joint Surg (Am) 60:** 1111-1112, 1978

34. Tator CH, Fehlings M, Thorpe K, et al: Current use and timing of spinal surgery for management of acute spinal cord injury in North America: results of a retrospective multicenter study. **J Neurosurg 91 (Suppl 1):**12-18, 1999

35. Taylor AS: Fracture dislocation of the neck. A method of treatment. **Arch Neurol Psychiatry 12:**625-627, 1924

36. Vinke TH: A skull-traction apparatus. **J Bone Joint Surg (Am) 30:**522-524, 1948

37. Walton GL: A new method of reducing dislocation of the cervical vertebrae. **J Nerv Ment Dis 20:**609-611, 1893

38. Waters RL, Adkins RH, Nelson R, et al: Cervical spinal cord trauma: evaluation and nonoperative treatment with halo-vest immobilization. **Contemp Orthop 14:** 35-45, 1987

39. Whitehill R, Richman JA, Glaser JA: Failure of immobilization of the cervical spine by the halo vest. **J Bone Joint Surg (Am) 68:**326-332, 1986

40. Yashon D, Tyson G, Vise WM: Rapid close reduction of cervical fracture dislocations. **Surg Neurol 4:** 513-514, 1975

CHAPTER 10

ANESTHESIA AND CRITICAL CARE MANAGEMENT OF SPINAL CORD INJURY

PERRY A. BALL, MD, RONALD E. CHICOINE, MD, AND ANDREW GETTINGER, MD

The airway, breathing, and circulation of the spinal cord injury (SCI) patient present unique challenges. This chapter focuses on the special considerations given to respiratory physiology, airway management, and circulatory support of SCI patients.

RESPIRATORY PHYSIOLOGY

The diaphragm is supplied by cervical nerve roots 3, 4, and 5. Injuries above C3 result in almost total respiratory paralysis, with patients requiring immediate ventilatory support for survival. Most frequently, patients with a cervical transection that leaves diaphragm function intact can initially ventilate effectively and may not require immediate intubation. These patients are often normocarbic but have some degree of hypoxia due to ventilation-perfusion mismatching, intrapulmonary shunting, or atelectasis.

In the acute phase, a patient with a cervical spinal cord injury (SCI) and intact diaphragm function has marked decrease in the vital capacity to about 25% of predicted value.[22] This is largely due to the paradoxical movement of the diaphragm and chest wall.[22,27,29,35,42] The negative intrathoracic pressure produced by diaphragm contraction causes the denervated flaccid chest wall to collapse, with the abdomen distending as the diaphragm compresses the abdominal contents. These patients cough poorly and have difficulty in clearing secretions. The resultant shallow breathing leads to a cascade of atelectasis and further reductions in forced vital capacity.

The decision regarding the need for intubation and mechanical ventilation needs to be individualized. Ominous signs include a rising respiratory rate, a rising PCO_2, a falling PO_2, or a forced vital capacity in the range of 15 cc/kg. It is often better to proceed with intubation under controlled circumstances than to wait until it is an emergent procedure. It should be kept in mind that while approximately one third of patients with cervical SCI will require mechanical ventilation at some point during the initial hospitalization,[9] the large majority of patients with injury levels of C4 and below can eventually be weaned from mechanical ventilation (Figure 1).

AIRWAY MANAGEMENT

Patients with acute cervical SCI require special precautions in the management of the airway: extension of the neck may result in further dam-

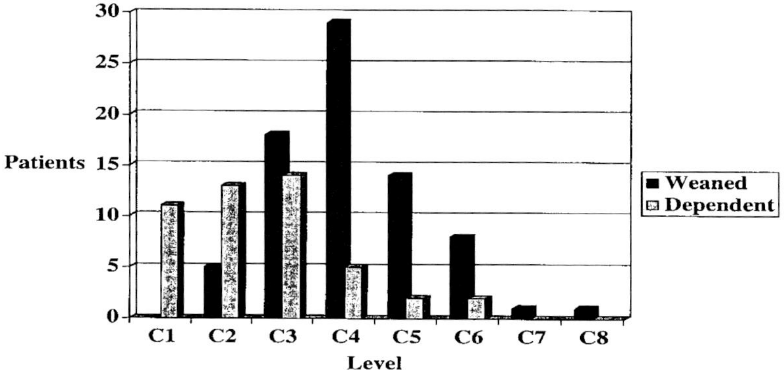

Figure 1: The number of patients with cervical cord injury who are ventilator-dependent vs. those who have been weaned from a ventilator at the time of discharge.

age to the spinal cord.[6,39,42,43] Alignment of the oral, pharyngeal, and laryngeal axes is more difficult than in patients without suspected spinal cord trauma (Figure 2A). Because the airway is harder to manage and intubating conditions are suboptimal, persons trained in handling this situation should be present, if possible. Various techniques are acceptable when attempting to intubate the larynx in patients who are spontaneously ventilating, but truly emergent intubations should be performed orally, utilizing cricoid pressure and manual in-line axial traction (Figure 2B). Regardless of the specific technique used to secure the airway, 100% oxygen should be administered via mask using a modified jaw-thrust technique (Figure 3) until laryngoscopy is performed and between attempts to intubate. All trauma patients should be considered to have a full stomach and be at risk for aspirating orogastric contents. Cricoid pressure should be applied when ventilating the patient and at any time in which the airway is unprotected.

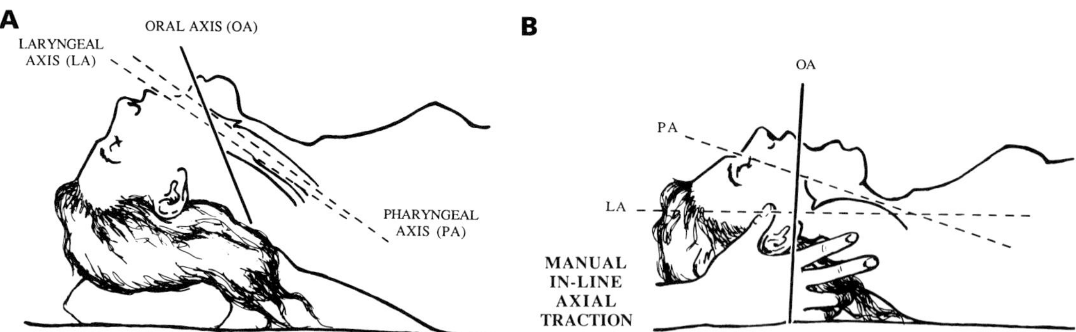

Figure 2: A) In patients without suspected SCI who require endotracheal intubation, the head and neck positioning can be optimized, allowing better alignment of the oral, pharyngeal, and laryngeal axes. **B)** In patients with suspected SCI, manual in-line axial traction is maintained throughout laryngoscopy and pillows are not used to elevate the head. Alignment of the three axes is not optimized, resulting in more difficult intubating conditions.

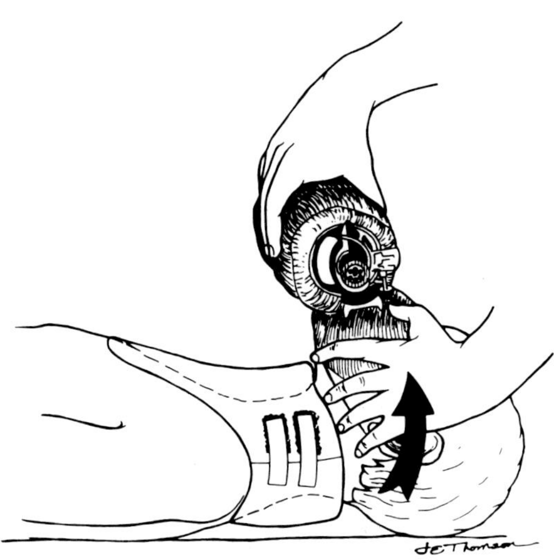

Figure 3: The modified jaw-thrust technique is performed with the cervical spine axis of the patient remaining neutral while the mandible is lifted toward the ceiling. This maneuver lifts the tongue out of the airway and allows for more effective mask ventilation without moving the neck.

Orotracheal Intubation

Oral intubation is a safe, feasible way to control the airway in suspected SCI patients.[12,16,39,43] Patients may be intubated when fully anesthetized, after sedation, or when fully awake. Careful intravenous titration of sedatives and analgesics is required to prevent precipitous drops in blood pressure, apnea, aspiration, and undesired change in the level of consciousness. Agents that allow for spontaneous ventilation and assist in support of blood pressure and heart rate, such as ketamine, may be useful in SCI patients. Ketamine is relatively contraindicated in patients with closed head injury because it increases cerebral blood flow and cerebral oxygen consumption. Although ketamine was once touted as an agent that kept airway reflexes intact, experience has shown that this is often not the case. In patients who cannot protect their airway and who are considered to have a full stomach, a rapid sequence induction with cricoid pressure should be performed. In all patients with suspected cervical SCI, manual in-line traction is maintained by an assistant while oral intubation is performed to prevent any further damage from extension of the neck. In a series reported from a major trauma center, no patient developed a change in spinal cord function after oral intubation using the manual in-line axial traction technique.[16]

Nasotracheal Intubation

Nasal intubation has the advantage that it can be performed with the patient breathing spontaneously and, thus, there is less risk of losing control of the airway. Topical anesthetics are usually all that is necessary to provide analgesia for the procedure. Because there may be less head and neck movement with nasal intubation, some authors prefer it over orotracheal intubation.[35]

Blind nasal intubations have a success rate of approximately 90%.[7,19] An appropriately sized nasal trumpet coated with a mixture of a local anesthetic agent and a vasoconstrictor is placed in the nares while the patient breathes spontaneously or is mask ventilated. The trumpet is then replaced with a well-lubricated endotracheal tube. While listening for breath sounds, the endotracheal tube is gently advanced into the trachea during inspiration when the vocal cords are abducted.

Fiberoptically guided nasotracheal intubation offers the advantage of direct visualization of the larynx without aligning the three axes described above. A lubricated endotracheal tube one size smaller than normally used for oral intubation is placed in the nares and into the nasopharynx. Atropine or glycopyrrolate are useful premedications as they aid in decreasing secretions that may obscure vision through the bronchoscope and may help prevent bradycardia associated with the parasympathetic stimulation from intubation. The bronchoscope is then placed through the endotracheal tube, the larynx is visualized, and the trachea is entered with the bronchoscope. Once the bronchoscope is in the trachea, the endotracheal tube is advanced over the bronchoscope until it is in the trachea, the cuff is inflated, and the bronchoscope removed. Insufflation of oxygen through the broncho-

1. Assess the likelihood and clinical impact of basic management problems:
   - A. Difficult Intubation
   - B. Difficult Ventilation
   - C. Difficulty with Patient Cooperation or Consent

2. Consider the relative merits and feasibility of basic management choices:
   - A. Non-Surgical Technique for Initial Approach to Intubation vs. Surgical Technique for Initial Approach to Intubation
   - B. Awake Intubation vs. Intubation Attempts After Induction of General Anesthesia
   - C. Preservation of Spontaneous Ventilation vs. Ablation of Spontaneous Ventilation

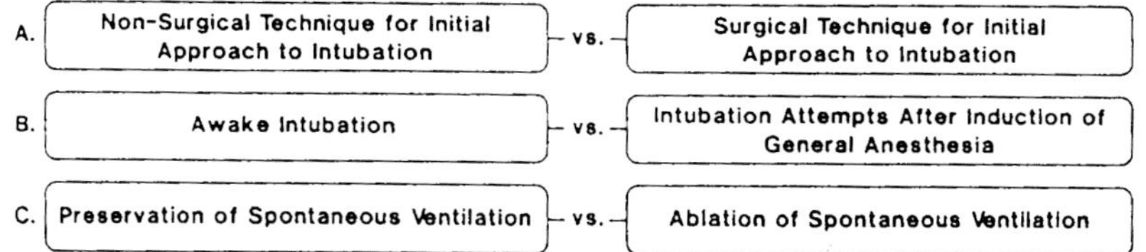

3. Develop primary and alternative strategies:

- CONFIRM INTUBATION WITH EXHALED CO_2

(a) Other options include (but are not limited to): surgery under mask anesthesia, surgery under local anesthesia infiltration or regional nerve blockade, or intubation attempts after induction of general anesthesia.

(b) Alternative approaches to difficult intubation include (but are not limited to): use of different laryngoscope blades, awake intubation, blind oral or nasal intubation, fiberoptic intubation, intubating stylet or tube changer, light wand, retrograde intubation, and surgical airway access.

(c) See awake intubation.

(d) Options for emergency non-surgical airway ventilation include (but are not limited to): transtracheal jet ventilation, laryngeal mask ventilation, or esophageal-tracheal combitube ventilation.

(e) Options for establishing a definitive airway include (but are not limited to): returning to awake state with spontaneous ventilation, tracheotomy, or endotracheal intubation.

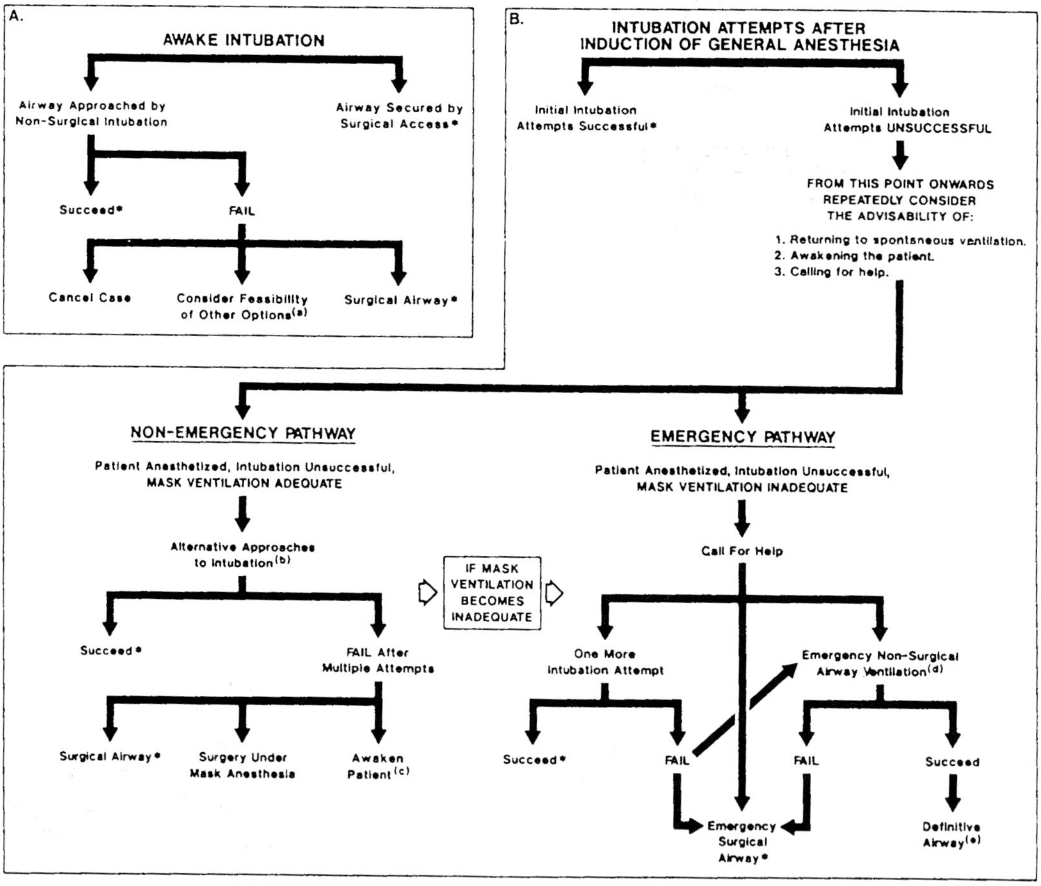

Figure 4: Difficult Airway Algorithm.
(Reprinted from the American Society of Anesthesiologists, with permission)

scope can augment oxygenation if the patient is ventilating spontaneously.

There are some drawbacks to nasotracheal intubation. The presence of midface injuries, sinusitis, and coagulopathies are contraindications. Nasotracheal intubation typically involves the use of a smaller diameter tube than is feasible with oral intubation, resulting in increased effort by the patient for breathing.

MUSCLE RELAXANTS

Occasionally, muscle relaxants are necessary to achieve intubation. Although they may make laryngoscopy technically easier by relaxing the jaw muscles, the patient will become apneic. The airway manager must be able to either intubate or mask ventilate the patient once neuromuscular block is achieved. Succinylcholine, a depolarizing neuromuscular blocker, offers the advantage of rapid onset of action (1 minute after intravenous administration) and short duration of action (3 to 5 minutes).[41] Due to its rapid onset, succinylcholine is the muscle relaxant of choice for the acute trauma patient who requires intubation. Succinylcholine should not be used in patients with SCIs of greater than 24 hours because of the potential for cardiac arrest. Succinylcholine may cause an exaggerated release of potassium in patients with SCI, beginning on approximately postinjury Day 4 and persisting for at least 3 to 6 months.[20,41] Cardiac arrest due to succinylcholine-induced hyperkalemia has been observed to occur as early as 7 days after SCI.[20] Peak release of potassium occurs when the injury is approximately 14 days old. The large amount of potassium released presumably reflects the proliferation of extra-junctional cholinergic receptors that are responsive to acetylcholine.

All of the nondepolarizing neuromuscular blockers are acceptable for the SCI patient, although neuromuscular blockers that induce histamine release (atracurium, curare, and mivacurium) may worsen hypotension. Pancuronium, with its sympathomimetic effects that increase blood pressure and heart rate, may be beneficial in patients with spinal shock who require muscle relaxation.

DIFFICULT AND SURGICAL AIRWAYS

Intubations that are difficult or impossible are not always predicted based on clinical criteria.[31] When SCI patients cannot undergo mask ventilation or translaryngeal intubation, other techniques need to be used to gain control of the airway. This situation is immediately life-threatening, and adequate contingency planning is crucial to prevent the adverse consequences of tissue hypoxia. The American Society of Anesthesiologists has developed a Difficult Airway Algorithm that can help guide decision-making (Figure 4).[1]

Laryngeal Mask Airway

The laryngeal mask airway is a device that consists of a tube to which an elliptical-shaped cuff resembling a miniature facemask is attached (Figure 5). General anesthesia is usually required for placement of this device, although obtunded or apneic patients are candidates if the airway cannot be secured by other means. The lubricated laryngeal mask airway is inserted blindly into the hypopharynx until it meets resistance. The cuff is inflated and, if in the proper position, forms a seal around the laryngeal perimeter. Positive-pressure ventilation is possible up to approximately 25 cm of water. This device has been used successfully in emergency situations when endotracheal intubation was impossible.[28]

The laryngeal mask airway does not protect against aspiration of gastric contents.[17] Addi-

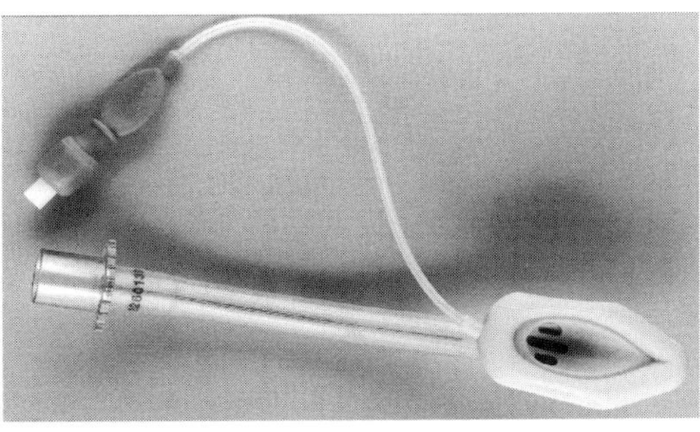

Figure 5: A laryngeal mask airway.

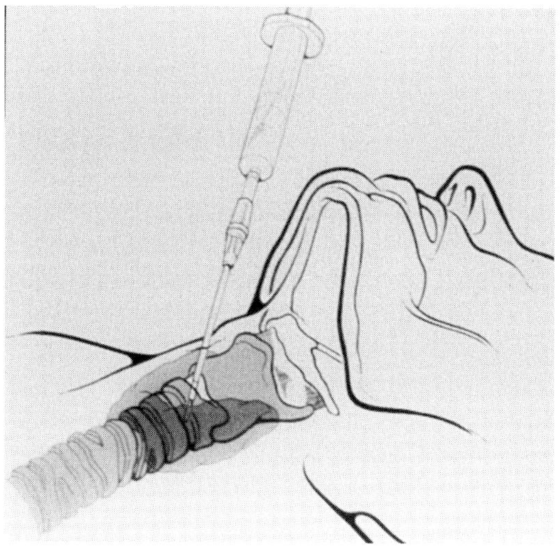

Figure 6: Needle cricothyroidotomy is performed through the cricothyroid membrane with a 14- or 16-gauge needle over the catheter followed by insufflation of 100% oxygen.

tional potential complications include laryngospasm and airway obstruction due to improper positioning of the device.[2,26]

Cricothyroidotomy

The American College of Surgeons[6] and others[25,34,45] support cricothyroidotomy as the standard surgical approach during emergencies when translaryngeal intubation is difficult, impossible, or contraindicated. The cricothyroidotomy can be an open procedure or performed percutaneously using the Seldinger technique.

Needle cricothyroidotomy can be performed by placing a large-bore intravenous catheter through the cricothyroid membrane. The patient is then oxygenated with insufflation of 100% oxygen (Figures 6 and 7). Although most patients can be oxygenated using this technique, ventilation is variable and a better airway should be established promptly.

Tracheostomy

Tracheostomy is less useful in the emergency setting due to the additional time needed to complete the procedure, but it is commonly used in the ventilatory management of the SCI patient. Controversy exists over the timing of conversion of translaryngeal intubation to tracheostomy. Proponents of early tracheostomy (<2 weeks after injury) state that tracheostomy offers better patient comfort, simplifies patient care, and decreases the risk of damage to the larynx.[4,8,45] Proponents of late tracheostomy (>2 weeks) argue that the procedure is risky and has a significant morbidity rate and a mortality rate

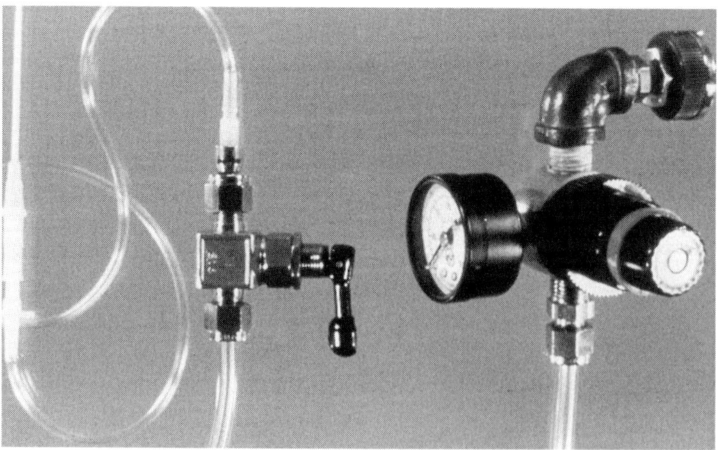

Figure 7: A jet ventilator can be attached to the cricothyroidotomy catheter and to wall oxygen. Insufflation is then performed until a more secure airway is established.

of 2% to 5%,[13,18,37] exposes the patient to unnecessary complications, promotes long-term tracheal damage, causes bacterial colonization of the airway, and prolongs intubation needlessly because of reluctance to discontinue a surgically placed airway.[3,8,38] The decision of when to place a tracheostomy should be individualized. For example, in patients who are able to be extubated in the near future, the risk of a surgically placed airway may outweigh the potential benefits of tracheostomy.

Because cervical stabilization is often performed through an anterior approach, a tracheostomy could hinder or delay definitive fixation due to concern about infection. One strategy is to separate the procedures by 2 weeks to allow healing of tissue planes.

An advantage of tracheostomy is that patients can be weaned from ventilatory support with a secure established airway. In this way, periods of spontaneous breathing can be alternated with periods of mechanical ventilatory assistance without repeated airway instrumentation. Tracheostomized patients also have slightly less "dead space" than those with a conventional endotracheal tube.

WEANING FROM VENTILATORY SUPPORT

Postural Dependence of Vital Capacity

A common belief is that patients with a cervical SCI are weaned from ventilatory support more quickly if early operative fixation allows them to sit up, thereby decreasing the abdominal pressure on the diaphragm.[21,35] This is not accurate in quadriplegic patients.[10,22,27] Early fixation may be beneficial for the management of secretions and pulmonary toilet, but patients should be placed in the supine position for weaning purposes. In a quadriplegic patient, the vital capacity increases when moved from the upright to the supine position.[10] In the upright position, the weakness of the abdominal muscles allows the diaphragm to passively descend, which overstretches its fibers. As a result, diaphragmatic contraction is less forceful. In the supine posi-

tion, the abdominal contents push the diaphragm cephalad into its normal position, allowing more forceful contraction. When the abdomen is tightly supported by binders, the postural dependence of vital capacity is lost.[27] Some investigators have documented vital capacity improvement in seated quadriplegic patients using abdominal binders, and suggest that the binders be used as adjuncts to breathing when a quadriplegic patient is mobilized.[15]

Ventilator Dependence and Weaning

Nearly all quadriplegic patients with intact diaphragm function should be able to be weaned from ventilatory support.[21-23,27,46] As the abdominal and thoracic muscles undergo reflex contraction and spasticity, the forced vital capacity increases. The chest wall, which initially collapses with negative intrathoracic pressure, becomes rigid and lung expansion improves (Figure 8). When the abdominal muscles become spastic, they facilitate expiration, in essence acting as an abdominal binder. The increase in forced vital capacity begins between 3 and 5 weeks postinjury and continues to rise until about 5 months postinjury, by which time it has approached 55% to 60% of the baseline predicted value.[22] Because pulmonary function improves slowly, weaning can be a lengthy process.[41]

Aggressive pulmonary toilet, the treatment of infections, and sufficient nutritional support should be maintained throughout the intensive care unit stay. Aggressive bronchial hygiene is of utmost importance regarding atelectasis and pneumonia prevention.[46] Changing the patient's position every few hours, deep-breathing exercises, incentive spirometry, chest percussion, and assisted coughing are strategies that should be used to prevent these complications.

Retention of secretions may be problematic. Intermittent positive-pressure breathing may be used (with or without bronchodilators) to help mobilize secretions. In patients with refractory lobar atelectasis, fiberoptic bronchoscopy and saline lavage for clearance of secretions are acceptable. An aggressive pulmonary toilet protocol improves survival in quadriplegic patients.[29]

No specific mode of weaning from ventilatory

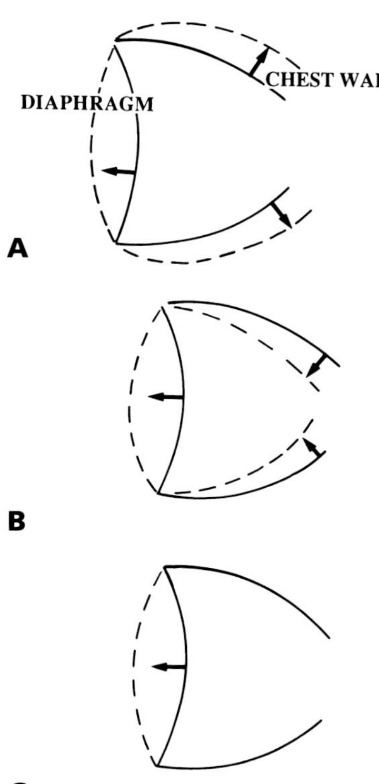

Figure 8: A) The normal patient has intact daphragmatic and chest wall excursions. **B)** The rcently injured quadriplegic patient with retained diaphragmatic function, has normal expansion of the diaphragm; the flaccid chest wall will collapse with negative inspiratory pressure and ventilation is impaired. **C)** At about 5 months after injury, when the chest wall muscle spasticity is complete, the chest no longer collapses with negative intrathoracic pressure and the forced vital capacity approaches 60% of predicted.

TABLE 1

LEVEL OF INJURY AND DISCHARGE VENTILATOR STATUS*

Level of Injury	Total Patients	No. Dependent	%	No. Weaned	%	No. Died
C1	13	11	85	0	0	2
C2	18	13	72	5	28	0
C3	35	14	40	18	51	3
C4	36	5	14	29	81	2
C5	18	2	11	14	78	2
C6	11	2	18	8	73	1
C7	2	0	0	1	50	1
C8	1	0	0	1	100	0
Total	134	47	35	76	57	11

*Adapted with permission from Wicks and Menter.[46]

support has proved to be superior.[11,14] Strategies that allow patients to do some of the work of breathing, without becoming fatigued, seem appropriate. The level of injury is of predictive value regarding weanability (Table 1). Patients with an SCI level of C4 or below have a high probability of ventilator weaning.[46]

MANAGEMENT OF SPINAL SHOCK

Patients who suffer from cervical spinal cord transection develop a condition known as spinal shock.[5,24,32,40] Spinal shock is caused by interruption of the sympathetic nervous system that arises from T1 to L2. Unopposed parasympathetic stimulation below the level of injury, along with a lack of sympathetic tone, leads to vascular pooling of blood, hypotension, and bradycardia.[27,35,42] The absence of sympathetic nervous system compensation makes these patients more likely to experience severe reductions in blood pressure in the presence of blood loss, changes in body position, and with the institution of positive-pressure ventilation.[35,42] In addition, the compensatory tachycardia that normally occurs in hypovolemic patients is not present.

SCI patients should be volume-resuscitated until blood pressure is adequate for tissue perfusion, with care taken to avoid volume overload. Fluid replacement can be guided by measurement of the central venous pressure (CVP), which, in patients with normal cardiac function, reflects left-ventricular filling pressure. In patients with pulmonary or cardiac disease, the CVP may not accurately reflect the left-sided filling pressures, and a pulmonary artery catheter may be needed for precise monitoring.[30,35,36] Accurate volume replacement is essential because the cardiac accelerators that emerge from the T1-4 spinal levels are interrupted in cervical spinal cord transection. This lack of innervation results in a decrease in cardiac chronotropy and inotropy. The myocardium may not be able to compensate for the increased work imposed by

TABLE 2

ACTIONS OF ADRENERGIC AGONISTS

Vasoactive Drug	Alpha 1	Alpha 2	Beta 1	Beta 2
Phenylephrine	+++++	?	+/-	0
Norepinephrine	+++++	+++++	+++	0
Dopamine	+ to +++++	?	++++	++
Epinephrine	+++++	+++	++++	++
Ephedrine	++	?	+++	++
Dobutamine	0 to +	?	++++	++
Isoproterenol	0	0	+++++	+++++

the excessive vascular volume, and heart failure may ensue.[27]

If patients have normal mental status, normal systemic pH, warm extremities, and good urine output, tissue perfusion is most likely adequate. If tissue perfusion does not appear adequate or refractory hypotension persists, alpha-adrenergic agonists and beta-adrenergic agonists may be required to support blood pressure and heart rate.[21,35]

Despite controversy over the use of pulmonary artery catheters to assist in the management of critically ill patients, catheters are helpful to determine the adequacy of perfusion in patients placed on adrenergic agonists.[30] For example, patients placed on phenylephrine or norepinephrine to support blood pressure may have a decrease in cardiac output (CO) secondary to increased cardiac afterload. This decrease in CO, even in the presence of adequate blood pressure, could be detrimental to tissue perfusion. Once a pulmonary artery catheter is inserted into patients being given alpha-adrenergic agents, the systemic vascular resistance should be calculated and maintained within the normal range (1200-1500 dynes/sec/cm^5 or less). Additional volume replacement can be administered as required to maintain the CO in the normal range (>2.5 liters/min/m^2). Vasoactive substances and their predominant effects are listed in Table 2.

In SCI patients in spinal shock, volume should first be employed until blood pressure is sufficient for organ perfusion. Once volume replacement is thought to be adequate, alpha-adrenergic agents are appropriate to support

blood pressure. The use of a pulmonary artery catheter may be helpful in assessing perfusion and CO in patients using alpha agents, and a catheter can document changes in the CO that result in the addition of beta-adrenergic agonists.

CONCLUSIONS

SCI patient management requires a thorough understanding of the physiology of spinal cord transection. Safe airway management, unique respiratory physiological changes, and the treatment of spinal shock are all important in the anesthetic and critical care management of SCI patients. Appropriate attention to these pathological changes is required to achieve a good outcome in these difficult-to-manage patients.

REFERENCES

1. American Society of Anesthesiologists Task Force on Management of the Difficult Airway: Practice guidelines for the management of the difficult airway. **Anesthesiology 78:**597-602, 1993
2. Brodrick PM, Webster NR, Nunn JF: The laryngeal mask airway. A study of 100 patients spontaneously breathing. **Anaesthesia 44:**238-241, 1989
3. Brooks R, Bartlet RH, Gazzaniga AB: Management of acute and chronic disorders of the trachea and subglottis. **Am J Surg 150:**24-31, 1985
4. Burns HP, Dayal VS, Scott A, et al: Laryngotracheal trauma: observations on its pathogenesis and its prevention following prolonged orotracheal intubation in the adult. **Laryngoscope 89:**1316-1325, 1979
5. Civetta JM, Gabel JC: Flow directed pulmonary artery catheterization in surgical patients: indications and

modifications of technic. **Ann Surg 176:**753-756, 1972

6. Collicot PA, Aprahamian C, Carrico CJ, et al: Upper airway management, in: **Advanced Trauma Life Support Course.** Chicago, Ill: American College of Surgeons, 1984, 155 pp

7. Danzl DF, Thomas DM: Nasotracheal intubations in the emergency department. **Crit Care Med 8:**677-682, 1980

8. Dayal VS, El Masri W: Tracheostomy in intensive care setting. **Laryngoscope 96:**58-60, 1986

9. DeVivo MJ, Rutt RD, Black KJ, et al: Trends in spinal cord injury demographics and treatment outcomes between 1973 and 1986. **Arch Phys Med Rehabil 73:**424-430, 1992

10. Estenne M, DeTroyer A: Mechanism of the postural dependence of vital capacity in tetraplegic subjects. **Am Rev Respir Dis 135:**367-371, 1987

11. Estenne M, DeTroyer A: Respiratory muscle involvement in tetraplegia. **Probl Respir Care 3:**360-374, 1990

12. Florette OG: Airway management, in Civetta JM, Taylor RW, Kirby RR (eds): **Critical Care. 2nd ed.** Philadelphia, Pa: JB Lippincott, 1992, pp 1419-1439

13. Frost EAM: Tracing the tracheostomy. **Ann Otol Rhinol 85:**618-624, 1976

14. Gardner BP, Watt JWH, Krishnan KR: The artificial ventilation of acute spinal cord damaged patients: a retrospective study of forty-four patients. **Paraplegia 24:**208-220, 1986

15. Goldman JM, Rose LS, Williams SJ, et al: Effect of abdominal binders on breathing in tetraplegic patients. **Thorax 41:**940-945, 1986

16. Grande CM, Barton CR, Stene JK: Appropriate techniques for airway management of emergency patients with suspected spinal cord injury. **Anesth Analg 67:**714-715, 1988 (Letter)

17. Griffin RM, Hatcher IS: Aspiration pneumonia and the laryngeal mask airway. **Anesthesia 45:**1039-1040, 1990

18. Heffner JE, Miller KS, Sahn SA: Tracheostomy in the intensive care unit. Part 2: Complications. **Chest 90:**430-436, 1986

19. IsersonKV: Blind nasotracheal intubation. **Ann Emerg Med 10:**468-471, 1981

20. John DA, Tobey RE, Homer LD: Onset of succinylcholine-induced hyperkalemia following denervation. **Anesthesiology 45:**294-299, 1976

21. Johnson GE: Spine injuries, in Hall JB, Schmidt GA, Wood LD (eds): **Principles of Critical Care.** New York, NY: McGraw-Hill, 1993, pp 715-726

22. Ledsome JR, Sharp JM: Pulmonary function in acute cervical cord injury. **Am Rev Respir Dis 124:**41-44, 1981

23. Lerman RM, Weiss MS: Progressive resistive exercise in weaning high quadriplegics from the ventilator. **Paraplegia 25:**130-135, 1987

24. Luce JM, Culver BH: Respiratory muscle function in health and disease. **Chest 81:**82-90, 1982

25. Mace SE: Cricothyrotomy. **J Emerg Med 6:**309-319, 1988

26. Maltby JR, Loken RG, Watson NC: The laryngeal mask airway: clinical appraisal in 250 patients. **Can J Anaesth 37:**509-513, 1990

27. Mansel JK, Norman JR: Respiratory complications and management of spinal cord injuries. **Chest 97:**1440-1452, 1990

28. McClune S, Regan M, Moore J: Laryngeal mask airway for caesarian section. **Anesthesia 45:**227-228, 1990

29. McMichan JC, Michel L, Westbrook PR: Pulmonary dysfunction following traumatic quadriplegia. Recognition, prevention and treatment. **JAMA 243:**528-531, 1980

30. Naylor CD, Sibbald WJ, Sprung CL, et al: Pulmonary artery catheterization: can there be an integrated strategy for guideline development and research promotion? **JAMA 269:**2407-2411, 1993

31. Norton ML, Brown ACD: **Atlas of the Difficult Airway.** St Louis, Mo: Mosby Year Book, 1991, pp 33-42

32. Osterholm JL Jr: The pathophysiological response to spinal cord injury. The current status of related research. **J Neurosurg 40:**5-33, 1974

33. Quimby CW, Williams RN, Greifenstein FE: Anesthetic problems of the acute quadriplegic patient. **Anesth Analg 52:**333-340, 1973

34. Roven AN, Clapham MC: Cricothyroidotomy. **Ear Nose Throat J 62:**489-493, 1983

35. Ruben BH, Greenberg J: Neurologic injury: prevention and initial care, in Civetta JM, Taylor RW, Kirby RR (eds): **Critical Care.** Philadelphia, Pa: JB Lippincott, 1992, pp 725-746

36. Samii K, Counseiller C, Viars P: Central venous pressure and pulmonary wedge pressure. A comparative study in anesthetized surgical patients. **Arch Surg 111:**1122-1125, 1976

37. Selecky PA: Tracheostomy: a review of present day indications, complications, and care. **Heart Lung 3:**272-282, 1974

38. Stauffer JL, Olsen DE, Petty TL: Complications and consequences of endotracheal intubation and tracheostomy. A prospective study of 150 critically ill adult patients. **Am J Med 70:**65-76, 1981

39. Stene JK: Anesthesia for critically ill trauma patients, in Siegel JH (ed): **Trauma: Emergency Surgery and Critical Care.** New York, NY: Churchill Livingstone, 1987

40. Stene JK, Grande CM: General anesthesia: management considerations in the trauma patient. **Crit Care Clin 6:**73-84, 1990

41. Stoelting RK: **Pharmacology and Physiology in Anesthetic Practice. 2nd ed.** Philadelphia, Pa: JB Lippincott, 1991, pp 172-225

42. Stoelting RK, Dierdorf SF, McCammon RL: **Anesthesia and Co-Existing Disease. 2nd ed.** New York, NY: Churchill-Livingstone, 1998, pp 263-254

43. **Upper Airway Management in Advanced Trauma Life Support.** Chicago, Ill: American College of Surgeons, Committee on Trauma, 1985

44. Walls RM: Cricothyroidotomy. **Emerg Med Clin North Am 6:**725-736, 1988

45. Whited RE: A prospective study of laryngotracheal sequelae in long-term intubation. **Laryngoscope 94:**367-377, 1984

46. Wicks AB, Menter RR: Long-term outlook in quadriplegic patients with initial ventilator dependency. **Chest 90:**406-410, 1986

CHAPTER 11

PATIENT SELECTION AND TIMING OF SURGICAL INTERVENTION

JAMES D. GUEST, MD, PHD, AND VOLKER K.H. SONNTAG, MD

> *"The brightest flashes in the world of thought are incomplete until they have proved to have their counterparts in the world of fact."* —John Tyndall

Arguments for the early or delayed surgical management of complete and incomplete spinal injuries were summarized based on the literature[66,91,120] as well as the authors' personal experience in the first edition of this book, in the chapter by Sonntag and Francis[97] entitled "Patient Selection and Timing of Surgery." The validity of these disparate arguments points out the continuing controversy among spinal surgeons regarding the safety of early surgical management and the ability of "early" surgery to influence neurological outcome, the incidence of complications, and the duration of hospitalization.

Since the publication of the first edition, there have been significant contributions to the literature on which these controversies are based. However, marked variation in opinion and practice remains,[52] and the optimal timing of surgical intervention is one of the most important unresolved questions in neurosurgery. We believe that early surgery can be performed safely in most cases and that surgical decompression can influence neurological recovery in some patients with spinal cord injury (SCI). Because there is currently no treatment that can restore lost spinal cord function, all reasonable efforts to preserve it seem justified.

This review discusses the currently accepted standards for the management of patients with SCI and vertebral trauma. Guidelines are provided for situations that have garnered a consensus. We believe that significant compression in association with an acute SCI should be considered an emergency. Because the efficacy and safety of acute surgical decompression are controversial, the evidence that early surgery is safe is summarized and the argument for early decompression is reviewed. It is not possible to describe all relevant studies in detail in a brief review, so we have focused on recent and key studies that illustrate findings with considerable support.

There is experimental evidence that the duration of spinal compression is related to neurological recovery.[21,29,31,35,53,99] There are also retrospective and anecdotal reports of unexpectedly favorable outcomes associated with clinically complete SCIs when decompression has been rapidly effected.[1,28,55] Nevertheless, controversy persists regarding the clinical issue of early surgical decompression after SCI. This concern is justified because a superior effect on neurological recovery has not been demonstrated in prospective and in many retrospective clinical studies assessing the efficacy of early (versus late) surgical decompression. Other studies have questioned the safety of this management strategy, and some have questioned whether surgery has any effect at all.[36,112] Because there has not been a satisfactory randomized prospective study of the efficacy of very early decompression (within 8 hours), no Class I clinical evidence exists.

Because significant recovery can be achieved if only a modest percentage of neurons and their processes survive, it is imperative that spinal injuries not be worsened by inappropriate therapy. The injured spinal cord is extremely vulnerable to exacerbation of insults.[18] Therefore, the onus is on surgeons who advocate early aggressive surgical management to establish the safety and efficacy of their treatments.

During the 1990s, evidence accumulated that early surgical decompression and stabilization can be performed safely, enable earlier mobilization, reduce complications, allow earlier entry to rehabilitation, and reduce hospital costs (see below). These findings have strengthened the argument for surgical intervention. Currently, the most promising experimental strategies in development require implementation during the acute injury phase. It is likely that these strategies will develop in concert with currently evolving techniques for surgical decompression and spinal stabilization.

MANAGEMENT OF SCI

The initial management of SCI is dictated by three general principles. First, further neurological injury should be prevented. Second, an optimum environment should be created for the recovery of spinal cord function to maximize the patient's return to functional independence. Finally, normal bony alignment should be achieved, compression relieved, the vertebral column stabilized, and the development of a late deformity prevented.

In terms of specific nonsurgical interventions, standard trauma resuscitation (airway, breathing, and circulation) should be instituted. Further neurological injury should be prevented by immobilization. Patients should be hemodynamically stabilized and maintained in a clinical environment where blood pressure can be closely monitored. Spinal shock is treated aggressively, with fluids and pressors as needed. All patients should receive methylprednisolone unless specifically contraindicated or the therapeutic window of 8 hours has been exceeded. The efficacy of this treatment has been established by Class I clinical evidence,[15,16] which, despite criticism,[80] has been widely accepted. Adequate diagnostic information is expeditiously obtained to classify the spinal cord, vertebral column, and associated injuries. Finally, closed anatomic reduction is achieved if possible.

Indications for Surgery

We advocate surgical decompression, fixation, or both in hemodynamically stable patients with acceptable systemic risk factors and the following indications. The first indication is the presence of an irreducible anatomic compressive lesion at the cervical, thoracolumbar, or lumbar level associated with a neurological deficit, particularly if the deficit is incomplete or progressing. We favor acute decompression of even complete injuries at these levels unless a magnetic resonance (MR) imaging study shows that the spinal cord is transected or severe hemorrhagic maceration is present.

Neurological deterioration after attempts at reduction is another indication. The third indication is vertebral instability that can be optimally managed by surgery, such as those associated with compressive lesions, predominantly ligamentous injuries, patients at a high risk for developing complications from prolonged recumbency, and those with a significant risk of malunion or nonunion. The need for multiple procedures and associated multiple trauma are also indications.

Several other conditions in the acute period

are controversial indications for surgical management: 1) a neurologically complete injury of the thoracic spinal cord with ongoing compression but a stable vertebral column; 2) anatomically stable incomplete neurological injury associated with modest degrees of compression (e.g., 25% of spinal canal compromised); and 3) the presence of a central SCI (see below) associated with stable cervical spondylosis.

Absolute contraindications to surgery include hemodynamic instability and/or insufficient resuscitation, severe head injury, and insufficient radiological information to classify injury. MR imaging evidence of transection or severe hemorrhagic maceration is a relative contraindication.

Hemodynamic Management of Acutely Injured Patients

In SCI, the autoregulation of blood flow is disturbed in the injured region. Spinal cord perfusion may be compromised if the systemic blood pressure is insufficient. The potential for surgical decompression to influence neurological recovery is contingent on optimal nonsurgical measures to enhance survival of the spinal cord. Experimental studies by Tator and others have shown a trauma dose-dependent decrease in spinal cord blood flow (SCBF), disturbed autoregulation,[96] and increased SCBF in response to therapy.[48,57,103,108] At least one study[34] has shown that volume expansion and pressors can increase SCBF and another[18] that somatosensory evoked potentials (SSEPs) can be improved by raising blood pressure during compression.

Vale et al[105] conducted a prospective uncontrolled study of the influence of an aggressive management strategy that included maintaining mean arterial pressure (MAP) >85 mm Hg for 7 days on neurological outcome. They employed volume and pressor support in combination with methylprednisolone, rapid closed reduction, and surgery when indicated. This strategy derived some support from clinical evidence that cerebral perfusion pressure during the acute phase of injury is an independent prognostic variable after severe closed head injuries.[92] Currently, there is no feasible method to correlate the SCBF in the injured human spinal cord with MAP; therefore,

any apparent positive effects do not necessarily directly correlate with the elevated MAP. Of 10 patients with a complete cervical SCI, four presented with established neurogenic shock and nine required both volume resuscitation and inotropes to maintain the MAP >85 mm Hg. Approximately one third of the patients with a complete thoracic SCI required pressor support and volume resuscitation.

Using this overall strategy, the extent of recovery significantly exceeded previously reported values.[65,109-111,113] More than 50% of the patients with complete cervical injuries and a third of those with thoracic injuries regained one or more grades on the American Spinal Injury Association (ASIA) scale. However, at a 1-year follow-up, none of the four patients with severe neurogenic shock had recovered neurological function and no patient with a complete injury above T9 had regained function. We believe that these clinical observations are consistent with the experimental literature and that, pending more definitive studies, all patients with acute SCI should undergo hemodynamic monitoring and volume-pressure support as needed. This support is particularly important during general anesthesia.

PROGNOSTIC FACTORS ASSOCIATED WITH ACUTE SCI

The severity of SCI varies significantly. Some patients sustain such severe primary injuries that all traversing axons are destroyed;[19] the long tracts cannot recover even with surgical decompression. Therefore, it would be helpful if prognostic indicators existed to guide the decision to undertake acute surgical management, particularly "urgent" surgical decompression. Several factors are considered to influence the potential for neurological recovery.

A careful neurological examination remains the most reliable predictor of the potential for neurological recovery and the most useful instrument for classifying injuries.[65] The occurrence of severe spinal shock in the presence of a complete cervical injury may indicate a massive primary anatomic injury with minimal potential for distal recovery.[55]

MR imaging definitely increases prognostic ability. Mascalchi et al[76] reviewed the MR imaging appearance of injured cervical spinal cords and found that no patient with low-intensity intramedullary signals (suggestive of hemorrhage) on T2-weighted images had shown significant clinical improvement. Ramón et al[86] obtained similar findings. Yamashita et al[121] found that the most important predictive factors for neurological recovery were the degree and extent of extrinsic spinal cord compression. In the presence of marked compression, intramedullary changes may be difficult to interpret.

Visualization of spinal cord compression is better on MR imaging than on computed tomography (CT). In a recent review for STASCIS (Surgical Treatment of Acute Spinal Cord Injury Study),[46] some patients with less than 25% narrowing of the spinal canal on CT were found to have spinal cord compression on MR imaging. A significant incidence of acute disc herniation is associated with cervical vertebral trauma.[38,42] The STASCIS pilot study II identified an incidence of 38%.[81]

Patient age is another factor that appears to be related to prognosis. Alander et al[2] correlated neurological outcome after complete cervical SCI with age and found that patients older than 50 years had a significantly worse prognosis for neurological recovery and survival than did younger patients. It is now accepted that subclinical function exists in some patients with chronic SCI that appears clinically complete. Electric potentials recorded across lesion sites demonstrate the presence of intact axons.[32] Unfortunately, neither motor evoked potentials (MEPs) nor SSEPs have proved to be more sensitive prognosticators of acute SCI than a proper clinical examination.[70] However, they may be of value in unconscious or uncooperative patients.

We believe that patients with an acute SCI whose MR images show persistent compression but no transection or significant intramedullary hemorrhage should be considered for urgent surgical decompression. There has been no information published about the impact of spinal cord hemorrhage on segmental or root recovery after decompression, but such recovery can most likely be obtained following later decompression.

ARGUMENTS FOR EARLY SURGERY

Safety of Early Surgery

Evidence for spontaneous deterioration during the first 72 hours postinjury has been discussed by Young and Dexter[122] and Herbison et al.[60] In the study by Herbison et al, losses in segmental motor power were recovered in the ensuing 6 months.

Several studies have questioned the safety of surgery during the acute phase of SCI,[41,45,58,74,75,106] citing an increased risk of neurological deterioration. The specific reasons for deterioration associated with early surgery have included an increased risk of blood loss, hemodynamic instability due to the presence of other injuries, and the vulnerability of the acutely swollen spinal cord to manipulation.

In a study by Marshall et al,[75] 5% of patients deteriorated, predominantly in association with treatment including surgery. Farmer et al[45] retrospectively reviewed 1031 SCI patients and found a 1.8% incidence of neurological deterioration. In that study, 40% of the patients deteriorated after surgery within 5 days of injury; in contrast, no patient deteriorated if surgery had been performed 5 or more days after injury. However, a 7.5% rate of spontaneous postinjury deterioration following incomplete cervical SCI has been observed in a series of conservatively managed patients.[64] Furthermore, a reduction by traction of cervical injuries is also associated with significant risk of neurological deterioration.[101] Our experience supports a 1% to 2% incidence of neurological deterioration.

Guttman[54] and Frankel et al[51] argued that postural reduction is safer than surgery following cervical spine injuries, and this philosophy dominated for several years. Frequently, however, traction reduction fails to achieve adequate decompression.[55,119] Other studies have challenged whether surgical procedures for decompression have any significant effect on neurological outcome.[36,37,112] These authors suggest that early surgery is not justified if it does not improve neurological recovery and if it is associated with increased risks.

Do these observations dictate a conservative attitude toward acute surgery? We believe that early surgery can be performed safely because, in the past two decades, there has been significant improvement in the level of pre-hospital care, pharmacological, systemic, and anesthetic management, intraoperative monitoring, diagnostic imaging, and techniques of decompression and instrumentation.

The following recent studies have shown that the risk of neurological injury is no greater in patients undergoing early surgery than in those undergoing delayed surgery in appropriately selected patients.[1,20,40,55,67,68,79,90,100,104,116,119] Cooper[26] pointed out that many of the original studies in which it was suggested that early surgery was unsafe employed laminectomy, which could not effect meaningful decompression and may even worsen the effect of anterior lesions. Furthermore, nonoperative management frequently fails to achieve alignment and stability and may lead to progressive deformity and increasing neurological deficits. We believe that early surgery should be performed only by experienced spinal surgeons and neuroanesthesiologists supported by expert intensive care facilities. We monitor SSEPs, MEPs, or both when operating on patients with incomplete SCI.

Early Surgery Reduces Complications

Delayed surgery may require prolonged immobilization, which can lead to increased complications such as pneumonia, decubiti, deep venous thrombosis, and pulmonary emboli. Several studies have examined the impact of surgery within the first 24 to 72 hours after SCI on the incidence of complications. Studies by Wilberger[116] and McBroom et al[79] have shown a significant decrease in complications in patients who undergo early surgery. Studies by Tator et al,[100,102] Levi et al,[68] and Campagnolo et al[20] have shown a decreased length of hospital stay and earlier mobilization. In these studies, early surgery was not associated with an increase in neurological or other complications. Studies by Fellrath et al[49] and Vaccaro et al[104] have suggested that overall hospitalization costs are reduced. Willén[117] found that the ability to reconstruct the sagittal diameter of the spinal canal is better if surgery is performed within 3 days of surgery.

Can Early Surgery Be Achieved?

Extrapolation from recent clinical trials using methylprednisolone (NASCIS 2 and 3)[15,16] and from several experimental studies (see below) led to the concept that the potential time for surgical decompression to influence secondary injury is limited to a period of a few hours after the injury. This "window of opportunity" has been estimated to be 8 hours or less. It is often difficult to achieve decompression within this time, particularly if the patient requires transfer from a triage facility to a Level 1 trauma center. This issue has been evaluated by the STASCIS group (pilot study 2) using a surgical window of 8 hours. Only a minority of the eligible patients underwent decompression within 8 hours.[81] The STASCIS study protocol requires MR imaging or CT myelography prior to closed decompression or surgery, and it can be difficult to obtain these studies rapidly in some centers.

A large randomized controlled trial in France is studying the impact of surgical decompression plus the N-methyl-D-aspartate antagonist gangcyclidine (or control) on SCI. Of approximately 200 patients who have been randomized, 86% underwent surgical decompression, stabilization, or both—one half of the study population within 8 hours (unpublished data). This remarkable achievement has involved organizing 26 centers into the study protocol and developing a national system of rapid trauma transfers. The STASCIS trial is needed to determine if access to imaging and spinal surgery should be organized to make decompression in less than 8 hours more universally possible. The study itself may be difficult to complete, however, unless these resources are more widely available.

CAN DECOMPRESSION SALVAGE NEUROLOGICAL FUNCTION?

It is currently accepted that many neurological functions are retained if even a fraction of normal axons are intact; there appears to be a threshold minimum number.[47,118] The goal of combining pharmacological and surgical treatment of SCI is to salvage this minimally sufficient fraction of axons to permit recovery, particularly in long-tract injuries.

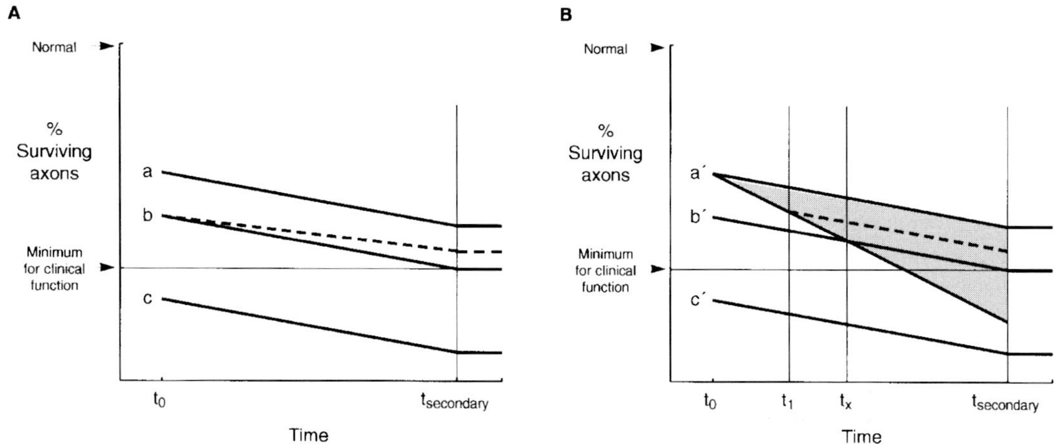

Figure 1: Theoretical basis of the concept that rapid spinal decompression may preserve neuronal function. **A)** Primary and secondary injuries without compression. Three magnitudes of primary injury are illustrated. Injuries *a* and *b* have a severity that could allow recovery while *c* is a primary injury of such severity that spontaneous recovery is impossible. All injuries are assumed to be followed by a secondary injury, shown here with a constant slope for simplicity. Because of increased axonal loss due to secondary injury, *b* will eventually cross the threshold for recovery of clinical function obviating recovery. The *dotted line* illustrates hypothetical attenuation of secondary injury to an extent that permits recovery of some function. **B)** Primary and secondary injuries with compression. Injury *a'* is now followed by a secondary injury with a steeper slope *(shaded region)* representing the exacerbation of secondary injury by compression. At t_x the injury will cross the secondary injury line for *b'* which, even without compression, crosses the threshold; decompression must be effected before this point. The *dotted line* illustrates the putative effect of decompression at t_1 on the slope of the secondary injury. Clinically, of course, it is difficult to separate those with anatomically complete primary injury *(c')* from those with a potentially significant anatomic preservation *(a', b')*. Patients with some preserved sensory or motor function with clear evidence of ongoing spinal cord compression after optimal closed reduction and stabilization are clearly those who fit the model at point *a'* and should be considered for urgent decompression.

The injury process has been conceptualized as an initial impact-mediated primary injury and a subsequent secondary injury (Figure 1). The magnitude of the secondary injury can be influenced by pharmacological agents that attenuate key molecular cascades,[4] and low blood pressure, hypoxia, and compression may worsen this injury.[18] Some primary injuries are overwhelming, effectively transecting the spinal cord.[19] In others, a smaller primary injury is significantly extended during the phase of secondary injury.[44,82] Because it has been difficult to accurately model human primary and secondary injuries, we do not know the extent to which the magnitude of the secondary injury is influenced by compression.

Experimental Evidence

Using a clip compression injury, Guha et al[53] concluded that the major determinant of the magnitude of an injury (and thus the potential for recovery) was the amount of force applied by the initial clip compression. The length of time until decompression also affected recovery, but only for animals injured with smaller compression forces.

Several other studies have demonstrated an association between the duration of a compressive injury and the potential for neurological recovery.[35,84,89,99] The hypothesis has been that spinal cord compression represents an ischemic injury that becomes irreversible after a period of time. Recent studies employing acutely delivered sustained compression have validated the premise that compression-related deficits are time dependent. Using a circumferential band-compression model, Delamarter et al[29] demonstrated complete recovery of SSEPs after 1 hour of compression despite moderate histological changes. After 6 hours of the same degree of compression, no meaningful recovery occurred.

Carlson et al[21] examined the relative contribution of mechanical and vascular factors to compression injury, and some of their findings challenge views that we previously held. After a precisely delivered and sustained noncontusive compression, the initially high interface pressure diminished markedly within 5 minutes but SSEPs did not recover. SSEPs recovered if decompression was effected at 60 minutes but not after 3 hours, even though SCBF recovered in all animals after decompression. Unexpectedly, the residual SCBF under compression was higher in the animals that did not recover. These animals also had smaller interface pressures. The authors concluded that residual blood flow during compression might cause an ischemic reperfusion-like injury, a concept supported by stroke literature.[88]

These studies have not actually modeled the effects of acute contusion followed by sustained compression but rather those of uniform compression. Contusive SCI is associated with progressive deterioration of local SCBF even without ongoing compression.[103] It remains unknown to what extent such postcontusion SCBF is affected by the added presence of compression.

A recent study by Dimar et al[31] employed a spinal cord impact injury model[5] followed by static compressive loads for relevant durations. Using this model, the authors determined that decompression was associated with improved recovery in a time-dependent fashion.

Additional experimental studies that accurately model contusive SCI with ongoing compression are required to determine if relief of compression at clinically relevant time points results in superior histological and functional outcomes, particularly of long-tract function. It would be valuable to determine if the duration of decompression windows can be increased by pharmacotherapy directed at secondary injury or by elevating MAP.

Appropriate Timing of Decompression: Correlation With Observations From NASCIS 2 and 3

The foregoing experimental studies demonstrated the existence of a window for spinal cord decompression. The therapeutic window derived from the NASCIS 2 and 3 pharmacological clinical studies is 8 hours. Several authors have extrapolated this observation to predict the time limit for efficacy of surgical decompression. This extrapolation requires the reasonable but unsubstantiated assumption that spinal compression exacerbates similar destructive processes to those attenuated by methylprednisolone. It is also possible that the use of methylprednisolone could extend the window for effective decompression. Young and Flam[123] demonstrated that high-dose methylprednisolone significantly improved SCBF after contusive SCI, but others have not reproduced this finding.[93]

The NASCIS 2 study demonstrated that methylprednisolone must be given within 8 hours of injury to have a beneficial effect on neurological recovery. This finding validated previous laboratory studies, which have shown that secondary injury can be attenuated by drugs such as methylprednisolone if they are administered soon after injury.[56] A further important review of NASCIS data revealed that in most instances, the recovery occurred below the level of the lesion and could be attributed more to preservation of long-tract function than to segmental function.[14]

Although compression can create injury by causing ischemia, it can injure the spinal cord by other mechanisms, including demyelination, apoptosis,[69] and the breakdown of the blood-brain barrier.[62] The time dependence of these effects is unknown, but they may be partly responsible for the benefits associated with delayed decompression.

Clinical Evidence

The following forms of clinical recovery after SCI have been described: root recovery,[7] segmental recovery in the zone of partial preservation,[33] and long-tract recovery.[10]

Unless studies employ randomization, it is difficult to determine if the degree of observed neurological recovery is spontaneous or attributable to an intervention such as surgical decompression. Several longitudinal studies have demonstrated that patients with any preserved function as defined by ASIA (sacral-sparing) have significant potential for recovery.[65] A greater potential for functional recovery is possible after a complete cervical injury than after a thoracic injury because the recovery of adjacent cervical roots below the level of injury can significantly improve clinical function.

Studies by Waters et al[109-111,113] and Katoh et al[64] have clarified the expected outcome for complete and incomplete cervical and thoracolumbar SCI. These studies provide a useful baseline against which to assess therapeutic interventions that appear to improve outcomes. No more than 10% of patients with initial complete motor and sensory quadriplegia recover any lower-extremity motor function. Some studies have indicated that approximately 3% of patients with initially complete motor and sensory injuries eventually ambulate.[120]

The ability to demonstrate a difference between groups that undergo different treatments depends on the sensitivity of the assessment methods. Motor assessment based on the ASIA scale is very reproducible in complete SCI.[25] However, this outcome measure may be insensitive to potentially significant changes and lead to Type II errors. While changes in manual muscle testing grades are clinically relevant, the change from Grade 3 to Grade 4 requires recovery of a disproportionately large number of motor neurons.[3] That is, the progress from Grades 1 to 5 does not represent recovery of uniform increments of functioning neurons. The handheld myometer can reliably detect more subtle improvements.[59]

Chronic Spinal Cord Compression

Recovery of neurological function after surgery for chronic spinal compression has been reported by several authors. The potential mechanisms for such recovery include remyelination and improved conduction in spinal roots, spinal cord tracts, recovery of the blood-brain barrier, and improved blood flow.

Benzel and Larson[6,8] documented clinical evidence that decompression of thoracolumbar and cervical fractures associated with spinal cord compression in patients with partial SCI could lead to significant improvement in neurological function. Some patients with only sensory function prior to surgery recovered long-tract motor

function. After decompression of complete cervical injuries, recovery was noted in nerve roots but not long tracts. Timing of decompression was not observed to affect the degree of recovery. These authors advocated allowing patients with incomplete injury to plateau before surgical intervention.

Similar observations have been reported by Maiman et al,[71,72] Horsey et al,[61] Stauffer,[98] Bohlman,[9] Bohlman and Anderson,[10] and Kaneda et al.[63] Bohlman and Anderson performed anterior decompression, stabilization, or both in 55 patients and observed long-tract neurological improvement in patients with incomplete injuries up to 12 months after injury. The authors advocated surgery for ongoing compression but suggested that delayed surgery offered equivalent benefits to acute surgery.

Acute Spinal Cord Decompression

The effect of acute spinal cord decompression on neurological recovery has the smallest body of substantive evidence. The most compelling evidence relates to numerous anecdotal cases of unexpectedly good neurological outcomes after early decompression was achieved with closed reduction or early surgery, particularly in patients who initially appeared to have a complete SCI but also in cases of severe incomplete injury.[1,22,27,28,39,55,90]

In the study by Aebi et al,[1] closed decompression within 6 hours of injury was associated with superior neurological outcomes. The neurological outcomes of patients undergoing surgical treatment in the NASCIS 2 study apparently were superior in those who underwent surgery within 25 hours or after 200 hours.[40] Wiberg and Hauge[115] also found that no postoperative neurological deterioration occurred if surgery was performed before 24 hours or after 7 days. These findings support the reasonable hypothesis that spinal cord edema and swelling, and hence, vulnerability to re-injury, is maximal during the first few days after injury.

Clohisy et al[24] and Krengel et al[67] retrospectively reviewed their experience with decompression of incomplete thoracolumbar spinal injury. They found that surgery within 48 hours of injury was safe and associated with a significantly better rate of neurological recovery.

Clinical Evidence That Neurological Outcome Following Early Spinal Cord Decompression is Not Superior to Delayed Decompression

Several studies, three of which are prospective, failed to determine that early surgery leads to improved neurological outcomes. Levi et al[68] conducted a nonrandomized prospective study of the effect of anterior decompression on outcome either before or after 24 hours. Whereas early surgery was associated with more rapid mobilization, easier patient care, and easier transfer to rehabilitation, it did not improve neurological outcome for patients with either complete or incomplete injuries. Vale et al[105] utilized the previously described intensive management protocol but found that patients treated surgically within 24 hours had similar neurological outcomes to those treated later.

Some studies found small but nonsignificant differences between early and delayed surgery. In 1997 Vaccaro et al[104] published a randomized prospective trial that compared the influence of surgical timing on several variables including neurological outcome. This study was conducted at one center and enrolled a relatively small number of patients with cervical SCI. Frankel grades and ASIA motor scores were used as outcome measures. All patients apparently received steroids within 8 hours but did not undergo closed reduction. All patients randomized to surgery had radiographically documented spinal cord compression. Surgery was undertaken either within 72 hours or after 5 days (mean 1.8 vs. 16.8 days). The data concerning the 34 early and 28 late patients were not segregated according to completeness of injury. Thus, there were large variations from the mean motor scores. The authors concluded that "there is no significant benefit in terms of neurologic or functional level in patients treated less than 72 hours, as opposed to those treated greater than 5 days."

This study illustrates the limitations of a small prospective study that reaches a negative conclusion. The authors' data did show higher ASIA motor scores (at last follow-up) for pa-tients who underwent early surgery. However, because of the large standard deviations, a much larger sample would be needed to demonstrate a statistically significant effect.

An important component of the design of randomized prospective trials is an estimate of sample size. This estimate is based on the smallest meaningful clinical difference to be detected, the acceptable alpha and beta errors, and the magnitude of the anticipated standard deviation. In the case of the study by Vaccaro et al,[104] the difference in the mean ASIA motor scores of the two groups at last follow-up was 9.8. If alpha is set at 0.05 and beta at 0.01, the estimated sample size needed to reach statistical significance is 280 patients per group. The actual sample size and standard deviations only permit a significant difference to be reached if the mean motor scores differed by 30 or greater. In the NASCIS 2 study,[15] 333 patients were randomized to either a methylprednisolone or a control group. At 6 months, a difference in ASIA scores of 6.3 achieved statistical significance (i.e., a smaller difference than in the study by Vaccaro et al).

The study by Wagner and Chehrazi[107] also illustrates this problem. The percentage of the potential neurological improvement derived from a 10-point scale were compared in groups undergoing decompression within 8 hours or 8 to 48 hours after SCI with persistent compression. No difference was found between the two groups. The treatment algorithm was pertinent to the current STASCIS study, although methylprednisolone had not yet become standard therapy. The difference in the neurological outcomes between the early and late treatment groups was 6%, but the standard deviations were 37%. This difference would only become significant with a sample size of 800. With their actual sample size of 44, the difference in percent neurological recovery would have to be 35% to reach significance. Thus, small studies have limited power to confirm small but potentially meaningful differences.

Other retrospective studies that have found no differences in neurological outcome between early or late surgical treatment include those by Bötel et al,[13] Wolf et al,[119] Dickson et al,[30] Epstein et al,[43] McAfee et al,[78] Weinshel et al,[114] and Petit-jean et al.[85] Maiman et al,[71] reviewed the outcome of their management strategy for neurologically complete and incomplete patients with bilateral locked facets and found no differences in neurological outcomes after early or late surgery. The study by Wagner and Chehrazi[107] is the only study that specifically examined the effect of surgery within 8 hours.

Some retrospective studies have determined that surgery (as compared to conservative management) has no clear impact on neurological outcome.[58,77,87,112] These studies included patients with complete and incomplete injuries and vary substantially in the timing of their determination of baseline neurological function (e.g., some studies used entry to rehabilitation as baseline) and the timing of surgery.

The current literature provides support for both conservative and aggressive treatment. Evidence that decompressive surgery can improve neurological function is substantial, but evidence that the timing of such surgery is important remains anecdotal. A large randomized prospective trial is needed to address more thoroughly the issue of surgical timing. The STAS-CIS pilot study has been designed to permit a significant difference to be detected with a unilateral ASIA motor score difference of 5 points. The sample size is estimated at about 160 patients per group.

Incomplete SCI: Central Cord Syndrome

The timing of surgery for incomplete SCIs has been controversial. After a cervical injury, the central cord syndrome is the most commonly observed pattern of incomplete injury. In 1954 Schneider et al[95] described the syndrome and advocated nonoperative management since most patients experience some degree of spontaneous recovery. Others such as Norell and Wilson,[83] who advocated early surgery for other injuries, believed that central cord syndrome unassociated with fracture or dislocation constituted "an absolute contraindication to operative intervention." However, Bosch et al[11] observed that many patients with central cord syndrome eventually develop worsening spasticity and deteriorating motor function. They characterized this myelopathic pattern as a "chronic central cord syndrome."

Brodkey et al[17] were also dissatisfied with the long-term outcome of patients with central cord syndrome. They performed surgical decompression on seven patients with compression visualized on myelography who subsequently improved rapidly and concluded that ongoing compression caused chronic central cord syndrome. In a retrospective review of the neurological outcome of surgically and conservatively treated patients, Bose et al[12] found that surgery improved outcome. Other studies have obtained similar conclusions.[50,73,94]

In a stable incomplete SCI, there is a risk of worsening the neurological deficit by performing inappropriate surgery. Patients with radiological compression whose neurological status worsens should undergo decompression. Patients with instability, particularly those with primarily ligamentous injury, are best managed surgically. In the past several years, we have practiced aggressive surgical intervention in patients with central cord injuries. We believe that patients with central cord injury with ongoing spinal compression from a fracture or disc herniation should undergo surgical decompression within 24 hours. Our approach to patients with a central cord injury and significant spinal stenosis is to perform an appropriate decompressive procedure soon after injury.[23] This decision is individualized. We treat all such patients with halo orthosis immobilization to reduce the potential for microtrauma and follow their neurological examination closely.

We do not immediately operate on patients who are showing a good rate of spontaneous neurological recovery. Patients who are not improving or who plateau early undergo what we consider the most appropriate anterior or posterior decompressive surgical procedure. The goal of this approach is to reduce the incidence of the chronic central cord syndrome. Frequently, this decompression is followed by renewed neurological improvement.

Conclusion

The large volume of literature on which this review is based does not support a rigid perspective on patient selection or timing of surgery after SCI. The important progress in this decade has been the consistent demonstration that early surgery can be performed safely and that it may reduce complications, facilitate early rehabilitation, and reduce the costs of care. We have attempted to develop a rational and consistent approach based these studies and the belief that the injuries of some patients (as seen in Figure 1B) can benefit substantially from early decompression. Like others, we have anecdotal clinical evidence of the validity of this approach and are frustrated by the persistent gap between what has been observed experimentally and what has been achievable clinically. We support the protocol designed by the STASCIS investigators and believe that this randomized study is essential to clarifying this clinical issue.

REFERENCES

1. Aebi M, Mohler J, Zäch GA, et al: Indication, surgical technique, and results of 100 surgically-treated fractures and fracture-dislocations of the cervical spine. **Clin Orthop 203:**244-257, 1986
2. Alander DH, Parker J, Stauffer ES: Intermediate-term outcome of cervical spinal cord-injured patients older than 50 years of age. **Spine 22:**1189-1192, 1997
3. Beasley WC: Quantitative muscle testing: principles and applications to research and clinical services. **Arch Phys Med Rehab 42:**398-425, 1961
4. Behrmann DL, Bresnahan JC, Beattie MS: Modeling of acute spinal cord injury in the rat: neuroprotection and enhanced recovery with methylprednisolone, U-74006F and YM-14673. **Exp Neurol 126:**61-75, 1994
5. Behrmann DL, Bresnahan JC, Beattie MS, et al: Spinal cord injury produced by consistent mechanical displacement of the cord in rats: behavioral and histologic analysis. **J Neurotrauma 9:**197-217, 1992
6. Benzel EC, Larson SJ: Functional recovery after decompressive operation for thoracic and lumbar spine fractures. **Neurosurgery 19:**772-778, 1986
7. Benzel EC, Larson SJ: Functional recovery after decompressive spine operation for cervical spine fractures. **Neurosurgery 20:**742-746, 1987
8. Benzel EC, Larson SJ: Recovery of nerve root function after complete quadriplegia from cervical spine fractures. **Neurosurgery 19:**809-812, 1986
9. Bohlman HH: Acute fractures and dislocations of the cervical spine. An analysis of three hundred hospitalized patients and review of the literature. **J Bone Joint Surg (Am) 61:**1119-1142, 1979
10. Bohlman HH, Anderson PA: Anterior decompression and arthrodesis of the cervical spine: long-term motor improvement. Part I—Improvement in incomplete traumatic quadriparesis. **J Bone Joint Surg (Am) 74:**671-682, 1992
11. Bosch A, Stauffer ES, Nickel VL: Incomplete traumatic quadriplegia. A ten-year review. **JAMA 216:**473-478, 1971
12. Bose B, Northrup BE, Osterholm JL, et al: Reanalysis of central cervical cord injury management. **Neurosurgery 15:**367-372, 1984
13. Bötel U, Gläser E, Niedeggen A: The surgical treatment of acute spinal paralysed patients. **Spinal Cord 35:**420-428, 1997
14. Bracken MB, Holford TR: Effects of timing of methylprednisolone or naloxone administration on recovery of segmental and long-tract neurological function in NASCIS 2. **J Neurosurg 79:**500-507, 1993
15. Bracken MB, Shepard MJ, Collins WF, et al: A randomized, controlled trial of methylprednisolone or naloxone in the treatment of acute spinal-cord injury. Results of the Second National Acute Spinal Cord Injury Study. **N Engl J Med 322:**1405-1411, 1990
16. Bracken MB, Shepard MJ, Holford TR, et al: Administration of methylprednisolone for 24 or 48 hours or tirilazad mesylate for 48 hours in the treatment of acute spinal cord injury. Results of the Third National Acute Spinal Cord Injury Randomized Controlled Trial. **JAMA 277:**1597-1604, 1997
17. Brodkey JS, Miller CF Jr, Harmody RM: The syndrome of acute central cervical spinal cord injury revisited. **Surg Neurol 14:**251-257, 1980
18. Brodkey JS, Richards DE, Blasingame JP, et al: Reversible spinal cord trauma in cats. Additive effects of direct pressure and ischemia. **J Neurosurg 37:**591-593, 1972
19. Bunge RP, Puckett WR, Becerra JL, et al: Observations on the pathology of human spinal cord injury. A review and classification of 22 new cases with details from a case of chronic cord compression with extensive focal demyelination. **Adv Neurol 59:**75-89, 1993
20. Campagnolo DI, Esquieres RE, Kopacz KJ: Effect of timing of stabilization on length of stay and medical complications following spinal cord injury. **J Spinal Cord Med 20:**331-334, 1997
21. Carlson GD, Minato Y, Okada A, et al: Early time-dependent decompression for spinal cord injury: vascular mechanisms of recovery. **J Neurotrauma 14:**951-962, 1997
22. Carol M, Ducker TB, Byrnes DP: Minimyelogram in cervical spinal cord trauma. **Neurosurgery 7:**219-224, 1980
23. Chen TY, Dickman CA, Eleraky M, et al: The role of decompression for acute incomplete cervical spinal cord injury in cervical spondylosis. **Spine 23:**2398-2403, 1998
24. Clohisy JC, Akbarnia BA, Bucholz RD, et al: Neurologic recovery associated with anterior decompression of spinal fractures at the thoracolumbar junction (T12-L1). **Spine 17 (Suppl 8):**S325-S330, 1992
25. Cohen ME, Ditunno JF Jr, Donovan WH, et al: A test of the 1992 International Standards for Neurological and Functional Classification of Spinal Cord Injury. **Spinal Cord 36:**554-560, 1998
26. Cooper PR: Injuries of the cervical spinal cord, in Clark CR (ed): **The Cervical Spine.** Philadelphia, Pa: Lippincott-Raven, 1998, pp 551-555
27. Cotler HB, Miller LS, DeLucia FA, et al: Closed reduction of cervical spine dislocations. **Clin Orthop 214:**185-199, 1987
28. Cotler JM, Herbison GJ, Nasuti JF, et al: Closed reduction of traumatic cervical spine dislocation using traction weights up to 140 pounds. **Spine 18:**386-390, 1993
29. Delamarter RB, Sherman J, Carr JB: Pathophysiology

of spinal cord injury. Recovery after immediate and delayed decompression. **J Bone Joint Surg (Am)** 77:1042-1049, 1995

30. Dickson JH, Harrington PR, Erwin WD: Results of reduction and stabilization of the severely fractured thoracic and lumbar spine. **J Bone Joint Surg (Am)** 60:799-805, 1978

31. Dimar JR, II, Glassman SD, Raque GH, et al: The influence of spinal canal narrowing and timing of decompression on neurologic recovery after spinal cord contusion in a rat model. **Spine** 24:1623-1633, 1999

32. Dimitrijevic MR, Dimitrijevic MM, Faganel J, et al: Suprasegmentally induced motor unit activity in paralyzed muscles of patients with established spinal cord injury. **Ann Neurol** 16:216-221, 1984

33. Ditunno JF Jr, Sipski ML, Posuniak EA, et al: Wrist extensor recovery in traumatic quadriplegia. **Arch Phys Med Rehabil** 68:287-290, 1987

34. Dolan EJ, Tator CH: The effect of blood transfusion, dopamine, and gamma hydroxybutyrate on posttraumatic ischemia of the spinal cord. **J Neurosurg** 56:350-358, 1982

35. Dolan EJ, Tator CH, Endrenyi L: The value of decompression for acute experimental spinal cord compression injury. **J Neurosurg** 53:749-755, 1980

36. Donovan WH: Operative and nonoperative management of spinal cord injury. A review. **Paraplegia** 32:375-388, 1994

37. Donovan WH, Cifu DX, Schotte DE: Neurological and skeletal outcomes in 113 patients with closed injuries to the cervical spinal cord. **Paraplegia** 30:533-542, 1992

38. Doran SE, Papadopoulos SM, Ducker TB, et al: Magnetic resonance imaging documentation of coexistent traumatic locked facets of the cervical spine and disc herniation. **J Neurosurg** 79:341-345, 1993

39. Ducker TB, Bellegarrigue R, Salcman M, et al: Timing of operative care in cervical spinal cord injury. **Spine** 9:525-531, 1984

40. Duh MS, Shepard MJ, Wilberger JE, et al: The effectiveness of surgery on the treatment of acute spinal cord injury and its relation to pharmacological treatment. **Neurosurgery** 35:240-249, 1994

41. Edwards CC, Levine AM: Early rod-sleeve stabilization of the injured thoracic and lumbar spine. **Orthop Clin North Am** 17:121-145, 1986

42. Eismont FJ, Arena MJ, Green BA: Extrusion of an intervertebral disc associated with traumatic subluxation or dislocation of cervical facets. Case report. **J Bone Joint Surg (Am)** 73:1555-1560, 1991

43. Epstein N, Speilholz N, Benjamin MV, et al: Evaluation of 200 patients with spinal cord injuries admitted to the NYU. Presented at the 47th Annual Meeting of the American Association of Neurological Surgeons, Los Angeles, California, 1979, p 128 (Abstract)

44. Falconer JC, Narayana PA, Bhattacharjee M, et al: Characterization of an experimental spinal cord injury model using waveform and morphometric analysis. **Spine** 21:104-112, 1996

45. Farmer J, Vaccaro A, Albert TJ, et al: Neurologic deterioration after cervical spinal cord injury. **J Spinal Disord** 11:192-196, 1998

46. Fehlings MG, Rao SC, Tator CH, et al: The optimal radiologic method to assessing spinal canal compromise and cord compression in patients with cervical spinal cord injury. Part II: Results of a multi-center study. **Spine** 24:605-613, 1999

47. Fehlings MG, Tator CH: The relationships among the severity of spinal cord injury, residual neurological function, axon counts, and counts of retrogradely labeled neurons after experimental spinal cord injury. **Exp Neurol** 132:220-228, 1995

48. Fehlings MG, Tator CH, Linden RD: The effect of nimodipine and dextran on axonal function and blood flow following experimental spinal cord injury. **J Neurosurg** 71:403-416, 1989

49. Fellrath RF Jr, Bohren B, Hanley EN Jr: Spinal injury and polytrauma: influence of surgical timing. **Orthopaedic Trauma Assoc** 19:149, 1995

50. Fox JL, Wener L, Drennan DC, et al: Central spinal cord injury: magnetic resonance imaging confirmation and operative considerations. **Neurosurgery** 22:340-347, 1988

51. Frankel HL, Hancock DO, Hyslop G, et al: The value of postural reduction in the initial management of closed injuries of the spine with paraplegia and tetraplegia. I. **Paraplegia** 7:179-192, 1969

52. Glaser JA, Jaworski BA, Cuddy BG, et al: Variation in surgical opinion regarding management of selected cervical spine injuries. A preliminary study. **Spine** 23:975-983, 1998

53. Guha A, Tator CH, Endrenyi L, et al: Decompression of the spinal cord improves recovery after acute experimental spinal cord compression injury. **Paraplegia** 25:324-339, 1987

54. Guttman L: Initial treatment of traumatic paraplegia and tetraplegia, in Harris P (ed): **Spinal Injuries Symposium.** Edinburgh: Morrison and Gibb, 1963, pp 80-92

55. Hadley MN, Fitzpatrick BC, Sonntag VKH, et al: Facet fracture-dislocation injuries of the cervical spine. **Neurosurgery** 30:661-666, 1992

56. Hall ED, Braughler JM: Effects of intravenous methylprednisolone on spinal cord lipid peroxidation and Na^+K^+-ATPase activity. Dose-response analysis during 1st hour after contusion injury in the cat. **J Neurosurg** 57:247-253, 1982

57. Hall ED, Yonkers PA, Horan KL, et al: Correlation between attenuation of posttraumatic spinal cord ischemia and preservation of tissue vitamin E by the 21-aminosteroid U74006F: evidence for an *in vivo* antioxidant mechanism. **J Neurotrauma** 6:169-176, 1989 (Abstract)

58. Heiden JS, Weiss MH, Rosenberg AW, et al: Management of cervical spinal cord trauma in Southern California. **J Neurosurg** 43:732-736, 1975

59. Herbison GJ, Isaac Z, Cohen ME, et al: Strength post-spinal cord injury: myometer vs manual muscle test. **Spinal Cord** 34:543-548, 1996

60. Herbison GJ, Zerby SA, Cohen ME, et al: Motor power differences within the first two weeks post-SCI in cervical spinal cord-injured quadriplegic subjects. **J Neurotrauma** 9:373-380, 1992

61. Horsey WJ, Tucker WS, Hudson AR, et al: Experience with early anterior operation in acute injuries of the cervical spine. **Paraplegia** 15:110-122, 1977

62. Jaeger CB, Blight AR: Spinal cord compression injury in guinea pigs: structural changes of endothelium and its perivascular cell associations after blood-brain barrier breakdown and repair. **Exp Neurol** 144:381-399, 1997

63. Kaneda K, Taneichi H, Abumi K, et al: Anterior decompression and stabilization with the Kaneda device for thoracolumbar burst fractures associated with neurological deficits. **J Bone Joint Surg (Am)** 79:69-83, 1997

64. Katoh S, El Masry WS, Jaffray D, et al: Neurologic outcome in conservatively treated patients with incomplete closed traumatic cervical spinal cord injuries. **Spine** 21:2345-2351, 1996

65. Kirshblum SC, O'Connor KC: Predicting neurologic recovery in traumatic cervical spinal cord injury. **Arch Phys Med Rehabil** 79:1456-1466, 1998

66. Kramer DL, Albert TJ: The spinal cord and its reaction to traumatic injury: implications for the timing of surgical intervention, in Capen DA, Haye W (eds): **Comprehensive Management of Spine Trauma.** St Louis, Mo: CV Mosby, 1998, pp 345-349

67. Krengel WF III, Anderson PA, Henley MB: Early stabilization and decompression for incomplete paraplegia due to a thoracic-level spinal cord injury. **Spine** 18:2080-2087, 1993

68. Levi L, Wolf A, Rigamonti D, et al: anterior decompression in cervical spine trauma: Does the timing of surgery affect the outcome? **Neurosurgery** 29: 216-222, 1991

69. Li GL, Brodin G, Farooque M, et al: Apoptosis and expression of Bcl-2 after compression trauma to rat spinal cord. **J Neuropathol Exp Neurol** 55:280-289, 1996

70. Macdonell RAL, Donnan GA: Magnetic cortical stimulation in acute spinal cord injury. **Neurology** 45: 303-306, 1995

71. Maiman DJ, Barolat G, Larson SJ: Management of bilateral locked facets of the cervical spine. **Neurosurgery** 18:542-547, 1986

72. Maiman DJ, Larson SJ, Benzel EC: Neurological improvement associated with late decompression of the thoracolumbar spinal cord. **Neurosurgery** 14: 302-307, 1984

73. Maroon JC, Abla AA, Wilberger JI, et al: Central cord syndrome. **Clin Neurosurg** 37:612-621, 1991

74. Marshall L, Garfin S: Incidence and causes of neurologic deterioration following spinal cord injury, in Peipmeier JM (ed): **The Outcome Following Traumatic Spinal Cord Injury.** Mt Kisco, NY: Futura, 1992, pp 13-130

75. Marshall LF, Knowlton S, Garfin SR, et al: Deterioration following spinal cord injury. A multicenter study. **J Neurosurg** 66:400-404, 1987

76. Mascalchi M, Dal Pozzo G, Dini C, et al: Acute spinal trauma: prognostic value of MRI appearances at 0.5 T. **Clin Radiol** 48:100-108, 1993

77. Maynard FM, Reynolds GG, Fountain S, et al: Neurological prognosis after traumatic quadriplegia. Three-year experience of California Regional Spinal Cord Injury Care System. **J Neurosurg** 50:611-616, 1979

78. McAfee PC, Bohlman HH, Yuan HA: Anterior decompression of traumatic thoracolumbar fractures with incomplete neurological deficit using a retroperitoneal approach. **J Bone Joint Surg (Am)** 67:89-104, 1985

79. McBroom R, Tucker W, Waddell J: Early versus delayed fixation of the thoraco-lumbar spine in polytrauma patients. **Orthop Trans** 19:149, 1995

80. Nesathurai S: Steroids and spinal cord injury: revisiting the NASCIS 2 and NASCIS 3 trials. **J Trauma** 45:1088-1093, 1998

81. Ng WP, Fehlings MG, Cuddy B, et al: Surgical treatment for acute spinal cord injury study pilot study #2: evaluation of protocol for decompressive surgery within 8 hours of injury. **Neurosurg Focus**

82. Noble LJ, Wrathall JR: Correlative analyses of lesion development and functional status after graded spinal cord contusive injuries in the rat. **Exp Neurol** 103: 34-40, 1989

83. Norrell H, Wilson CB: Early anterior fusion for injuries of the cervical portion of the spine. **JAMA** 214:525-530, 1970

84. Nyström B, Berglund JE: Spinal cord restitution following compression injuries in rats. **Acta Neurol Scand** 78:467-472, 1988

85. Petitjean ME, Mousselard H, Pointillart V, et al: Thoracic spinal trauma and associated injuries: should early spinal decompression be considered? **J Trauma** 39:368-372, 1995

86. Ramón S, Domínguez R, Ramírez L, et al: Clinical and magnetic resonance imaging correlation in acute spinal cord injury. **Spinal Cord** 35:664-673, 1997

87. Raynor RB: Severe injuries of the cervical spine treated by early anterior interbody fusion and ambulation. **J Neurosurg** 28:311-316, 1968

88. Rehncrona S, Mela L, Siesjö BK: Recovery of brain mitochondrial function in the rat after complete and incomplete cerebral ischemia. **Stroke** 10:437-446, 1979

89. Rivlin AS, Tator CH: Effect of duration of acute spinal cord compression in a new acute cord injury model in the rat. **Surg Neurol** 10:39-43, 1978

90. Rizzolo SJ, Vaccaro AR, Cotler JM: Cervical spine trauma. **Spine** 19:2288-2298, 1994

91. Rosenfeld JF, Vaccaro AR, Albert TJ, et al: The benefits of early decompression in cervical spinal cord injury. **Am J Orthop** 27:23-28, 1998

92. Rosner MJ, Rosner SD, Johnson AH: Cerebral perfusion pressure: management protocol and clinical results. **J Neurosurg** 83:949-962, 1995

93. Ross IB, Tator CH: Spinal cord blood flow and evoked potential responses after treatment with nimodipine or methylprednisolone in spinal cord–injured rats. **Neurosurgery** 33:470-477, 1993

94. Roth EJ, Lawler MH, Yarkony GM: Traumatic central cord syndrome: clinical features and functional outcomes. **Arch Phys Med Rehabil** 71:18-23, 1990

95. Schneider RC, Cherry G, Pantek H: The syndrome of acute central cervical spinal cord injury. With special reference to the mechanisms involved in hyperextension injuries of cervical spine. **J Neurosurg** 11: 546-577, 1954

96. Senter HJ, Venes JL: Loss of autoregulation and posttraumatic ischemia following experimental spinal cord trauma. **J Neurosurg** 50:198-206, 1979

97. Sonntag VKH, Francis PM: Patient selection and timing of surgery, in Benzel EC, Tator CH (eds): **Contemporary Management of Spinal Cord Injury.** Park Ridge, Ill: American Association of Neurological Surgeons, 1994, pp 97-108

98. Stauffer ES: Neurologic recovery following injuries to the cervical spinal cord and nerve roots. **Spine** 9: 532-534, 1984

99. Tarlov IM, Klinger H: Spinal cord compression studies. II. Time limits for recovery after acute compression in dogs. **Arch Neurol Psychiatry** 71:271-290, 1954

100. Tator CH, Duncan EG, Edmonds VE, et al: Comparison of surgical and conservative management in 208 patients with acute spinal cord injury. **Can J Neurol Sci 14:**60-69, 1987

101. Tator CH, Duncan EG, Edmonds VE, et al: Complications and costs of management of acute spinal cord injury. **Paraplegia 31:**700-714, 1993

102. Tator CH, Fehlings M, Thorpe K, et al: Current use and timing of spinal surgery for management of acute spinal cord injury in North America: results of a retrospective multicenter study. **Neurosurg Focus 91 (Spine Suppl 1):**12-18, 1999

103. Tator CH, Fehlings MG: Review of the secondary injury theory of acute spinal cord trauma with emphasis on vascular mechanisms. **J Neurosurg 75:**15-26, 1991

104. Vaccaro AR, Daugherty RJ, Sheehan TP, et al: Neurologic outcome of early *versus* late surgery for cervical spinal cord injury. **Spine 22:**2609-2613, 1997

105. Vale FL, Burns J, Jackson AB, et al: Combined medical and surgical treatment after acute spinal cord injury: results of a prospective pilot study to assess the merits of aggressive medical resuscitation and blood pressure management. **J Neurosurg 87:**239-246, 1997

106. Verbiest H: Anterior operative approach in cases of spinal-cord compression by old irreducible displacement or fresh fracture of cervical spine. Contribution to operative repair of deformed vertebral bodies. **J Neurosurg 19:**389-400, 1962

107. Wagner FC Jr, Chehrazi B: Early decompression and neurological outcome in acute cervical spinal cord injuries. **J Neurosurg 56:**699-705, 1982

108. Wallace MC, Tator CH: Successful improvement of blood pressure, cardiac output, and spinal cord blood flow after experimental spinal cord injury. **Neurosurgery 20:**710-715, 1987

109. Waters RL, Adkins RH, Yakura JS, et al: Effect of surgery on motor recovery following traumatic spinal cord injury. **Spinal Cord 34:**188-192, 1996

110. Waters RL, Adkins RH, Yakura JS, et al: Motor and sensory recovery following complete tetraplegia. **Arch Phys Med Rehabil 74:**242-247, 1993

111. Waters RL, Adkins RH, Yakura JS, et al: Motor and sensory recovery following incomplete paraplegia. **Arch Phys Med Rehabil 75:**67-72, 1994

112. Waters RL, Adkins RH, Yakura JS, et al: Motor and sensory recovery following incomplete tetraplegia. **Arch Phys Med Rehabil 75:**306-311, 1994

113. Waters RL, Yakura JS, Adkins RH, et al: Recovery following complete paraplegia. **Arch Phys Med Rehabil 73:**784-789, 1992

114. Weinshel SS, Maiman DJ, Baek P, et al: Neurologic recovery in quadriplegia following operative treatment. **J Spinal Disord 3:**244-249, 1990

115. Wiberg J, Hauge HN: Neurological outcome after surgery for thoracic and lumbar spine injuries. **Acta Neurochir 91:**106-112, 1988

116. Wilberger JE: Diagnosis and management of spinal cord trauma. **J Neurotrauma 8 (Suppl 1):**S21-S30, 1991

117. Willén J, Lindahl S, Irstam L, et al: Unstable thoracolumbar fractures. A study by CT and conventional roentgenology of the reduction effect of Harrington instrumentation. **Spine 9:**214-219, 1984

118. Windle WF, Smart JO, Beers JJ: Residual function after subtotal spinal cord transection in adult cats. **Neurology 8:**518-521, 1958

119. Wolf A, Levi L, Mirvis S, et al: Operative management of bilateral facet dislocation. **J Neurosurg 75:**883-890, 1991

120. Wolf A, Wilberger JE Jr: Timing of surgical intervention after spinal cord injury, in Narayan RK, Wilberger JE Jr, Povlishock JT (eds): **Neurotrauma.** New York, NY: McGraw-Hill, 1996, pp 1193-1199

121. Yamashita Y, Takahashi M, Matsuno Y, et al: Acute spinal cord injury: magnetic resonance imaging correlated with myelopathy. **Br J Radiol 64:**201-209, 1991

122. Young JS, Dexter WR: Neurological recovery distal to the zone of injury in 172 cases of closed, traumatic spinal cord injury. **Paraplegia 16:**39-49, 1978

123. Young W, Flamm ES: Effect of high-dose corticosteroid therapy on blood flow, evoked potentials, and extracellular calcium in experimental spinal injury. **J Neurosurg 57:**667-673, 1982

CHAPTER 12

SURGICAL TECHNIQUES: CRANIOCERVICAL FIXATION AND STABILIZATION

DAVID PETERSON, BSC, FRCS, AND H. ALAN CROCKARD, FRCS

The atlanto-occipital and atlantoaxial joints form a complex articulation whose freedom of movement inherently predisposes to destabilizing injury. As with injury elsewhere, the principles of anatomic reduction, adequate stabilization, and early mobilization apply. A number of additional factors, however, must be considered:

- Craniocervical injuries are frequently associated with compression of the high cervical spinal cord or brain stem, or with threatened compression due to instability. Decompression is a treatment priority that may be achieved most simply by vertebral alignment restoration. This may be difficult to achieve due to the complexity of the normal anatomy, which is often considerably distorted by the original injury.
- Most current techniques of surgical stabilization limit the normal mobility of the craniovertebral junction by fixation and fusion of more vertebral levels than are injured. The ultimate goal of surgical management should be to restore stability without extensive fixation in order to preserve movement.
- The role of soft-tissue injury is frequently underestimated in craniocervical injury. Ligament interposition is almost always responsi-

ble for difficult reduction or fusion failure. Even with perfect osseous realignment, ligament damage permits movements that may compromise the neuraxis, either in a sudden devastating manner or by repeated minor impacts.

- Malunion of craniocervical junction fractures affect the biomechanics of the area, and late complications may arise where stress loading is excessive. The atlas is a ring structure with inward beveled articular surfaces interposed between the head and the vertebral column. If the atlas ring is disrupted, the weight of the head will force the lateral masses outward with subluxation of the atlanto-occipital and atlantoaxial joints.
- Injuries in adults and children differ due to anatomic differences and the relatively greater mass of a child's head.[1] Because the articular surfaces are flatter in children, in association with ligamentous laxity, it is more likely that rotational or subluxation and dislocation injuries will occur. In addition, children may survive injuries (such as atlanto-occipital dislocation) that are fatal in adults. The distribution of injuries, therefore, is different in pediatric practice. In terms of management, early reduction is essential in children. For many, surgery will not be necessary. However,

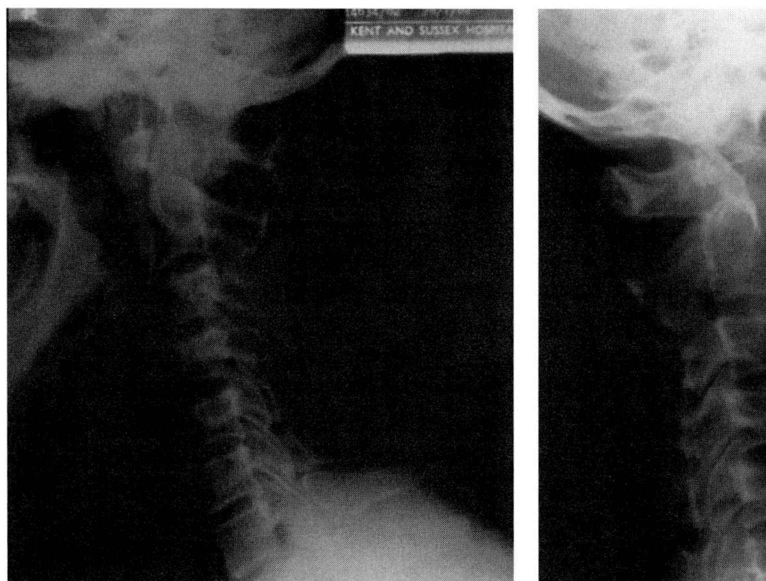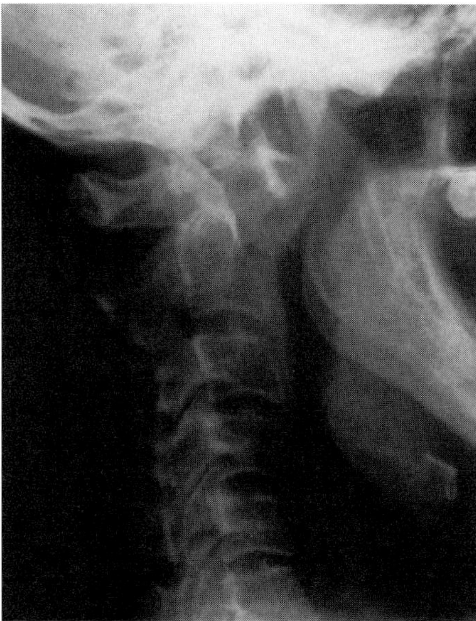

Figure 1: Plain lateral radiographs taken in extension *(left)* and flexion *(right)*. Atlantoaxial subluxiation is clearly seen using dynamic imaging.

when surgery is undertaken, the future growth of the epiphyses must be considered when contemplating fixation and fusion.

GENERAL PRINCIPLES OF INVESTIGATION AND MANAGEMENT

Investigation

Modern techniques of dynamic imaging have advanced the understanding of craniocervical anatomy, biomechanics, mechanisms of injury, and the role of soft-tissue components. In addition, they lead to more accurate assessment of craniocervical injury.

Plain radiograph cervical spine examination is an important first-line investigation for craniocervical trauma. Further information regarding upper cervical spine stability is obtained with supervised flexion and extension views of the area in question. Although much is gained from these static views, screening of the moving cervical spine under fluoroscopy is recommended to obtain a dynamic view of the injured area (Figure 1).

Computed tomography (CT) provides useful detail on the extent of bony injury (Figure 2). Imaging of the neuraxis is obtained increasingly by magnetic resonance imaging (MRI) rather than contrast injection techniques, and important information is provided concerning ligaments and the presence or absence of neuraxial contusion (Figure 3). As with plain radiographs, functional images can be acquired in flexion and extension. In terms of follow-up, it is desirable that the instrumentation chosen for fixation is compatible with MRI.[4]

Management

The first stage in the treatment of craniocervical fracture or dislocation is reduction. Although manipulation under anesthesia may be required, reduction is more commonly achieved by skull traction. This may be adjusted to provide flexion or extension and the traction weight altered as necessary. Overdistraction is an under-recognized complication of cervical traction and

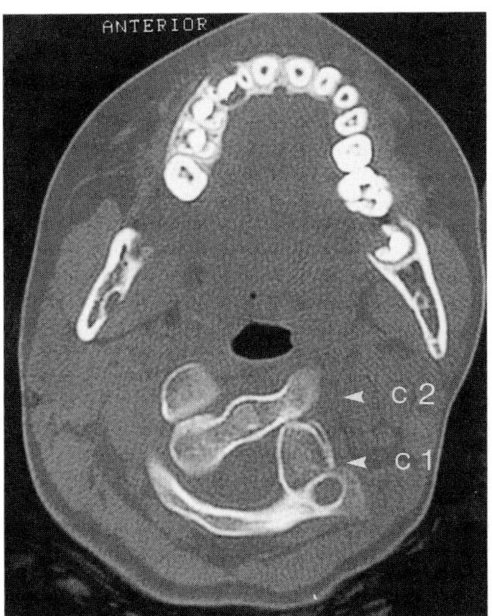

Figure 2: CT scan through the C1-2 junction illustrating a case of atlantoaxial rotatory dislocation. Valuable information is gained regarding bony alignment and the likely position of the vertebral arteries.

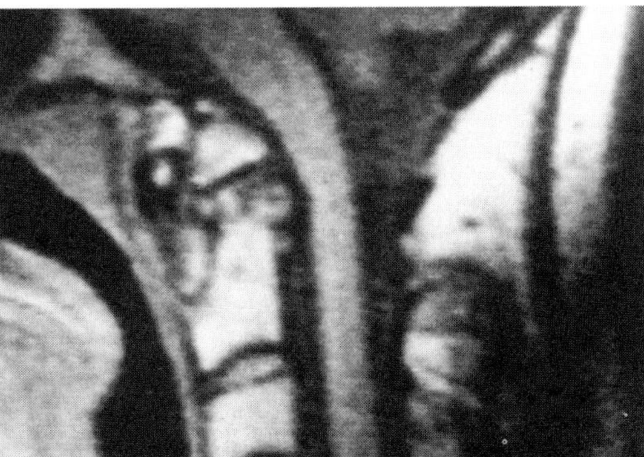

Figure 3: Midsagittal MRI demonstrating a type II odontoid fracture with interposition of the transverse ligament between the odontoid process and the body of C2.

may cause permanent neurological deficit; it can be avoided by clinical diligence and serial radiographs. Atlanto-occipital injuries require only 1 or 2 kg to reduce and maintain alignment, where atlantoaxial subluxation may require 10 to 20 kg. Traction is maintained during surgery, and the skull tongs provide a means of manual distraction to assist open reduction and realignment.

Surgical intervention is not indicated in all traumatic lesions of the craniocervical junction and, for many injuries, more than one form of treatment will apply. As with other diseases, the clinician must assess the relative certainty of good outcome with the inconvenience to the patient. Halo body jackets are a well-established method of conservative treatment for many patients with these injuries. However, they present a formidable inconvenience to the patient who may be immobilized for 6 months or longer. The advantages of internal fixation are that the joint is stable at the end of surgery, and mobilization and rehabilitation of the patient can be commenced immediately. Nursing care and subsequent anesthesia are simplified. The disadvantages are the risks of anesthesia and major surgery in the ill patient and, in the long-

term, the effects of the internal fixation on adjacent cervical segments. In addition, internal fixation of the spine may immobilize uninjured levels and this is of potentially greater significance in the mobile upper cervical spine.

When surgery is required for craniocervical trauma, it is necessary to involve a skilled anesthetist because of the imposed limitation of head and neck movement during intubation. Awake intubation under endoscopic visualization is mandatory when there is instability, and close preoperative monitoring of the patient must be maintained when spinal cord damage may impair homeostatic responses to blood loss.

In operative cases in which compression of the neuraxis is in question, useful preoperative information may be obtained from somatosensory recordings or motor evoked potentials.

The methods of occipitocervical fixation may be classified according to the direction of surgical approach and the levels of fixation. Although many methods of fixation have been outlined in the surgical literature, the management of every injury in this region is beyond the scope of this chapter, as are the relative merits of all the described forms of treatment. Set out below are the operative techniques that the authors of this chapter use. No attempt is made to cover all the surgical possibilities. A summary of conservative and surgical treatment options for a variety of craniocervical injuries is shown in Table 1.

TABLE 1

SUMMARY OF CONSERVATIVE AND SURGICAL TREATMENT OPTIONS
FOR A VARIETY OF CRANIOCERVICAL INJURIES

Injury	Preoperative Reduction	External Orthosis	Comment	Open Reduction	Comment
Atlanto-occipital dislocation	Yes	Yes		Not usually	
Atlantoaxial rotatory subluxation and dislocation	Early reduction	Yes		Late presentation necessitates open reduction	
Atlantoaxial subluxation (rheumatoid)	Often not possible	Inadequate		Open reduction TI-FRAME Transoral surgery Transarticular screw	
Atlantoaxial subluxation (non-rheumatoid)	Occasionally not possible	Inadequate		Open reduction TI-FRAME Transoral surgery Transarticular screw	
Jefferson's fracture	No	Yes	Nonunion	Miniplate fixation	Vertebral artery
Odontoid fracture I	No	Yes			
II	—	Yes	Transverse ligament interposition	Transoral surgery Posterior fixation Odontoid screw	
III	Yes	Yes			
Crushed lateral mass	Yes	Yes			
C2-3 acute disc	No	—		Anterior discectomy	
C2-3 dislocation	Yes	—		Titanium cervical locking plate	

SURGICAL TECHNIQUES IN CRANIOCERVICAL JUNCTION TRAUMA

Dorsal Approach

Occipitocervical Instability

Acute ligamentous injury rarely occurs in isolation and is made worse by all but the most gentle skull traction. A more chronic situation develops in the rheumatoid patient in whom there is inevitably atlantoaxial instability as well. The authors' approach is TI-FRAME occipitocervical fixation and bone grafting (vide infra).

C1-2 Instability

A number of methods of treatment for C1-2 instability are available and the merits of each technique are discussed.

Gallie Fusion

This established method is particularly resistant to flexion forces.[6] It is indicated when there is atlantoaxial instability that may follow fracture of the odontoid process or rupture of the C1 transverse ligament. It has the advantage of relative simplicity and may assist in the reduction of ventral atlantoaxial subluxation. It is not, however, suitable for fractures that involve the C1 arch and provides only minimal protection

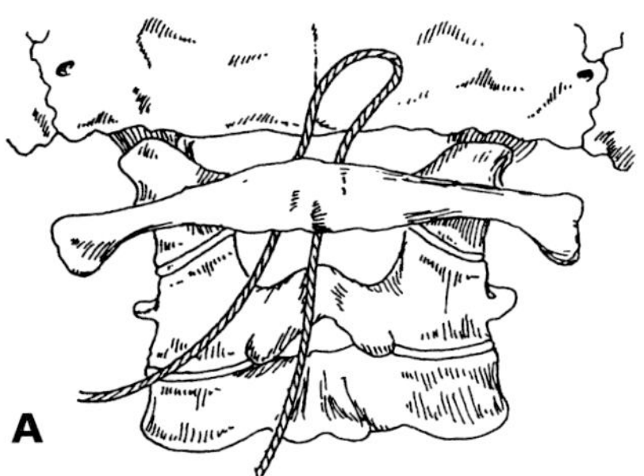

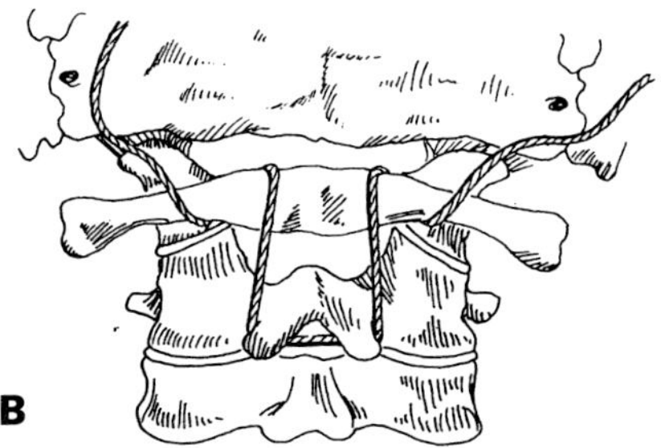

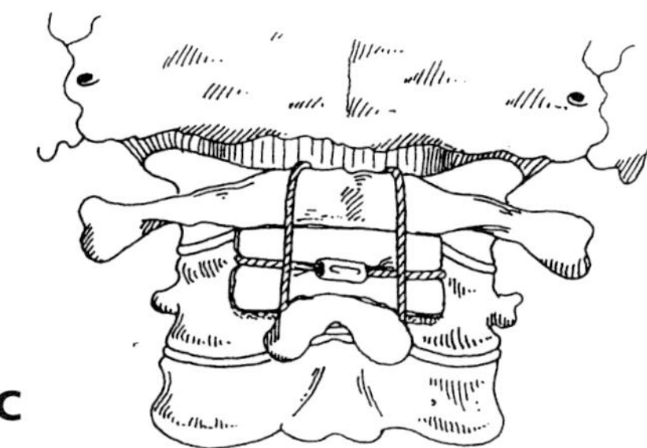

Figure 4: Dorsal fusion. A cable is passed beneath the posterior arch of C1 **(A)** and looped over the spinous process of C2 **(B)**. The cable is then tightened and secured over a shaped iliac crest bone graft applied to decorticated bone surfaces **(C)**.

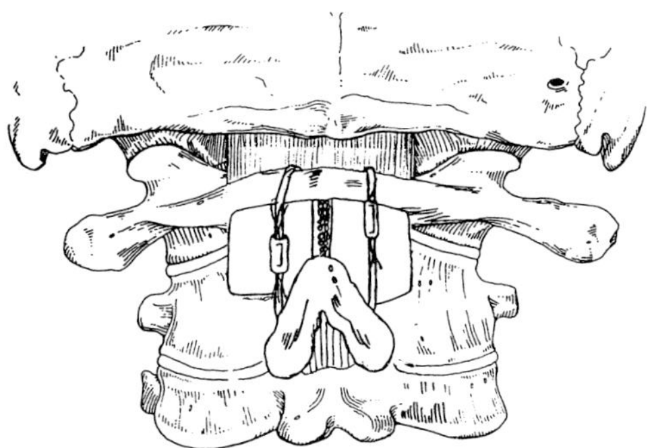

Figure 5: Brooks fusion using bilateral sublaminar wires to secure the bone graft.

from recurrent translocation movements of C1 on C2. In addition, all of the dorsal wiring techniques require sublaminar cable passage that may compress an already compromised high cervical spinal cord or cervicomedullary junction where the subluxation has occurred.

The patient is placed in the prone position and reduction is confirmed using lateral image intensification. A midline incision is made, extending from the occiput to C4. At C1-2, soft tissue is cleared in the midline to permit atraumatic sublaminar wire passage deep to the ligamentum flavum. A loop of wire is passed in a rostral direction beneath C1, and is then brought up and passed over the dorsal arch of C1 to hook around the spinous process of C2 (Figure 4). The exposed dorsal elements of C1 and C2 are decorticated using a high-speed drill. A 2 × 3-cm corticocancellous bone graft is taken from the dorsal iliac crest and fashioned to conform to the dorsal elements of C1 and C2 to provide maximum area of contact. With the graft in place, the two free ends of wire are brought from laterally to secure the graft when tightened. Further reduction may be achieved during tightening.

Sublaminar wire passage is a technique common to many of the methods of dorsal fixation. It is economical and provides a strong fixation. Meticulous technique is demanded, however, if complications such as dural penetration or spinal cord damage are to be avoided.[7] It is the authors' preference to use multifilament stainless steel or titanium cable in wiring techniques. Advantage is gained in ease of sublaminar passage without the risk of elbowing into the spinal canal as may occur with conventional malleable wire. Fixation is achieved using a malleable crimp instead of twisting the wire. Some training is recommended to develop the skills necessary to use the crimping tools.

Brooks Wedge-Compression Technique

This modification of Gallie fusion provides greater rotational strength[2] (Figure 5). A similar exposure is performed with clearance of soft tissue deep to the lamina of C2 in addition to C1. Cable loops are then passed from above, beneath the arch of C1 and the lamina of C2, and brought out at C2-3. Loops are passed on both sides. Two corticocancellous grafts are fashioned into a wedge with the cortex positioned dorsally and secured onto the decorticated surfaces of C1 and C2 with the double wires.

Atlantoaxial Arthrodesis Using Interlaminar Clamps

Interlaminar clamp arthrodesis affords greater stability than the wiring techniques described above by limiting C1-2 subluxation. The reported rates of fusion are good. However, the clamps are vulnerable to dislocation or loosening caused by rotational movements of the head. It is felt that the technique has been superseded by the screw techniques detailed below.

Transarticular Screw Fixation of C1-2

Although more technically demanding, screw fixation through the lateral masses is biomechanically more stable than the techniques described above.[8] The wiring and interlaminar clamp techniques rely on the integrity of the dorsal arch of the atlas and may be inappropriate after trauma. The transarticular screw technique allows the stable fixation of C1-2 and is not contraindicated when fractures disrupt the dorsal arch of C1. Preoperative assessment by CT is mandatory to provide information on the integrity of the lateral masses as well as the size and position of the vertebral artery canal. In 20% of cases, screw insertion is contraindicated on anatomical grounds because the course of the vertebral artery interrupts the proposed screw trajectory through C2.[11]

The patient is placed prone, and position and reduction are confirmed using lateral image intensification. A midline incision is made extending from the occiput to C7. The cervical laminae are exposed. The arch of C1 and the laminae and articular masses of C2 and C3 are cleared using subperiosteal dissection. Atlantoaxial subluxation may be reduced by repositioning or upward traction on a C1 sublaminar wire. Under image intensification, a Kirschner wire is drilled parallel to the sagittal plane entering at the inferior articular process of C2 and in the

direction of the anterior tubercle of C1 shown by the image intensifier. The wire passes through the lamina of C2 and the C1-2 articular surfaces, and enters the lateral mass of the atlas. A second K-wire is drilled parallel to the first on the opposite side; the first K-wire is then overdrilled using a 2.7-mm cannulated bit. The depth is ascertained, and a solid 3.5-mm screw of appropriate length is inserted. The second K-wire is kept in place to maintain position until the first screw is secure; it is then overdrilled and screwed. Compression may be achieved by overdrilling C2 to 3.5 mm or by the use of a lag screw. A Gallie-type dorsal fusion is commonly performed to provide three-point fixation and to increase the fusion rate (Figures 6 and 7).

Occipitocervical Fusion

Although it remains a principle of internal fixation to avoid uninjured areas in fusion, instability between the occiput and atlas may require stabilization across the craniocervical junction because of the difficulties encountered in fixing implants to the atlas alone. In cases where the ring of the atlas has been disrupted, there is a tendency for the lateral masses of C1 to be splayed laterally. The effect of this is to allow translocation and subluxation at the atlanto-occipital joint. To prevent this phenomenon, the occiput must be included in the fixation by a technique that will minimize or reduce translocation. Indications for post-traumatic occipitocervical fusion are uncommon, but include an unstable Jefferson's fracture, a dislocated fracture of the lateral mass of the atlas or of the occipital condyle, and atlanto-occipital dislocation. Three principal types of fusion in current use are: 1) onlay bone grafting, 2) bone grafting with internal fixation, and 3) fixation with methylmethacrylate cement.

The first methods described for occipitocervical fusion involved onlay bone graft positioned over the occiput and upper cervical vertebrae. Fibular, tibial, and, subsequently, iliac crest grafts were used. These methods have the inherent disadvantage of providing no immediate postoperative stability and they have been superseded by instrumentation techniques that provide early primary stability and avoid the need for halo

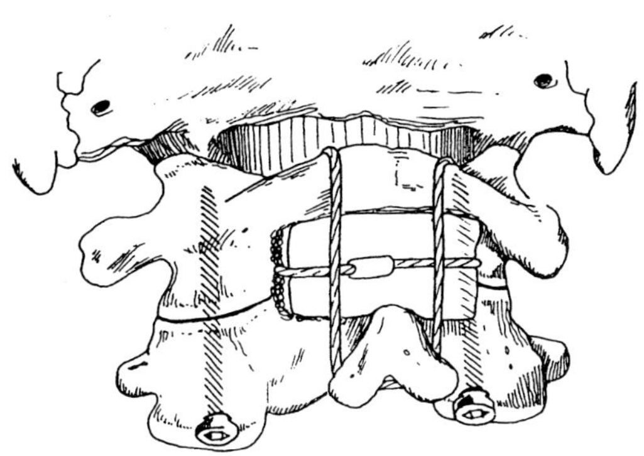

Figure 6: C1-2 lateral mass screw fixation; the intra-osseous position of the screws is shaded. An extremely solid construct is achieved combining this with a Gallie fusion to provide "three-point fixation."

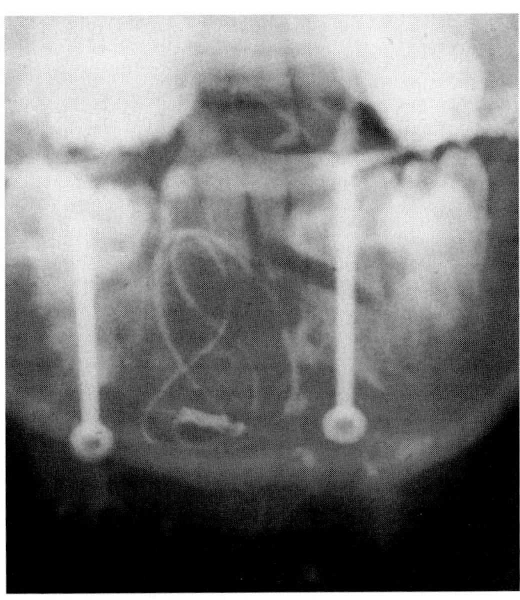

Figure 7: Plain anteroposterior radiograph of C1-2 lateral mass screw fixation.

jacket or Minerva cast immobilization. Cement fixation has been used to achieve immediate stability. However, a significant rate of complications precludes its routine clinical use.

Dorsal Occipitocervical Fusion Using Contoured Loop Fixation

A variety of fixation techniques have been developed using molded Steinmann pins and Wisconsin and Luque rods for immediate postoperative stability. To achieve a good fit, these require a great deal of practice and three-dimensional skills. The majority employ sublaminar wiring or cable, although methods using screw-and-plate fixation are available. A preformed titanium loop is available (TI-FRAME, Codman and Shurtleff) for the purpose of craniocervical fixation. This has the advantage of MRI compatibility. It is preformed, avoiding the need for complicated rod bending which may itself induce points of fatigue within the implant. The loop is notched, preventing cable migration and providing a force for maintaining regular vertebral spacing.

The patient is placed prone and the occipital bone and laminae are exposed as far laterally as the facet joints. The ligamentum flavum is removed in order to avoid inadvertent cord damage and sublaminar cables passed. The interspinous ligament is preserved from below

C2 to avoid postoperative kyphosis. A TI-FRAME of suitable size is selected and adjusted to the contour of the bone. For craniocervical instability, fixation to the occiput, C1, and C2 is sufficient and the loop legs are cut to an appropriate length. With the head in a neutral position, the occipital wires are passed through drill holes adjacent to the loop; the occipital and cervical wires are then tightened and secured. Onlay bone graft from the iliac crest is applied to the decorticated surface of the occiput, C1, and C2.

A prerequisite for fixation using sublaminar cables is intact laminae at the levels of fixation. In cases of laminar fracture or where laminectomy is performed, segmental fixation can be achieved using a screw-based system. Craniocervical junction fixation is performed with screws into the occipital bone in conjunction with C1-2 lateral mass screws, and fixation is extended inferiorly into the subaxial lateral masses as required.

Osteoplastic Repair of Dorsal C1 Arch Fractures

Fractures of the atlas comprise between 4% and 12% of bone injuries affecting the cervical

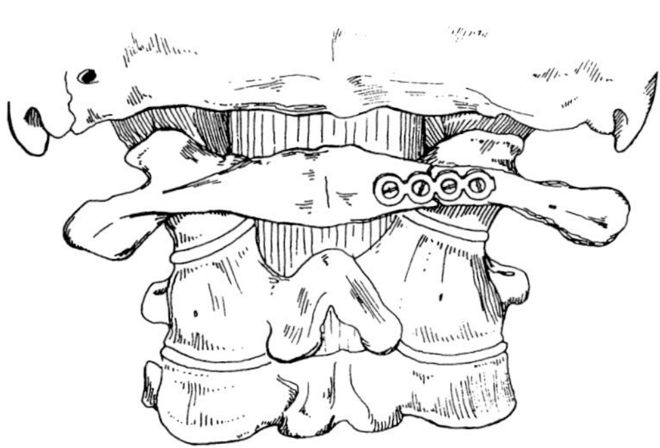

Figure 8: Osteoplastic repair of an atlas fracture using titanium miniplate and screws.

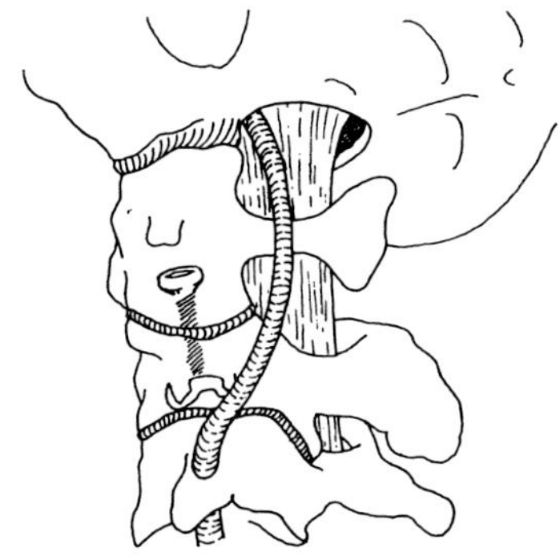

Figure 9: Lateral mass screw fixation from the lateral approach. The vertebral artery is mobilized after opening the foramen transversaria.

spine. Although most are successfully treated by cervical orthosis, nonunion may be associated with pain on movement and methods of internal fixation may restrict movement. A method of direct repair of the dorsal arch has been described in which the full range of neck movement is preserved without the need for external support[12] (Figure 8).

The patient is placed prone and the craniocervical junction is approached in the midline. The fracture site is exposed using careful subperiosteal dissection in consideration of the course of the vertebral artery. Rotation of the head presents the fracture site nearer to the midline; the fracture may then be reduced under direct vision, interposed soft tissue excised, bone graft applied, and the fracture fixed using an appropriate plating system.

Lateral Approach

Atlantoaxial Rotatory Dislocation

Atlantoaxial rotatory dislocation defines a complete and persistent displacement of adjacent articular surfaces at the C1-2 lateral mass joint. It is preferentially treated by early closed reduction and external bracing to restore the normal anatomy of the joint surfaces. The dislocation may be irreducible, and fusion in malalignment may result in significant torticollis and facial asymmetry in the growing child.[5]

The dislocated C1-2 joint may be reduced using the extreme lateral approach first described in 1957 by Henry.[9] The patient is placed in the lateral position and a 10-cm incision is made from the mastoid process along the dorsal border of the sternomastoid muscle. The deep cervical fascia is divided deep to the dorsal border of the muscle, and a plane can then be followed down to the transverse processes of the upper cervical vertebrae through blunt dissection. In this region, the vertical segment of the vertebral artery is crossed superficially by the ventral ramus of the C2 nerve root. The vertebral artery may take an abnormal course between the dislocated axis and atlas, dictated by the relative positions of the C2 foramen transversarium and the transverse process of C1 (Figure 9).

Irreducible atlantoaxial rotatory dislocation is associated with the interposition of soft tissue between articular surfaces. Established cases may be further complicated by ankylosis and extensive scar tissue that require release before reduction is achieved. Division of the base of the odontoid has been described where fusion to the ventral arch of atlas prevented reduction. Bilateral exploration may be required.

Transarticular Screw Fixation of C1-2

In addition to the dorsal approach described above, atlantoaxial screw arthrodesis may be performed laterally having exposed the lateral mass joint as above. With the vertebral artery located medial and dorsal, a screw may be passed from above downward to transfix the joint (Figure 9).

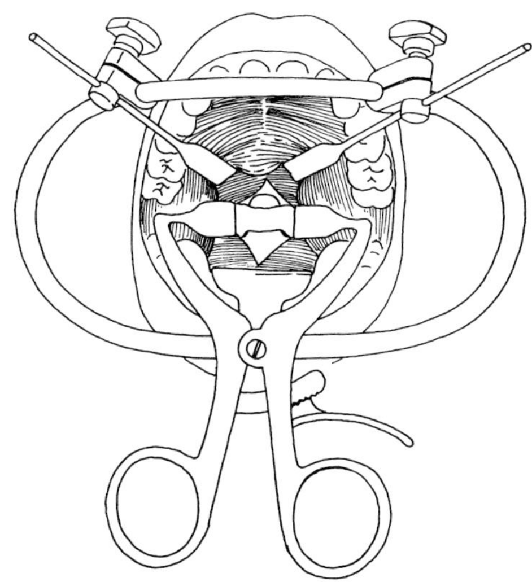

Figure 10: Transoral exposure of the ventral tubercle of C1 and odontoid.

Ventral Approach

Compression Osteosynthesis of Odontoid Fractures

Transverse fractures of the odontoid peg may be treated by compression osteosynthesis screw fixation.[10] This procedure preserves the atlanto-axial motion segment and removes the need for prolonged immobilization. It is a demanding technique and requires biplanar fluoroscopic imaging. The technique may not be possible in the short-necked patient or in cases in which extension of the cervical spine is limited. If there is wide separation of the fragments, it is likely that the transverse ligament is interposed, and, unless the soft tissue is removed, there will be no bony union.

The patient is placed supine and the head extended to reduce the fracture. The body of C2 is approached ventrally via an incision along the ventral border of the sternomastoid muscle. The ventral-caudal border of the C2 body is identified and, under biplanar imaging, a 2.7-mm drill is angled dorsally to exit the dorsal half of the odontoid tip. The drill is angled 5° to 10° medially. The odontoid fracture is fixed with one or two 3.5-mm screws passed into the tip of the dens, avoiding dural penetration. Compression of the fracture is achieved using lag screws or by overdrilling C2.

Ventral Atlantoaxial and Craniocervical Decompression and Fusion

In keeping with the general principle that ventral neuraxis compression requires a ventral operation, it is more appropriate to perform ventral transoral decompression and fusion procedures in certain cases of irreducible and nonunited odontoid fracture or where trauma has exacerbated a pre-existing craniocervical anomaly.

For transoral procedures, the patient is supported in the lateral position with the head immobilized in the Mayfield retractor. This allows for ventral decompression with the option of progressing to dorsal stabilization in the same position.[3] The dorsal oropharynx is exposed using a transoral retractor, and C1 and C2 may be exposed through a midline incision (Figure 10).

Decompression, if required, may be performed using a high-speed drill. In a very unstable situation, it may be necessary to steady the odontoid with forceps while drilling. Remaining bone and ligament can then be removed using punches and dissectors. It is not always essential to remove the transverse ligament deep to the odontoid process. Preservation of this structure will prevent splaying of C1 with malalignment of the lateral mass joints.

Odontoid fracture nonunion is frequently caused by the interposition of soft tissue, such as the transverse ligament, between the fracture surfaces. After removing the interposed ligament, the fracture edges can be roughened and grafted.

CONCLUSION

The management of craniocervical junction traumatic lesions is challenging, with a complexity dictated by the unique anatomy of the vertebral column in this area and the close proximity of the brain stem and high cervical cord. In each case, actual or threatened compression of the neuraxis is a priority in treatment. Having achieved decompression, adequate stabilization is necessary without excessive function impairment. There are many available treatment options, each having particular advantages and disadvantages dependent on the nature of the injury, the characteristics of the patient, the skill of the surgical team, and the facilities available.

REFERENCES

1. Adams VI: Neck injuries, II: Atlantoaxial dislocation–a pathologic study of 14 traffic fatalities. **J Forensic Sci 37:**565-573, 1992
2. Brooks AL, Jenkins EB: Atlantoaxial arthrodesis by the wedge compression method. **J Bone Joint Surg (Am) 60:**279-284, 1978
3. Crockard HA, Calder I, Ransford AO: One-stage transoral decompression and posterior fixation in rheumatoid atlanto-axial subluxation. **J Bone Joint Surg (Br) 72:**682-685, 1990
4. Crockard HA, Tammam A, Mendoza ND: Magnetic resonance imaging-compatible posterior cervical implant for occipitocervical stabilization. **J Neurosurg 89:**852-856, 1998
5. Fielding JW, Hawkins RJ: Atlanto-axial rotatory fixation. **J Bone Joint Surg (Am) 59:**37-44, 1977
6. Gallie W: Fractures and dislocations of the cervical spine. **Am J Surg 46:**495-499, 1939
7. Geremia GK, Kwang SK, Cerullo L, et al: Complications of sublaminar wiring. **Surg Neurol 23:**629-634, 1985
8. Grob D, Jeanneret B, Aebi M, et al: Atlanto-axial fusion with transarticular screw fixation. **J Bone Joint Surg (Br) 73:**972-976, 1991
9. Henry AK: **Extensile Exposure. 2nd ed.** Baltimore, Md: Williams & Wilkins, 1957
10. Jeanneret B, Vernet O, Frei S, et al: Atlantoaxial mobility after screw fixation of the odontoid: a computed tomographic study. **J Spinal Disord 4:**203-211, 1991
11. Madawi AA, Casey ATH, Solanki G, et al: Radiological and anatomical evaluation of the atlantoaxial transarticular screw fixation technique. **J Neurosurg 86:**961-968, 1997
12. Rogers MA, Ransford AO, Crockard HA: Osteoplastic repair of the atlas. **J Bone Joint Surg (Br) 74:**880-882, 1992

CHAPTER 13

SURGICAL TECHNIQUES: CERVICAL SPINE STABILIZATION

MARC E. EICHLER, MD, CHARLES B. STILLERMAN, MD, AND RANJAN S. ROY, MD, PHD

The yearly incidence of cervical spine injuries in North America is 15 per 1 million population.[45] In a majority of these, significant spinal column disruption occurs. Managing these injuries surgically has become increasingly popular for a variety of reasons, including better fusion rates, earlier patient mobilization, improvement in deformity correction, the prevention of bone graft migration, and diminished postoperative bracing requirements. During the past decade, new spinal fixators have been developed to improve patient management.

This chapter provides insight into the principles and techniques of cervical stabilization and fusion. Emphasis is placed on contemporary methods; however, several earlier techniques are also evaluated. The advantages and disadvantages of these devices are analyzed, as are the general indications for fusion and stabilization. Prior to performing these procedures, a surgeon must have a solid understanding of the anatomical and biomechanical operatives; therefore, our discussion begins with these fundamental issues.

RELEVANT ANATOMY AND BIOMECHANICS

Rational treatment of traumatic cervical spine instability requires an understanding of normal anatomy, biomechanics, and kinematics. The mechanism of injury frequently influences the surgical approach selected to reduce subluxations, decompress neural structures, counteract the forces that produced the injury, and stabilize the spinal column.

The upper cervical spine consists of the foramen magnum, paired occipital condyles, and the atlas and axis, and is often referred to as the cervicocranium (Figure 1). Craniocervical articulation provides protection to the lower medulla and the upper cervical cord; occipitoatlantal articulation is supported by the anterior and posterior atlanto-occipital membrane, the joint capsule, and the ligamentum nuchae. Additional stability is provided by ligaments, which extend from the occiput directly to the axis. This includes the paired alar ligaments, the apical liga-

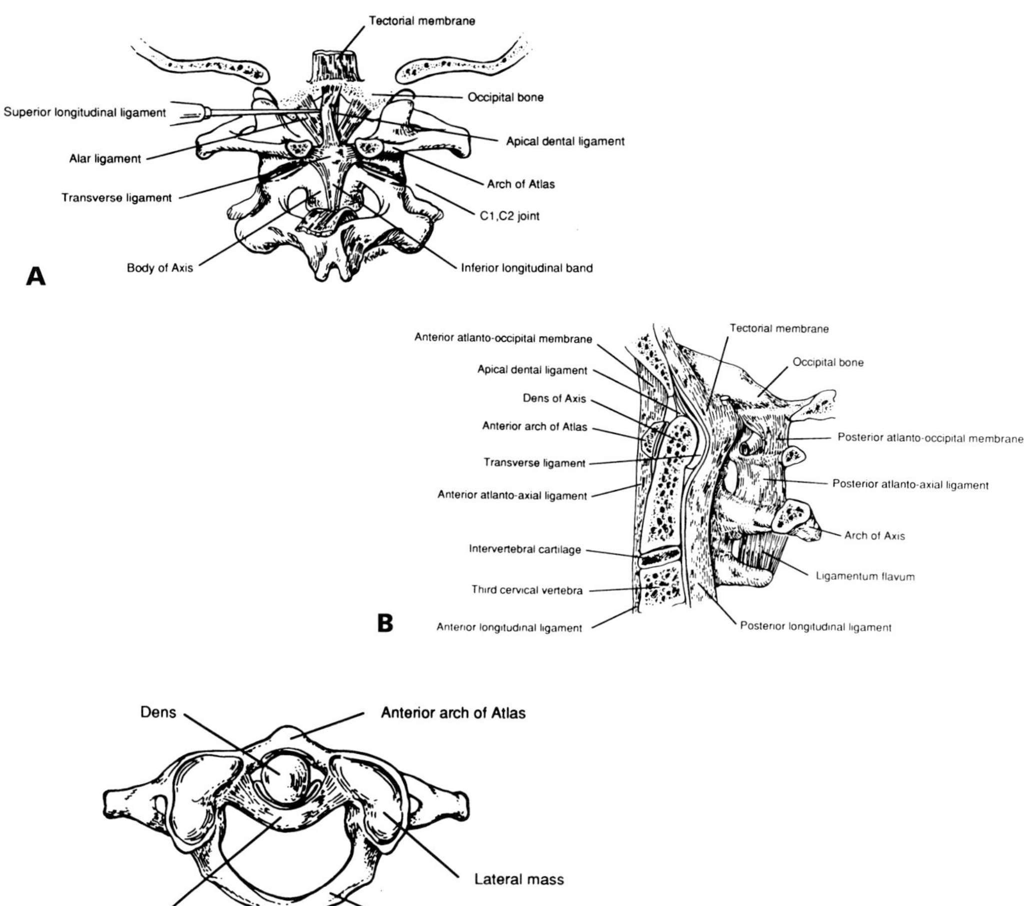

Figure 1: Diagram of the craniocervical junction. **A)** Dorsal view illustrating the major internal cranial cervical ligaments including the tectorial membrane, the transverse atlantal ligament, and the paired alar ligaments. Minor internal ligaments in this region include the apical and accessory ligaments. **B)** Lateral view, including major external cranial cervical ligaments. The external ligaments illustrated are the anterior atlanto-occipital membrane, the posterior atlanto-occipital membrane, and the anterior and posterior atlantoaxial membranes. The articular capsules and ligamentum nuchae are not included. **C)** Axial view of the atlantoaxial region. The major contributor to stability here is provided by the transverse ligament, which inserts onto the medial portion of the lateral masses of C1. (Reproduced with permission from Stillerman et al.[104])

ment, and the tectorial membrane.

Stability at the atlantoaxial articulation is provided by both bony and ligamentous structures. The transverse ligament, which inserts onto the medial tubercles of the lateral masses of C1 and passes dorsal to the odontoid dens, is most important in maintaining atlantoaxial stability (Figure 1C). The dens and the ventral arch of C1 are also stabilizing structures. Hyperflexion is limited by the tectorial membrane and hyperextension is limited by the ventral arch of C1 contacting the process. Ventral translation of the C1-2 articulation is limited by the transverse ligament, and excessive rotation is held in check by the paired alar ligaments. Radiographically, an interval of >3 mm in adults and >5 mm in the pediatric population between the dorsal surface of C1 and the ventral surface of the dens is generally considered consistent with incompetence of the transverse ligament and atlantoaxial instability.

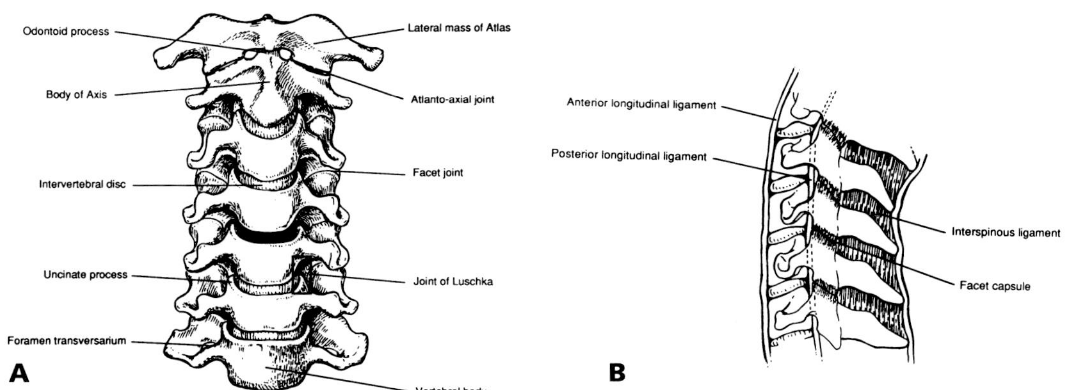

Figure 2: Cervical spine. **A)** Frontal view; note how the uncinate process from the vertebrae below and the lateral portion of the body above form the joints of Luschka. The size of the vertebral bodies increase moving down the cervical spine with the exception that the height of the C6 vertebrae may be less than at the adjacent levels. **B)** Lateral view, illustrating the anterior and posterior longitudinal ligaments, facets and their capsules, and the interspinous ligaments. These structures play an important role in maintaining stability. (Reproduced with permission from Stillerman et al.[104])

Analysis of the degree of motion in various planes at the occipitoatlantal junction revealed 13° in flexion-extension, 8° in lateral bending, and a complete absence of axial rotation. At the atlantoaxial articulation, ligaments allowed 47° in axial rotation and 10° in flexion-extension movements (Table 1).[112] No appreciable lateral bending occurs here. The greater range of motion exhibited by the C1-2 articulation correlates with this joint being more susceptible to pathology than the occiput-C1 junction.

The third through the seventh cervical vertebrae are similar in most respects. Although uniform in configuration, there is a gradual increase in size, moving caudally down the spine. The C6 vertebrae, however, may be smaller in height than either C5 or C7 (Figure 2).[13] Soft-tissue structures are present throughout the cervical spine. Interposed between two adjacent vertebrae are intervertebral discs that attach to end plates through dense Sharpey's fibers, a component of the annulus fibrosis. Discs distribute weight over the entire vertebral body surface during bending movements and function as "shock-absorbers" during direct axial loading. The aging process may lead to disc desiccation, producing loss of disc space height. A consequence of this change is that the dorsal elements, particularly the facet joints, are subjected to greater load-bearing capacity. This accelerates hypertrophic degenerative changes of the articular facets. Such changes may potentiate a neurological deficit in the presence of traumatic cervical injury.

Fibers of the anterior longitudinal ligament are closely adherent to the discs and end plates but not to the ventral vertebral body; it functions to maintain stability during cervical extension. Along the dorsal surface of the vertebral bodies and discs lie the posterior longitudinal ligament, broad over the disc space and narrower over the body. Like its ventral counterpart, it adheres to the disc and end plate and provides considerable stability to the cervical spine. The dorsal ligamentous margin of the spinal canal is the ligamentum flava, which connect adjacent lamina. Hypertrophy of this ligament can significantly contribute to spinal cord injury in the face of trauma. Additional dorsal column soft-tissue structures that contribute to stability include the joint capsule, interspinous and supraspinous ligaments, and ligamentum nuchae. These structures provide their greatest resistance to flexion and torsional forces.

Motion in the subaxial spine is greatest at C4-5 and C5-6, making these levels more susceptible to trauma (Table 1).[112] Flexion is limited largely by contact of the chin to the chest, although the dorsal ligaments and musculature also play a significant role. Ventral neck muscles and fascia, as well as the anterior longitudinal ligament, restrict hyperextension. Lateral bending and axial rota-

TABLE 1

REPRESENTATIVE ANGLE (°) OF ROTATION OF THE CERVICAL SPINE*

Interspace	Combined Flexion-Extension (x-axis rotation)	One Side Lateral Bending (z-axis rotation)	One Side Axial Rotation (y-axis rotation)
Upper			
Occiput-C1	13°	8°	0
C1-2	10°	0	47°
C2-3	10°	10°	3°
Middle			
C3-4	15°	11°	7°
C4-5	20°	11°	7°
C5-6	20°	8°	7°
Lower			
C6-7	17°	7°	6°
C7-T1	9°	4°	2°

*Adapted from White and Panjabi. Reproduced from Stillerman et al[104] with permission.

tion are also prominent in the midcervical region. Extreme lateral bending is held in check by the articular pillars and intertransverse ligaments.

Classification of traumatic injuries, based on the mechanism of injury, is facilitated by depicting the cervical spine as consisting of two columns. Although a three-column anatomy of the spine has been described,[98] the two-column concept is sufficient to explain patterns of fractures and subluxations.[5,56] All structures located ventral to the posterior longitudinal ligament comprise the ventral column. The vertebral arch and the dorsal ligamentous complex, including the ligamentum flavum and facet capsule, constitute the dorsal column. The ventral column serves as a tension band that limits extension, and the dorsal column as a tension band that limits flexion.[114] Flexion forces produce compression of the ventral column and distraction of the dorsal column, whereas extension forces accomplish the opposite. Thus, flexion and extension forces reciprocally affect the two columns.[56]

INDICATIONS FOR AND GOALS OF SURGERY

The overall goals of surgery are to decompress neural elements and prevent further injury, maintain or produce anatomic alignment, and provide long-term stability.[57] Internal fixation and fusion should be restricted to only unstable motion segments, since extension of the fusion to uninvolved regions promotes nonunion and instrument failure as well as additional loss of normal motion in the various planes.[39,76] An additional point of concern is the increased stress to which the adjacent motion segments are exposed. Segments above and below an arthrodesis are more susceptible to fracture and instability.[66]

Demonstration of traumatic instability of the cervical spine is a prime indication for surgical intervention. Several guidelines may be used alone or in tandem to help clarify whether instability exists (Table 2). In the absence of a complete spinal cord injury, when neural structures are compressed, a decompression procedure is frequently combined with stabilization and fusion. In patients in whom instability is the sole issue, bone grafting followed by internal fixation may be all that is required. Operative treatment should take into account the patient's neurological status, the pattern and level of injury, the degree of spinal deformity, the feasibility of safely achieving intraoperative reduction, and the patient's age and medical condition.

Spinal instrumentation as an adjunct to bony fusion is indicated for complex spinal instability,

TABLE 2

ESTABLISHING THE PRESENCE OF INSTABILITY[**]

Level	Signs of Instability
Occiput-C1	AP translation on flexion-extension views >1 mm[*] BC/AO ratio >1, same in children[†] Axial rotation to one side on AP view >8° Neurological deficit
C1-2	Total overhang of C1-2 on AP open-mouth view >7 mm Atlanto-dental interval on static lateral film >4 mm in adults,[§] >5 mm in children Axial rotation to one side on AP view >45° Widened interspinous space on lateral view Axial rotation of vertebra on AP view Neurological deficit

C3-7	Signs of spine trauma
	    Retropharyngeal space swelling >7 mm in adult or child
	    Retrotracheal space >14 mm in adults; ≥22 mm in children
	    Abnormal vertebral alignment on lateral view
	    Widened interspinous space on lateral view
	    Axial rotation of vertebra on AP view
	Signs used to establish diagnosis of instability[#]
	    Anterior or posterior elements destroyed or unable to function
	    Sagittal plane translation on lateral view >3.5 mm
	    Sagittal plane rotation on lateral view >11°
	    Spinal cord or nerve root damage
	    Abnormal disc narrowing
	    Positive stretch test
	Neurological deficit

[*] Assuming intact transverse ligament; accepted dens tip to basion interval is 4 to 5 mm.

[†] Powers ratio: BC/AO where B is basion, C is posterior arch of atlas, O is opisthion, and A is anterior arch of atlas.

[§] Accepted interval ranges from 2.7 to 4 mm in adults.

[#] A combination of these objective criteria is used to decide whether clinical instability exists.

[**] Table adapted from White and Panjabi.[113]

multilevel fusions, and malalignment or nonunion of fractures despite prolonged immobilization in a rigid cervical orthosis. Internal fixation should be considered for patients with spinal deformity from previous extensive surgery[58,80] and patients with instability who prefer to avoid long-term immobilization with a halo or Minerva brace. Internal fixation allows for immediate and multidirectional stability of unstable motion segments, while the osseous fusion matures. Conventional wisdom holds that the hardware will fatigue and then fail without the establishment of this fusion.

Indications for a particular implant are multifactorial, being influenced by the level of the injury, the mechanical forces resulting in the instability, the need to further destabilize the column with a decompression, and the quality of the patient's bone. Additional considerations include the desire to avoid rigid external bracing, the cost of the device, and the ease and safety with which the implant is assembled.

VENTRAL VS. DORSAL PROCEDURES

Once the decision is made for operative stabilization, the surgeon must decide whether the approach should be ventral, dorsal, or by a combination. Prior to the availability of instrumentation, the ventral approach was often accompanied by high rates of fusion failure, graft extrusion, and recurrent spinal deformity.[12,23,110] This was especially prevalent in cases of traumatic instability. It was often necessary to use either prolonged postoperative immobilization as an adjunct to the ventral surgery or additional surgery for stabilization of the dorsal elements. With the development of various ventral and dorsal fixators, the need for long-term postoperative immobilization has been reduced.

In general, the ventral approach is utilized for ventral pathology and the dorsal approach for when dorsal elements are primarily involved. The dorsal cervical approach provides a more-limited access to the vertebral body, the ventral spinal canal, and the ventral spinal cord. The ventral approach, alone or in concert with dorsal surgery, is becoming popular for traumatic cervical spine injuries that involve the ventral column.[82] Ventral decompression and stabilization are indicated for persistent ventral cord compression in patients exhibiting at least partial neurological function. The offending agent may be bony fragments, osteophytic spurs, or traumatically herniated disc fragments. Vertebral body fractures with resultant kyphosis and canal compromise from bony fragments are best approached ventrally for decompression and correction of the deformity.

A dorsal approach may be indicated for patients requiring exposure of the dorsal spinal canal and bony elements and for the treatment of fractures or dislocations. Additionally, it allows for decompression over a large length of the spinal canal via multilevel laminectomies. Dorsal stabilization is often preferred for the patient with complete injury, despite ventral spinal cord compression due to the limited likelihood of functional improvement following direct decompression of a persistent ventral mass. It is frequently used for dorsal ligamentous disruption without bony injury and for facet fracture-dislocations. In such cases, ventral stabilization may also be effective.

Controversy arises regarding the management of the grossly unstable three-column injury and in clinical situations of vertebral collapse without neural compromise. In the former, surgeons remain divided between ventral stabilization alone and the need for both ventral and dorsal procedures to achieve adequate fixation.[2,23,26,87,110] In the latter, either approach may be satisfactory although, with dorsal stabilization, progressive loss of correction of the kyphos can occur at the injured level and produce subopti-

mal results. Consistently safe and effective management requires individualization of strategies, combined with the expertise to facilitate reconstruction of the spinal canal, direct removal of lesions deforming neural structures, and/or optimal construct design for stabilization and fusion.

UPPER CERVICAL SPINE

Overall, 25% of cervical trauma occurs in the region of the occiput, atlas, and axis.[17,56,96,104] Of patients with upper cervical lesions, up to 20% of fractures involve the axis[6,52,68] and between 3% and 13% occur in the atlas.[11,32,52,53] A combination of occiput, atlas, and axis fractures occur in the remainder. Many upper cervical spine fractures are treated nonoperatively. Only those lesions that require surgery are discussed in this chapter.

OCCIPITAL-ATLANTOAXIAL DISLOCATION

Recent literature reflects an increase in the number of occiput-C1 dislocations occurring in survivors of accidents.[18,61] A distractive force, with the neck hyperflexed, appears to be the predominant mechanism of injury. Rupture of the anterior occipitoatlantal ligaments, the tectorial membrane, and the alar ligaments leads to disruption and dislocation of the occipital condyles on the lateral masses of the atlas.[109] Traynelis et al[107] classified occiput-C1 dislocations into three subgroups:

- Type I: Ventral translation of the cranium relative to the cervical spine. This is the most common variety.
- Type IIA: Longitudinal distraction between the occiput and the atlas.
- Type IIB: Vertical distraction between the occiput and atlas, as well as between the atlas and the axis.
- Type III: Dorsal displacement of the cranium with respect to the cervical spine.

Atlantoaxial instability may accompany occiput-C1 dislocations if there is associated incompetence of the transverse ligament. The symptoms and signs of patients surviving these

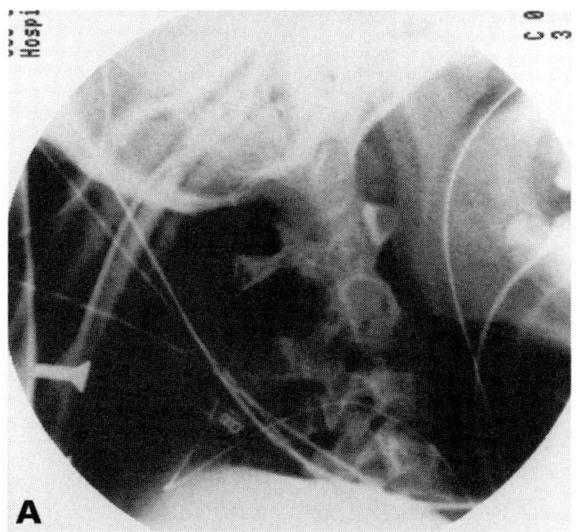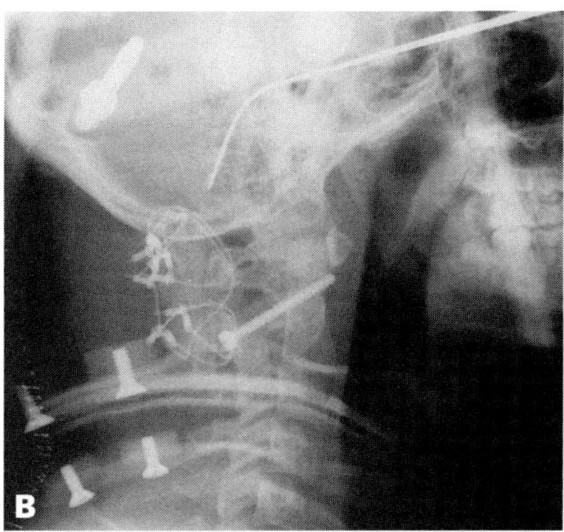

Figure 3: Occipital-atlantoaxial dislocation. **A)** Lateral x-ray of a Type IIB occipital-atlantoaxial dislocation. In addition to the longitudinal distraction of the occiput relative to the atlas, there is injury involving the C1-2 region. **B)** This patient was neurologically intact. He underwent an occiput-C2 fusion and stabilization using a screw-cable-rib construct. Dorsal C1-2 transarticular screwing was used to maximize support at this level (especially in rotation) following the atlantoaxial disruption. The rib onlay graft was secured to the occiput, C1, and C2 using sublaminar cables. (Reproduced with permission from Stillerman et al.[104])

injuries vary. Neurological deficits, when present, may result from upper cervical and lower cranial nerve injuries, vertebral artery damage, and brainstem and spinal cord dysfunction.[72]

Treatment has generally been directed toward reduction, followed by occipitocervical fusion and stabilization. The authors closely monitor the application of traction either by serial neurological examination in the awake patient or by somatosensory evoked potentials. Occipitocervical fusion is usually performed via a dorsal approach, although ventral procedures for occiput-C1-2 fusion have been described (Figure 3).[31,95]

Exposures

Ventral Approach

Ventral exposure of the craniocervical region presents a formidable challenge. The options include transoral exposure[29,97] or rostral extension of the ventrolateral approach of Smith and Robinson,[92] as described by DeAndrade and MacNab.[31] The transoral route permits excellent extradural decompression of ventral pathology. However, it is not a suitable approach for performing a stable arthrodesis. Bone grafts are fitted in a lock-and-key fashion from the clivus down to C2 without instrumentation.[36] This provides architectural support and resists axial load-ing to some extent, but it does not prevent axial rotation, flexion-extension, and lateral bending motion. Thus, immediate postoperative stability is not accomplished and the patient is required either to undergo supplemental dorsal fixation and fusion or to remain immobilized with a halo device for several months. Ventral fusion using the ventrolateral approach fares no better than the transoral approach in providing immediate stability and is therefore not recommended.[95]

Dorsal Approach

Occipitocervical fusion is the preferred method for arthrodesis. The patient is turned prone on a Stryker Frame and the operation is performed while on the frame. The relationship of the occiput to the atlas and axis is confirmed either by fluoroscopy or by a lateral x-ray. Surgically, a midline dorsal approach is used to expose from the external occipital protuberance down to the dorsal elements of the axis, but avoiding damage to the C2-3 interspinous ligament. Caudal dissection can be extended should the need to fuse a segment below the axis become necessary. The atlas is exposed, being easily recognized by its prominent and bifid spinous process. Subperiosteal dissection is performed to expose the squamous portion of the occipital bone and the dorsal rim of the foramen magnum, atlas, and

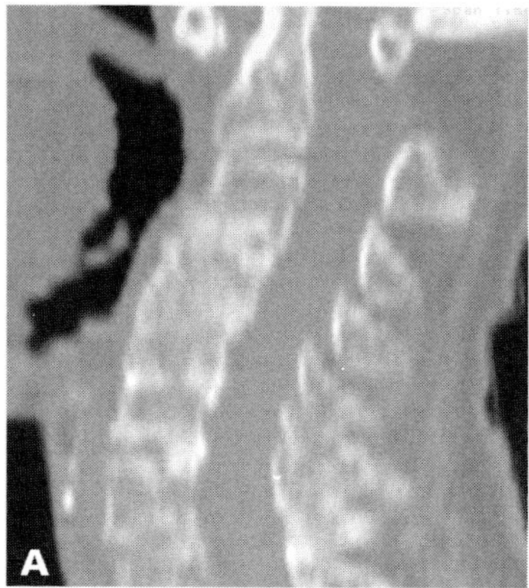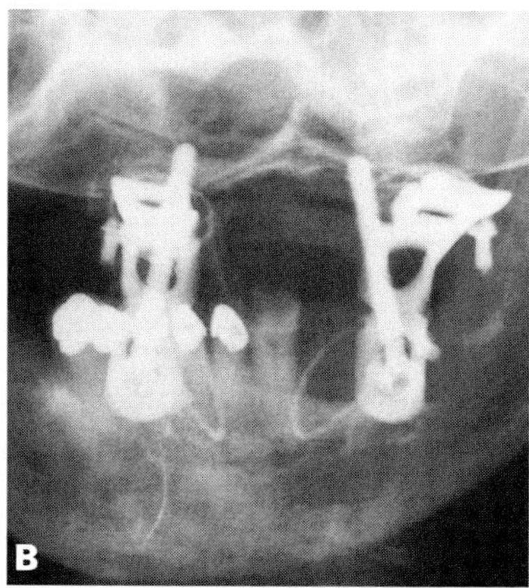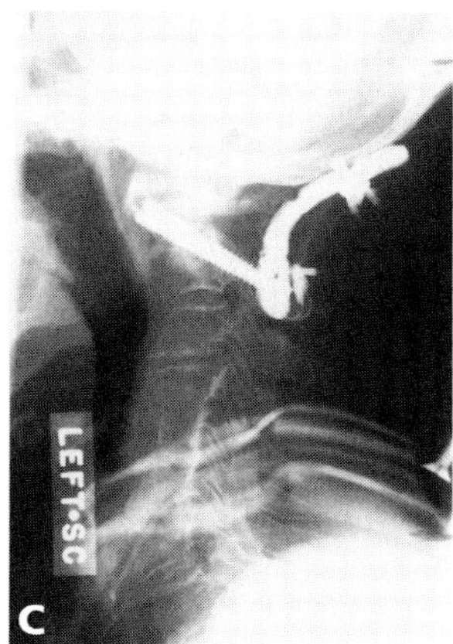

Figure 4: Occipital-atlantoaxial (OAA) instability. **A)** Sagittal reformat of CT bone window. Patient had myelopathy secondary to OAA instability caused by rheumatoid arthritis. Note significant cranial settling. **B** and **C)** Postoperative AP and lateral radiographs. Patient underwent a course of skeletal traction for reduction. Subsequently, OAA stabilization and fusion were performed using C1-2 screw-plate-cable fixation. This construct design included plates to maintain the reduction and C1-2 transarticular screws to maximize stability at the atlantoaxial level. The patient's myelopathy and neck pain improved following surgery. (Reproduced with permission from Stillerman et al.[104])

axis down to the subaxial level to be fused. Caution is exercised as one approaches dissection along the lateral aspect of the atlas to avoid injuring the vertebral artery.

Occipital Stabilization and Fusion Techniques

Dorsal fusion of the occiput to the cervical spine is the goal of surgery. The traditional methods of simple onlay grafts or bone grafts wired into position do not provide immediate stability and often lead to an unacceptable rate of nonunion, despite prolonged external immobilization.[47,55,63,78,105] Internal fixation as an adjunct to bony fusion allows for immediate rigid fixation without the need for long-term postoperative bracing and a better opportunity for long-term arthrodesis.[50,51,59,81,89] Newer techniques of fusing the occiput to the cervical spine, in conjunction with bone grafting, include the use of contoured rods, threaded pins, or plates secured with wires, screws, or cables alone or in combination. In several cases of occipitoatlantal instability, the authors secured reconstruction plates to the occiput with cables instead of screws and used atlantoaxial transarticular screws for fixation to the cervical spine (Figure 4).

Rods: Straight and Rectangular

Malleable rods from one of several Universal Spinal Instrumentation sets,[38,101,102] rectangular rods,[81,89] Luque/Hartshill rectangles,[65] or wide-diameter threaded Steinmann pins may be contoured and secured to the occiput (Figure 5).

Plates: Screws and Cable

Coupling of the occiput to the cervical spine with screw-plate fixation was first reported by Roy-Camille (Figure 6). Premolded plates, with an angulation of 105°, were designed to maintain lordosis of the occipitocervical junction.[88] The technique required fixation of two plates laterally and symmetrically. They are secured to the occiput with 13-mm long cancellous screws and to the cervical spine with transarticular screws at C2 or, if necessary, lateral mass screws subaxially. Heywood et al[59] described using T-shaped plates affixed to the axis by a screw in the spinous process and to the occipital bone with 8- to 10-mm screws. Grob et al[50] further modified this technique by designing inverted atlanto-occipital reconstruction Y-shaped plates secured to the occiput using one or two 10- to 12-mm screws into the midline crest and to C2 using transarticular screws. These plates are cut to the appropriate length and can be easily molded to

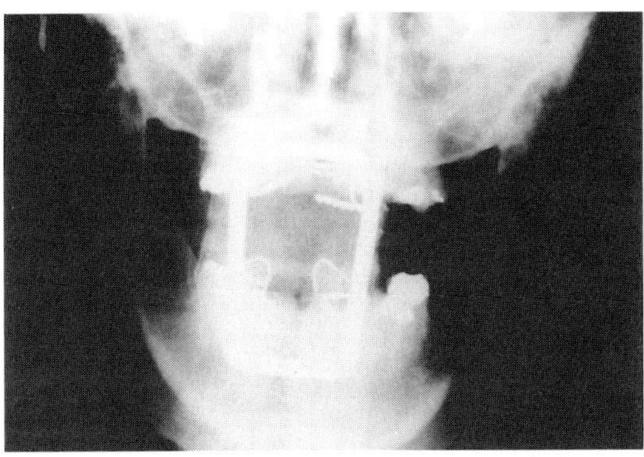

Figure 5: Luque rectangle and wires used for occipital cervical fusion. The major limitation of using this device for stabilization of this region is the difficulty encountered with rod bending.

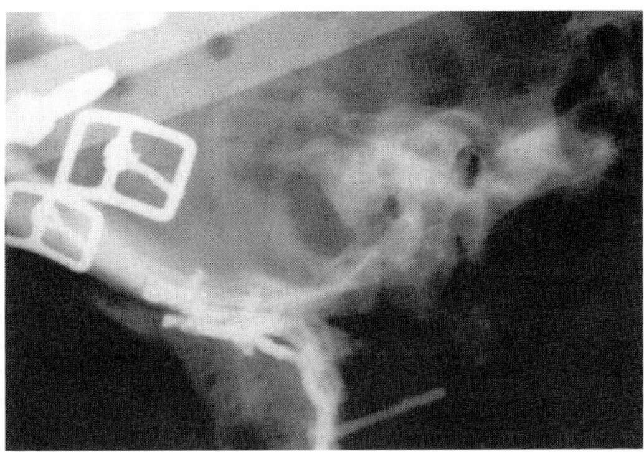

Figure 6: Screw-plate fixation for occiput-C2 stabilization. Reconstructive axis plates are contoured to the occipital cervical angle and anchored to the skull using fully threaded screws. Cervical fixation was achieved using a screw passed along the C2 pars interarticularis.

the contour of the dorsal surface. Tightening of the screws allows for excellent contact between the corticocancellous bone graft and the decorticated surface of the occiput, atlas, and axis. Because occipital bone is thicker and stronger in the midline than it is laterally, midline fixation provides more stability and fewer complications of screw penetration through the skull than those placed laterally.[88]

Advantages of the screw-plate techniques over those requiring the use of wire or cable include the avoidance of complications related to the passage of sublaminar wires and the increased stability provided by C1-2 transarticular screws, with respect to rotation. On the other hand, occipital screws can loosen and pull out, especially when shorter screws are used to avoid complications of intradural penetration.[50] Both techniques can potentially produce cerebrospinal fluid (CSF) leaks, although no leaks were reported with the screw-plate technique in the series of either Roy-Camille or Grob.

The fixation of rods or reconstruction plates with cables requires drilling holes into the occiput. The size and configuration of holes are arbitrary and depend on the preference of the surgeon. Wires can be passed through holes in the outer table of the occiput along the midline[111] or through bilateral burr holes. The passage of single- or double-stranded epidural cables or wires between the burr hole and the foramen magnum is facilitated by drilling holes

1-cm lateral to the midline and 0.5 cm rostral to the rim of the foramen magnum. Fixation with rods can also be performed by passing wires through two paramedian suboccipital burr holes or double grooves with at least 1 cm of bone between them to ensure bony arthrodesis. Complications of passing wires through the epidural space include the development of intracranial hematoma and CSF leak.

ATLANTOAXIAL INSTABILITY

Many causes of atlantoaxial instability have been recognized. Atlantoaxial subluxation with the potential for damage to the cervical spinal cord, can occur due to trauma, rheumatoid arthritis, neoplastic disease, degenerative disease, basilar invagination, occipitalization of the atlas, os odontoideum, aplasia or dysplasia of the dens, Down's syndrome, ankylosing spondylitis, and retropharyngeal infections.[72,109] Treatment must be based on individual pathology, and the technique chosen to achieve atlantoaxial arthrodesis must be suitable to that particular condition. Rupture of the transverse ligament associated with fractures of the atlas (C1 arch or classic Jefferson's fracture), rotatory subluxation of higher grades, or odontoid fractures will not heal spontaneously and require surgical fusion. Ligamentous insufficiency, without evidence of bony fractures, or fractures that have failed conservative management also require surgical treatment.

In the presence of atlantoaxial subluxation with normal occipitoatlantal integrity, fusion of C1-2 is the treatment of choice. The occiput is included in the fusion mass only when evidence of occipitoatlantal pathology co-exists. In doing so, approximately 13° of flexion-extension and 8° of lateral bending movements are eliminated in the upper cervical spine (Table 1). The techniques of surgical fixation to the occiput have already been described.

Exposures

Ventral Approach

In most cases of atlantoaxial instability, stabilization is performed via a dorsal approach. Surgery for ventral decompression may be indicated for irreducible odontoid fractures causing symptomatic spinal cord compression. In such cases, the ventral transoral approach is used for extradural decompression. However, instability created by removal of the ventral arch of the atlas and the fractured dens is difficult to stabilize via this approach. The use of transoral bone grafts fitted between the clivus and C2 has been described.[36] Immediate stability is not achieved and, postoperatively, the patient will require either dorsal fusion or halo immobilization.

Dorsal Approach

In general, patients are already in cervical traction prior to the operation. Patients are induced while awake, with fiberoptic intubation and evoked potential monitoring. They are then turned prone with the head resting in a horseshoe-shaped headrest, affixed to a table-mounted head holder, or secured on the Stryker table. A lateral radiograph or fluoroscopy imaging is obtained to check the alignment of the upper cervical spine. The length and position of the midline incision are dictated by the procedure performed. The nuchal fascia and the paraspinous muscles are subperiosteally dissected to expose the dorsal rim of the foramen magnum and the dorsal elements of the atlas and axis. Spinal fixation techniques for atlantoaxial instability include bone grafting with wiring procedures between C1 and C2, Halifax clamp fixation of the C1-2 lamina when bony fractures of the dorsal elements are absent, and transarticular screw fixation of the lateral mass of the atlas and C2.

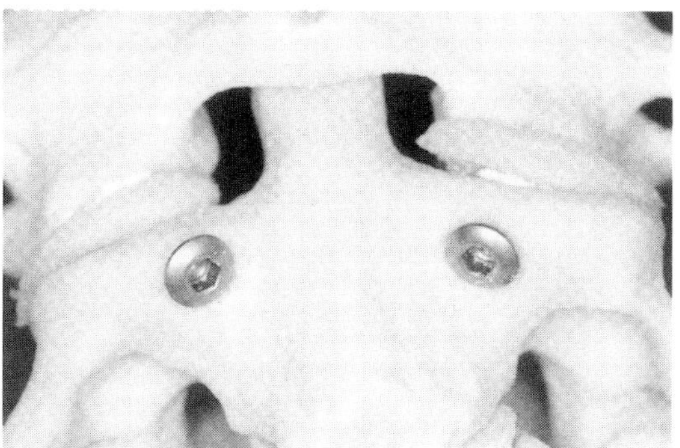

Figure 7: Ventral C1-2 transarticular screws used for stabilization of the atlantoaxial region.

Stabilization and Fusion Techniques

Ventral C1-2 Transarticular Screw Fixation

Ventral transarticular screw fixation of C1-2 for instability has been reported (Figure 7).[10,95] Its use is not common since high cervical exposure is technically difficult and may require bilateral exposure. Screws 3.5 mm in diameter are passed under fluoroscopic guidance from the caudal-medial aspect of the lateral mass of C2, extending through the C1-2 junction and ending into the C1 lateral masses. The dorsal approach for C1-2 screw fixation is technically easier and poses less operative risk to the patient.

Bone-Wire Constructs: Gallie, Brooks, and Modified Techniques

Traditional dorsal atlantoaxial fusion utilizes a combination of wiring and a corticocancellous bone graft. Membranes and ligaments from the undersurface of dorsal elements of the atlas and axis are removed to facilitate the passage of sublaminar wires. In the Gallie fusion, a bone graft is interposed between the dorsal arch of C1 and the spinous process of C2. This is held in place by one wire passed sublaminarly at C1 and looped around the spinous process of C2 (Figure 8).[43] Recently, cables have been introduced and may be used instead of wires to provide more strength and safety during these procedures.[94] Brooks' modification of this technique includes the insertion of two wedge-shaped bone grafts placed bilaterally between the dorsal arch and the lam-

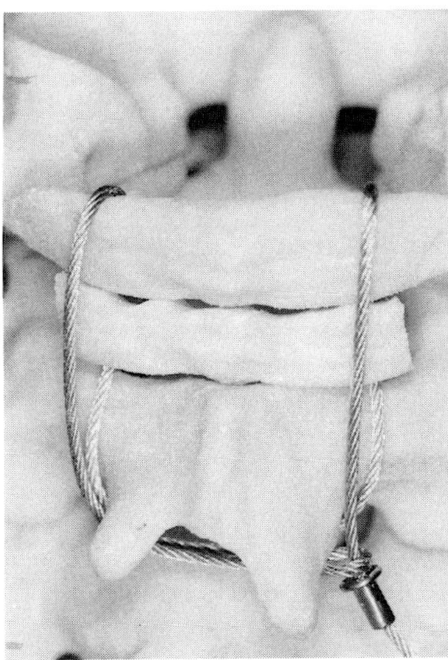

Figure 8: Gallie fusion. Cables are passed under the lamina of C1 and wrapped around the spinous process of C2.

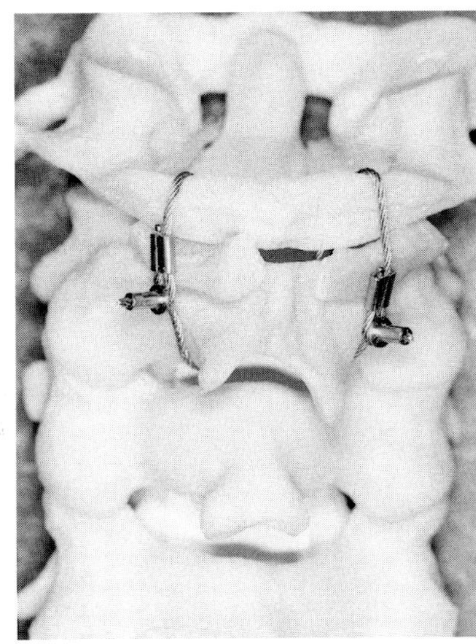

Figure 9: Brooks fusion. Two sublaminar cables are used, one on each side of midline, to secure two wedges of bone. For illustrative purposes, the size of the bone graft is smaller than actually used.

ina of the axis. In addition, a pair of wires (instead of one) is passed beneath both the dorsal arch and the lamina of C2, securing each bone graft in position (Figure 9).[20] Other modifications have involved changes in the shape of the bone graft or variations of wiring techniques, all with the intention of enhancing bony fusion and improving fixation strength.

Biomechanical evaluation *in vitro* reveals that wiring procedures significantly decreased motion in all planes compared to that exhibited by intact and injured spines.[48,49,54] It also indicated that Brooks' modification provides more stability in flexion, extension, axial rotation, and lateral bending movements than does the Gallie technique. Although wiring procedures are that simple and relatively easy to perform, they do have the disadvantages of sublaminar wiring. This is especially significant when there is spinal canal compromise due to ventrally located lesions, making the passage of wires unsafe. Additionally, the rate of nonunion with wiring techniques exceeds 10%.[41,91,93,105] A further disadvantage of wiring procedures is that the patient usually undergoes external immobilization in a halo or Minerva fixation for a period of 8 to 12 weeks postoperatively.[68,91]

The development of alternative internal fixation techniques has been stimulated by the de-

sire for increased safety, decreased postsurgical bracing needs, increased mechanical strength of C1-2 fixation without fusion of the occiput, and improvement in fusion rates. Methods of dorsal atlantoaxial fusion developed in an attempt to meet these needs include fixation with clamps or hooks and transarticular screws.

Halifax Clamp

The use of Halifax interlaminar clamps, in combination with bone grafting, is a relatively new technique for C1-2 fixation (Figure 10).[3,4,30,60] Following subperiosteal exposure, bilateral clamps are placed snugly over the rostral edge of the atlas and under the caudal edge of the lamina of the axis. A screw of appropriate length is then selected and applied to couple the hooks together and tightly compress the lamina so that no movement occurs at the fused level. Sequential screw tightening is performed with a specially designed 90° angled wrench, followed by crimping of the distal threads to prevent screw loosening. Corticocancellous bone graft is inserted between the dorsal arch of C1 and C2. The overall rate of atlantoaxial fusion by this technique is 80%-90%, yielding slightly better results in patients with instability due to trauma.[3] Mechanical studies comparing dorsal atlantoaxial fixation techniques revealed that the sta-

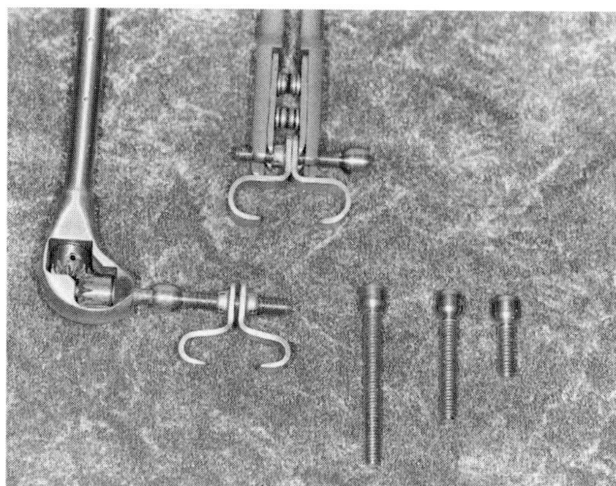

Figure 10: Halifax clamps and instrumentation. A variety of clamps exist for sublaminar placement in different areas of the cervical spine. Screw lengths also vary to accommodate different fusion lengths. The hooks are interconnected by threading a screw through a hole at the top of the hook. Special right-angle screwdrivers have greatly improved the ease of screw placement *(far left)*. Once the screw is placed, a crimping device is used to help prevent screw backout *(top center)*.

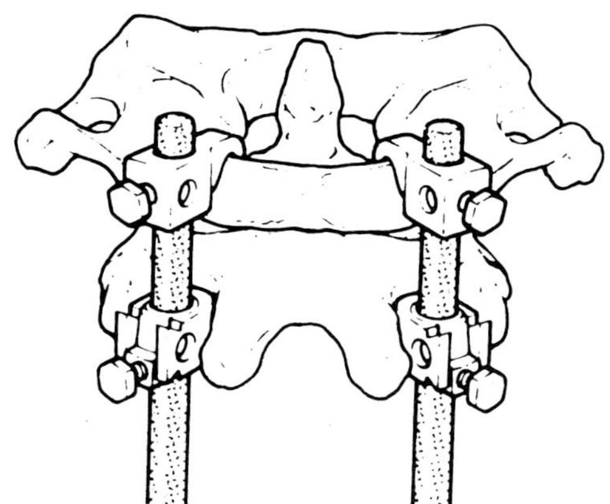

Figure 11: Diagram of pediatric Universal Spinal Instrumentation hooks and rods used for cervical stabilization. Migration of hooks into spinal canal may result in significant neurological complications.

bility provided with clamps is equal to that observed with the Brooks' wiring procedure, but with less rotational control than that attained with transarticular screws.[49] Clamps are magnetic resonance imaging (MRI)-compatible and may be easier to apply than wires or cables. The use of clamps also avoids some of the risks of sublaminar wiring. These implants are relatively bulky within the spinal canal, however, and may contribute to neurological injury by compressing the spinal cord. This is especially true in the presence of ventral intracanalicular soft tissue or incompletely reduced subluxations. An additional problem using clamps in the atlantoaxial region is screw loosening, with a resultant loss of fixation. To reduce the incidence of screw loosening, newer clamps have been designed. Postoperatively, immobilization is recommended for at least 6 weeks in a Philadelphia collar.

Universal Spinal Instrumentation Hooks: Pediatric

Pediatric or specially designed narrow-bladed hooks have been used as anchors and coupled to rods to achieve fixation in the upper cervical spine (Figure 11). Extreme caution must be maintained to avoid hook migration into the spinal canal.

Dorsal C1-2 Transarticular Screw Fixation

Dorsal screw fixation with rigid coupling of the axis and atlas is frequently regarded as the method of choice for atlantoaxial arthrodesis.[51,67,69,105] The technique involves bilateral placement of screws, beginning directly above the C2-3 facet joint, across the C2 pars interarticularis and C1-2 joint space, and terminating in the lateral mass of C1. In the original report of the procedure by Magerl and Seeman,[67] transarticular screw fixation of C1-2 was supplemented with a Gallie-type bone-wire fusion. A true three-point fixation was thus achieved. This was believed to provide greater multidirectional stability than either procedure alone. Stillerman and Wilson,[105] on the other hand, provided evidence against the need for supplemental wiring with transarticular screw fixation. In their series of patients who underwent C1-2 screw fixation and bone grafting without simultaneous wiring procedures, 95% demonstrated solid bony union. Complications were minimal and no neurological, vascular, or hardware-related problems have been reported.

In addition to improved fusion rates, other characteristics make this technique desirable. Biomechanical testing in human cadaver specimens has shown transarticular screw fixation to be superior in providing immediate three-dimensional stability.[49] It provides the greatest stability in axial rotation and lateral bending and, compared to the wiring methods of Gallie and

Brooks or with Halifax clamps, is slightly better in prohibiting ventral/dorsal translation. Since this procedure may eliminate sublaminar wiring and intraspinal placement of bulky implants such as Halifax clamps, it is well suited for patients with C1-2 instability in the face of spinal canal compromise. In situations that preclude the use of wiring or clamp fixation, as with fractures of the dorsal elements of C1 and/or C2, transarticular screw fixation can stabilize atlantoaxial motion, obviating the need to extend the fusion to the occiput. Thus, atlanto-occipital motion is preserved and the risk of nonunion, reportedly as high as 23%, is avoided.[40,48,91,105] An additional advantage of dorsal atlantoaxial facet screws is that they can be combined with metallic plates for fusion to the occiput or to the subaxial spine, if necessary.

Technique

Following awake fiberoptic nasotracheal intubation in the supine position, the patient is turned prone on a Stryker or similar bed. Radiolucent sponges are packed in the mouth to obtain adequate real-time fluoroscopic visualization of anteroposterior (AP) and lateral images. Baseline somatosensory evoked potentials are obtained, and monitoring is continued throughout the operation. The patient is placed either in a halo ring or in Gardner-Wells tongs for intraoperative traction. To obtain proper alignment of C1 and C2 for drilling and screwing, the position of the neck is neutral or slightly flexed and placed in a manner that permits intraoperative manual flexion. A midline incision is made from the level of the inion to T1, followed by subperiosteal exposure from C1 to C7. A wide rostral-caudal exposure further facilitates the angulation that is required for insertion of drills and screws.

Subperiosteal dissection is used to expose the dorsum of the isthmus of C2 and the C1-2 articular surface. Coagulation of the vascular plexus and retraction of the C2 nerve root in the rostral direction provide direct visualization of the C1-2 joint. Prior to the drilling of holes, cartilage from the joint space is removed with small curettes, and the entire dorsum of the C2 pars interarticularis is exposed (Figure 12). This minimizes the risk of damage to the vertebral artery laterally and the spinal cord medially. An entry site is

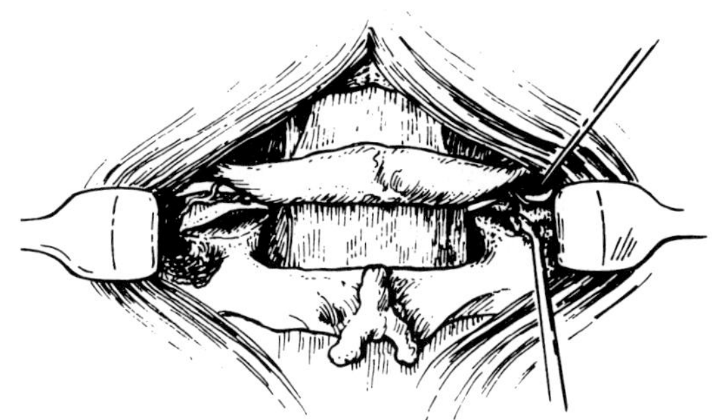

Figure 12: The C2-3 facet joint is identified. Dissection is then carried in the rostral direction to expose the entire dorsum of the C2 pars interarticularis. This exposure minimizes the likelihood of unsatisfactory screw placement by enabling better appreciation of where instruments are in relation to the C2 isthmus during the hole preparation and screw placement. Caudal to the C1-2 joint, a neurovascular plexus containing the C2 nerve and veins is encountered. The vascular plexus may be coagulated and cut, and the C2 nerve may be gently elevated with a nerve hook. A small curette directed medially away from the vertebral artery is shown here removing the cartilage from the joint. (Reproduced with permission from Stillerman et al.[105])

selected. This is generally 2 mm above the center of the C2-3 facet joint and 2 mm medial to the middle of the joint. This is decorticated using a high-speed drill. A pilot hole is then made using a 2.7-mm drill bit powered by a mini-screwdriver. Biplanar real-time fluoroscopic imaging is essential to visualize the optimal path for passage through the C1-2 joint space and entry into the lateral mass of C1 (Figure 13). Drilling is stopped once the dorsal cortical surface of the ventral arch of C1 is reached. In some cases, the trajectory may be directed too far ventrally into the retropharynx and drilling may completely miss the lateral mass of C1. This risk can be reduced by elevating the spinous process of C2 using a Kocher clamp, with simultaneous displacement of C1 ventrally to facilitate drilling at a greater angle relative to the sagittal plane. Caution must be exercised, however, since excessive pulling of C2 may produce abnormal flexion with loss of normal alignment. A 3.5-mm self-tap is used to continue the hole preparation before placement of permanent titanium nonself-tapping screws (Figure 14). In most patients, cortical screws measuring 3.5 mm in major diameter are used (Figure 15). Screws of smaller diameter are avail-

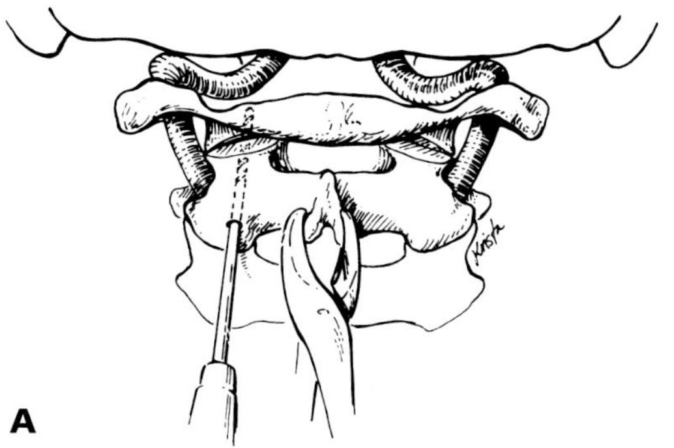
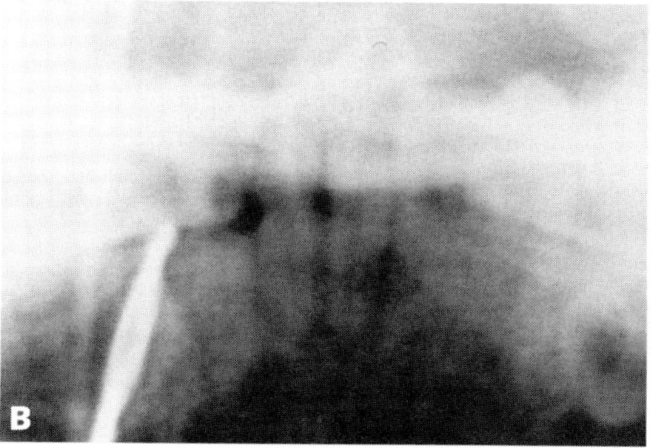

Figure 13: Hole preparation–pilot hole. **A)** The screw entry site is located directly above the C2-3 facet joint and 2 mm medial to the center of the joint. Exposure of the dorsum of the C2 isthmus allows direct monitoring during drilling. Drilling is carried out along the center of the pars, with great care taken to avoid angling lateral into the vertebral artery. The drill bit is advanced until the dorsal surface of the ventral arch of C1 is reached. Biplanar real time imaging facilitates safety during hole preparation and screw placement. **B)** Modified open-mouth fluoroscopic view. A non-reinforced nasotracheal tube is used. The mouth has been packed open with radiolucent sponges. This allows excellent visualization of the C1-2 region, which enables appreciation of coronal plane orientation. This helps avoid lateral placement with vertebral artery damage as well as medial injury to the spinal cord. Additionally, the AP view helps provide information regarding the number of screw threads that are capturing the lateral mass of C1. (Reproduced with permission from Stillerman et al.[105])

able and may be required if the transverse diameter of the isthmus directly below the C1-2 joint is a limiting factor. Permanent screw lengths range from 35 to 45 mm, with the average measuring 39 mm; the screw length is determined by measuring the depth of the hole with a depth gauge. After placing the initial screw, a second hole is drilled on the other side and another screw is threaded into place. The dorsal arch of the C1 and C2 lamina and spinous process is decorticated using a high-speed drill, and an onlay bone graft is placed. In addition, the bone graft is packed into the C1-2 facet joints. Postoperatively, the patient is kept in a soft collar or a Philadelphia collar for up to 3 months.[69,105]

Percutaneous modification of the dorsal transarticular procedure has made possible a much smaller skin incision with less soft-tissue dissection, requiring exposure of only C1-3. Small stab wounds are made on either side of C7 or T1 for insertion of a drill guide through the subcutaneous tissue and muscle extending rostral to the caudal border of C2. Extended drill bits, taps, depth gauges, and screwdrivers are used for hole preparation and permanent screw placement (Figure 16).

Complications directly related to the technique of C1-2 fixation are attributed to improper trajectory for screw insertion and malposition of the screws.[48,51] Screws directed too far laterally can potentially injure the vertebral artery with consequent ischemic damage to the brainstem and upper cervical cord. A small number of patients have aberrant vertebral artery anatomy, and transarticular screw fixation may not be the method of choice for such patients. Preoperative computed tomography (CT) and/or MRI studies are needed to carefully evaluate the course of the artery around the atlantoaxial region so as to avoid vascular complications that, although quite rare, have been reported. Injury to the spinal cord or CSF fistulas can result with screws that are aimed too far medially. Screws that are too long can project beyond the lateral mass of the atlas ventrally with resultant neurological sequelae. Grob et al[51] reported the development of unilateral paresis of the hypoglossal nerve in a patient who had undergone transarticular screw fixation. They attributed this injury to a long screw that projected ventral to the occipital condyle, most likely causing hypoglossal nerve irritation; once the screw was replaced with one of appropriate length, recovery of the deficit followed. Long screws penetrating beyond C1 and into the region of the occipital condyle have been reported to cause erosion of the atlanto-occipital joint, with subsequent instability and pain.[51] Reoperation was required to remove the screw and

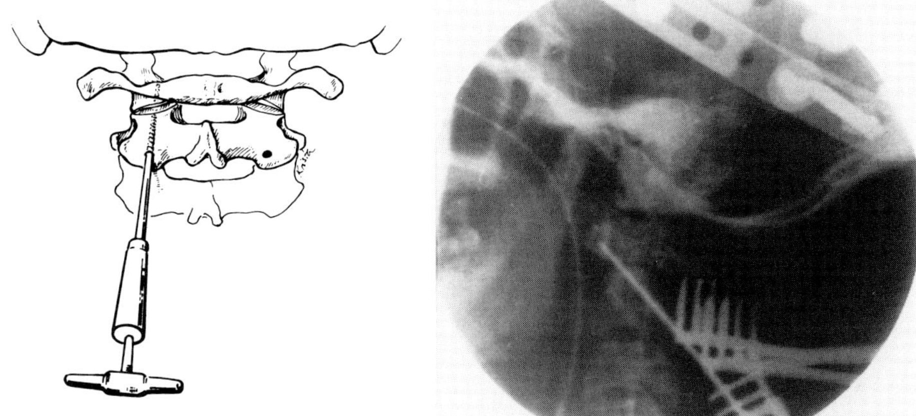

Figure 14: Hole preparation and tapping. A 3.5-mm tap is used to continue the preparation. The tap is advanced to the dorsal surface of the ventral arch of C1. (Reproduced with permission from Stillerman et al.[105])

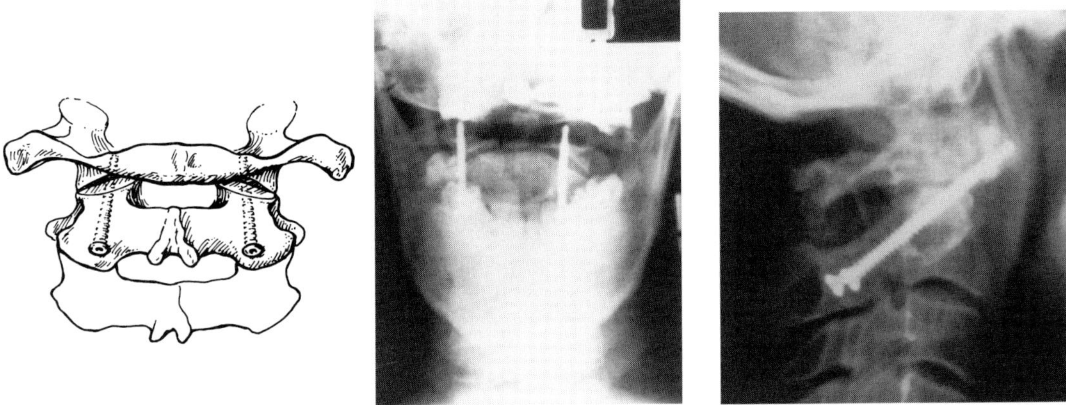

Figure 15: Screw placement. After the tapping is completed, a depth gauge is inserted to measure the length of the permanent screw. The C1-2 joint is packed with bone. Permanent screws are then placed. Optimally, several screw threads should enter the lateral mass of C1. This enhances resistance to screw pull-out. (Reproduced with permission from Stillerman et al.[105])

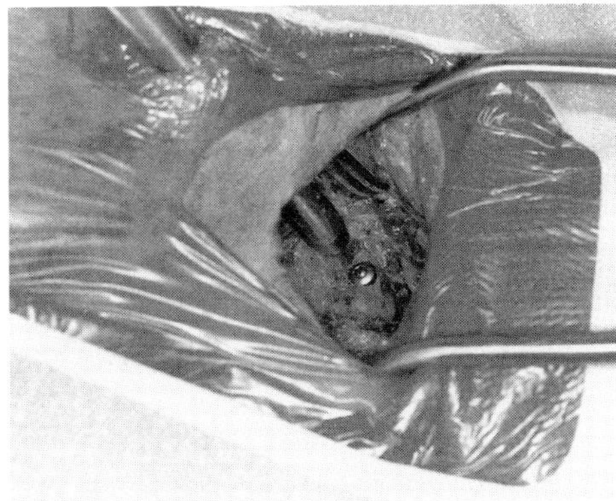

Figure 16: Percutaneous modification of the dorsal transarticular procedure. A small incision exposing C1-3 only is combined with percutaneous hole preparation and screw placement. This technique is intended to diminish postoperative pain and the length of hospitalization without sacrificing safety. (Reproduced with permission from Stillerman et al.[104])

extend the fusion to the occiput for stabilization and relief of pain. Obviously, screws that are too short will not provide adequate stability.

A comminuted fracture of the lateral mass of C1 or the C2 pars interarticularis on the ipsilateral side may preclude bilateral screw placement. For maximal rotational stability, both lateral masses of C1 should be engaged. If one is successfully coupled and the other is not, rotational stability may be inadequate with an increased potential for screw breakage and loss of fixation. However, this has not been substantiated in clinical cases.[51] The inadequate reduction with improper alignment of the C1-2 complex is another indication for atlantoaxial fusion by techniques other than that of transarticular screw placement.[69]

When performed by surgeons experienced with the nuances of this technique, dorsal C1-2 transarticular screw fixation provides superior fixation of the atlantoaxial level with enhanced fusion rates and a reduced incidence of postoperative bracing, hardware failures, and complications.[51,67,69,105]

ODONTOID FRACTURES

Fractures of the axis comprise approximately 17% of cervical spine injuries, with the majority of these injuries being odontoid fractures.[6,9,18,52,68] The most widely accepted classification for these fractures is that proposed by Anderson and D'Alonzo.[7] Their scheme divides fractures of the odontoid into three subtypes, based on the anatomic location of the fractured site.

- Type I: This fracture type involves only the tip of the odontoid process. These are stable fractures and require bracing for 12 weeks. This type is rare.
- Type II: This fracture pattern involves the synchondrosis where the body of C2 fuses with the odontoid process. A consequence of this fracture pattern is disruption of the blood supply to the dens, which results in a poor prognosis for fracture healing. Nonunion rates for Type II fractures without operation range from 10% to 100%.[7] Two major criteria that predispose a patient to nonunion is advanced age and significant AP translation. It is generally agreed that subluxation of greater than 4-6 mm significantly enhances the likelihood of non-osseous union.[9] When these criteria are met, most surgeons advocate operative stabilization for Type II fractures. This type is the most commonly seen.
- Type III: Fractures of this type extend into the body of the axis and have a 95% chance of a solid osseous union with external immobilization.

This classification scheme has been criticized because of a lack of anatomical precision. A new classification scheme for C2 vertebral body fractures has been proposed by Benzel et al.[14] Unlike the scheme of Anderson and D'Alonzo, there is distinction between the odontoid process and the C2 vertebral body fractures. The scheme accepts Anderson Type II as the only true odontoid process fracture and subclassifies C2 vertebral body fractures as Type 1 (coronally oriented fractures), Type 2 (sagittally oriented fractures), and Type 3 (horizontal fractures through the rostral aspect of the body). Type 3 is the previously described Anderson Type III. This system clearly represents an improvement in terms of identification of the injured regions and the mechanism whereby these injuries occurred. It is hoped that this information will enable improvement in treatment algorithms for these patients.

Odontoid Stabilization and Fusion Techniques

Ventral Transodontoid Screw Fixation

Surgical options for odontoid fractures include ventral transodontoid screw fixation and dorsal C1-2 arthrodesis. Transodontoid screw fixation may be the optimal treatment for acutely unstable Type II fractures if the transverse ligament is intact. This technique was initially described by Nakanishi et al[77] and has subsequently been used by other authors.[1,19,35,42,44,73] Apfelbaum[8] refined the procedure and has been instrumental in developing retractors and instrumentation to facilitate the technique of screw fixation. One major advantage of this procedure over dorsal fusion is that it preserves atlantoaxial motion.

Technique

An absolute requirement of transodontoid screw fixation the availability of high-resolution fluoroscopic imaging. Biplanar real-time AP and

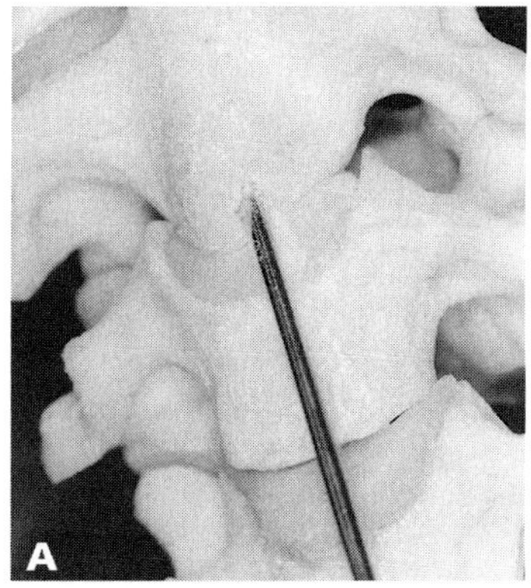
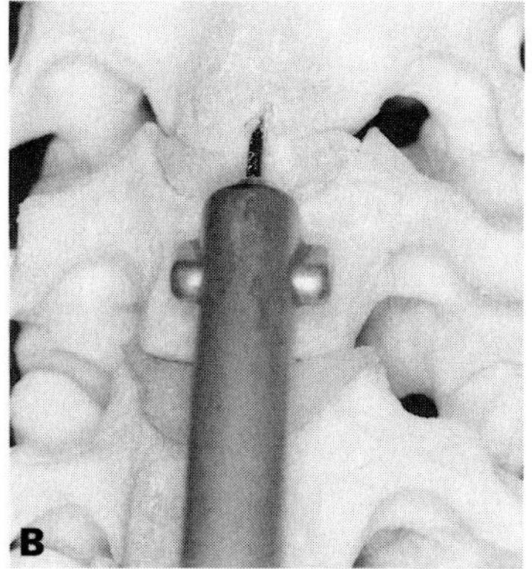
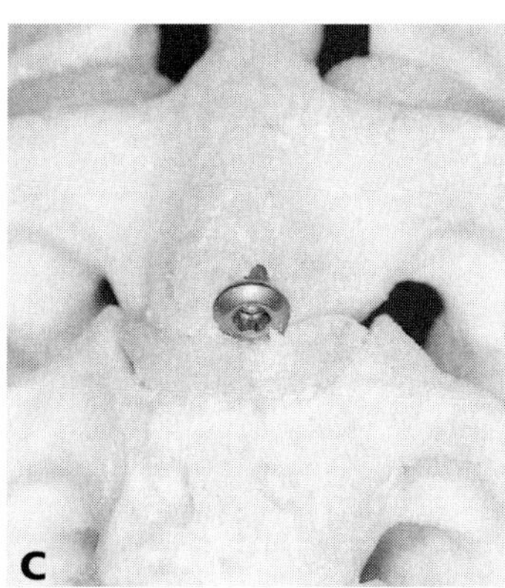
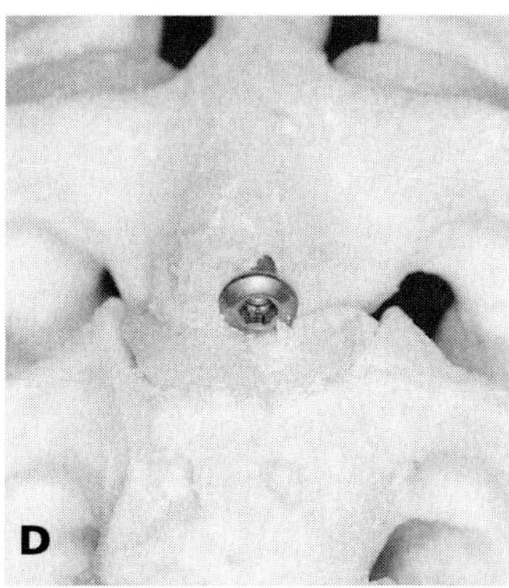

Figure 17: Transodontoid screw fixation. **A)** K-wire placement. K-wire is inserted under fluoroscopic guidance into the caudal portion of the C2 vertebrae. A coring instrument is then placed over the K-wire to create a trough in the ventral rostral portion of C3 and C2-3 disc. This trough enables drilling at an appropriate angle to capture the odontoid process. **B)** Insertion of the drill guide. A drill guide is placed over the K-wire. This guide consists of an outer tube that is secured to the C3 vertebrae via spikes. The inner tube (partially seen in this photograph) is advanced to contact the inferior portion of C2. **C)** Tapping. After drilling to the tip of the dens, the drill is removed and the hole is tapped. **D)** Screw placement. After tapping, the hole is measured using a depth gauge. A permanent screw is selected. A lag screw, which only has distal threads, is used to enable compression of the fractured odontoid onto the body of C2.

lateral imaging is optimal. The patient is placed in the supine position with the head extended to facilitate the attainment of the trajectory required for odontoid screw placement. A small transverse skin incision is made above the level of the C5-6 disc space. Dissection is carried down to the longus coli muscle, which is elevated and reflected laterally. Self-retaining retractors are carefully seated under the muscle bellies. Blunt dissection is performed until the anterior longitudinal ligament at the caudal margin of the C2 body is reached. The C2-3 disc space is identified, and the ventral ligament is sharply cut. C2 transodontoid screw fixation involves the passage of a screw, beginning 2-3 mm lateral to the midline at the ventral-caudal body of C2. A K-wire is placed into the caudal portion of C2 under fluoroscopic guidance (Figure 17A). A hollow coring instrument is then passed over the wire and is used to create a trough in the C3 vertebral body and C2-3 disc. This trough enables drilling at an angle favorable for screw capture of the odontoid process. The coring instrument is removed and the drill guide, which

consists of inner and outer tubes, is introduced over the K-wire (Figure 17B). The outer guide tube is secured to the C3 vertebral body by fixation spikes. This minimizes the potential for drill-guide slippage and enables manipulation of the spinal column to improve the angle of drilling. The inner tube is advanced to contact the caudal portion of the C2 vertebral body. The K-wire is removed and a drill bit is introduced and used to drill the pilot hole that extends from the C2 vertebral body across the fracture to the tip of the dens. Rostral migration of the dens during drilling will not occur in the absence of ligamentous injury. Once drilling is complete, the inner drill guide is removed and a tap is inserted through the outer guide (Figure 17C). Following tapping, the length of the hole is determined. This can be accomplished using either a depth gauge or the calibrated markers found on the drill and tap. A permanent lag screw is selected and threaded into place through the outer guide (Figure 17D). The screw passes across the C2 synchondrosis and into the tip of the fractured odontoid process. A partially

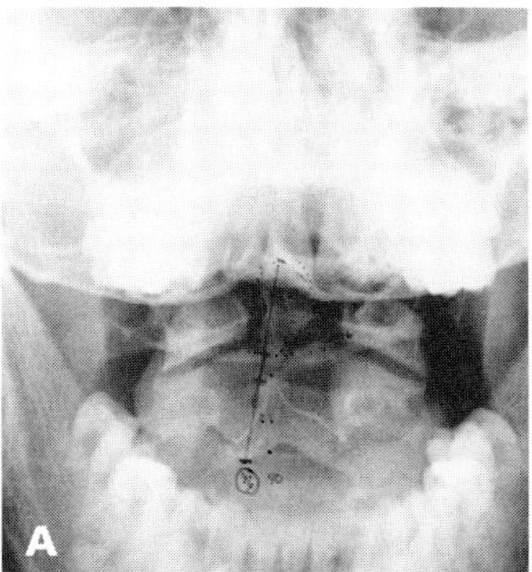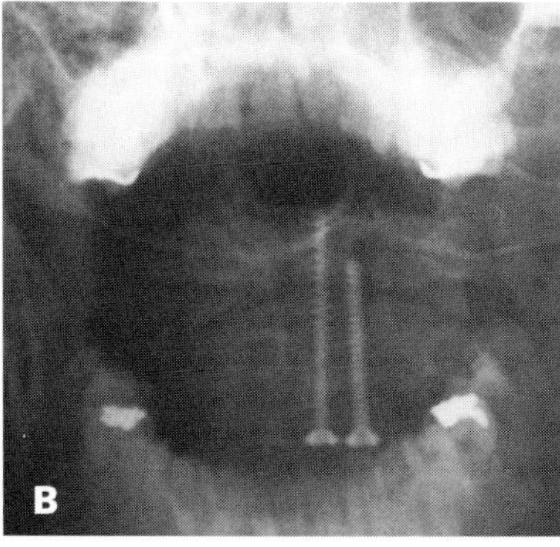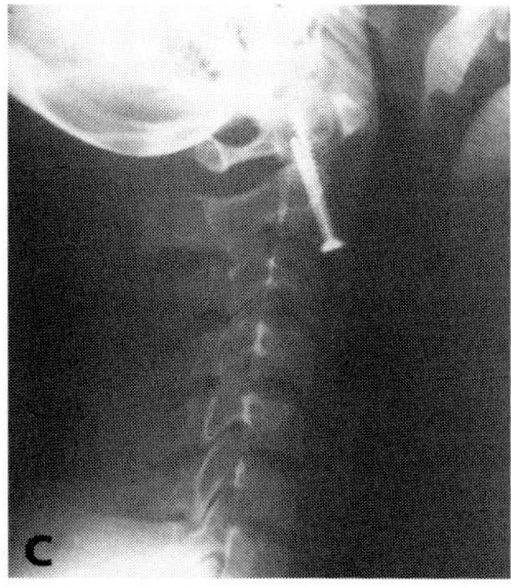

Figure 18: A) Nonunion of Type II odontoid fracture in a 16-year-old patient. X-ray after placement in a halo device for over 4 months. **B** and **C)** Anteroposterior and lateral postoperative x-rays. Transodontoid screw fixation was used to stabilize the fracture. Despite being a chronic injury, the fractured odontoid was compressed onto the C2 body with the lag screw. Prior to screw placement, the fibrous tissue at the synchondrosis was curetted. The second screw was fully threaded and provides additional mechanical strength. Used with permission from Stillerman et al.[104]

threaded screw (lag screw) is selected as the first screw is placed. This screw design helps pull the fractured dens down, compressing it against the body of C2. The screw should penetrate the tip of the odontoid process with one full thread turn. The size of the odontoid process dictates the feasibility of safely placing more than one screw. When two screws are used, the second screw can be a fully threaded screw (Figure 18). The second screw functions to provide mechanical strength and rotational stability, not compression. For this reason, not all of the threads need to pass beyond the fractured site.[35]

Contraindications

Absolute

When there is evidence of rupture of the transverse ligament in addition to a Type II fracture, a dorsal atlantoaxial fusion is indicated. Direct ventral screw fixation of the dens in this situation does not address instability at the C1-2 level.

Relative

Chronic nonunion of an odontoid fracture may not heal with ventral screw fixation. This is attributed to the development of scar tissue and sclerosis around the fractured fragment, which interferes with reduction and bony fusion. However, nonunions have been successfully treated up to 24 months following injury with this technique (Figure 18).[1,18,41,43,72,76] In chronic fractures, curetting the fibrous tissue prior to screw passage has been advocated.[8] Patients with radiographic evidence of osteoporosis secondary to advanced age or generalized bone atrophy may experience failure with this technique because of inadequate bone purchase. Ventral screw fixation is not ideal for barrel-chested patients or those with short necks because of the technical difficulties encountered with screw placement. Patients in whom fracture reduction cannot be achieved with ventrally translated dens are also poor candidates for this procedure.

SUBAXIAL INSTABILITY

Approximately 75% of cervical spine injuries involve the subaxial cervical region (C3-7).[17] Injury in this region occurs most commonly in the skeletally mature patient and involves several distinct failure patterns. A number of surgical options exist because of modern developments in this area. The following section focuses on the contemporary fixation methods, while emphasizing principles, techniques, and limitations of each procedure. This section begins with the evaluation of a classification scheme, which attempts to define the failure forces that have created the injury. This information provides the foundation for optimal implant selection, design, and application.

Mechanistic Classification of Injuries

The determination of spinal instability relies on the understanding of normal spinal kinematics (Table 1). In an attempt to organize a broad spectrum of injuries affecting the cervical spine, several classification schemes have been proposed. In 1982, Allen et al[5] introduced their mechanistic classification scheme. The hypothesis of this classification is that injuries can be grouped into specific patterns based on major and minor forces, or "injury vectors," that create anatomic disruption. The severity of the spinal disruption is a function of the magnitude of the vectors, and similar vectors produce similar injury patterns.

Six common patterns of indirect injury to the mid and lower cervical spine were identified: 1) compressive-flexion; 2) compressive-extension; 3) distractive-flexion; 4) vertical-compression; 5) lateral-flexion; and 6) distractive-extension. The most common patterns seen are compressive-flexion, compressive-extension, and distractive-flexion. Lateral-flexion and distractive-extension are seen least often, with vertical-compression patterns being intermediate in frequency. Each pattern of injury can be further subdivided into stages, depending upon the severity of fractures and vertebral displacement. Thus, a particular force vector gives rise to a family of injuries within a specific pattern, with each new stage of injury being added onto the injury incurred in the prior stage. There is usually a strong correlation between the magnitude of the force required for each injury pattern and the consequent neurological damage.

Compressive-flexion, compression-extension, and vertical-compression injuries share a common feature in that all undergo an axial load that contributes to their failure. A result of the axial forces is shortening of the injured portion of the spine. Distraction injuries (distractive-flexion and distractive-extension), on the other hand, result from supraphysiological distractive forces that cause tension failure and lengthening of the injured segment. Lateral-flexion injuries result from an asymmetrically applied compressive injury vector toward the side of flexion and a minor distractive injury vector along the opposite side.

Advantages of this classification scheme include: 1) a systematic evaluation of radiographic studies in search of evidence for anatomic disruption; 2) categorization of injuries into specific patterns based on the mechanism of injury facilitates interobserver consistency; and 3) knowledge of the failure forces that created the injury enables a thoughtful and appropriate stabilization procedure, designed to counteract these forces.

Specific Injury Patterns

Compressive-Flexion

This group comprises approximately 20% of subaxial injuries and results from vector forces directed caudally and ventrally. Early stages of compressive-flexion (CF) injuries may show only loss of vertebral body height to less than 30% without compromising either ventral or dorsal ligamentous structures. The spine in this stage is considered stable and management is conservative. In higher grades of injuries, as seen with increasing compressive loading of a flexed spine, significant vertebral body collapse and displacement of the body into the spinal canal may result. In the most severe cases, there may be incompetence of the posterior longitudinal ligament and dorsal ligamentous complex with distraction of the facet joints.

Surgery is required to treat severe CF injuries. The approach is influenced by factors that include the patient's neurological status, compression of neural elements from bone or disc, and integrity of the dorsal ligamentous complex. Decompression is essential only for patients with incomplete deficits, since it is unclear whether removing compressive lesions provides neurological benefit in the patient with complete cord injury. If a corpectomy is performed to decompress neural structures, an interbody bone graft is used for load-bearing and ultimate fusion.

To ensure immediate mechanical stability, techniques using internal fixation have been developed as adjuncts to bone grafting. Both ventral and dorsal techniques are described in the literature. However, controversy remains as to which is the better approach. Ventral screw-plate fixation provides immediate stability to the injured segment and helps prevent subluxation and graft dislodgement. In select CF injuries, ventral plating may obviate the need for dorsal stabilization and/or reduce the need for postoperative bracing, even in the presence of dorsal ligamentous disruption. In the presence of pancolumn disruption, a circumferential fusion may be indicated, combining ventral cervical plating with dorsal wiring or plating procedures.[24,25]

Vertical-Compression

In contrast to CF injuries where the axial loading is oblique, vertical-compression injuries occur when axial loading is applied to the center of the vertebrae, with the spine in a neutral position at the time of impact. This may result in "bursting" of the vertebral body with retropulsion of bone fragments into the spinal canal. In less severe injuries, ligamentous structures are intact and the spine remains stable. In more-severe injuries, the vertebral arch may be comminuted with failure of the dorsal ligamentous complex, rendering the spine unstable. Surgery is indicated for decompression of neural elements and spinal stabilization. Fractures may be stabilized from either a ventral or dorsal approach with satisfactory results. The ventral procedure involves vertebrectomy followed by cervical plating, while the dorsal approach relies on wired bone grafts and/or lateral mass plating. When dorsal ligament disruption is present, both approaches may be necessary to achieve adequate fixation.

Compressive-Extension

The major compressive force in compressive-extension injuries is concentrated on the dorsal elements while the neck is extended. Low grades of injury consist of unilateral vertebral arch fracture, with bilateral laminar fractures present in injuries of greater severity. The most severe injuries consist of bilateral vertebral arch fractures with displacement of the vertebral body ventrally. Many of these injuries heal following reduction and external bracing.

Distractive-Flexion

Distractive-flexion injuries comprise up to 40% of cervical spine injuries. This is the result of major force vectors being directed toward the occiput with the neck in flexion. This produces tension on the dorsal elements, with secondary compression of the ventral elements. A unique feature of this group of injuries is the early failure of ligaments with minimal loss of bony integrity. Failure of the dorsal ligamentous complex results in widening of the spinous processes and facet subluxation in flexion. As the severity of the major vector force increases, unilateral and bilateral facet dislocations can occur, with translation in the AP direction approaching the full width of the vertebral body in the most severe cases.

The management of these patients depends largely on the neurological status, the degree of spinal column injury, MRI, the ability to achieve reduction, and the patient's medical condition. Treatment algorithms for unilateral and bilateral dislocations have previously been reported (Tables 3-5).[101]

Distractive-Extension

The major force vector of distractive-extension injuries is tension along the ventral elements resulting in failure of the anterior longitudinal ligament with an avulsion fracture of the injured vertebral body. With increasing tension, there may also be failure of the dorsal ligamentous complex, with retrodisplacement of the rostral vertebral body into the canal. Decompression is indicated for injuries with compressive pathology. Significant panligamentous disruption generally requires surgical stabilization and fusion.

Lateral-Flexion

Lateral-flexion injuries are extremely rare. The major force vector is compression along the side of the spine that is flexed laterally, and the minor force vector is tension or distraction along the opposite side. Usually, there is ipsilateral compression fracture of the vertebral body and neural arch with displacement of the neural arch or ligamentous injury in the more severe cases. Surgery is generally not necessary in lateral-flexion injuries that do not manifest instability.

OPERATIVE TECHNIQUES
Ventral Subaxial Instrumentation

Internal fixation using ventral plates and screws for the treatment of instability is a relatively new concept. The earliest plating systems

TABLE 3

A New Management Scheme for the Treatment of Unilateral Facet Dislocation*

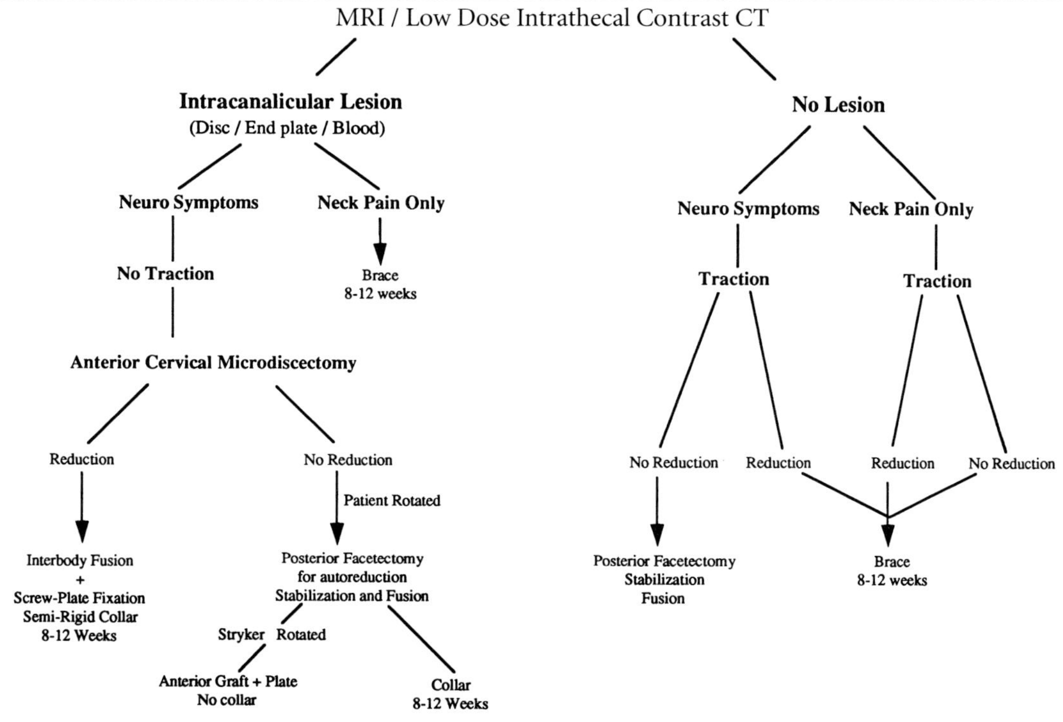

*Reproduced from Stillerman et al[104] with permission.

involved coupling of a long bone fracture plate to the ventral spine, with a single screw into each vertebral body.[16,62] Subsequently, a variety of plating systems specially designed for ventral osteosynthesis have been developed.[79] These systems may be divided based on whether the screws are locked to the plate. Regardless of the screw design, all available systems provide immediate stability and help maintain fixation while bone fusion occurs. They decrease the incidence of non-union and graft migration and also shorten the time required for bony fusion. In many instances, cumbersome external bracing may be avoided.

Caspar Plating

This nonlocking ventral cervical screw-plate system gained popularity in the late 1980s with the introduction of a standardized step-by-step protocol as well as instruments designed to facilitate cervical fusion and screw-plate fixation.[26] Although plating systems developed over the last

10 years have made the Caspar system antiquated, the system is worth describing, since it was the first widely utilized screw-plate system.

Plates. The plates are trapezoidal in shape and come with oval holes of different lengths, in the rostral-caudal direction, to allow for versatility during screw placement (Figure 19). Selection of the appropriate plate is essential for successful stabilization. A plate of correct length should not extend beyond the vertebral body being fixated. Screws placed across a nonfused disc space may lead to movement of the plate with normal flexion and extension movements. This may result in early degenerative changes at the nonfused level as well as screw loosening. The plate is contoured to fit flush with the ventral cortex, avoiding preloading the screws with distractive forces. All soft tissue must be removed from the ventral vertebral body to allow direct contact between cortical bone and the construct. The orientation of the construct over the vertebral body in the mediolateral direction is important and should

TABLE 4

"Conventional" Management for Bilateral Facet Dislocation in the Intact
Patient or the Patient with Incomplete Injury*

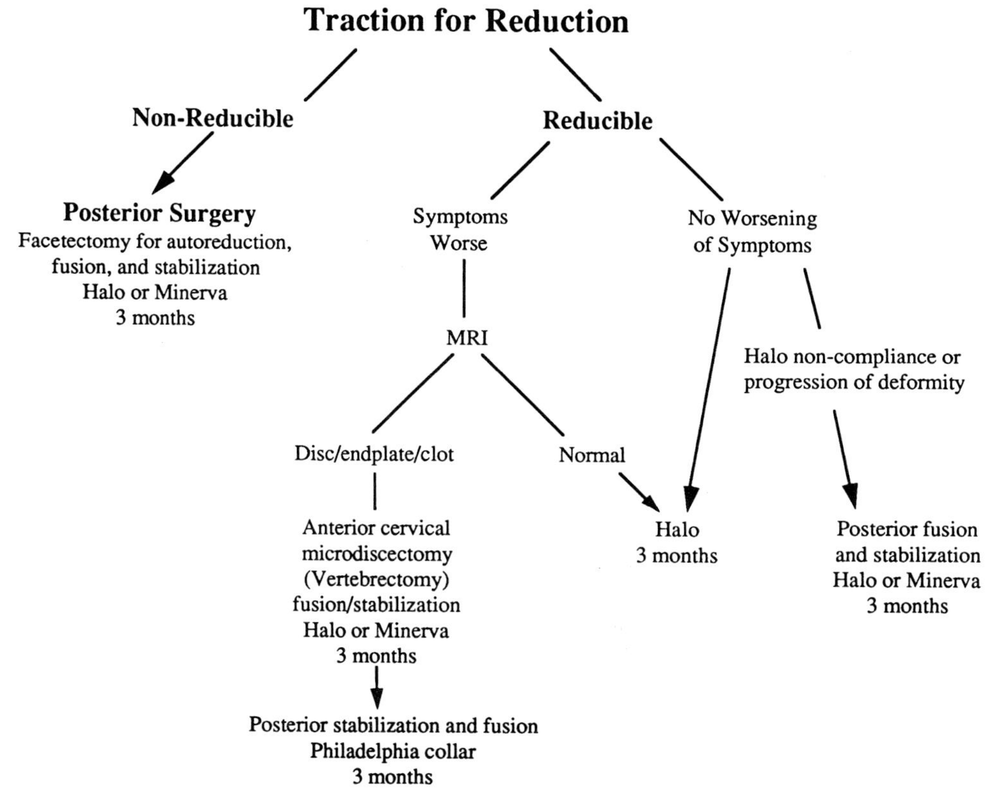

*Reproduced from Stillerman et al[104] with permission.

be confirmed using intraoperative fluoroscopy. Screws placed too far laterally may penetrate the neural foramen and produce nerve root injury. Intervening tissue may promote delayed loosening and migration of the plate, with resultant instability. Similarly, all osteophytic spurs must be drilled out to provide bone-plate contact over the entire length of the construct.

Screws. Lateral intraoperative fluoroscopy is essential to the Caspar technique for drilling and tapping of holes and the final insertion of screws. Because the system uses nonlocking screws (Figure 19), purchase through the dorsal cortex is mandatory to obtain maximum holding power and prevent screw loosening. Screws of the appropriate length must be selected. Short screws will not engage the dorsal cortex and will loosen, resulting in spinal instability and, possi-

bly, esophageal irritation. Long screws may penetrate the dura mater and spinal cord, producing disastrous consequences. Optimal screw length is based on the depth of the dorsal cortex, which is determined with a special gauge. Holes are then tapped and the final screws are inserted and tightened alternately to "two-finger" tightness.

Screw loosening by one or two thread lengths is clinically insignificant. A greater "pull-out" may produce symptoms of dysphagia requiring reoperation for removal of that particular screw. Caspar does not recommend either retightening or replacing a single loose screw, as long as the plate is firmly affixed to the vertebral body. However, plate motion in the absence of graft incorporation is an indication for complete re-plating and refusion.[26] In the event that excessive tightening leads to screw stripping, the screw

TABLE 5

A NEW MANAGEMENT SCHEME FOR BILATERAL FACET DISLOCATION IN THE INTACT PATIENT
OR THE PATIENT WITH INCOMPLETE INJURY*

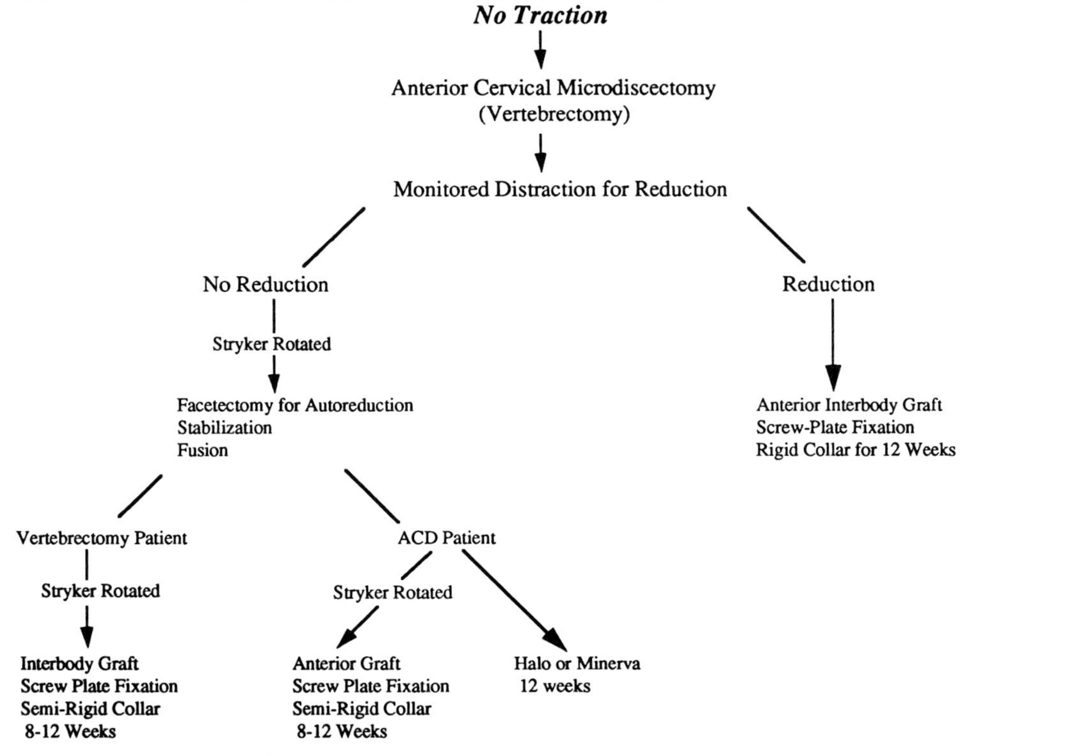

*Reproduced from Stillerman et al[104] with permission.

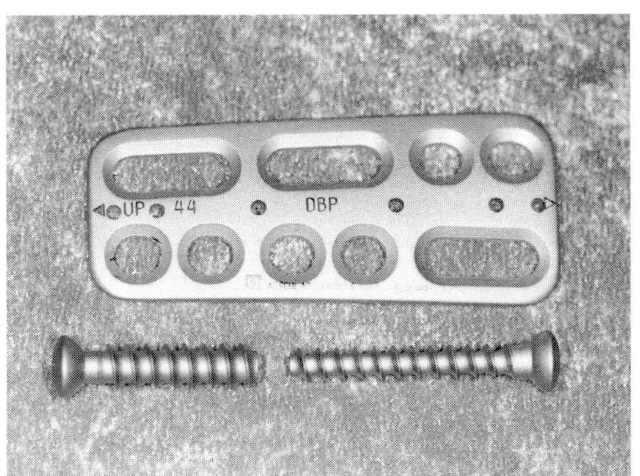

Figure 19: Caspar nonlocking ventral cervical screw-plate fixator.

should be removed. To salvage the incompetent hole, bone chips or pressurized methylmethacrylate can be placed in the hole prior to reinsertion with a "rescue" screw (i.e., a screw with a larger major diameter).[26,82,106] It is critical to avoid inserting bone chips or cement through the dorsal cortical defect into the spinal canal. Another option is to insert a second screw through an adjacent fresh hole (Figure 20).

Instrumentation. The Caspar set contains special instruments for retraction of soft tissue, distraction of adjacent vertebral bodies, and plates and screws of various sizes. Because of its unique function, the vertebral body distractor deserves special mention. The instrument is slipped over screw shafts that are inserted into vertebral bodies above and below the vertebrectomy, allowing distraction of the vertebral bodies and widening of the interspace. Distraction facilitates discectomy and/or vertebrectomy, preparation of the graft site, and placement of the bone graft. Re-

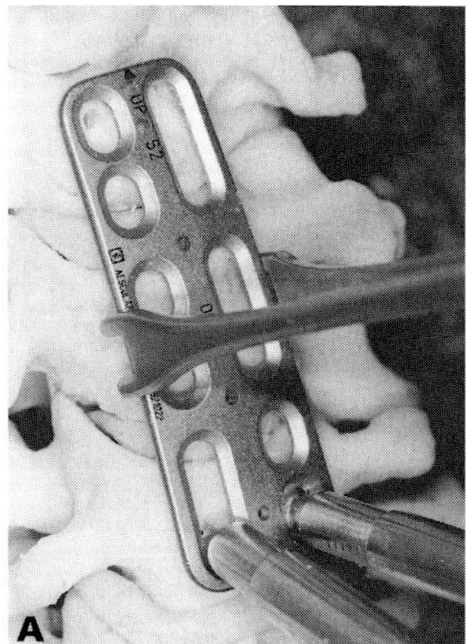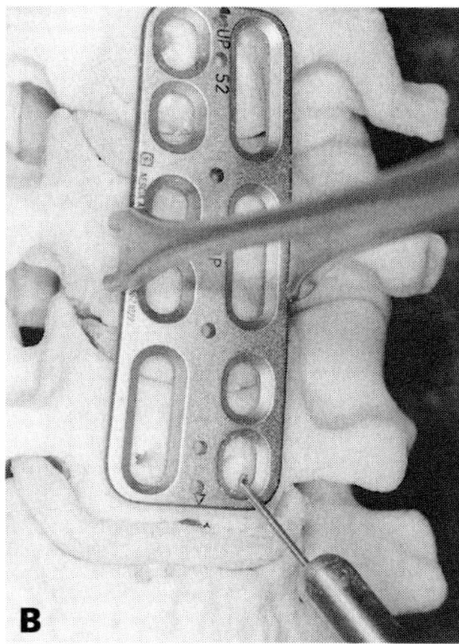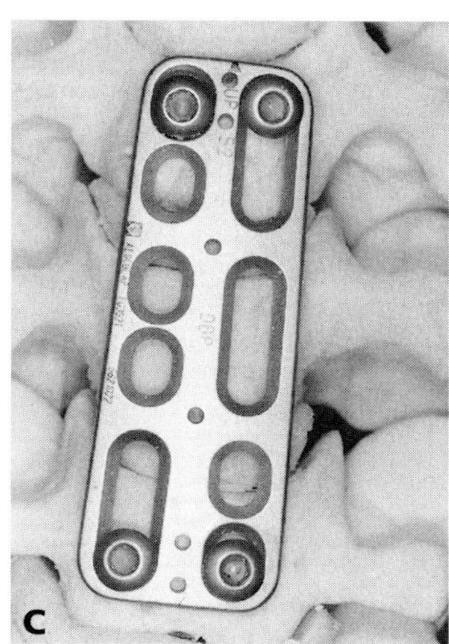

Figure 20: The Caspar technique. **A)** The surface of the ventral column has been flattened with a high-speed drill. A plate holder is used to secure the plate. A double-barrel drill guide with an adjustable distal tip is placed through the plate holes and drilling is carried out under fluoroscopy. **B)** After tapping the holes, a depth gauge (shown here) is introduced and used for determination of permanent screw length. **C)** Nonlocking permanent screws have been placed.

lease of the distraction causes the bone graft to be compressed against the vertebral endplates, thereby providing maximal bone surface contact and, hence, the optimal chance for fusion. The distraction screw shafts are then removed and plate stabilization is performed (Figure 21). The major limitations of the Caspar system include the need to drill and place screw threads into the spinal canal and the nonlocking screw design.

Synthes Cervical Spine Locking Plate System

The Synthes cervical spine locking plate system was one of the first systems designed to permit unicortical screw purchase (Figure 22). The screw head expands and locks to the plate once an insert screw is engaged, allowing unicortical screw purchase without increasing the risk of screw backout and subsequent injury to prevertebral structures. The initial popularity of this system reflected the desirability to avoid bicortical screw purchase, which increases the risk of drilling and placement of permanent screw threads into the spinal canal. Recent advances in the system, including the introduction of titanium plates and "small stature" plates, has made this system one of the most widely used systems on the market.

Plates. Synthes plates are designed to provide a "toenail" (toe-in) orientation with regard to screw placement. This theoretically enhances the resistance of the screws to pull-out forces (Figure 22). The rostral holes allow the screws to be directed medially and angled 6° or 12° rostrally using the standard or small stature plate, respectively. The rostral screw orientation makes it easier to prepare screw holes in the upper cervical spine by avoiding the need to drill perpendicular to the plate. At the caudal hole, screws enter perpendicular to the plate and are directed medially. When using this system at the cervicothoracic junction, the plate can be reversed. This maneuver places the angled screw holes caudally, simplifying hole preparation and screw placement. Although fluoroscopy is not mandatory because of the avoidance of bicortical purchase, most surgeons use imaging to optimize plate and screw positioning relative to the disc space. The plates are available in lengths ranging from 24 to 92 mm, and the screws are available in lengths of 12, 14, and 16 mm. All screws measure 4 mm in major diameter with an expanding head and are locked to the plate when an insert screw 1.8 mm in diameter is inserted into the screw head (Figure 23).

Disadvantages of the system include its lack of versatility with respect to screw angulation during placement and the ability to contour the

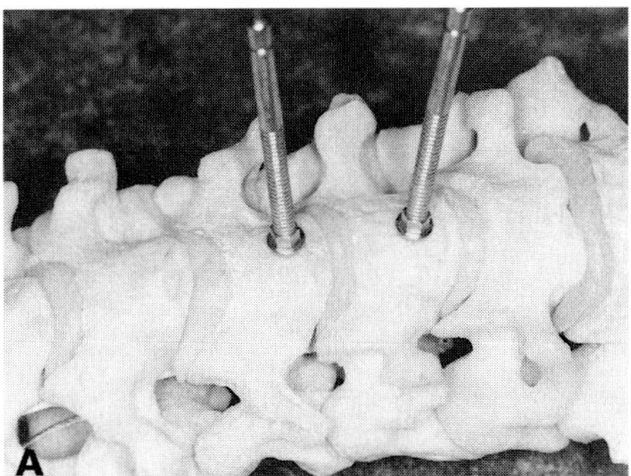

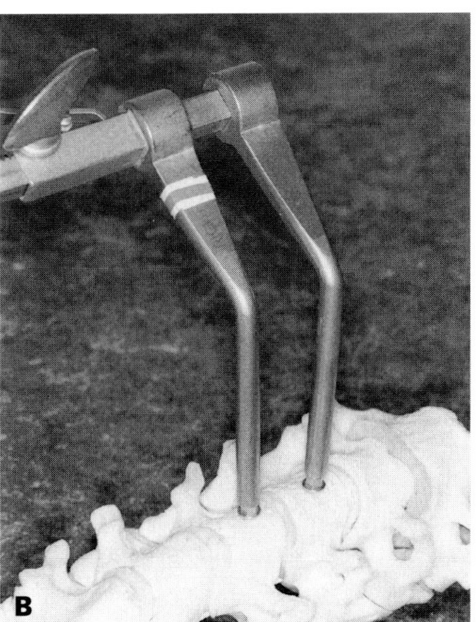

Figure 21: The Caspar distraction system. **A)** The distraction posts are in place. These were screwed into the vertebral bodies after a pilot hole was drilled. **B)** The distractor is slipped over the posts and gentle distraction may be applied. This system simplifies interbody bone graft placement.

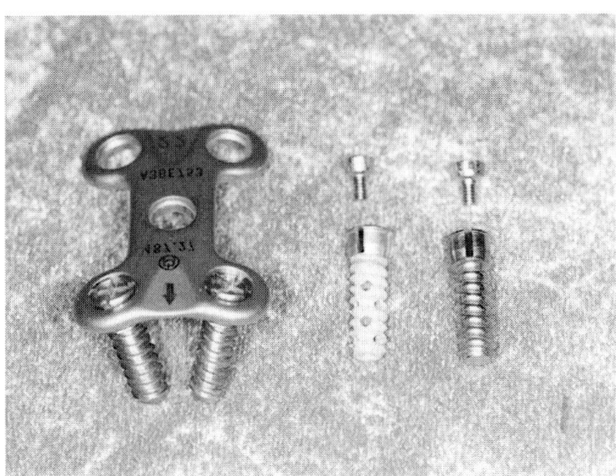

Figure 22: The Synthes cervical spine locking plate system. The expansion head screw and locking insert screw as well as the "toenail" orientation of the expansion head screws can be visualized.

plate with the plate benders only in the area between the screw holes. In addition, despite an included plate holder that secures the plate to the bone during its application, movement of the plate during hole preparation often occurs, even with the aid of an assistant (Figure 23).

Since the advent of the Synthes system, many newer systems have been developed that also utilize titanium plates, unicortical screw purchase, and locking screw designs to help prevent screw pull-out. Many of these newer systems are more versatile than the Synthes system, allowing placement of screws at more variable angles and improved screw to plate locking mechanisms.

Codman Ventral Cervical Plate System

The titanium Codman ventral cervical plate system enables the surgeon to select various angles of screw placement to better conform to the individual patient anatomy, providing a non-fixed cantilever beam construct, while still allowing a mechanism for locking the screws to the plate (Figure 24). With this system, 12- and 15-mm screws with corresponding depth drill guides are available. Although typical screw placement is 10° medial angulation with the screw parallel to the disc space, the ability to lock the screws to the plate in a nonfixed manner allows variable rostral and caudal angulation of the screws. In order to avoid confusion during application of the plate, the 12- and 15-mm screws and the corresponding drill bits and taps are color-coded. In addition, an easy-to-use plate bender can be utilized to optimally contour the plate to ensure maximum bone plate interface, and a plate holder is available to help maintain alignment of the plate while drilling and tapping the pilot holes. The disadvantages of this system

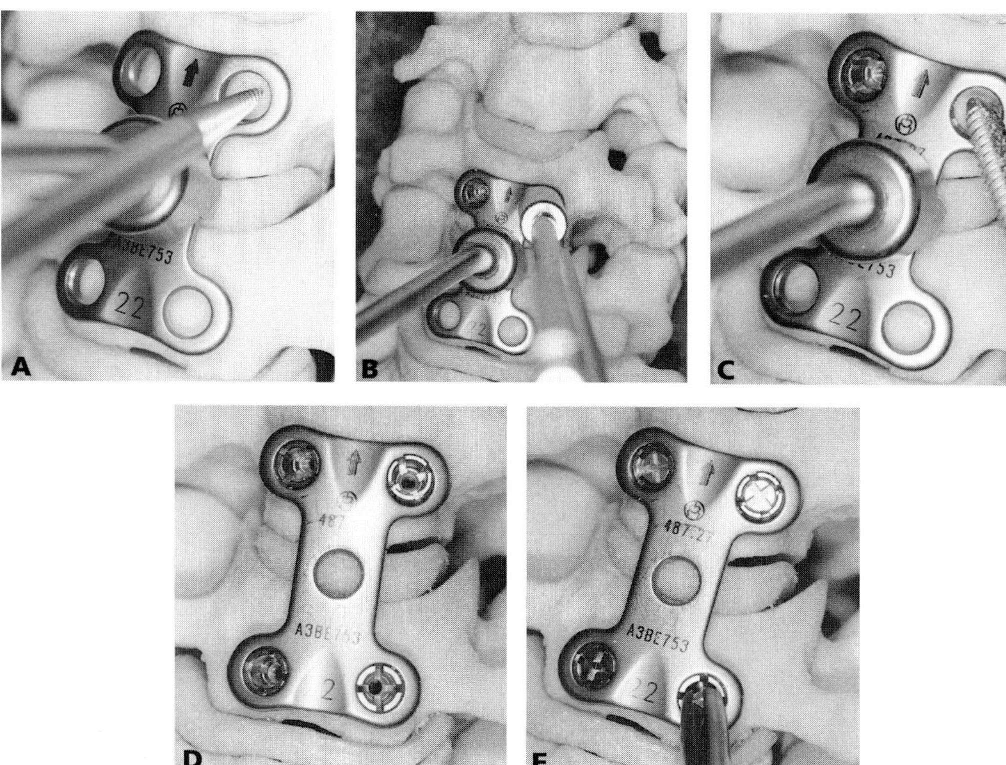

Figure 23: The Synthes cervical spine locking plate technique. **A)** The surface of the ventral column has been flattened with a high-speed drill. A plate holder is used to secure the plate. The surface of the vertebrae is decorticated. **B)** The drill guide is introduced and drilling is carried out. **C)** The holes are tapped to a length of 1.4 cm. **D)** Screws of 4 mm in major diameter are threaded through the plate. **E)** The anchor screws are locked to the plate by inserting a 1.8-mm diameter short screw through the plate into the head of the anchor screw. This expands the screw head and locks it to the plate.

include the inability to adequately lock the screws to the plate with placement of the bone screws at angulations greater than 16°; additionally, the plate holder furnished with the system does not grip the plate adequately, often allowing movement of the plate while drilling the pilot holes (Figure 24A). Also, the narrow lumen of the variable-angle drill guide does not allow the surgeon to both drill and tap the pilot hole through the same drill guide (Figure 24C and D).

Surgical Dynamics

The Aline ventral cervical plating system produced by Surgical Dynamics is a titanium plate system that allows unicortical screw placement with a screw-plate locking mechanism similar to the Synthes system (Figure 25). The plate holder supplied with the system can be used to stabilize the plate, while drilling pilot holes or plate loca-

tion tacks can be used to further prevent movement of the plate during application (Figure 26A and C). Medial holes within the plate allow placement of a third screw into the superior and/or inferior vertebrae, and a variable-angle drill guide permits screw angulation of 15° in any direction about the central axis (Figure 26B); a fixed-angle drill guide is also included. Further, the design of the drill guide allows both drilling and tapping of the pilot holes through the same guide. Disadvantages of the system include its plate holder (similar to the Synthes Cervical Spine Locking Plate system), which does not adequately engage the plate during application, and the inability to place bone screws at angles greater than 15°.

Sofamor-Danek

The Atlantis cervical plating system (Figure 27) produced by Sofamor-Danek is an addition

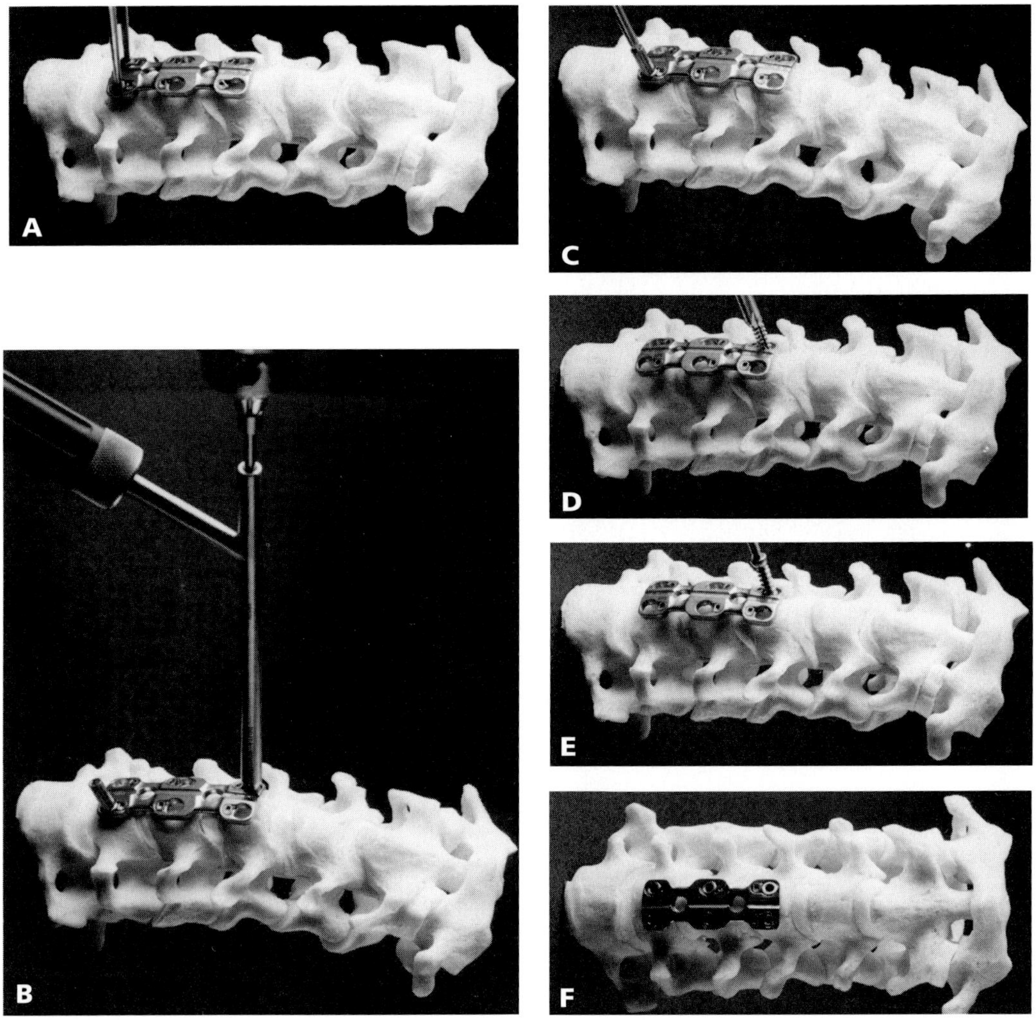

Figure 24: The Codman ventral cervical plate system. **A)** The Codman plate is positioned on the cervical spine using the forceps plate holders. **B)** The plate can be secured to the cervical spine using a temporary fixation pin. **C)** Utilizing the drill guide and plate holder to secure the implant, screw trajectory is selected and a drill bit placed through the drill guide is used to place an initial pilot hole. **D)** The pilot hole is tapped at the appropriate angle. **E)** After tapping of the pilot hole, an appropriate diameter and length screw is placed. In this view, the temporary fixation pin has been removed. **F)** The cam tightener is utilized to lock all the cams into position preventing screw backout.

to their existing system, the Orion anterior cervical plate. The titanium Atlantis system allows unicortical and/or bicortical bone screw purchase, fixed cantilever beam constructs for significant spinal instability, and nonconstrained variable-angle cantilever beam constructs to facilitate bone fusion by allowing physiological loading in more stable clinical scenarios. In addition, hybrid constructs can be performed by using a combi-

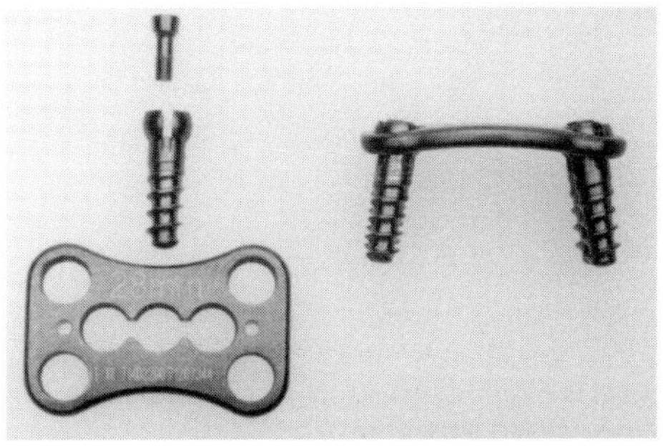

Figure 25: The Aline implant with variable-angle bone screw and locking screw.

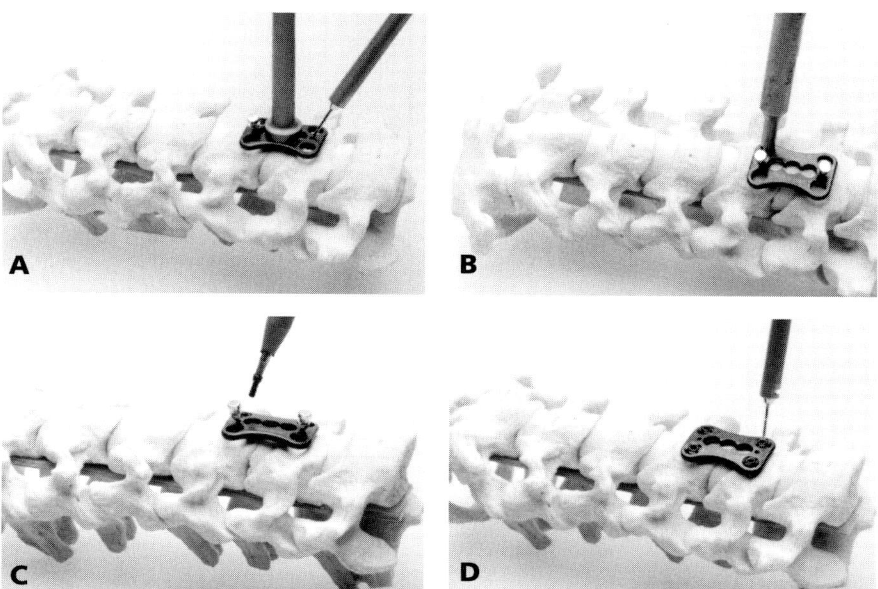

Figure 26: A) The Aline plate is positioned with a plate holder and is temporarily secured to the bone using a tack inserter to insert plate tacks. **B)** The crew depth is set on the variable-angle drill guide. The drill and tap are placed through the same drill guide. **C)** After placement of the appropriate bone screws, a locking screw is placed into each bone screw using a tapered hex driver. The hex driver's counter torque prongs engage the Aline bone screws to prevent movement while the locking screws are torque in place. **D)** Once all screws are in place, the temporary plate tacks can be removed with the tack inserter.

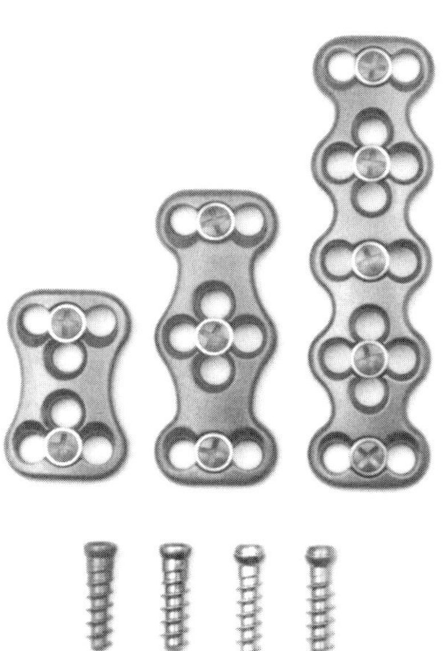

Figure 27: The Atlantis anterior cervical plating system with both fixed- and variable-angle bone screws.

nation of fixed- and variable-angle screws within the same plate (Figure 28). This type of construct allows flexibility for a patient's aberrant anatomy or for suboptimal screw positions or purchases. The fixed- and variable-angle screws and the corresponding drill guides and taps are color-coded. Like other systems, the bone screws can be securely locked to the plate after the implant is in place and the plate is pre-cast with a lordotic curve for the cervical spine, which may be increased or decreased with the accompanying plate bender. The system comes with a plate holder that securely engages the plate, as do the drill guides, to prevent migration of the plate while drilling the pilot holes (Figure 28). As with other systems, the narrow lumen of the drill guide does not allow tapping of the pilot hole through the drill guide (Figure 28). In addition, the shallow slots on the head of the locking screws allow some stripping to occur if the screws are overtightened and, similar to the Codman system, marked rostral, caudal, medial, or lateral angulation of the screws will prevent adequate locking of the screws to the plate.

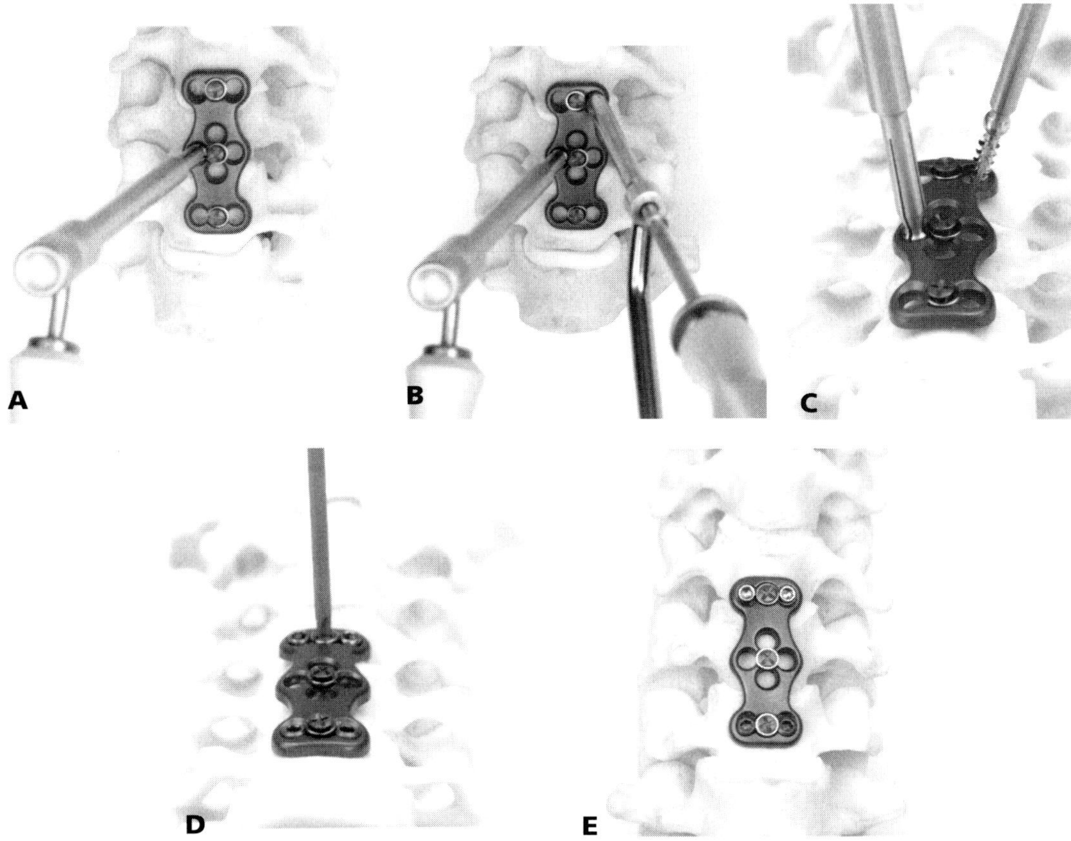

Figure 28: The Atlantis technique. **A)** A plate holder or pin can be placed into any of the bone screw holes to provide temporary fixation while drilling. **B)** A fixed- or variable-angle drill guide is seated within the screw hole and a pilot hole is drilled at the appropriate angle. **C)** The pilot holes are taped at the appropriate angles (color-coded taps) before placing the fixed- or variable-angle bone screws. **D)** Once all bone screws have been securely seated into the plate, the lock screwdriver is engaged into each lock screw and tightened. The lock screw centers the washer and covers the portion of the bone screw head. **E)** A hybrid construct with fixed-angle screws locked in place inferiorly and variable-angle screws locked in place rostrally.

DePuy-AcroMed

A new plating system manufactured by De-Puy-AcroMed, the Peak polyaxial ventral cervical plate (Figure 29), is innovative in its design in that the plate is manufactured with a rotational locking bushing that allows placement of unicortical screws at more extreme cranial, caudal, medial, and lateral angles while still achieving a rigid locking interface between the plate and the screw. This is accomplished without additional lock screws, caps, or cams. The system incorporates temporary compressor pins, which can be inserted into the caudal and rostral aspects of the plate to prevent migration of the plate while

drilling the pilot holes (Figure 30A). In addition, by removing either the rostral or caudal compressor pin after insertion of the corresponding rostral or caudal bone screws, a compression device, which is supplied with the set, allows compression of the intervening bone plug (Figure 30C). Screws are 4 mm in diameter and self-tapping. Unfortunately, the rotational locking bushing, while allowing even marked cranial, caudal, medial, or lateral angulation of the screws while still allowing a rigid locking interface, can be problematic in that the "thread through" design of the plate does not allow the screw to be used to pull the plate down to the bone. There-

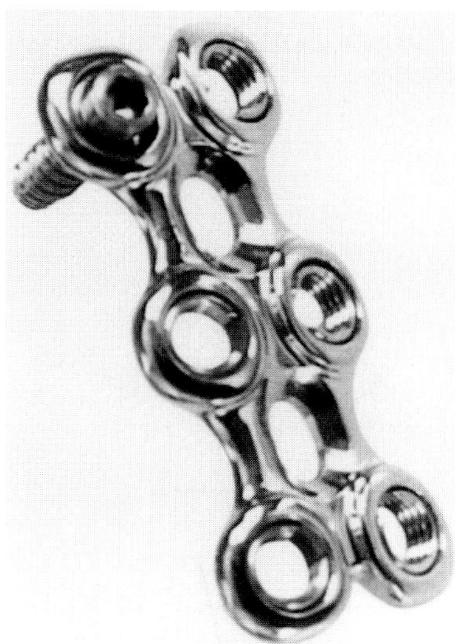

Figure 29: The Peak polyaxial ventral cervical plate. A rotational locking bushing can be seen located within each screw hole of the plate.

fore, great care must be exercised to not push the screw into the bone, as this will elevate the plate off the bony surface during the surgical procedure. Further, although the compressor pins allow good fixation of the plate to the bone while drilling the pilot holes, they can at times prevent significant lateral angulation of the superior and inferior screws because the pins may get in the way of medial to lateral angulation of the drill guide (Figure 30B).

A new system by DePuy-AcroMed, the DOC ventral cervical stabilization system, is the first rod-screw system utilized for the cervical spine as compared to the standard plate-screw systems (Figure 31). This system is unique in that its rod configuration allows significant axial settling (dynamism) to occur between the adjacent vertebral bodies and the intervening bone implant. The ability of the system to allow axial settling may enhance bone fusion by preventing stress shielding. Construct-securing pins, a well-designed rod holder, and a drill guide that securely seats in the screw hole prevent migration of the rods while drilling the pilot holes (Figure 32A and B). The bone screws lock to the system utilizing an inner screw, which inserts into the head of the bone screws, expanding the screw tip in a fashion similar to the Synthes system (Figure

32C). The system has some disadvantages in that is has a slightly higher profile then many of the cervical screw-plate systems and the complexity of the system makes for a steep learning curve.

Manny-Stillerman and EBI Systems

Two other titanium cervical systems are worth mentioning because of their singular design. The Manny-Stillerman system (Figure 33) and the EBI SpineLink system (Figures 34 and 35) both allow screw-hole preparation and anchor screw placement without drilling through the plate. These systems allow for larger screw diameters, provide improved bone purchase, and eliminate the predicament of plate migration while drilling the pilot holes. Further, the modular links utilized in the EBI system allow easy extension of the instrumentation should fusion cranial or caudal to the original site be necessary and allow greater postoperative visualization of the intervertebral space and graft site as no overlying solid plate is used (Figure 35C). Biomechanical testing in cadaver models has demonstrated that the Manny-Stillerman and the EBI systems are as capable as the other cervical systems mentioned previously with respect to axial load to failure and cyclic loading trials.

Dorsal Instrumentation

Dorsal cervical stabilization historically involved placement of onlay bone grafts over the site to be fused. However, because of a lack of immediate stability, fusion was often augmented with some form of internal fixation. A number of implants have been used for this purpose. The early techniques involved wiring of the dorsal elements. With advances in technology and the discovery of biomechanical principles, stabilization is now performed using rectangular rods, sublaminar clamps, and lateral mass plates and screws. Simple wiring techniques, however, remain an extremely efficient method of achieving immediate postoperative stability and anatomic alignment.

Wiring Techniques

Anatomic structures accessible to wiring include the spinous process, facets, and, when

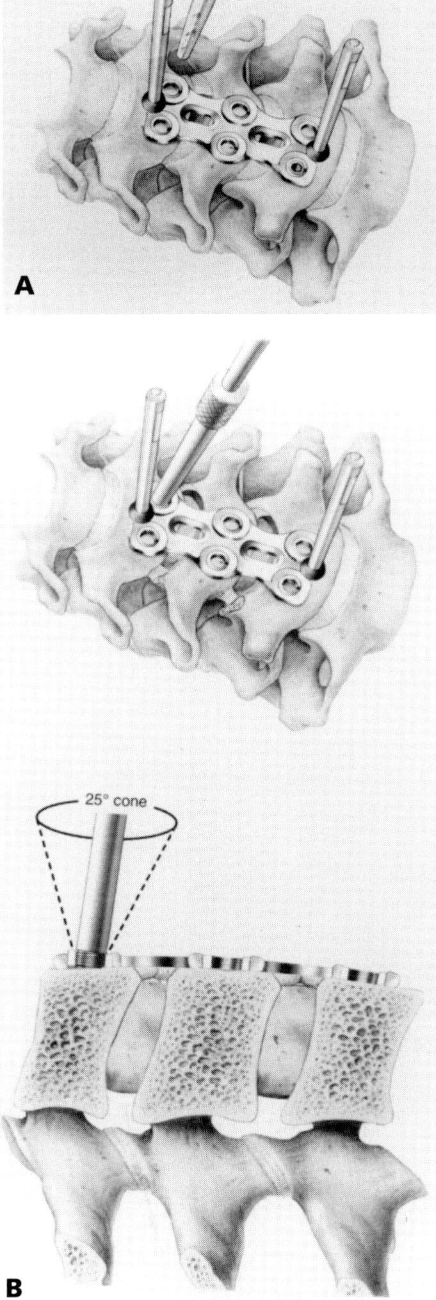

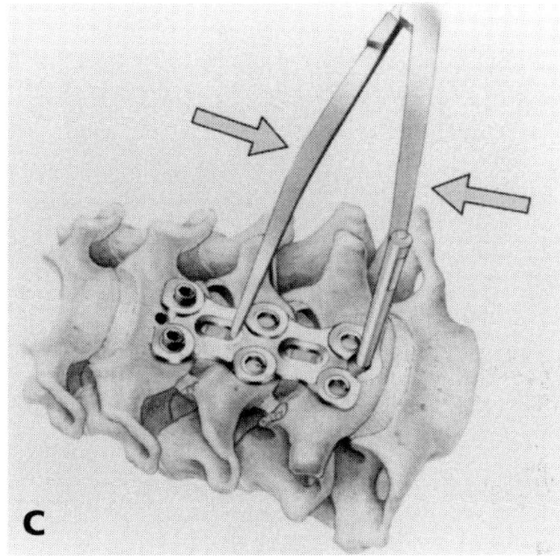

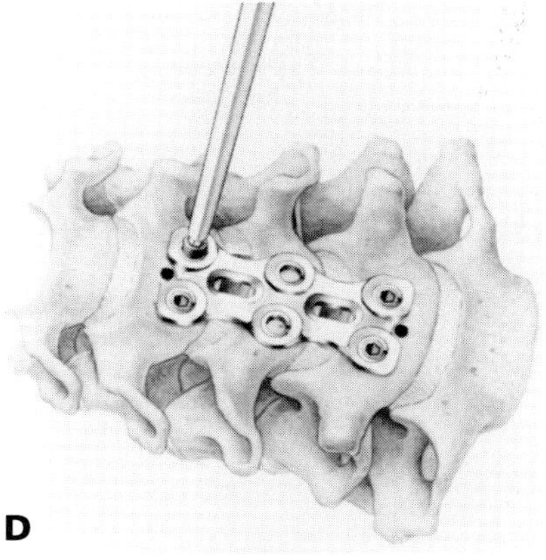

Figure 30: The Peak polyaxial ventral cervical plate by DePuy-AcroMed. **A)** Temporary compressor pins have been inserted into the rostral and caudal aspects of the Peak plate to prevent migration while drilling. A 2.8-mm drill with its sleeve is directed into the bushing of the screw hole. **B)** Once the 2.8-mm drill with sleeve is fully seated within the bushing, it can be rotated to any position within a 25° cone before drilling is performed. **C)** Once the rostral or caudal screws are in place, the corresponding compressor pin can be removed and a compression device utilized to place the intervening bone plug under compression. **D)** The final construct with inferior and superior screws in place and the temporary compressor pins removed.

Figure 31: The DePuy-AcroMed DOC ventral cervical stabilization system.

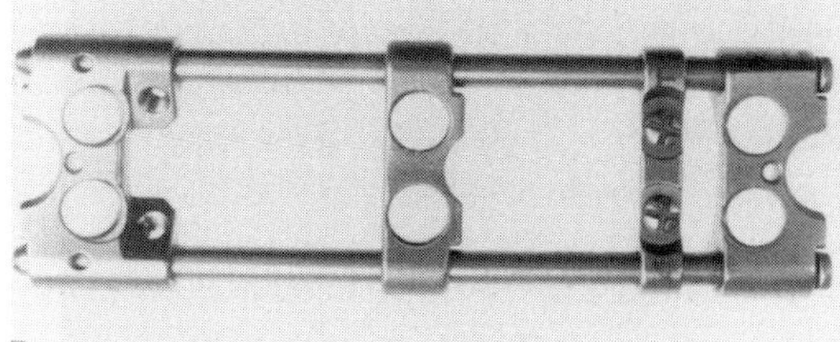

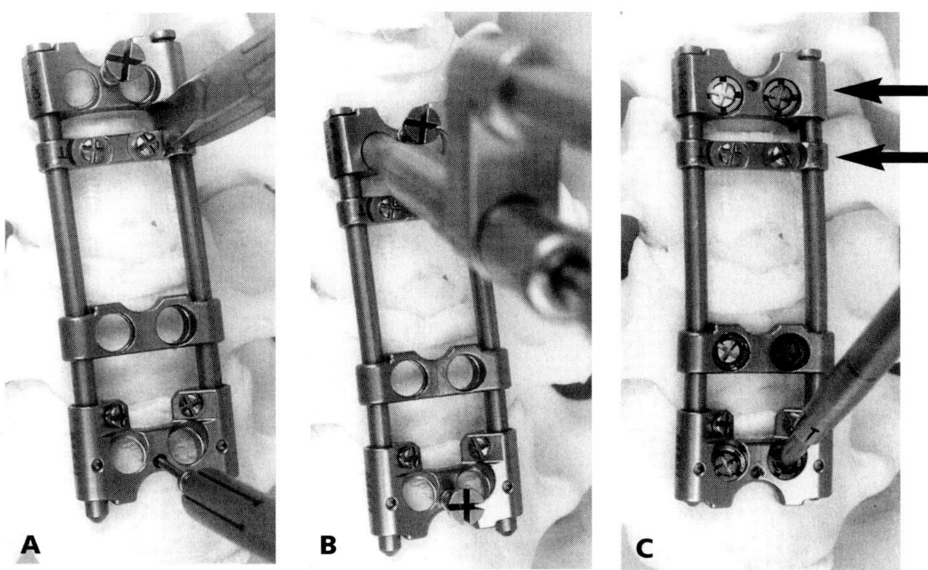

Figure 32: The DOC ventral cervical stabilization system by AcroMed. **A)** Construct securing pins of the DOC system are temporarily inserted into the caudal and rostral aspects of the construct to hold the implant in position. **B)** The drill guide is placed in the screw hole. It seats in the screw hole to provide the appropriate screw trajectory. **C)** Once all outer bone screws have been placed, the small screwdriver is used to insert the inner bone screws into the outer bone screws, thereby locking the screws to the plate. The amount of axial settling (dynamism) permitted by the construct is limited to the distance between the cross-connector and the nonlocking angled platform *(arrows)*.

indicated, the lamina. Wiring through the spinous process is best suited for cases with dorsal ligamentous and facet capsule disruption, without bony injury. Interspinous wiring has largely evolved from the original method described by Rogers.[84,85] A 22-gauge or 24-gauge stainless steel wire is passed through a hole made at the rostral end of the base of the spinous process. The wire is looped over the rostral border and back through the hole to completely encircle the spinous process. Wire ends are passed in a similar fashion through a hole made in the adjacent spinous process that is being fused. The ends are tightly twisted at the inferior border of the lower segment, forming a tension band over the dorsal elements. The procedure is repeated at adjacent levels for patients who require multilevel fusion. Bone is harvested from the iliac crest, and onlay grafts are placed in and around the wires over the decorticated lamina being fused.

Since Rogers' original description, many variations of interspinous wiring have been utilized.[15,75,83,84,98,113,115] Modifications have included

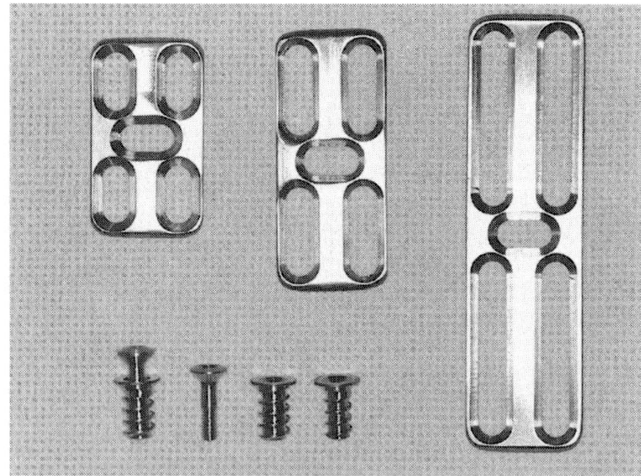

Figure 33: The Manny-Stillerman locking ventral cervical screw-plate fixator. (Reproduced with permission from Stillerman et al.[104])

the use of multiple wires to stabilize adjacent segments, changes in the configuration of wiring,[90] and improvement in ways to better secure bone grafts to the dorsal elements. Increasing the number of wires to secure vertebral segments, as for example with Bohlman's triple wire technique,[70,71,99] add greater strength to the cervical construct. This has been confirmed with biome-

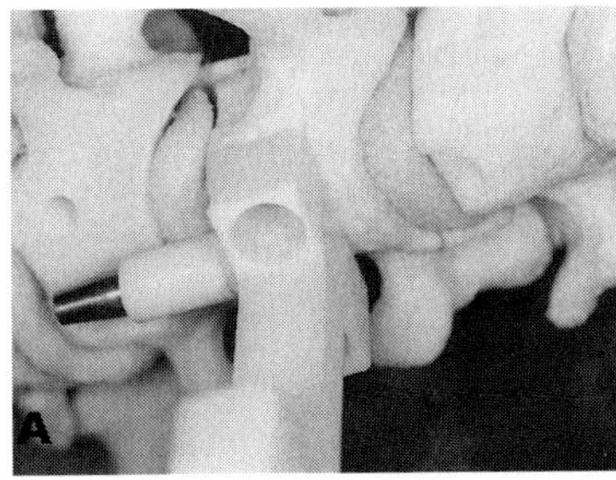

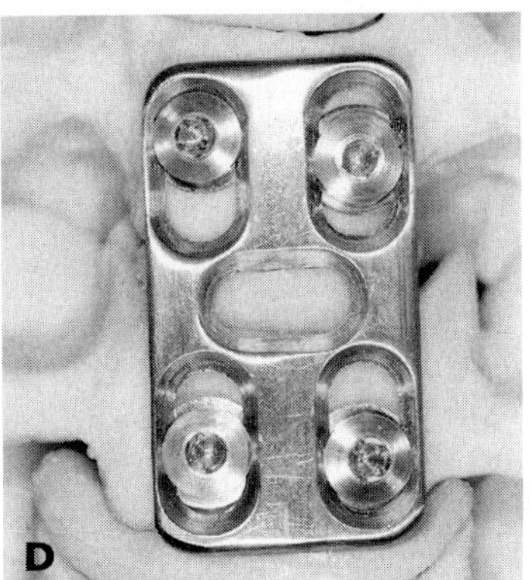

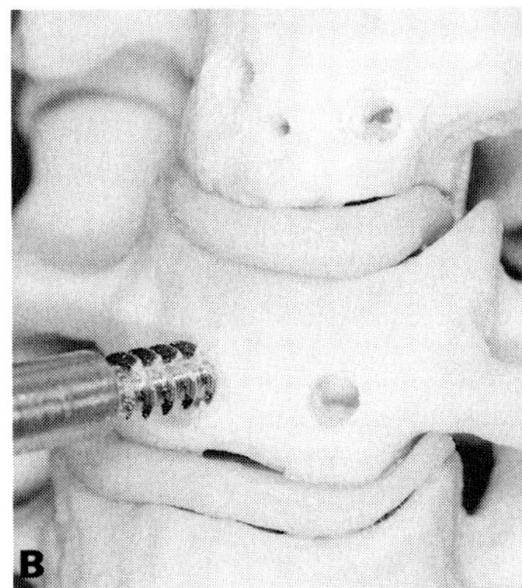

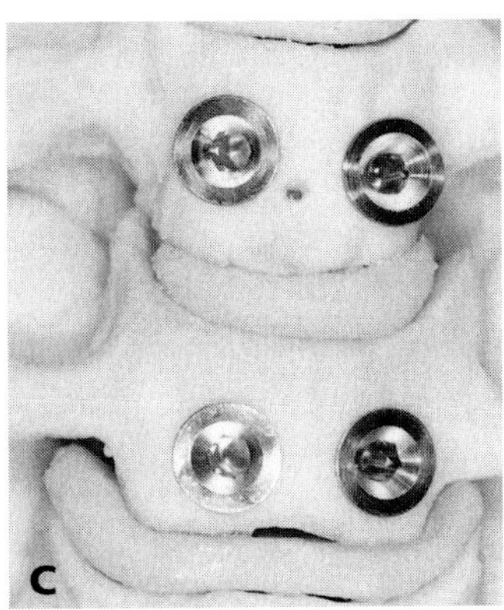

Figure 34: The Manny-Stillerman technique. **A)** A double-barrel guide is secured to the vertebral body with a small spike. An orientation post helps evaluate coronal plane alignment. Drilling is carried out to a depth of 1.1 cm. **B)** The holes are then tapped. **C)** Anchor screws of a large diameter are threaded into place. **D)** A plate is selected and then placed over the anchor screws. Universally engaging insert screws are threaded through the plate into the anchors to lock the plate to the anchors.

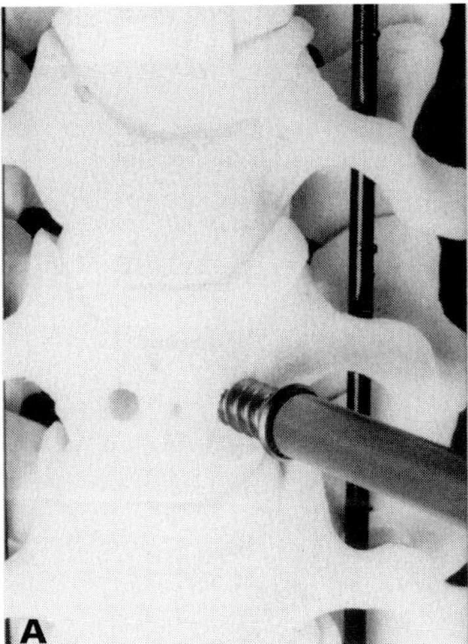

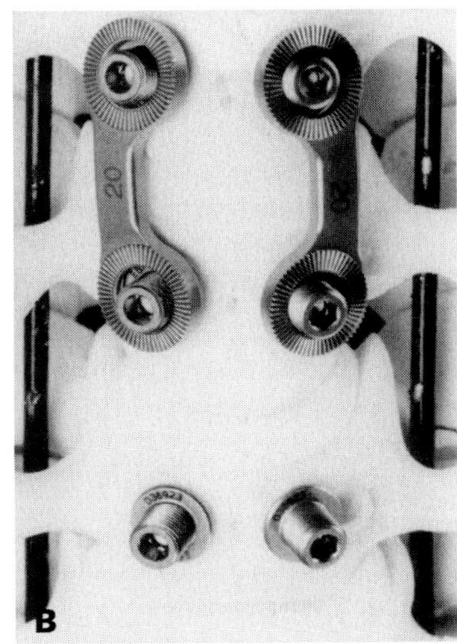

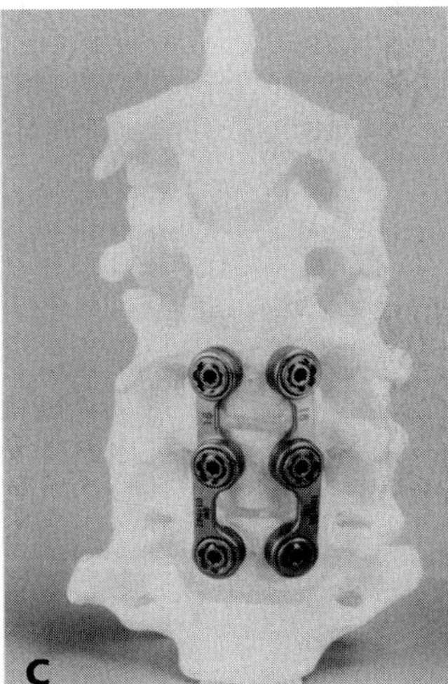

Figure 35: The EBI SpineLink ventral cervical spine system. **A)** Large self-tapping screws are placed independently into each vertebral body after pilot holes have been drilled using a fixed-width drill guide. **B)** Appropriate length links are used to connect each self-tapping bone screw over the length of the construct. **C)** A two-level spinal construct using the EBI SpineLink ventral cervical spine system.

chanical results showing that triple wire fixation provided superior strength compared to other dorsal fusion techniques.[27,70,71] An early technique of bone grafting involved the placement of simple onlay grafts over the lamina being fused. Newer methods involve splitting the corticocancellous bone graft into halves. The bone graft is then laid down with the cancellous bone along the decorticated spinous process and medial borders of the lamina. Longitudinal splitting of the bone graft provides maximal medullary bone surface contact with the vertebral elements and likely promotes early bone fusion. Wiring the graft to the dorsal elements further optimizes stability and the potential for osseous union.

The prerequisite for successful interspinous wiring is that the dorsal elements be completely intact and stable. In the event of a fractured lamina, pedicle, or spinous process, it is reasonable to bypass that level and wire the spinous process of the next intact segment. A longer construct further restricts cervical motion and increases the chance of failure of bony fusion. In cases where interspinous wiring is not possible or greater rotational stability is needed, bilateral facet-to-spinous process wiring (oblique wiring) can provide adequate stabilization.[21] A facet-to-facet fusion is useful in instances where the lamina and spinous process are incompetent.[22,83] In brief, holes are drilled through the inferior facets of the segments to be fused and wires are passed through the hole. Following removal of articular cartilage and decortication of the bone surface, long corticocancellous struts are secured with wires to the dorsal articular surface.

Wiring techniques provide a relatively stable cervical construct. The procedure is simple and straightforward and requires no complicated instruments or equipment to perform. A major limitation of wiring is that fixation strength is not as good as that provided by rigid devices. Hence, postoperative rigid external bracing is required, ranging from a Philadelphia collar to a halo vest. The lower fusion rates associated with wiring may reflect their relatively poor strength as a construct. Potential dangers of wiring include injury during sublaminar dissection and wire passage, wire fatigue with loosening or breakage, wire pulling through the bone (particularly in patients with osteoporotic bone or metabolic bone disease), and loss of reduction that may occur requiring reoperation.

The recent development of the Songer cable system, now used in place of monofilament wires, represents a major advance in dorsal cervical stabilization. Biomechanical testing results have shown that cables have greater fatigue resistance than wires, thereby reducing the incidence of revision procedures due to breakage.[94] The system contains specially designed instruments that allow controlled measured tensioning of the cable, further reducing the likelihood of break-

age. Additionally, titanium cables are MRI-compatible and much more flexible than wires. This latter property reduces the chance of injury to the spinal cord during insertion under the lamina. Finally, cable ends secured with top hats and crimped to a specific tension are less likely to loosen than twisted wire (see Figures 8 and 9).

Luque Loop and Rectangles

Luque[64] was the first to describe a method of dorsal segmental spinal fixation using L-shaped metal rods and sublaminar wires. Modification of the Luque rod led to the development of preformed rectangular loops, the Hartshill rectangle, which provided greater control of spinal rotation.[33] The rectangular loop, initially designed for lumbar stabilization, has been used in other areas of the spine including the cervical spine.[34] Use of the Luque/Hartshill rectangle to successfully produce craniocervical fusion has been previously described.[65] For cervical stabilization, a rectangle of appropriate length is selected to fit above the upper spinous process and below the lower spinous process to be stabilized. It is secured to the spinal column by multiple sublaminar or interspinous wires or cables. Advantages of the loop rectangle system include a low profile, relative ease of application, and low cost. Its major disadvantage lies in the need to contour the rectangle, especially when used in the occipitocervical region (see Figure 5).

Halifax Clamps

Halifax interlaminar clamps for atlantoaxial instability were described earlier in this chapter. Clamps have also been used to achieve fixation of the mid and lower cervical spine, with even more favorable results.[3,4,60,108] The application of the system is essentially the same as in the upper cervical spine. Sublaminar clamps are positioned in a compressive mode and interconnected with a threaded rod. Controversy arises with respect to the use of unilateral versus bilateral clamps for traumatic dorsal cervical instability.[60] Some advocate using unilateral clamps in cases of unilateral laminar and facet fractures. Others believe that the severity of the trauma is sufficient to produce contralateral facet instability and, therefore, recommend using bilateral clamps.[3,4] Multilevel clamping spanning two levels has been reported.[4] Other than ease of the technique, Halifax clamps offer no advantages over other systems. Biomechanically, they provide less rotational stability and resistance to flexion than offered by other techniques. Clamp hooks also have the disadvantage of requiring an intact lamina, and the incidence of hook dislodgement is reported to be high in some series. Additionally, hooks lie within the spinal canal and have the potential for spinal cord injury (see Figure 10).

Lateral Mass Plates

For more than a decade, metal plates and screws have been widely used for stabilization of cervical fractures and subluxations.[28,37,86] Their usefulness is largely due to the biomechanical strength of the construct and the disadvantages inherent in other techniques. Unlike fixation with wiring and Halifax clamps, the application of lateral mass plates does not require intact lamina or spinous process. Because it avoids intraspinal instrumentation, dorsal plating avoids some of the dangers associated with sublaminar wiring and intraspinal hook placement. Biomechanically, plates provide greater flexion-extension stability than dorsal wiring or interlaminar clamp fixation.[27,46,86] Cadaveric models of stress during flexion showed that plate fixation increased stability by 92%, compared to 33% with interspinous wiring and 88% with facet-facet wiring. With respect to extension, dorsal wiring was insufficient to stabilize the spine; however, plates increased stability by 60%.[86] Immobilization of the facet joints with plates also prevents rotational movements. It is therefore ideal for injuries with rotational or facet instability and compares favorably with midline wiring or fixation with clamps. Lastly, plate fixation produces immediate stability, thereby eliminating the need for complex and long-term external orthosis. Large clinical series have demonstrated the efficacy of this technique.[37]

The original plates, designed by Roy-Camille, are 1 cm wide, 2 mm thick, and have a slight concavity that conforms to the normal cervical lordosis. Plates with up to five holes are commercially available, with the most common ones having two or three holes to stabilize one or two motion segments, respectively. The inter-hole distance is 13 or 15.5 mm, which represents the average distance between two articular pillars. The longer spacing of holes may be more appropriate for larger patients. Screws 15.5 mm in length and 3.5 mm in diameter secure the plates to the lateral masses.

Newer plating systems are now available with greater versatility than that provided by the original Roy-Camille system. Of particular significance is the development of the Axis fixation system by Danek. The system offers a wide range of cortical and cancellous screws, as well as plates of various lengths with two-, four-, six-, and eight-hole segments. Specially designed instruments are also provided to contour plates to fit the anatomy without distorting the screw-plate interface. A unique feature of the plate is the "figure 8" screw-hole design which permits numerous screw placement options with variable angles in both the longitudinal and transverse directions.

Two-hole plates are indicated for single-level dorsal ligamentous injury, with or without lamina or spinous process fractures, and unilateral or bilateral facet dislocation. Stabilization of two motion segments with three-hole plates is performed when there is evidence of instability at two adjacent levels. It is particularly suitable for patients with lateral mass (facet) fractures or pedicle disruption. In such situations, levels above and below the fractured articular mass or pedicle are stabilized with plates. On the contralateral side, all three lateral masses are secured. Dorsal plating is contraindicated in patients with osteoporosis, metabolic bone disease, and ankylosing spondylitis. In all three conditions, the bone may be too soft to permit adequate bone-metal purchase.

A standard midline incision and subperiosteal exposure is performed bilaterally over the levels to be instrumented. Muscle dissection must extend far laterally to completely expose the lateral masses. Unreduced subluxations and dislocations are reduced by standard techniques prior to instrumentation. After removal of soft tissue and articular cartilage, the center of the facets being plated are identified. The entry site for screw placement is 1 mm medial to the center of the lateral mass (Figure 36B). An awl or high-speed drill is used to pierce the cortical surface to ensure drill purchase. This is followed by drilling to a depth of approximately 10 mm with

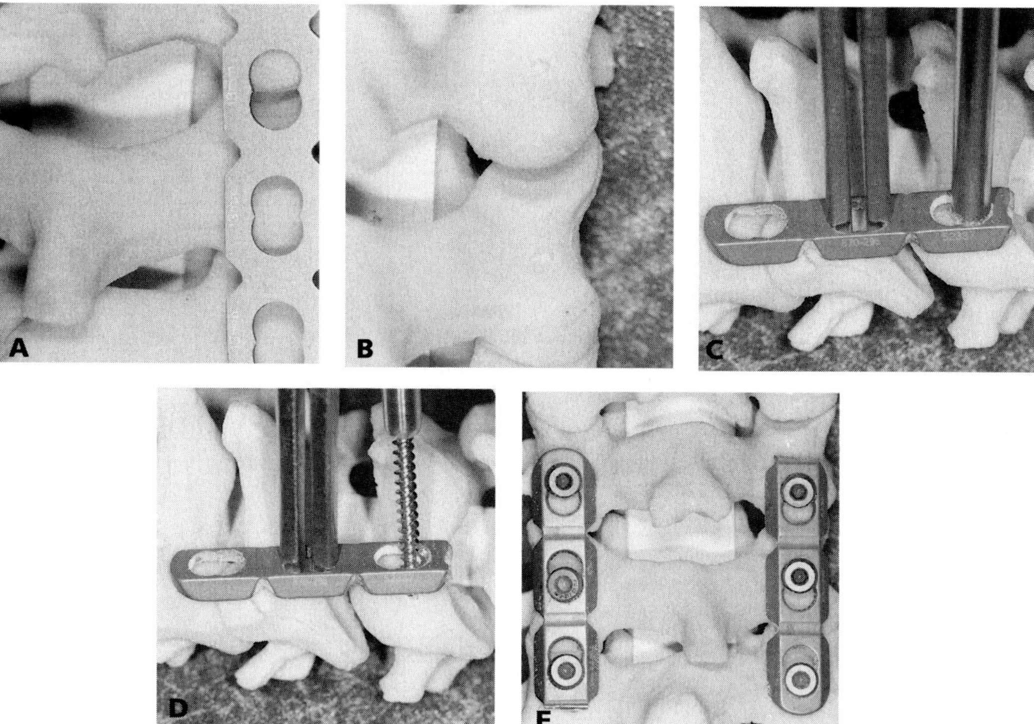

Figure 36: Lateral mass plating–the axis technique. **A)** A template is used for decortication of the entry site and to establish spinal contour. **B)** The entry sites are generally 1 mm medial to the center of the lateral mass. These have been decorticated with a high-speed drill. **C)** The plate has been contoured and may be secured with a plate holder. A drill guide is used to drill the pilot hole. The orientation of drilling is controversial. An orientation 30° lateral and 10°-20° rostral helps minimize nerve root and vertebral artery injury. **D)** After drilling is completed, the guide is removed and the holes are tapped and measured with a depth gauge. The lateral masses are decorticated, cartilage is removed from the facet joints, and permanent screws are selected. Bone graft is placed into the joints and on the lateral masses. The plates are seated. **E)** The permanent screws are threaded into place. The procedure is repeated on the opposite side.

a 2.5-mm diameter drill bit. Permanent screws of 3.5 or 4.0 mm in diameter and variable lengths secure the plates to the lateral masses. The authors generally use shorter screws, between 12 and 14 mm. This sacrifices bicortical screw purchase, but helps avoid nerve root and vertebral artery injury (Figures 36 and 37). When midline structures are intact, the lateral mass plates may be augmented with an interspinous cable.

Several trajectories for drilling and screw placement have been described for the Axis plates. Roy-Camille et al[87] advocate placing the drill directly perpendicular to the bone in the sagittal direction and angled 10° laterally in the transverse direction. The major disadvantage of this technique is the potential risk of damaging the vertebral artery and the exiting nerve root. A

safer trajectory angles the drill 10° to 20° rostrally and 30° laterally, with the starting point for screw placement 1 mm medial to the center of the lateral mass. Rostral angulation places the screw nearly parallel to the facet joint, thus avoiding injury to the nerve root. Lateral angulation of 30° provides more assurance that drilling and screw placement will avoid the vertebral artery. It also permits the use of longer screws, thereby enhancing bone-screw interface and maximizing bone purchase. Finally, biomechanical testing in cadaver spines demonstrated that the latter technique provides a much stronger and rigid construct.[74]

Recently, Synthes has developed a titanium screw-rod system, CerviFix, for dorsal stabilization in the cervical spine (Figure 38). The system is a modular tension band system that utilizes

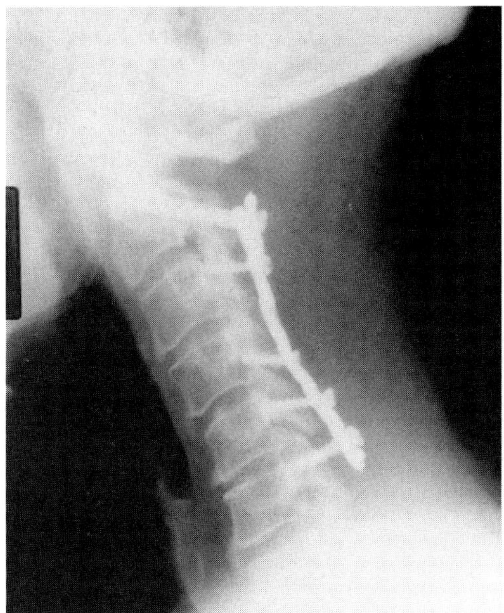
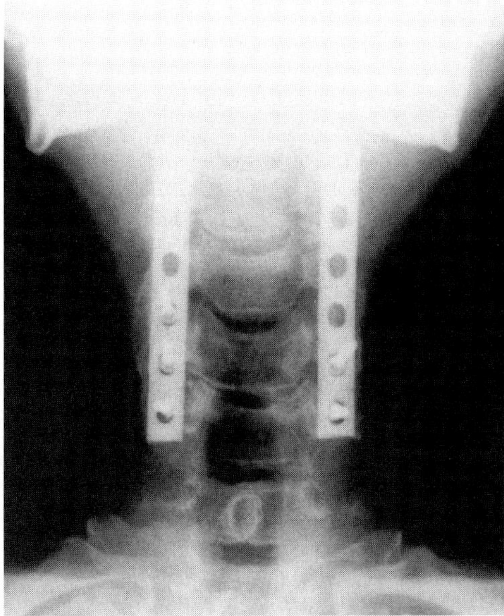

Figure 37: Postoperative radiographs of multilevel lateral mass screw-plate fixation used in the management of a patient with degenerative instability.

lateral mass screws and sublaminar hooks fixed to titanium rods by means of set screws. The system allows placement of crosslinks to connect both rods to provide more torsional support; a rod with one end shaped like a reconstruction plate is furnished for fixation to the occiput (Figure 38).

CONCLUSION

The current era in modern spine stabilization has ushered in many new implants and techniques for cervical stabilization. These include isolated screw fixation for odontoid and atlanto-axial fixation, screw-plate devices for ventral and dorsal subaxial stabilization, and cables that are stronger yet provide increased safety because of greater flexibility.

In appropriately selected patients, when performed by surgeons familiar with the nuances of each technique, these new methods offer decided advantages over older methods. Better outcomes relating to fusion, pain, and postoperative bracing without sacrificing safety or ease of application are advantages that these new methods can offer patients.

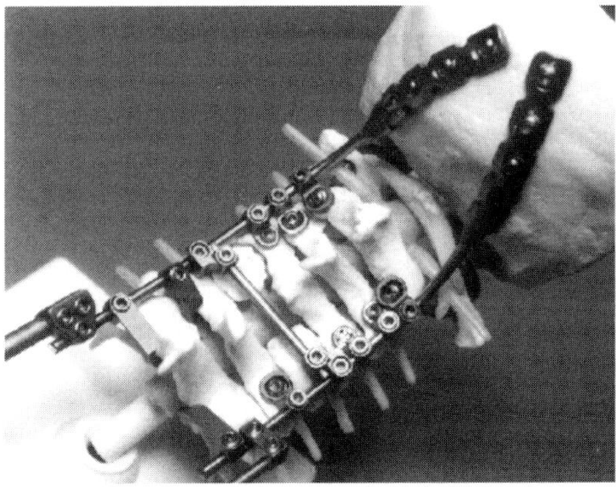

Figure 38: The Sofamor-Danek modular cervical spine rod system, CerviFix, used for dorsal cervical fixation. Cross fixators can be utilized for improved torsional support, and special rods are available for fixation to the occiput.

REFERENCES

1. Aebi M, Etter C, Coscia M: Fractures of the odontoid process. Treatment with anterior screw fixation. **Spine 14**:1065-1070, 1989
2. Aebi M, Zuber K, Marchesi D: Treatment of cervical spine injuries with anterior plating. Indications, techniques, and results. **Spine 16 (Suppl 3)**:S38-S45, 1991
3. Aldrich EF: Halifax interlaminar clamps: indications and operative technique. **Contemp Neurosurg 15**: 1-6, 1993
4. Aldrich EF, Weber PB, Crow WN: Halifax interlaminar clamp for posterior cervical fusion: a long-term follow-up review. **J Neurosurg 78**:702-708, 1993
5. Allen BL Jr, Ferguson RL, Lehmann TR, et al: A mechanistic classification of closed, indirect fractures and dislocations of the lower cervical spine. **Spine 7**: 1-27, 1982
6. Anderson LD, Clark CR: Fractures of the odontoid process of the axis, in Sherk HH, Dunn EJ, Eismont FJ, et al (eds): **The Cervical Spine. 2nd ed.** Philadelphia, Pa: JB Lippincott, 1989, pp 325-343
7. Anderson LD, D'Alonzo RT: Fractures of the odontoid process of the axis. **J Bone Joint Surg (Am) 56**: 1663-1674, 1974
8. Apfelbaum RI: Anterior screw fixation of odontoid fractures in Camins MS, O'Leary (eds): **Disorders of the Cervical Spine.** Baltimore, Md: Williams & Wilkins, 1992, pp 603-608
9. Apuzzo MLJ, Heiden JS, Weiss MH, et al: Acute fractures of the odontoid process. An analysis of 45 cases. **J Neurosurg 48**:85-91, 1978
10. Barbour JR: Screw fixation in fracture of the odontoid process. **South Aust Clin 5**:20, 1971
11. Bauer DR, Errico TJ: Cervical spine injuries, in Errico TJ, Bauer DR, Waugh T (eds): **Spinal Trauma.** Philadelphia, Pa: JB Lippincott, 1991, pp 71-121
12. Bell GD, Bailey SL: Anterior cervical fusion for trauma. **Clin Orthop 128**:155-158, 1977
13. Benzel EC: **Biomechanics of Spine Stabilization. Principles and Clinical Practice.** New York, NY: McGraw-Hill, 1994, p 3
14. Benzel EC, Hart BL, Ball PA, et al: Fractures of the C2 vertebral body. **J Neurosurg 81**:206-212, 1994
15. Benzel EC, Kesterson L: Posterior cervical interspinous compression wiring and fusion for mid to low cervical spine injuries. **J Neurosurg 70**:893-899, 1989
16. Bohler J: Sofort- und Fruhbehandlung traumatischer Querschnittlähmungen. **Z Orthop 103**:512-528, 1967
17. Bohlman HH: Acute fractures and dislocations of the cervical spine. An analysis of three hundred hospitalized patients and review of the literature. **J Bone Joint Surg (Am) 61**:1119-1142, 1979
18. Borges LF: Clinical assessment of posttraumatic spinal instability, in Cooper PR (ed): **Management of Posttraumatic Spinal Instability.** Park Ridge, Ill: American Association of Neurological Surgeons, 1990, pp 37-49
19. Borne GM, Bedou GL, Pinaudeau M, et al: Odontoid process fracture osteosynthesis with a direct screw fixation technique in nine consecutive cases. **J Neurosurg 68**:223-226, 1988
20. Brooks AL, Jenkins EB: Atlantoaxial arthrodesis by the wedge compression method. **J Bone Joint Surg (Am) 60**:279-283, 1978
21. Cahill DW, Bellegarrigue R, Ducker TB: Bilateral facet to spinous process fusion: a new technique for posterior spinal fusion after trauma. **Neurosurgery 13**:1-4, 1983
22. Callahan RA, Johnson RM, Margolis RN, et al: Cervical facet fusion for control of instability following laminectomy. **J Bone Joint Surg (Am) 59**:991-1002, 1977
23. Capen DA, Garland GE, Waters RL: Surgical stabilization of the cervical spine. A comparative analysis of anterior and posterior spine fusion. **Clin Orthop 196**:229-237, 1985
24. Capen DA, Nelson RW, Zigler J, et al: Surgical stabilization of the cervical spine: a comparative analysis of anterior and posterior spine fusions. **Paraplegia 25**:111-119, 1987
25. Capen DA, Zigler J, Garland D: Surgical stabilization in cervical spine trauma. **Contemp Orthop 14**:25-32, 1987
26. Caspar W, Barbier DD, Klara PM: Anterior cervical fusion and Caspar plate stabilization for cervical trauma. **Neurosurgery 25**:491-502, 1989
27. Coe JD, Warden KE, Sutterlin CE III, et al: Biomechanical evaluation of cervical spinal stabilization methods in a human cadaveric model. **Spine 14**: 1122-1131, 1989
28. Cooper PR, Cohen A, Rosiello A, et al: Posterior stabilization of cervical spine fractures and subluxations using plates and screws. **Neurosurgery 23**:300-306, 1988
29. Crockard HA: Anterior approaches to lesions of the upper cervical spine. **Clin Neurosurg 34**:389-416, 1988
30. Cybulski GR, Stone JL, Crowell RM, et al: Use of Halifax interlaminar clamps for posterior C1-2 arthrodesis. **Neurosurgery 22**:429-431, 1988
31. DeAndrade JR, MacNab I: Anterior occipito-cervical fusion using an extra-pharyngeal exposure. **J Bone Joint Surg (Am) 51**:1621-1626, 1969
32. Dickman CA, Hadley MN, Browner C, et al: Neurosurgical management of acute atlas-axis combination fractures. A review of 25 cases. **J Neurosurg 70**:45-49, 1989
33. Dove J: Internal fixation of the cervical spine. The Hartshill system, in Louis R, Weidner A (eds): **Cervical Spine II.** New York, NY: Springer-Verlag, 1989, pp 79-86
34. Dove J: Internal fixation of the lumbar spine. The Hartshill rectangle. **Clin Orthop 203**:135-140, 1986
35. Etter C, Coscia M, Jaberg H, et al: Direct anterior fixation of dens fractures with a cannulated screw system. **Spine 16 (Suppl 3)**:S25-S32, 1991
36. Fang HSY, Ong GB: Direct anterior approach to the upper cervical spine. **J Bone Joint Surg (Am) 44**: 1588-1604, 1962
37. Fehlings MG, Cooper PR, Errico TJ: Posterior plates in the management of cervical instability: long-term results in 44 patients. **J Neurosurg 81**:341-349, 1994
38. Fehlings MG, Errico T, Cooper P, et al: Occipitocervical fusion with a five-millimeter malleable rod and segmental fixation. **Neurosurgery 32**:198-208, 1993
39. Fielding JW: The status of arthrodesis of the cervical spine. **J Bone Joint Surg (Am) 70**:1571-1574, 1988
40. Fielding JW, Hawkins RJ, Ratzan SH: Spine fusion for atlantoaxial instability. **J Bone Joint Surg (Am) 58**: 400-407, 1976

41. Fried LC: Atlanto-axial fracture dislocations. Failure of posterior C-1 to C-2 fusion. **J Bone Joint Surg (Br)** 55:490-496, 1973

42. Fujii E, Kobayashi K, Hirabayashi K: Treatment in fractures of the odontoid process. **Spine 13:**604-609, 1988

43. Gallie WF: Fractures and dislocations of the cervical spine. **Am J Surg 46:**495-499, 1939

44. Geisler FH, Cheng C, Poka A, et al: Anterior screw fixation of posteriorly displaced Type II odontoid fractures. **Neurosurgery 25:**30-38, 1989

45. Gerhart K: Spinal cord injury outcomes in a population-based sample. **J Trauma 31:**1529-1535, 1991

46. Gill K, Paschal S, Corin J, et al: Posterior plating of the cervical spine. A biomechanical comparison of different posterior fusion techniques. **Spine 13:** 813-816, 1988

47. Grantham SA, Dick HM, Thompson RC Jr, et al: Occipitocervical arthrodesis. Indications, techniques and results. **Clin Orthop 65:**118-129, 1969

48. Grob D: Complications and pitfalls of spinal fusion, in Grob D (ed): **Spine. State of the Art Reviews.** Philadelphia, Pa: Hanley and Belfuse, 1992, Vol 6, pp 615-627

49. Grob D, Crisco JJ III, Panjabi MM, et al: Biomechanical evaluation of four different posterior atlantoaxial fixation techniques. **Spine 17:**480-490, 1992

50. Grob D, Dvorak J, Panjabi M, et al: Posterior occipitocervical fusion. A preliminary report of a new technique. **Spine 16 (Suppl 3):**S17-S23, 1991

51. Grob D, Jeanneret B, Aebi M, et al: Atlanto-axial fusion with transarticular screw fixation. **J Bone Joint Surg (Br)** 73:972-976, 1991

52. Hadley MN, Browner C, Sonntag VKH: Axis fractures: a comprehensive review of management and treatment in 107 cases. **Neurosurgery 17:**281-290, 1985

53. Hadley MN, Dickman CA, Browner CM, et al: Acute traumatic atlas fractures: management and long term outcome. **Neurosurgery 23:**31-35, 1988

54. Hajek PD, Lipka J, Hartline P, et al: Biomechanical study of C1-2 posterior arthrodesis techniques. **Spine** 18:173-177, 1993

55. Hamblen DL: Occipito-cervical fusion. Indications, techniques and results. **J Bone Joint Surg (Br) 49:** 33-45, 1967

56. Harris JH Jr: Radiographic evaluation of spinal trauma. **Orthop Clin North Am 17:**75-86, 1986

57. Heiden JS, Weiss MH, Rosenberg AW, et al: Management of cervical spinal cord trauma in Southern California. **J Neurosurg 43:**732-736, 1975

58. Herman JM, Sonntag VKH: Cervical corpectomy and plate fixation for postlaminectomy kyphosis. **J Neurosurg 80:**963-970, 1994

59. Heywood AWB, Learmonth ID, Thomas M: Internal fixation for occipitocervical fusion. **J Bone Joint Surg (Br) 70:**708-711, 1988

60. Holness RO, Huestis WS, Howes WJ, et al: Posterior stabilization with an interlaminar clamp in cervical injuries: technical note and review of the long term experience with the method. **Neurosurgery 14:** 318-322, 1984

61. Hosono N, Yonenobu K, Kawagoe K, et al: Traumatic anterior atlanto-occipital dislocation. A case report with survival. **Spine 18:**786-790, 1992

62. Krag MH: Biomechanics of the cervical spine, in Fry-moyer JP (ed): **The Adult Spine.** New York, NY: Raven Press, 1991, pp 929-965

63. Lee PC, Chun SY, Leong JCY: Experience of posterior surgery in atlanto-axial instability. **Spine 9:**231-239, 1984

64. Luque ER: The anatomic basis and development of segmental spinal instrumentation. **Spine 7:**256-259, 1982

65. MacKenzie AI, Uttley D, Marsh HT, et al: Craniocervical stabilization using Luque/Hartshill rectangles. **Neurosurgery 26:**32-36, 1990

66. MacMillan M, Stauffer ES: Traumatic instability in the previously fused cervical spine. **J Spinal Disord 4:** 449-454, 1991

67. Magerl F, Seemann PS: Stable posterior fusion of the atlas and axis by transarticular screw fixation, in Kehr P, Weidner A (eds): **Cervical Spine I.** New York, NY: Springer-Verlag, 1987, pp 322-327

68. Maiman DJ, Larson SJ: Management of odontoid fractures. **Neurosurgery 11:**471-476, 1982

69. Marcotte P, Dickman CA, Sonntag VKH: Posterior atlantoaxial facet screw fixation. **J Neurosurg 79:** 234-237, 1993

70. McAfee PC, Bohlman HH, Wilson WL: The triple wire fixation technique for stabilization. **Orthop Trans 9:**142, 1985 (Abstract)

71. McAfee PC, Bohlman HH, Wilson WL: The triple wire fixation technique for stabilization of acute cervical fracture dislocations: a biochemical analysis. **Orthop Trans 10:**455, 1986 (Abstract)

72. Menezes AH, Muhonen M: Management of occipitocervical instability, in Cooper PR (ed): **Management of Posttraumatic Spinal Instability.** Park Ridge, Ill: American Association of Neurological Surgeons, 1990, pp 65-76

73. Montesano PX, Anderson PA, Schlehr F, et al: Odontoid fractures treated by anterior odontoid screw fixation. **Spine 16 (Suppl 3):**S33-S37, 1991

74. Montesano PX, Jauch E, Jonsson H Jr: Anatomic and biomechanical study of posterior cervical spine plate arthrodesis: an evaluation of two different techniques of screw placement. **J Spinal Disord 5:**301-305, 1992

75. Murphy MJ, Daniaux H, Southwick WO: Posterior cervical fusion with rigid internal fixation. **Orthop Clin North Am 17:**55-65, 1986

76. Murphy MJ, Southwick WO: Posterior approaches and fusions, in Sherk HH, Dunn EJ, Eismont FJ, et al (eds): **The Cervical Spine. 2nd ed.** Philadelphia, Pa: JB Lippincott, 1989, pp 775-791

77. Nakanishi T, Sasaki T, Tokita N, et al: Internal fixation for the odontoid fracture. **Orthop Trans 6:**176, 1982

78. Newman P, Sweetnam R: Occipito-cervical fusion. An operative technique and its indications. **J Bone Joint Surg (Br) 51:**423-431, 1969

79. Orozco R, Llovet J: Osteosintesis en las fracturas del raquis cervical. **Rev Ortop Traumatol 14:**285-288, 1970

80. Papadopoulos SM: Anterior cervical stabilization. **Clin Neurosurg 40:**273-285, 1993

81. Ransford AO, Crockard HA, Pozo JL, et al: Craniocervical instability treated by contoured loop fixation. **J Bone Joint Surg (Br) 68:**173-177, 1986

82. Ripa DR, Kowall MG, Meyer PR Jr, et al: Series of ninety-two traumatic cervical spine injuries stabilized with anterior ASIF plate fusion technique. **Spine 16 (Suppl 3):**S46-S55, 1991

83. Robinson RA, Southwick WO: Indications and techniques for early stabilization of the neck in some fracture dislocations of the cervical spine. **South Med J 53:**565-579, 1960

84. Rogers WA: Fractures and dislocations of the cervical spine. An end-result study. **J Bone Joint Surg 39:** 341-376, 1957

85. Rogers WA: Treatment of fracture-dislocation of the cervical spine. **J Bone Joint Surg 24:**245-258, 1942

86. Roy-Camille R, Mazel CH, Saillant G: Treatment of cervical spine injuries by a posterior osteosynthesis with plates and screws, in Kehr P, Weidner A (eds): **Cervical Spine I.** New York, NY: Springer-Verlag, 1987, p 163

87. Roy-Camille R, Saillant G, Laville C, et al: Treatment of lower cervical spinal injuries—C3 to C7. **Spine 17 (Suppl 10):**S442-S446, 1992

88. Roy-Camille R, Saillant G, Mazel C: Internal fixation of the unstable cervical spine by a posterior osteosynthesis with plates and screws, in Sherk HH, Dunn EJ, Eismont FJ, et al (eds): **The Cervical Spine. 2nd ed.** Philadelphia, Pa: JB Lippincott, 1989, pp 390-403

89. Sakou T, Kawaida H, Morizono Y, et al: Occipito-atlantoaxial fusion utilizing a rectangular rod. **Clin Orthop 239:**136-144, 1989

90. Segal D, Whitelaw GP, Gumbs V, et al: Tension band fixation of acute cervical spine fractures. **Clin Orthop 159:**211-222, 1981

91. Sherk HH, Snyder B: Posterior fusions of the upper cervical spine: indications, techniques, and prognosis. **Orthop Clin North Am 9:**1091-1099, 1978

92. Smith GW, Robinson RA: The treatment of certain cervical spine disorders by anterior removal of the intervertebral disc and interbody fusion. **J Bone Joint Surg (Am) 40:**607-624, 1958

93. Smith MD, Philips WA, Hensingen RN: Complications of fusion to the upper cervical spine. **Spine 16:** 702-705, 1991

94. Songer MN, Spencer DL, Meyer PR Jr, et al: The use of sublaminar cables to replace Luque wires. **Spine 16 (Suppl 8):**S418-S421, 1991

95. Sonntag VKH, Dickman CA: Craniocervical stabilization. **Clin Neurosurg 40:**243-272, 1993

96. Sonntag VKH, Hadley MN: Management of non-odontoid upper cervical spine injuries, in Cooper PR (ed): **Management of Posttraumatic Spinal Instability.** Park Ridge, Ill: American Association of Neurological Surgeons, 1990, pp 99-110

97. Spetzler RF, Dickman CA, Sonntag VKH: The transoral approach to the anterior cervical spine. **Contemp Neurosurg 13:**1-6, 1991

98. Stauffer ES: Management of spine fractures C3 to C7. **Orthop Clin North Am 17:**45-53, 1986

99. Stauffer ES: Wiring techniques of the posterior cervical spine for the treatment of trauma. **Orthopedics 11:**1543-1548, 1988

100. Stillerman CB, Chen TC, Gruen JP, et al: Anterior cervical fixation using the Manny fixator: clinical experience and follow-up on 32 patients. Poster presented at the Annual Meeting of the American Association of Neurological Surgeons, April 1994, San Diego, California

101. Stillerman CB, Gruen JP: Universal Spinal Instrumentation fixation, in Benzel EC (ed): **Spinal Instrumentation.** Park Ridge, Ill: American Association of Neurological Surgeons, 1994, pp 147-174

102. Stillerman CB, Gruen JP, Roy RS: Thoracic and lumbar fusion: techniques for posterior stabilization, in Menezes AH, Sonntag VKH (eds): **Principles of Spinal Surgery.** New York, NY: McGraw-Hill, 1994

103. Stillerman CB, Mueller W, Baker G: Clinical and biomechanical characteristics of a new anterior cervical screw-plate fixation device. The Manny fixator. Poster presented at the Annual Meeting of the American Association of Neurological Surgeons, April 1993, Boston, Massachusetts

104. Stillerman CB, Roy RS, Weiss MH: Cervical spine injuries, in Wilkins RH, Rengachary SS (eds): **Neurosurgery. 2nd ed.** New York, NY: McGraw Hill, YEAR?

105. Stillerman CB, Wilson JA: Atlanto-axial stabilization with posterior transarticular screw fixation: technical description and report of 22 cases. **Neurosurgery 32:** 948-955, 1993

106. Tippets RH, Apfelbaum RI: Anterior cervical fusion with the Caspar instrumentation system. **Neurosurgery 22:**1008-1013, 1988

107. Traynelis VC, Marano GD, Dunker RO, et al: Traumatic atlanto-occipital dislocation. Case report. **J Neurosurg 65:**863-870, 1986

108. Tucker HH: Technical report: method of fixation of subluxed or dislocated cervical spine below C1-2. **Can J Neurol Sci 2:**381-382, 1975

109. VanGilder JC, Menezes AH, Dolan KD: **The Craniovertebral Junction and its Abnormalities. Traumatic Lesions.** Mt Kisco, NY: Futura, 1987, pp 195-215

110. Van Peteghem PK, Schweigel JF: The fractured cervical spine rendered unstable by anterior cervical fusion. **J Trauma 19:**110-114, 1979

111. Wertheim SB, Bohlman HH: Occipitocervical fusion. Indications, technique and long-term results in thirteen patients. **J Bone Joint Surg (Am) 69:**833-866, 1987

112. White AA III, Panjabi MM: **Clinical Biomechanics of the Spine.** Philadelphia, Pa: JB Lippincott, 1990, p 110

113. White AA III, Panjabi MM: The role of stabilization in the treatment of cervical spine injuries. **Spine 9:** 512-522, 1984

114. White AA III, Panjabi MM, Saha S, et al: Biomechanics of the axially loaded cervical spine: development of a clinical test for ruptured ligaments. **J Bone Joint Surg (Am) 57:**582, 1975 (Abstract)

115. Whitehill R, Schmidt R: The posterior interspinous fusion in the treatment of quadriplegia. **Spine 8:** 733-740, 1983

CHAPTER 14

SURGICAL TECHNIQUES: THORACIC AND LUMBAR

ZIYA L. GOKASLAN, MD, AND PAUL McCORMICK, MD

No consensus presently exists on the surgical treatment of thoracic and lumbar fractures.[65] In the past, a nonoperative approach has been emphasized in the treatment of these injuries.[4,5,48] It was believed that if patients were kept at bed rest long enough, removal of the axial compression force from the spine would eventually lead to the achievement of osseous stability. It is now known that an acceptable level of stability against the forces of axial distraction, rotation, and hyperextension cannot be achieved by bed rest alone. In addition, imprudent handling during the early post-injury period can lead to the displacement of unstable fractures, possibly resulting in further damage to delicate neural elements.[74,102] To avoid these and additional risks from prolonged immobilization, operative reduction and stabilization of the injuries have been proposed.

Single-wire techniques and the use of plates fixed to the spinous processes above and below the level of a spinal fracture are among the early, frequently unsuccessful, surgical methods employed to treat spinal fractures and fracture dislocations. The Harrington distraction system overcame many of the limitations seen with these methods.[40,61,75] It has proved to be a landmark development in spinal surgery, offering excellent spinal stabilization and an acceptable level of morbidity.[1,13,40] Subsequently, we have seen the development and satisfactory clinical performance of several additional dorsal and ventral instrumentation systems.[86] In this chapter, the treatment of traumatic thoracolumbar spinal injuries is discussed with special emphasis on surgical options and indications.

GENERAL CONSIDERATIONS

Although there is no consensus regarding indications for the surgical treatment of thoracic and lumbar injuries, surgical intervention is unquestionably indicated in certain instances. These include situations where there is great risk of further neurological injury from additional compression of neural elements and fragment displacement such as fractures with excessive distraction and separation of fragments or those with gross translation and unopposed fragments. Nevertheless, in the majority of cases the need for surgery is not obvious. The most important determinants of the need for surgical intervention are whether there is acute spinal instability or compression of the neural elements. Also important when making the decision is the possible risk of delayed complications, including neurological deterioration, pain, or progressive deformity.

Several criteria have been established for determining spinal stability because it is a complicated process.[22,23,54,55,63,84] The classification of Ferguson and Allen,[37] which is based on mechanism of injury, has proved to be the most clinically useful, but it is still necessary for the surgeon to make a judgment as to the predominant mechanism that produced the injury, as many spinal injuries are the result of a combination of forces. Because compression of neural elements occurs with some injuries, the need for neural decompression must be addressed as well as spinal stability.

Classification of Thoracolumbar Injuries

There are three major categories of injury to the thoracolumbar spine: flexion-axial compression; flexion-distraction; and shear fractures and/or dislocation.

Flexion-Axial Compression

Approximately 80% of all patients with spinal injury undergoing surgical stabilization are represented within the following combinations of flexion-and-axial compression injury categories:[1,4,22,37,99,100] "compression fracture," "flexion-compression fracture," and "burst fracture." In many patients with these injuries, conservative treatment using an orthosis may be instituted. A loss of more than 50% of the vertebral body height is frequently associated with disruption of the dorsal ligamentous complex.[16,67] In cases of disruption of the dorsal elements, several region-specific instrumentation methods are available to correct the resulting spinal instability.[17,19,91,96,l05]

Flexion-Distraction

Fifteen percent of all injuries that require surgery are produced by flexion and distraction.[47] Logic dictates the use of extension and compression to reverse the deformity caused by flexion and distraction;[13,35,37,57] however, this should be approached cautiously in cases of bilateral facet dislocation because compression and extension can potentiate disc retropulsion,[43,62] despite its ability to restore normal sagittal alignment of bony elements. Other types of flexion-distraction injuries include bony-type injuries (Chance[18]) and combinations of bony and ligamentous injuries. When surgery is required, the deformity is reduced by the application of extension and compression to the injured spinal segment.[81,92]

Shear Fractures and/or Dislocation

Mixed injuries constitute approximately 3% to 5% of deformities, which typically have an element of shear.[58,73] These injuries may necessitate a complex configuration of surgical reconstruction to bring about a reduction of all deformities.

Decompressive Procedures

Significant partial neurological deficits must be present before undertaking decompression of the spinal cord and neural elements. Decompressive procedures in patients with complete paraplegia after 48 hours are not necessary because at that point there is no chance for neurological improvement. Surgery is usually recommended for patients who retain partial spinal neurological function. However, because most such incomplete lesions tend to improve without intervention, it is hard to prove the benefit of surgical decompression.[9,56,97] Either direct or indirect means of surgical decompression may be carried out, employing either a dorsal or ventral approach to the spine.

Dorsal Techniques: Exposure

After placement in the prone position on the operating table, the patient is prepped from the nape of the neck down to the iliac crest. An incision is begun at the midline at approximately three levels above the level of injury and is carried to three levels below it. Electrocautery is then used to carry the incision down the spinous processes. After exposure of the spinous processes, a localizing radiograph is obtained. Subperiosteal dissection is then carried out using cautery to expose the spinous processes, laminae, and transverse processes. Dorsal element fractures are carefully exposed and loose pieces of spinous process removed.

Indirect Decompression

Several types of dorsal instrumentation systems are available to provide indirect decompression by correcting kyphosis and ligamentotaxis. Once vertebral height and spinal alignment are restored, the spinal canal can be brought back to its normal configuration, provided that the posterior longitudinal ligament is intact and that comminuted fragments are not present.[21,31,33,38,40,80] Indirect decompression using Harrington instrumentation with distraction rods has been attempted but is usually found to be ineffective in relieving compression by intraoperative myelography.[39] Furthermore, there have been reports of neurological deterioration after indirect decompression with this instrumentation.[27,28,38] Recently, better results with spinal canal decompression have been obtained using the internal spinal fixator and other methods of pedicle screw fixation.[6,9,17,71,91,105]

Direct Decompression

Methods of direct decompression are laminectomy, dorsolateral transpedicular decompression, and ventral decompression.

Laminectomy. Laminectomy is rarely indicated in the surgical treatment of thoracolumbar fractures. The only indication for laminectomy is significant dorsal impingement by fragments of the neural arch.[90] Laminectomy has been shown to adversely affect spinal stability and to increase neurological damage.[82] In most cases, it has not been shown to either relieve the myelographic block or improve the neurological status of the patient.[4,8,43,53] Additionally, the repair of a dural tear seen on a computed tomography (CT) myelogram cannot be done using laminectomy because the ventral location of most tears makes them very hard to repair via a dorsal approach.

Irrespective of these disadvantages, until recently, laminectomy has been used to treat approximately 30% of thoracolumbar fractures.[3] The risks and limited benefits have since been recognized, and unilateral or bilateral posterolateral decompressive procedures, as well as ventral surgical approaches, have been advocated.

Dorsolateral Transpedicular Decompression. Dorsolateral transpedicular decompression involves the partial or complete removal of the pedicle via a costotransverse approach (Figure 1) in order to incise fragments of bone or soft tissue compressing the dura ventrally.[28,35,41,51,57, 72,77] A benefit of this procedure is that the patient does not have to be moved on the table in order to carry out a dorsal stabilization at the same time.[35,38,41,77,82,92] It also permits the use of intraoperative ultrasonography for confirmation that spinal canal decompression is sufficient, as posterolateral decompression of fragments in the canal and dorsal reduction are undertaken. Among the major limitations to this approach is the potential for spinal cord retraction injury because some retraction of the dura mater, conus, and adjacent nerve root is required. If tethering or scarring exists at the fracture site, retraction of the dura mater may be difficult.[15] Furthermore, in most patients the dorsolateral approach fails to provide sufficient visualization across the entire length of the canal.[20,29,59,64,79] An additional problem can result if the already injured spine is rendered unstable by removal of the pedicle.[13,38] Using this approach, some improvement in somatosensory evoked potentials has been observed;[72] however, patient recovery rates are comparable to those for conservatively treated patients,[41] and postoperatively, inadequate decompression and persisting compromise of the spinal canal are commonly found on CT.[41,46,81] Because of the limitations of this approach, ventral decompression has become the procedure of choice for these patients.

Ventral Decompression and Exposure

Neurological improvement is commonly noted in patients undergoing ventral decompression procedures[30,70,78,85] and, in most patients,

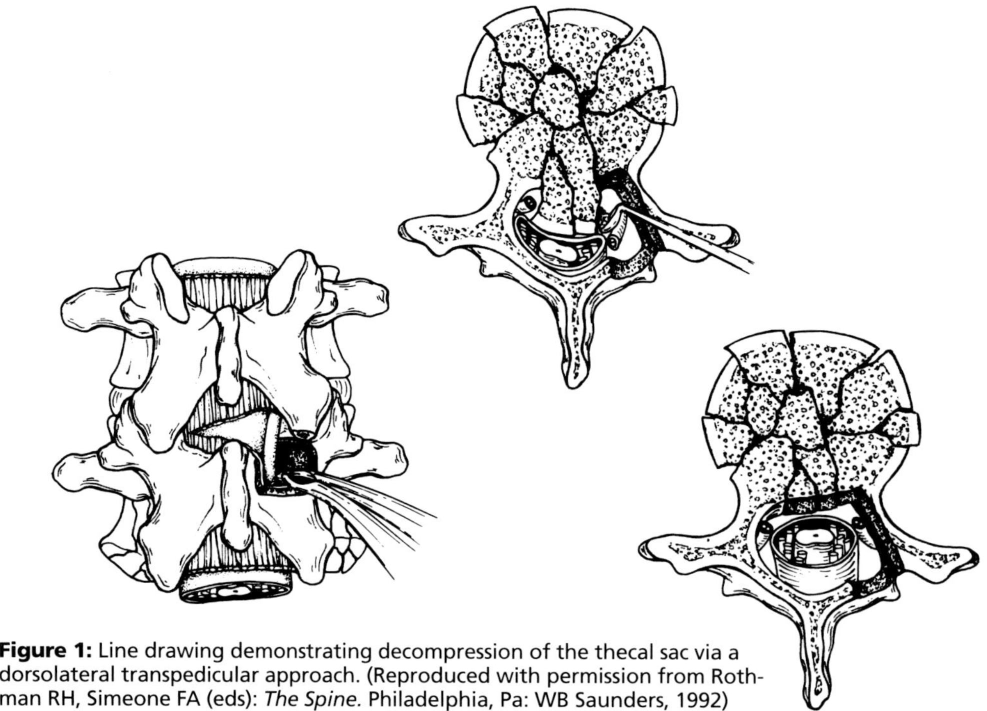

Figure 1: Line drawing demonstrating decompression of the thecal sac via a dorsolateral transpedicular approach. (Reproduced with permission from Rothman RH, Simeone FA (eds): *The Spine.* Philadelphia, Pa: WB Saunders, 1992)

progressive deficits are halted.[59] On postoperative CT, residual canal stenosis with the ventral approach is usually found to be less than 1%, whereas with the dorsal approach, a canal compromise of approximately 25% is associated (Figure 2).[15]

Ventral decompression procedures increase the risk of spinal instability. Decompression necessitates surgical disruption of the ventral elements, and the bone graft placed in the site of decompression often fails to provide sufficient stability until fusion occurs.[56,79] Therefore, proper stabilization is often indicated.[98] Other potential complications include retrograde ejaculation,[14] failure to obtain primary union,[30] blood loss averaging approximately 1800 ml,[30,87] the need for tube thoracostomy, and prolonged ileus.[33]

Exposure

Depending on the level at which the injury occurs, there are three commonly employed approaches: via the thoracic spine for injuries occurring from approximately T3 to T10, via the thoracolumbar spine from T11 to L1, and via the lumbar spine from L2 to L4. Initial patient

preparation varies only slightly among these approaches, with the patient having a high thoracotomy undergoing intubation with a double-lumen tube, so that the lung on the side of the approach can be selectively deflated, making exposure easier.

The upper thoracic spine approach requires elevation of the scapula on the central and lateral borders, thereby allowing exposure of the third through sixth thoracic ribs. Scapula elevation generally requires a division of the rhomboid and part of the trapezius muscles. The spine should be approached through the rib lying one or two levels above the fractured vertebra.

There are two possibilities for approaching fractures in the thoracolumbar area at the T11, T12, and L1 levels. Excellent exposure can be achieved via a thoracoabdominal approach, involving splitting of the diaphragm; however, this is not always necessary, and exposure of T12 and L1 can often be carried out using a retroperitoneal approach involving a caudal-to-rostral dissection with elevation of the crus of the diaphragm.

In the lumbar spine from L2 to L4, a retro-

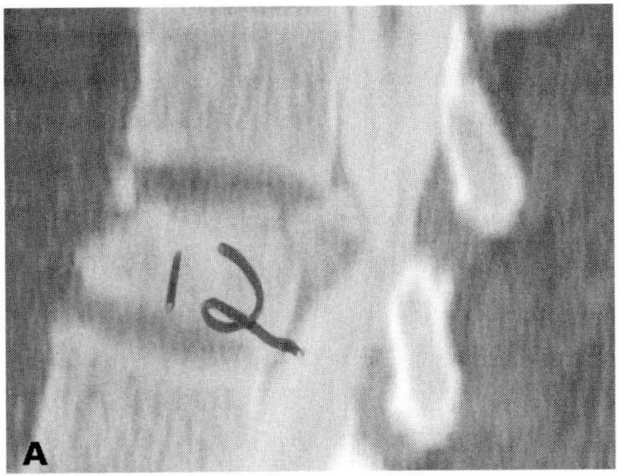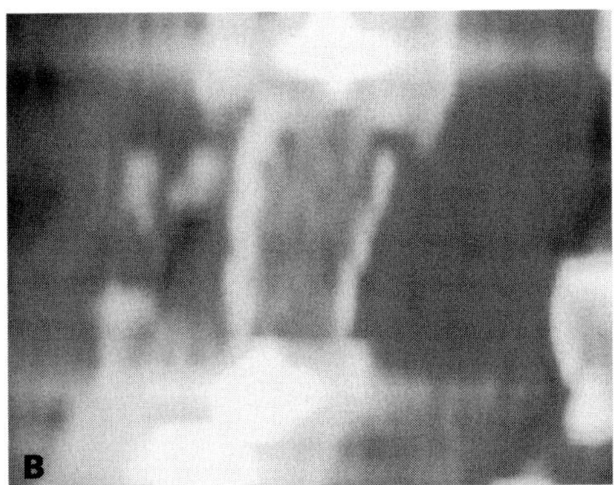

Figure 2: CT scans of a patient with T12 burst fracture. **A)** Sagittal reconstruction following a myelogram showing significant compression of the thecal sac (conus) due to a retropulsed fragment in a T12 burst fracture. **B)** Postoperative scan with sagittal reconstruction demonstrating excellent decompression of the neural elements and iliac crest strut, spanning the space from T11 to L1.

peritoneal approach provides excellent exposure. For L4 and L5, fixation ventrally is difficult and it is easier to perform neural root decompression via a dorsal (laminectomy) approach.

The use of instrumentation also dictates the side of approach, such that high-profile implants should be placed from the right side to avoid contact with the pulsating aorta. Low-profile instrumentation, on the other hand, is preferably placed via a left-sided approach because it is easier to repair the aorta than the inferior vena cava, if a vascular injury were to occur.

After exposure of a level, the disc on either end should be removed, isolating the fractured body. Loose fragments can be removed initially with a curet or an osteotome; however, a high-speed burr is usually necessary to remove the remaining bone. Bone removal proceeds gradually toward the spinal canal. After the thinning of the dorsal cortex, dissection begins at the inferior edge of the vertebral body and is carried proximally toward the pedicles. Finally, any remaining fragments are gently eased away from the posterior longitudinal ligament and/or the dura using a small angled curette.

Combined Procedures

Another surgical option is to perform an initial dorsal reduction of the fracture with Harrington distraction rods or other similar techniques and to assess whether protruding fragments of bony or disc material are compressing the neural structures to a significant degree.[95] If there is significant compression as well as no evidence of neural recovery, ventral decompression can be performed via a separate approach.[44] Translational injuries, flexion-compression fractures, fractures with angular displacement, and complete injuries are usually treated via dorsal approaches.[14,44] However, it should always be kept in mind that a potential risk of iatrogenic injury is associated with these procedures. As a solution to this problem, many surgeons advocate a simultaneous ventral decompression with dorsal instrumentation.[98] Ventral thoracolumbar plates have recently become available, and it is now possible to obtain decompression and instrumentation at the same time, through the same incision, with an acceptable degree of stability (Figure 3).[12,49,103] No long-term studies are presently available to satisfactorily assess the applicability of this instrumentation method in treating thoracolumbar fractures.

Instrumentation Methods

Instrumentation is selected for a given patient with respect to an understanding of the mechanism that caused the injury and, consequently, the forces that have produced the deformity. Once this is understood, subsequent selection of the approach can be based on the knowledge of which instrumentation system allows appropriate forces to be applied to the spine.

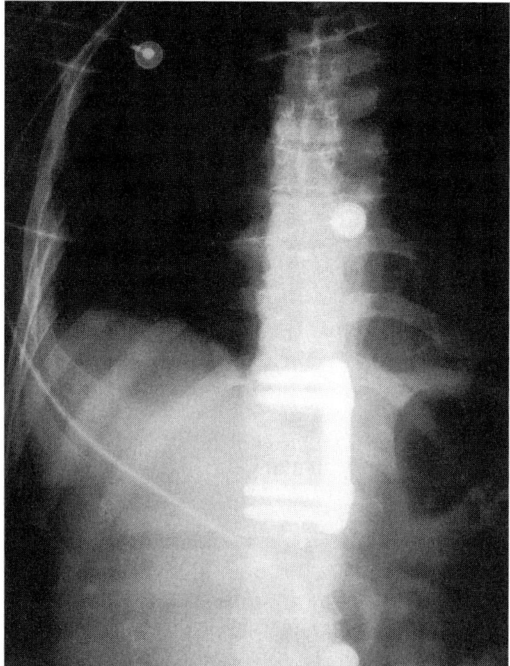

Figure 3: Postoperative anteroposterior thoraco-lumbar spine radiograph showing ventral instrumentation using a Synthes locking plate/screw construct following a T12 vertebrectomy.

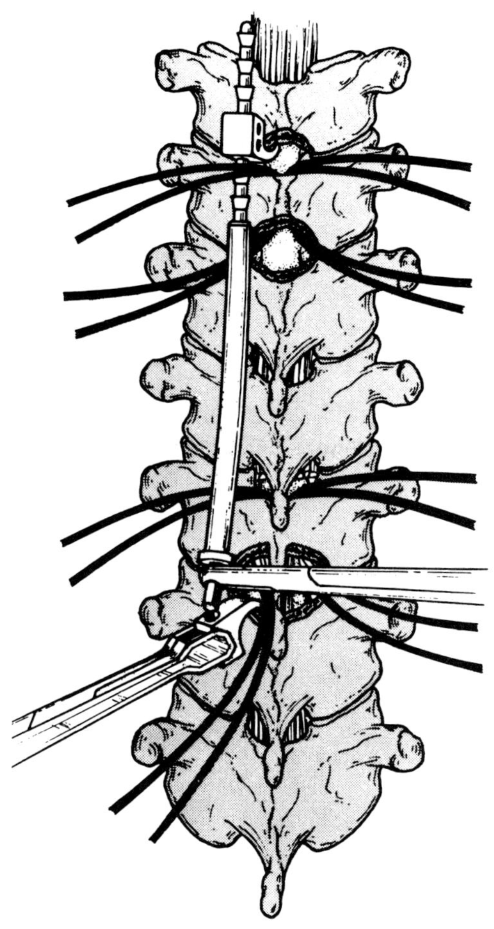

Figure 4: Line drawing showing placement of a Harrington distraction rod on the left side. In this instance, sublaminar wires are also being used to supplement the system. (Reproduced with permission from Rothman RH, Simeone FA (eds): *The Spine.* Philadelphia, Pa: WB Saunders, 1992)

Dorsal Techniques

Harrington Distraction Rod Technique

Harrington instrumentation with distraction rods is a simple system that provides excellent corrective forces for reduction of a thoracolumbar fracture (Figure 4).[7,33,50,93,101] A limitation of the system is its reliance on distraction for hook fixation and correction. Overdistraction, decreased lumbar lordosis (flat back), and loss of correction are problems associated with the use of this method.[70,78,106] Nevertheless, Harrington instrumentation has played a significant role in establishing the basic principles for the surgical treatment of spinal deformities.

Irrespective of the type of injury, the hooks of the Harrington distraction system are typically placed at three levels above and two levels below the injury site. The most-rostral hook sites are prepared for Harrington 1253 hooks by squaring the inferomedial edge of the laminae bilaterally. The rostral hooks are then seated symmetrically

in the sublaminar position. Next, the inferior hook sites two levels below the fractured vertebral body are prepared. This usually requires removal of the inferior edge of the laminae above. The hooks are then placed on the superior laminar edge of the vertebra as shown in the drawing (Figure 4). The rods are contoured in standard fashion to maintain lordosis at the thoracolumbar junction and kyphosis in the thoracic region. In the thoracic spine, contouring is especially important to prevent prominence of the rod tips. The rod is then passed up through the proximal hook and distracted into the distal hook. A con-

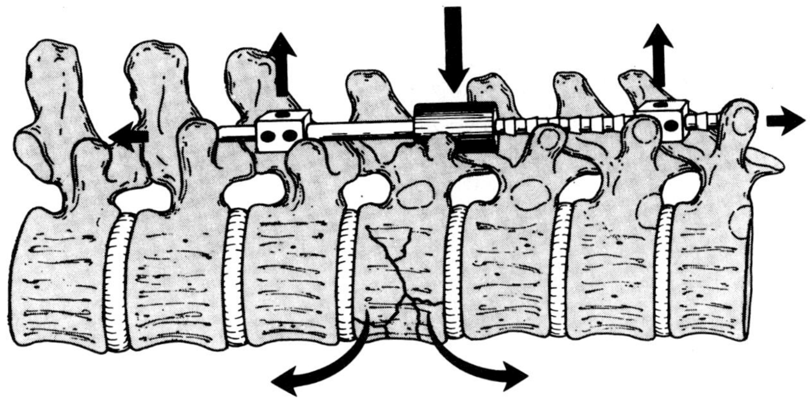

Figure 5: Line drawing showing the rod-sleeve technique and the application of various corrective forces to the spine for fracture reduction. (Reproduced with permission from Rothman RH, Simeone FA (eds): *The Spine.* Philadelphia, Pa: WB Saunders, 1992)

stant downward force is necessary to reduce the kyphosis during contouring of the rod so that the tip of the rod can be inserted into the distal hook. The distal hook is grasped with a hook holder and the end of the rod with a rod holder, thus allowing a downward force to be achieved. The tip of the rod is inserted into the hook while an assistant uses a spreader to distract the rod into the appropriate position. The distal end is then advanced until the nipple of the rod is fully inserted into the hook. Sublaminar wires can be used to supplement the system (Figure 4).[76] Bone grafting is performed in the usual manner. An additional one or two ratchets of distraction can be achieved after viscoelastic relaxation. Two C-washers are then placed below the proximal hooks to maintain distraction.

Rod-Sleeve Techniques

Rod-sleeve techniques are similar to the Harrington distraction system; however, they have the advantage of applying a ventrally directed force to counteract the flexion moment found with most spinal injuries (Figure 5). Moreover, the application of sleeves wedged between the facets and spinous processes on either side provides greater rotational stability than is obtained with Harrington rods.

A sleeve of proper size is selected and placed over the rod on one side of the spine. The rod is advanced through the rostral hook proximally until the end of the nipple is cephalad to the distal hook. The surgeon then grasps the distal hook with a hook holder and the nipple with a rod holder. By applying continuous downward pressure, the surgeon can reduce the kyphosis before distracting the nipple into the distal hook. The rod should be distracted just enough to engage the distal hook. Once the rod is engaged within the distal hook and sufficient distraction has been achieved to simply hook the system in place, the sleeve is moved to its proper location over the facet joints and pedicles using a rod spreader distally, thus completing the reduction. After placement of the second rod, the sleeve on that side is placed making the entire construct symmetrical. Bone grafting is performed in the usual manner. After about 10 to 15 minutes have elapsed, one or two additional ratchets of distraction can be obtained. C-washers are then placed below the upper hooks to prevent loosening of the construct.

Spinal Rod/Hook Systems

Unstable thoracic and lumbar fractures may be treated effectively using Cotrel-Dubousset instrumentation (Figure 6);[34,36,83] however, it is essential to employ a sufficient number of skeletal fixation sites and to be sure that the construct is long enough. Satisfactory results can usually be obtained using the multiple-hook, standard-length constructs (six segments) in the thoracic

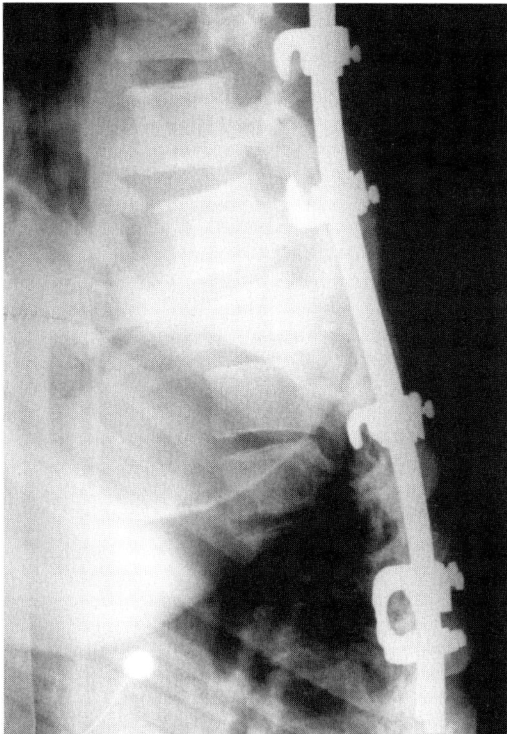

Figure 6: Lateral thoracolumbar spine radiograph showing the Cotrel-Dubousset instrumentation (spinal rod/hooks) for T12 flexion-compression fracture.

spine. However, early experience with the use of short constructs, especially at the thoracolumbar junction and high lumbar spine, has been less than satisfactory.

Cotrel-Dubousset instrumentation is assembled in the form of claw configurations above and below the level of injury. A combination of closed and open lumbar, thoracic, transverse process, and pedicle hooks is used to create claws above and below the level of injury. The ends of the construct are secured by closed hooks. First, a rod is contoured to the physiological norms of the spine and is passed through the proximal claw. It is then advanced rostrally until it extends above the level of the most-caudal closed hook, simultaneously engaging the two intermediate open hooks. Two blockers are engaged through the two open hooks. Beginning at the rostral end of the construct, the nut on the most-proximal hook is tightened. A hook approximator is used to tighten the upper claw. The open hook at the level above the fracture is advanced rostrally

using a spreader; its blocker is then tightened into place. Insertion of the appropriately contoured rod should theoretically have reduced the kyphosis at this point, necessitating only slight distraction between the hooks above and below the level of injury. The distal claw can then be approximated by compressing the hooks together. A symmetrical construct is placed on the contralateral side. Cross fixators (transverse traction devices) are placed at the proximal and distal ends of the construct, and all nuts are broken off in the hooks and devices.

Universal rod/hook systems have been introduced recently, and most of the basic principles of fracture reduction and fixation are similar to the Cotrel-Dubousset instrumentation. However, most Universal systems rely more on distraction-compression forces than on the contouring of the rod to obtain reduction. The assembly of hooks and rods varies with each system, making a detailed description of each system beyond the scope of this chapter. Thoracic and lumbar fractures have been treated using several Universal systems, such as the modular spinal system by Edwards[32] and the Texas Scottish Rite Hospital (TSRH) rod instrumentation.[11] Short-segment compression instrumentation (the short rod/two-claw technique) with the TSRH has been shown to be effective in treating selected thoracic and lumbar injuries.[10]

Segmental Pedicle Screw Fixation

There are several advantages to segmental pedicle screw fixation beyond those of the previously described spinal rod/hook systems (Figure 7). It provides a very stable construct with fusion extending only above and below the level of injury, and it includes both distraction and compression capabilities, allowing anatomic reduction with preservation of lordosis.

Most pedicle screw systems limit surgical exposure to one level above and one level below the fracture site. Spinous processes, laminae, facets, and transverse processes are exposed bilaterally through a midline incision. The placement of pedicle screws is performed using radiological guidance, either with plain x-rays or with an image intensifier. The pedicles are localized at the junction of transverse processes and the facet joints. The starting hole, as advocated by Roy-Camille et al,[88] is found at the intersection of a

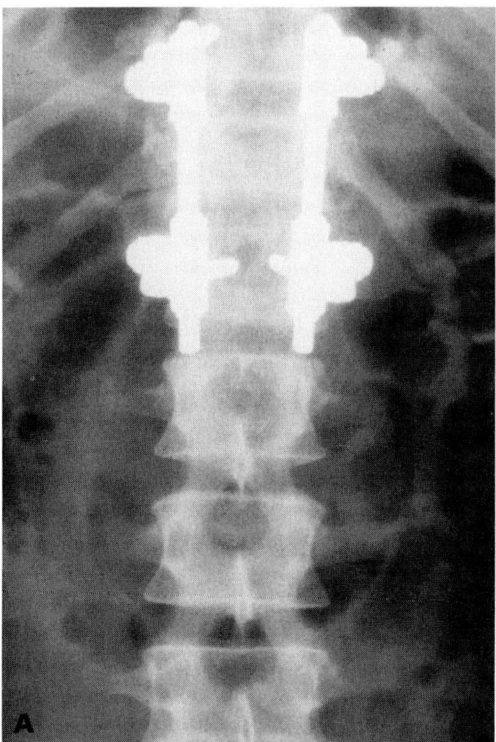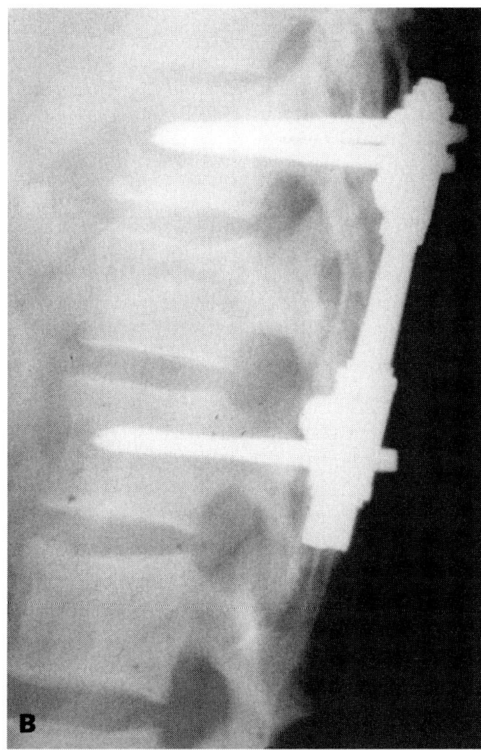

Figure 7: Anteroposterior **(A)** and lateral **(B)** thoracolumbar spine radiographs showing the use of an "internal spinal fixator" for reduction of a T12 flexion-compression fracture.

line drawn transversely through the midportion of the transverse process and vertically through the facet joints. The entry hole is placed 1 to 2 mm laterally to this point, which places the screw in the axis of the pedicle (Figure 8A). The relative orientation of the screws in a rostral-caudal direction changes depending on the level of the lumbar spine and can be estimated from plain films (Figure 8B). An awl or high-speed burr is used to start the screw holes, entering through the dorsal cortical bone. A slowly rotating power drill can be used to feel the cancellous bone of the pedicle. A pedicle probe is then used to check the integrity of the pedicle walls and to verify overall pedicle integrity. The holes are then tapped and the screws are inserted while the position of the screws is confirmed using imaging studies.[96]

The screw design, the connecting construct (plates vs. rods), and the assembly vary depending on the system used.[6,8,9,17,19,66,71,88,89,91,94,105] In selected cases, the segmental pedicle fixation system employing the "internal spinal fixator" has proved to be useful in indirect decompression of the spinal canal by ligamentotaxis[6,25,26,71] (Figure 7).

Ventral Techniques

Ventral decompression is frequently indicated in patients with incomplete neurological injury following thoracolumbar trauma.[52] The indications for ventral implants are not yet established, but these implants may be advantageous in allowing single-stage decompression, stabilization, and short-segment fusion of spinal injuries. Either compressive or distractive forces may be applied across an injured segment using rod-screw systems.

Several types of ventral implants have been designed during the last 35 years. Zielke instrumentation was initially used for ventral fixation but was found to be biomechanically unsuitable for fracture management.[42] Ventral fixation with AO plates was believed to be associated with a high nonunion rate.[100] This was also found to be true for Dunn instrumentation, which was with-

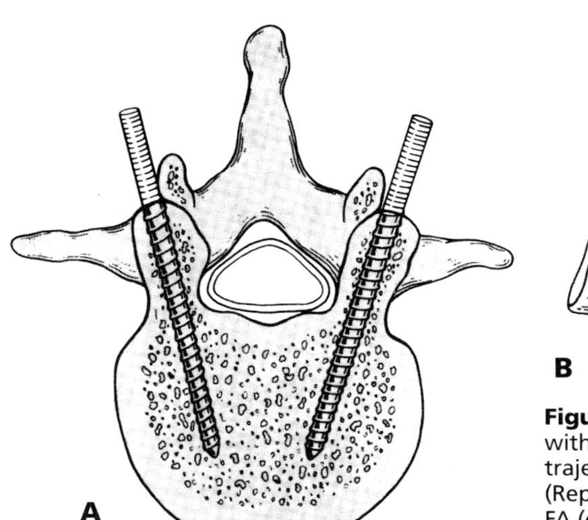

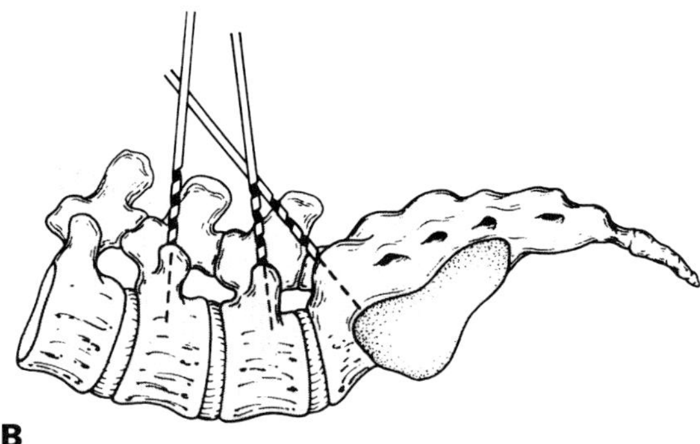

Figure 8: Line drawings showing the position of screws within pedicles and the vertebral body **(A)** and variable trajectory of the screws depending upon the level **(B).** (Reproduced with permission from Rothman RH, Simeone FA (eds): *The Spine.* Philadelphia, Pa: WB Saunders, 1992)

drawn from the market due to the potential risk of vascular injury.[29,64] Rod-screw devices, such as the Kostuik-Harrington[59,68-70] and Kaneda[60] implants, are advantageous in allowing either compression or distraction across the injured segment; however, because of their bulk, they are difficult to cover with soft tissue, causing concerns for potential vascular injury. Because of this, the use of various low-profile plates has been suggested in place of rod-screw implants. The Syracuse I-plate, the Armstrong plate, and recently available ventral plates such as the University plate and the Z-plate are low-profile constructs that are nearly as rigid as the Kaneda system, but they vary in their ability to employ reduction forces across the injured segment.

Kostuik-Harrington Ventral Distraction System

The only requirement for this system is standard Harrington distraction instrumentation. A crimper is needed if heavy compression rods are to be used in conjunction with distraction.[59,69,70] Following decompression, the distraction system requires the placement of two vertebral screws, one above and one below the level of fracture. Screw holes are begun using an awl at the vertebral midbody or slightly ventrally. Both cortices must be penetrated, as these are bicortical fixation screws. In addition, staples should be used where possible. The screw length is deter-

mined using a depth gauge. The distraction rod is inserted first rostrally, then caudally until the nipple is advanced into the screw head. Distraction is obtained while maintaining manual pressure dorsally. After a satisfactory amount of distraction has been achieved, a bone graft is placed. A heavy second compression rod is then added and the screw heads are slightly crimped.

Kaneda Ventral Spinal Instrumentation

The components of the Kaneda ventral spinal device (Figure 9) include the vertebral plate, vertebral screw, paravertebral rod and nut, and transverse fixator. Tetra-spikes on the vertebral plate are anchored to the lateral vertebral body. The vertebral screws are tapered and self-tapping, and they require bicortical purchase for fixation. The ventral and dorsal paravertebral rods connect the vertebral screws above and below and are coupled with the transverse fixators. The nuts on the rod are capable of applying both compressive and distractive force. Biomechanically, the transverse fixators are important for the elimination of rotatory and flexion-extension instability.[60]

The Syracuse Ventral I-Plate

The Syracuse ventral I-plate[103] is an I-shaped vertebral plate with four holes, two located ventrally and two dorsally. The plate is angled so

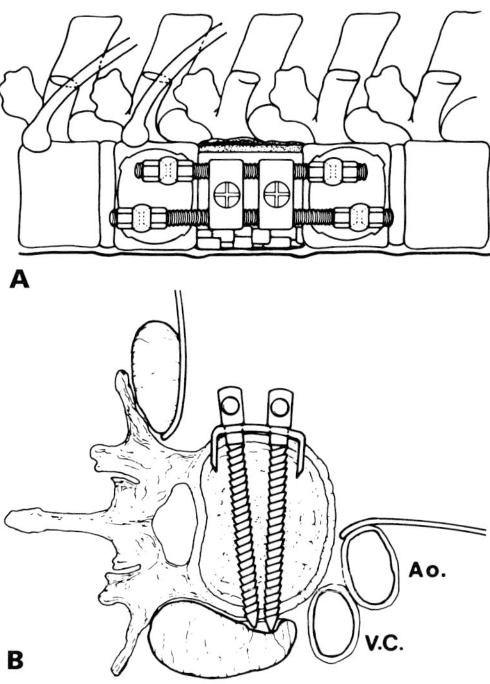

Figure 9: A) Axial view of the vertebral body with bicortical screws through a vertebral plate (Kaneda device). **B)** Sagittal view of the final Kaneda construct across the injured segment. (Reproduced with permission from An HS, Cotler JM (eds): *Spinal Instrumentation.* Baltimore, Md: Williams & Wilkins, 1992)

that there is 60° of curvature between the ventral and dorsal holes. It is applied with one pair (ventral and dorsal) of screws inserted into each intact vertebral body above and below the involved vertebra. Plates come in three sizes and the screw length is variable. The I-plate functions as a neutralization plate after compression has been applied across the bone graft. The screws require bicortical purchase for fixation. After ventral decompression, a large spreader clamp is used between the vertebrae above and below the level of injury for distraction in order to restore the spinal alignment and achieve placement of the bone graft. Once alignment of the vertebral column has been established, the distance between the midpoints of the vertebral bodies is measured and the appropriate plate length chosen. The I-plate is placed as dorsolaterally as possible on the vertebrae, and the dorsal holes are drilled with a drill bit. The holes are not tapped. The depth is measured to the oppo-

site cortex, and a screw of the appropriate length is tightened in the two dorsal holes. Both ventral holes are then drilled and measured, and the screws are placed. The shape of the plate causes each ventral and dorsal pair of screws to converge, providing good translational and rotational stiffness.

Many of the more recently developed low-profile ventral fixation devices share the design and application features of the Syracuse I-plate. In a few, such as the Synthes thoracolumbar locking plates/screws (Figure 3), the screws are able to lock to the plate to prevent screw back-out, and they require only unicortical vertebral body fixation, which avoids the potential penetration of the opposing cortex and consequent vascular injury. Most recently, the Z-plate[104] (Figure 10) and the University plate have been introduced for ventral thoracolumbar spinal fixation. These two plate designs not only allow the application of compressive and/or distractive forces across the vertebrectomy defect but have the torsional stiffness of a plate-based construct. In addition, these devices have a lower profile than the Kaneda device, but their vertebral body screws cannot be locked to the plate to prevent screw back-out, as can be done with the AO plate. The Z-plate has been used successfully in the treatment of thoracolumbar burst fractures[45] (Figure 11). Biomechanical testing of ventral thoracolumbar constructs has revealed comparable stiffness in most planes except for minor differences in the fatigue life of certain designs.[2,24] In the clinical setting, almost all of the ventral thoracolumbar devices provide satisfactory support to withstand the usual physiological loads.

CONCLUSION

Modern management of thoracolumbar fractures should include early mobilization and ambulation, reduction of acute deformity, restoration of spinal canal dimensions (especially in neurologically injured patients), and long-term stabilization to prevent late-onset deformity, pain, or neurological deficits. All of these should be accomplished while sacrificing as few motion segments as possible and without causing iatrogenic neurological injury. To achieve these goals, the surgeons dealing with these injuries should

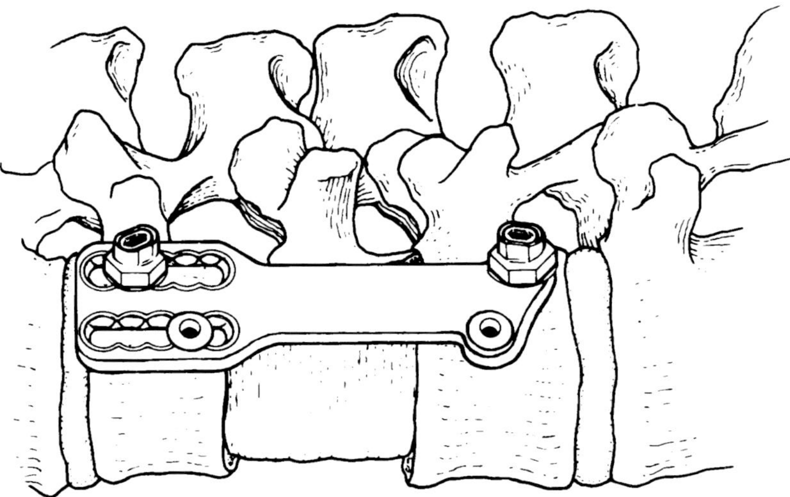

Figure 10: The Z-plate device. (Reproduced with permission from Zdeblick TA: Z-plate anterior thoracolumbar instrumentation, in Fessler RG, Haid RW (eds): *Current Techniques in Spinal Stabilization.* New York: McGraw-Hill, 1996, pp 211-224)

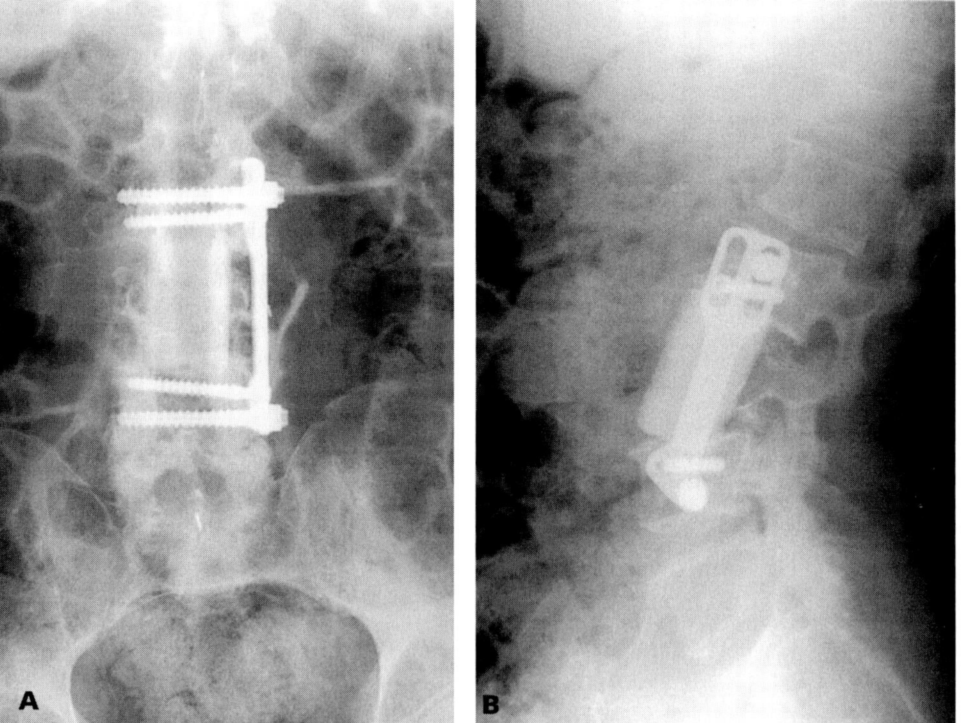

Figure 11: Anteroposterior **(A)** and lateral **(B)** radiographs of a patient with a traumatic spinal injury who underwent an L3 vertebrectomy, reconstruction with a femoral allograft, and ventral lumbar fixation with the Z-plate. The design of the plate, which allows both distraction and compression of the involved segments, is clearly seen in addition to the bicortical screw fixation.

be familiar with the various approaches to the spine, the methods of decompression, and both ventral and dorsal instrumentation techniques. Only then can one select the optimum treatment option for a patient and provide the best chance for recovery.

REFERENCES

1. Akbarnia BA, Fogarty JP, Smith KR Jr: New trends in surgical stabilization of thoracolumbar spinal fractures with emphasis for sublaminar wiring. **Paraplegia 23:**27-33, 1985

2. An HS, Lim TH, You JW, et al: Biomechanical evaluation of anterior thoracolumbar spinal instrumentation. **Spine 20:**1979-1983, 1995

3. Bauer RD, Errico TJ: Thoracolumbar spine injuries, in Errico TJ, Bauer RD, Waugh T (eds): **Spinal Trauma.** Philadelphia, Pa: JB Lippincott, 1991, 195-269

4. Bedbrook GM: Spinal injuries with tetraplegia and paraplegia. **J Bone Joint Surg (Br) 61:**267-284, 1979

5. Bedbrook GM: Treatment of thoracolumbar dislocations and fractures with paraplegia. **Clin Orthop 112:**27-43, 1975

6. Bednar DA: Experience with the "fixateur interne:" initial clinical results. **J Spinal Disord 5:**93-96, 1992

7. Beerman R, Batt HD, Green BA: Lumbar vertebral reformation after traumatic compression fracture. **AJNR 6:**455-456, 1985

8. Benli IT, Tandogan NR, Kis M, et al: Cotrel-Dubousset instrumentation in the treatment of unstable thoracic and lumbar spine fractures. **Arch Orthop Trauma Surg 113:**86-92, 1994

9. Benson DR, Burkus JK, Montesano PX, et al: Unstable thoracolumbar and lumbar burst fractures treated with the AO fixateur interne. **J Spinal Disord 5:**335-343, 1992

10. Benzel EC: Short-segment compression instrumentation for selected thoracic and lumbar spine fractures: the short-rod/two-claw technique. **J Neurosurg 79:**335-340, 1993

11. Benzel EC, Kesterson L, Marchand EP: Texas Scottish Rite Hospital rod instrumentation for thoracic and lumbar spine trauma. **J Neurosurg 75:**382-387, 1991

12. Black RC, Eng P, Gardner VO, et al: A contoured anterior spinal fixation plate. **Clin Orthop 227:**135-142, 1988

13. Bradford DS, Akbarnia BA, Winter RB, et al: Surgical stabilization fracture and fracture dislocations of the thoracic spine. **Spine 2:**185-196, 1977

14. Bradford DS, McBride G: Surgical management of thoracolumbar spine fractures with incomplete neurologic deficits. **Clin Orthop 218:**201-216, 1987

15. Bradford DS, McBride G: Thoracic/lumbar spine fractures with incomplete neurologic deficit: a correlative study on the adequacy of decompression vs. neurologic return. **Orthopaed Trans 8:**159-160, 1984

16. Cantor JB, Lebwohl NH, Garvey T, et al: Nonoperative management of stable thoracolumbar burst fractures with early ambulation and bracing. **Spine 18:**971-976, 1993

17. Carl AL, Tromanhauser SG, Roger DJ: Pedicle screw instrumentation for thoracolumbar burst fractures and fracture-dislocations. **Spine 17 (Suppl 8):** S317-S324, 1992

18. Chance CQ: Note on a type of flexion fracture of the spine. **Br J Radiol 21:**452-453, 1948

19. Cigliano A, de Falco R, Scarano E, et al: A new instrumentation system for the reduction and posterior stabilization of unstable thoracolumbar fractures. **Neurosurgery 30:**208-216, 1992

20. Cook WA: Transthoracic vertebral surgery. **Ann Thorac Surg 12:**54-68, 1971

21. Cotler JM, Vernace JV, Michalski JA: The use of Harrington rods in thoracolumbar fractures. **Orthop Clin North Am 17:**87-103, 1986

22. Denis F: Spinal instability as defined by the three-column spine concept in acute spinal trauma. **Clin Orthop 189:**65-76, 1984

23. Denis F: The three column spine and its significance in the classification of acute thoracolumbar spinal injuries. **Spine 8:**817-831, 1983

24. Dick JC, Brodke DS, Zdeblick TA, et al: Anterior instrumentation of the thoracolumbar spine. A biomechanical comparison. **Spine 22:**744-750, 1997

25. Dick W: The 'fixateur interne" as a versatile implant for spine surgery. **Spine 12:**882-900, 1987

26. Dick W, Kluger P, Magerl F, et al: A new device for internal fixation of thoracolumbar and lumbar spine fractures: the "fixateur interne." **Paraplegia 23:** 225-232, 1985

27. Dickson JH, Harrington PR, Erwin WD: Harrington instrumentation in the fractured, unstable thoracic and lumbar spine. **Tex Med 69:**91-98, 1973

28. Dickson JH, Harrington PR, Erwin WD: Results of reduction and stabilization of the severely fractured thoracic and lumbar spine. **J Bone Joint Surg (Am) 60:**799-805, 1978

29. Dunn HK: Anterior spine stabilization and decompression for thoracolumbar injuries. **Orthop Clin North Am 17:**113-119, 1986

30. Dunn HK: Neurologic recovery following anterior spinal canal decompression in thoracic and lumbar injuries. **Orthopaed Trans 8:**160, 1984

31. Durward QJ, Schweigel JF, Harrison P: Management of fractures of the thoracolumbar and lumbar spine. **Neurosurgery 8:**555-561, 1981

32. Edwards CC: Thoracolumbar trauma: posterior reduction and fixation with the modular spinal system. **Semin Spine Surg 2:**8-18, 1990

33. Edwards CC, Levine AM: Early rod-sleeve stabilization of the injured thoracic and lumbar spine. **Orthop Clin North Am 17:**121-145, 1986

34. Engler GL: Cotrel-Dubousset instrumentation for reduction of fracture dislocations of the spine. **J Spinal Disord 3:**62-66, 1990

35. Erickson DL, Leider LL, Brown WE: One-stage decompression: stabilization for thoracolumbar fractures. **Spine 2:**53-56, 1977

36. Farcy JP, Wiedenbaum M, Michelson CB, et al: A comparative biomechanical study of spinal fixation using Cotrel-Dubousset instrumentation. **Spine 12:** 877-881, 1987

37. Ferguson RL, Allen BL Jr: A mechanistic classification of thoracolumbar spine fractures. **Clin Orthop 189:** 77-88, 1984

38. Flesch JR, Leider LL, Erickson DL, et al: Harrington

instrumentation and spine fusion for unstable fractures and fracture dislocations of the thoracic and lumbar spine. **J Bone Joint Surg (Am) 59**:143-153, 1977

39. Fountain SS: A single-stage combined surgical approach for vertebral resections. **J Bone Joint Surg (Am) 61**:1011-1017, 1979

40. Gaines RW, Humphreys WG: A plea for judgment in management of thoracolumbar fractures and fracture-dislocations. A reassessment of surgical indications. **Clin Orthop 189**:36-42, 1984

41. Garfin SR, Mowery CA, Guerra J Jr, et al: Confirmation of the posterolateral technique to decompress and fuse thoracolumbar spine burst fractures. **Spine 10**:218-223, 1985

42. Gelderman PW: The operative stabilization and grafting of thoracic and lumbar spinal fractures. **Surg Neurol 23**:101-120, 1985

43. Gertzbein SD, Court-Brown CM: Flexion-distraction injuries of the lumbar spine. Mechanism of injury and classification. **Clin Orthop 227**:52-60, 1988

44. Gertzbein SD, Court-Brown CM, Marks P, et al: The neurologic outcome following surgery for spinal fractures. **Spine 13**:641-644, 1988

45. Ghanayem AJ, Zdeblick TA: Anterior instrumentation in the management of thoracolumbar burst fractures. **Clin Orthop 335**:89-100, 1997

46. Golimbu C, Firooznia H, Raffi M, et al: Computed tomography of thoracic and lumbar spine fractures that have been treated with Harrington instrumentation. **Radiology 151**:731-733, 1984

47. Gumley G, Taylor TKF, Ryan MD: Distraction fractures of the lumbar spine. **J Bone Joint Surg (Br) 64**: 520-525, 1982

48. Guttmann L: Spinal deformities in traumatic paraplegics and tetraplegics following surgical procedures. **Paraplegia 7**:38-58, 1969

49. Haas N, Blauth M, Tscherne H: Anterior plating in thoracolumbar spine injuries. Indication, technique, and results. **Spine 16 (Suppl 3)**:S100-S111, 1991

50. Hannon KM: Harrington instrumentation in fractures and dislocations of the thoracic and lumbar spine. **South Med J 69**:1269-1273, 1976

51. Hardaker WT Jr, Cook WA Jr, Friedman AH, et al: Bilateral transpedicular decompression and Harrington rod stabilization in the management of severe thoracolumbar burst fractures. **Spine 17**:162-171, 1992

52. Harris MB: The role of anterior stabilization with instrumentation in the treatment of thoracolumbar burst fractures. **Orthopedics 15**:347-350, 1992

53. Hazel WA, Jones RA, Morrey BF, et al: Vertebral fractures without neurological deficit. A long-term follow-up study. **J Bone Joint Surg (Am) 70**:1319-1321, 1988

54. Holdsworth F: Fractures, dislocations and fracture dislocations of the spine. **J Bone Joint Surg (Am) 52**: 1534-1551, 1970

55. Holdsworth FW, Hardy A: Early treatment of paraplegia from fractures of thoracolumbar spine. **J Bone Joint Surg (Br) 35**:540-550, 1953

56. Jacobs PR, Casey MP: Surgical management of thoracolumbar spinal injuries. General principles and controversial considerations. **Clin Orthop 189**:22-35, 1984

57. Jacobs RR, Asher MA, Snider RK: Thoracolumbar spinal injuries. A comparative study of recumbent and operative treatment in 100 patients. **Spine 5**: 463-477, 1980

58. Jeanneret B, Ho PK, Magerl F: Burst-shear flexion-distraction injuries of the lumbar spine. **J Spinal Disord 6**:473-481, 1993

59. Johnson JR, Leatherman KD, Holt RT: Anterior decompression of the spinal cord for neurological deficit. **Spine 8**:396-405, 1983

60. Kaneda K, Abumi K, Fujiya N: Burst fractures with neurologic deficits of the thoracolumbar-lumbar spine. Results of anterior decompression and stabilization with anterior instrumentation. **Spine 9**: 788-795, 1984

61. Kaufer H, Hayes JT: Lumbar fracture-dislocation. A study of twenty-one cases. **J Bone Joint Surg (Am) 48**:712-730, 1966

62. Keene JS: Thoracolumbar fractures in winter sports. **Clin Orthop 216**:39-49, 1987

63. Kelly RP, Whitesides TE Jr: Treatment of lumbodorsal fracture-dislocations. **Ann Surg 167**:705-717, 1968

64. King AG: Burst compression fractures of the thoracolumbar spine. Pathologic anatomy and surgical management. **Orthopedics 10**:1711-1719, 1987

65. King AG: Spinal column trauma, in Anderson LD (ed): **Instructional Course Lectures. Vol 35**. St Louis, Mo: CV Mosby, 1986, pp 40-51

66. Kinnard P, Ghibely A, Gordon D, et al: Roy-Camille plates in unstable spinal conditions: a preliminary report. **Spine 11**:131, 1986

67. Kinoshita H, Nagata Y, Ueda H, et al: Conservative treatment of burst fractures of the thoracolumbar and lumbar spine. **Paraplegia 31**:58-67, 1993

68. Kostuik JP: Anterior fixation for burst fractures of the thoracic and lumbar spine with or without neurological involvement. **Spine 13**:286-293, 1988

69. Kostuik JP: Anterior fixation for fractures of the thoracic and lumbar spine with or without neurologic involvement. **Clin Orthop 189**:103-115, 1984

70. Kostuik JP: Anterior spinal cord decompression for lesions of the thoracic and lumbar spine, techniques, new methods of internal fixation results. **Spine 8**: 512-531, 1983

71. Kuner HE, Kuner A, Schlickewei W, et al: Ligamentotaxis with an internal spinal fixator for thoracolumbar fractures. **J Bone Joint Surg (B) 76**:107-112, 1994

72. Larson SJ, Holst RA, Hemmy DC, et al: Lateral extracavitary approach to traumatic lesions of the thoracic and lumbar spine. **J Neurosurg 45**:628-637, 1976

73. Levine A, Bosse M, Edwards CC: Bilateral facet dislocations in the thoracolumbar spine. **Spine 13**:630-640, 1988

74. Levine A, Edwards CC: Lumbar spine trauma, in Camins M, O'Leary P (eds): **The Lumbar Spine**. New York, NY: Raven Press, 1987, pp 183-212

75. Lewis J, McKibbin B: The treatment of unstable fracture-dislocations of the thoracolumbar spine accompanied by paraplegia. **J Bone Joint Surg (Br) 56**: 603-612, 1974

76. Louw JA: Unstable fractures of the thoracic and lumbar spine treated with Harrington distraction instrumentation and sublaminar wires. **S Afr Med J 71**: 759-762, 1987

77. Maiman DJ, Larson SJ, Benzel EC: Neurological improvement associated with late decompression of the thoracolumbar spinal cord. **Neurosurgery 14**:

302-307, 1984

78. McAfee PC, Bohlman HH: Complications following Harrington instrumentation for fractures of the thoracolumbar spine. **J Bone Joint Surg (Am) 67:** 672-686, 1985

79. McAfee PC, Bohlman HH, Yuan HA: Anterior decompression of traumatic thoracolumbar fractures with incomplete neurological deficit using a retroperitoneal approach. **J Bone Joint Surg (Am) 67:** 89-104, 1985

80. McAfee PC, Werner FW, Glisson RR: A biomechanical analysis of spinal instrumentation systems in thoracolumbar fractures. Comparison of traditional Harrington distraction instrumentation with segmental spinal instrumentation. **Spine 10:**204-217, 1985

81. McAfee PC, Yuan HA, Fredrickson BE, et al: The value of computed tomography in thoracolumbar fractures. An analysis of one hundred consecutive cases and a new classification. **J Bone Joint Surg (Am) 65:**461-473, 1983

82. McAfee PC, Yuan HA, Lasda NA: The unstable burst fracture. **Spine 7:**365-373, 1982

83. Moreland DB, Egnatchik JG, Bennett GJ: Cotrel-Dubousset instrumentation for the treatment of thoracolumbar fractures. **Neurosurgery 27:**69-73, 1990

84. Nicoll EA: Fractures of the dorso-lumbar spine. **J Bone Joint Surg (Br) 31:**376-394, 1949

85. O'Laoire SA, Thomas DGT: Surgery in incomplete spinal cord injury. **Surg Neurol 17:**12-15, 1982

86. Rimoldi RL, Zigler JE, Capen DA, et al: The effect of surgical intervention on rehabilitation time in patients with thoracolumbar and lumbar spinal cord injuries. **Spine 17:**1443-1449, 1992

87. Riska EB, Myllynen P, Böstman O: Anterolateral decompression for neural involvement in thoracolumbar fractures. A review of 78 cases. **J Bone Joint Surg (Br) 69:**704-708, 1987

88. Roy-Camille R, Saillant G, Berteaux D, et al: Osteosynthesis of thoracolumbar spine fractures with metal plates screwed through vertebral pedicles. **Reconstr Surg Traumatol 15:**2-16, 1976

89. Roy-Camille R, Saillant G, Mazel C: Internal fixation of the lumbar spine with pedicle screw plating. **Clin Orthop 203:**7-17, 1986

90. Roy-Camille R, Saillant G, Mazel C: Plating of thoracic, thoracolumbar and lumbar injuries with pedicle screw plates. **Orthop Clin North Am 17:**147-159, 1986

91. Simpson JM, Ebraheim NA, Jackson WT, et al: Internal fixation of the thoracic and lumbar spine using Roy-Camille plates. **Orthopedics 16:**663-672, 1993

92. Sullivan JA: Sublaminar wiring of Harrington distraction rods for unstable thoracolumbar spine fractures. **Clin Orthop 189:**178-185, 1984

93. Svensson O, Aaro S, Öhlén G: Harrington instrumentation for thoracic and lumbar vertebral fractures. **Acta Orthop Scand 55:**38-47, 1984

94. Viale GL, Silvestro C, Francaviglia N, et al: Transpedicular decompression and stabilization of burst fractures of the lumbar spine. **Surg Neurol 40:**104-111, 1993

95. Weber SC, Sutherland GH: An unusual rotational fracture-dislocation of the thoracic spine without neurologic sequelae internally fixed with a combined anterior and posterior approach. **J Trauma 26:** 474-479, 1986

96. Weinstein JN, Rydevik BL, Rauschning W: Anatomic and technical considerations of pedicle screw fixation. **Clin Orthop 284:**34-46, 1992

97. Weitzman G: Treatment of stable thoracolumbar spine compression fractures by early ambulation. **Clin Orthop 76:**116-122, 1971

98. Whitesides TE, Shah SGA: On the management of unstable fractures of the thoracolumbar spine: rationale for the use of anterior decompression and fusion and posterior stabilization. **Spine 1:**99-107, 1976

99. Willén JA: Unstable thoracolumbar injuries. **Orthopedics 15:**329-335, 1992

100. Willén JA, Gaekwad UH, Kakulas BA: Acute burst fractures. A comparative analysis of a modern fracture classification and pathologic findings. **Clin Orthop 276:**169-175, 1992

101. Yosipovitch Z. Robin GC, Makin M: Open reduction of unstable thoracolumbar spinal injuries and fixation with Harrington rods. **J Bone Joint Surg (Am) 59:**1003-1015, 1977

102. Young B, Brooks WH, Tibbs PA: Anterior decompression and fusion for thoracolumbar fractures with neurological deficits. **Acta Neurochir 57:**287-298, 1981

103. Yuan HA, Mann KA, Found EM, et al: Early clinical experience with the Syracuse I-plate: an anterior spinal fixation device. **Spine 13:**278-285, 1988

104. Zdeblick TA: Z-plate anterior thoracolumbar instrumentation, in Fessler RG, Haid RW (eds): **Current Techniques in Spinal Stabilization.** New York, NY: McGraw-Hill, 1996, pp 211-224

105. Zindrick MR, Lorenz MA: The use of intrapedicular fixation systems in the treatment of thoracolumbar and lumbosacral fractures. **Orthopedics 15:**337-341, 1992

106. Zou D, Yoo JU, Edwards WT, et al: Mechanics of anatomic reduction of thoracolumbar burst fractures. Comparison of distraction versus distraction plus lordosis in the anatomic reduction of the thoracolumbar burst fracture. **Spine 18:**195-203, 1993

CHAPTER 15

SURGICAL TECHNIQUES: LUMBOSACRAL AND SACROPELVIC FIXATION

NEVAN G. BALDWIN, MD, AND CATHLEEN S. VAN BUSKIRK, MD

Achieving rigid sacral fixation is, in many cases, a crucial factor in improving fusion rates at the lumbosacral junction.[21,28] Fusion procedures in this region are frequently required for the treatment of traumatic spinal injury at, or caudal to, the third lumbar vertebra. Other conditions that may lead to a need for lumbosacral stabilization include degenerative disease, tumor, congenital deformity such as scoliosis, or acquired deformity such as spondylolisthesis.

In most instances, fixation to the sacrum is adequate for immobilizing the lumbosacral junction. However, additional security of fixation may be required in a number of situations. If sacral integrity is lost (e.g., in tumor resection) or if bone quality is inadequate for the implants to maintain sufficient hold using the sacrum alone, then instrumentation across the sacroiliac joint may be necessary to rigidly immobilize the lumbosacral junction. In constructs with a very long moment arm, such as a multilevel scoliosis correction procedure, fixation across the sacroiliac joint is also a common consideration.

To surgically secure the sacrum in a rigid manner can be difficult, due mainly to its anatomical features and location. The sacral pedicles are broad and provide less of a cylinder-like configuration of cortical bone for screw purchase than lower lumbar pedicles (Figure 1). The bone of the dorsal sacrum is often thin and may provide an inadequate bone-metal interface for sublaminar wires or laminar hooks. Specialized techniques for sacral fixation are occasionally required to overcome these limitations. Finally, the anatomy of the sacrum, with large vessels and neural structures in immediate juxtaposition, affords substantial risk for surgical misadventure if caution is not exercised with procedures in this region.

To address the aforementioned issues, this chapter presents an overview of lumbosacral and sacropelvic fixation including relevant surgical anatomy, biomechanics, indications, techniques, and complications.

ANATOMIC AND BIOMECHANICAL CONSIDERATIONS

In the region of the lumbosacral junction, a number of important anatomical relationships exist with respect to spinal anatomy and that of the surrounding structures. The sacrum consists of five fused vertebrae whose transverse processes

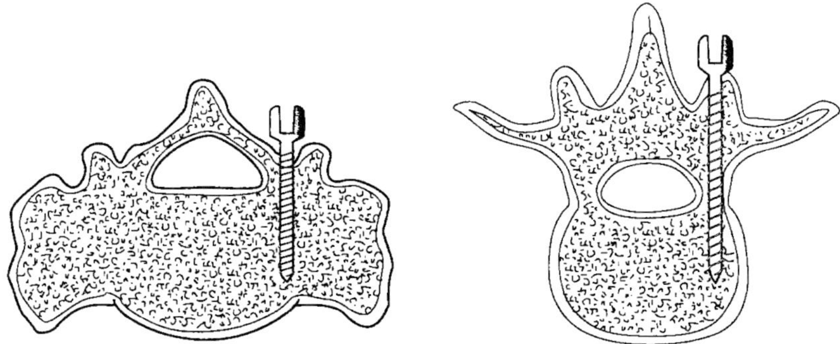

Figure 1: *Left:* A cross section of the sacrum demonstrating the broad channel of cancellous bone into which bone screws are placed. Although the medial aspect of the S1 pedicle looks similar to those of the lumbar pedicles, the sacral pedicle has no distinct lateral margin. *Right:* A cross section of the lumbar vertebra demonstrating the cylindrical nature of the pedicles.

do not exist as such, but instead are fused into large lateral masses forming the sacral ala. At the lateral margins, the alar surfaces contain smooth and irregular-shaped contours that interdigitate with the medial surface of the iliac bone on each side to form the sacroiliac joint. The matching contours of the sacrum and ilium create an interlocking mechanism that serves to stabilize the sacroiliac joint. Due to its triangular shape (in the coronal plane), the sacrum is essentially wedged between the iliac bones. This helps to stabilize the sacroiliac joint as well as transfer loads placed upon the spine.

The sacroiliac joint acts primarily as a shock absorber for the axial column. It is predominantly a fibrocartilaginous joint without a synovial lining or a true joint capsule (amphiarthrodial portion). In its ventral aspect, there is a small area lined by synovium (diarthrodial portion). The primary stabilizer of the joint is the interosseous sacroiliac ligament that bridges the two bones along their dorsal surface and forms a capsule-like array over the surface of the sacroiliac joint (Figure 2). In a normal anatomic configuration, the sacrum is tilted ventrally and is loaded ventral to the sacroiliac joint (Figure 3). This results in a tendency toward ventral rotation of the sacrum. The sacroiliac joint is centered around the area of the S2 vertebra; therefore, the S2 level represents the location of the axis for this rotational tendency.

The sacrum is stabilized and rotation prevented by the ligamentous attachments. The sacrotuberous and sacrospinous ligaments attach to the caudal end of the sacrum. The interosseous and dorsal sacroiliac ligaments (the strongest lig-

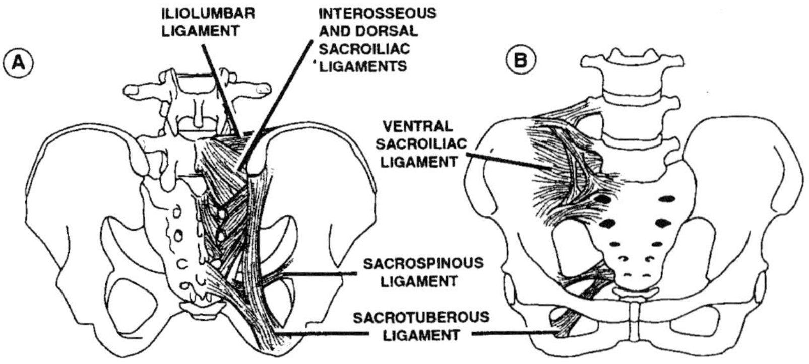

Figure 2: The primary stabilizer of the sacroiliac joint is the ligamentous complex along the dorsal surface of the joint **(A).** There is also a significant ligamentous array along the ventral surface **(B).** The ligaments of the sacropelvic region provide enormous load-bearing capacity and shock absorption to protect the lumbar spine from injury.

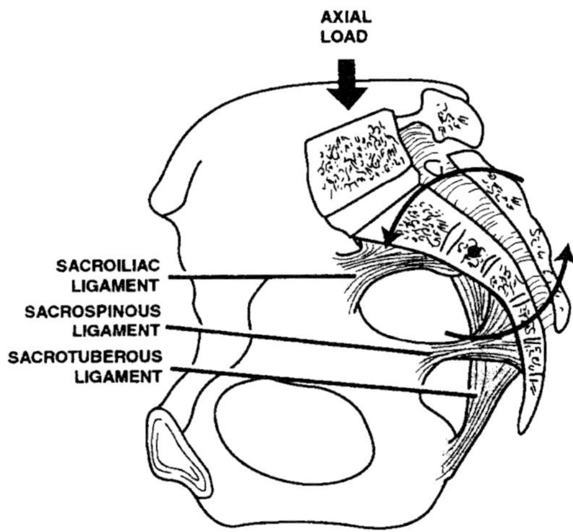

Figure 3: The normal anatomic position of the sacroiliac joint is dorsal to the axial load applied via the lumbar spine. This results in a rotational force at the sacrum *(circular arrows)*. The axis of the rotational force is located at the center of the sacroiliac joint (the S2 vertebra). The various ligaments depicted, as well as the ligaments of the dorsal sacral surface, serve to prevent rotation from actually occurring.

aments of the pelvis) bind the rostral sacrum to the rostral aspect of the ilium dorsally (Figure 3).

The motion of the sacroiliac joint and its relationship to hip and lumbar spine function is poorly understood. Classical studies of sacroiliac motion in cadavers have suggested that little or no motion existed in the joint. Brooke[7] found that no motion was present in 75% of adults aged 50 years or older. In a study by White et al,[40] 1 mm of motion was present in the pediatric population and no appreciable movement was observed in adults. In a recent and more sophisticated study by Smidt et al,[36] digitized computed tomography (CT) data were used to evaluate sacroiliac motion, with the hips forced to the extremes of their range of motion. They found significant sacroiliac motion (average 7-8 degrees rotation in the sagittal plane) in fresh adult cadavers and postulated that this motion was sufficient to influence motion at the lumbosacral junction.

Although recent evidence demonstrated that the sacroiliac joint is a mobile structure, clinical experience has shown that it can be compromised with instrumentation when necessary. Kostuik et al[22] observed no substantial increase

in morbidity with instrumentation constructs that crossed the sacroiliac joint, either immediately following surgery or in long-term follow-up. Therefore, when additional security of fixation is needed, crossing the sacroiliac joint is both justified and prudent.

The anatomy of the sacral spinal canal differs somewhat from that of the other spinal regions. In most individuals, the dorsal and ventral branches of the sacral nerves exit the spinal canal through four sets of paired dorsal and ventral foramina. The canal contains the thecal sac and the terminal portions of the cauda equina. The subarachnoid and subdural spaces usually terminate at the caudal margin of the second sacral vertebral body. In that region, the dural sheath narrows to invest the filum terminale. The filum terminale internum is the continuation of the pia mater, extending from the conus medullaris to the termination of the subarachnoid space. The filum terminale externum fuses with the investing dural layers and extends throughout the remainder of the sacral canal to attach at the dorsal surface of the upper portion of the coccyx.

Vascular and visceral anatomic relationships in the sacropelvic region are relatively consistent. Usually only minor variations are observed. The common and internal iliac veins lie lateral and dorsal to their corresponding iliac arteries. The common iliac veins converge on the right side of the fifth lumbar vertebra to form the inferior vena cava. The internal iliac veins lie directly ventral to the sacral ala and medial to the sacroiliac joint. The internal iliac arteries do not contact the bony sacrum due to their position anterior and medial to the iliac veins. The lumbosacral trunk, formed by the exiting anterior branches of L4 and L5 and then joined by the sacral nerves, is situated on the anterior surface of the sacral ala lateral to the internal iliac vein and medial to the sacroiliac joint. The third sacral vertebra is the landmark for the rectosigmoid junction. The sigmoid colon is quite mobile at the upper sacrum. However, at approximately S3, it comes into contact with the ventral sacral surface and loses its mesentery, thereby becoming less mobile (Figure 4).

The lumbosacral junction (L5-S1 level) represents a unique spinal segment with respect to its range of motion, ligamentous attachments, and load-bearing characteristics.[16] It has the

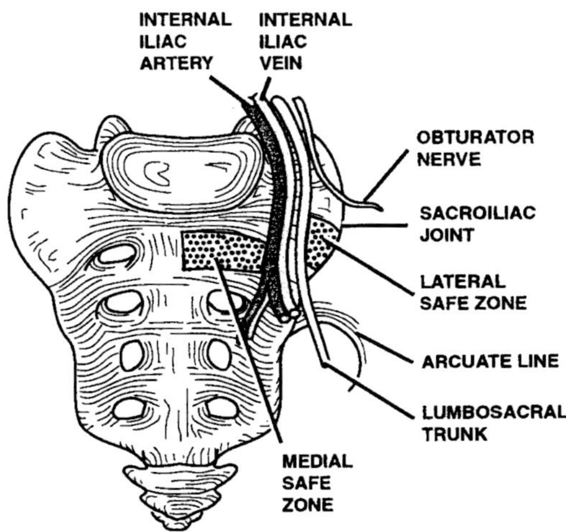

Figure 4: The anatomical position of the vital structures ventral to the sacrum creates a danger zone for screw placement. By directing dorsally placed screws either medially (the medial safe zone) or laterally (the lateral safe zone), vital structures can be avoided.

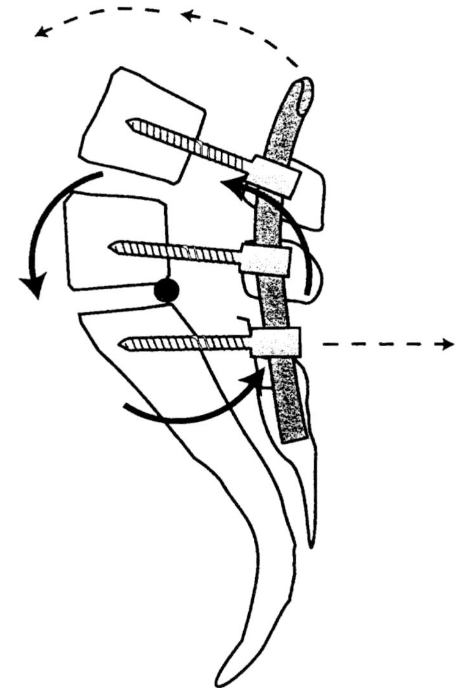

Figure 5: During flexion, there is a tendency for motion to occur at the lumbosacral junction. The axis of rotation for this motion is shown by the *black dot*. The use of long constructs creates a tendency for sacral screws to dislodge due to the cantilever effect created by flexion forces.

largest amount of flexion/extension motion in the lumbar region (averaging approximately 17 degrees) while also having the most restricted ranges of lateral bending (approximately 3 degrees) and axial rotation (approximately 1 degree).[41] Because of the summation effect of spinal loading, the lumbosacral junction is exposed to large applied force vectors. The lordotic curvature of the lumbar spine, the tilted orientation of the L5-S1 intervertebral disc, the relatively small size of the L5-S1 disc, and the position of the sacroiliac joint dorsal to the lumbosacral junction all play a role in the load-bearing mechanics of this spinal region.[12,13,16]

Instrumentation at the lumbosacral junction can include bone screws, hooks, or sublaminar cables, and interbody devices. These devices provide adequate bone-metal interface strength in most cases. The holding strength of bone screws at the sacrum is limited somewhat by the bony anatomy of the sacrum. The sacral pedicles are broader than the lumbar pedicles. Screw purchase in the sacral pedicle is therefore obtained largely in a broad channel of cancellous bone that extends laterally into the ala. The narrower lumbar pedicle, with its cylindrical shape, provides greater resistance to pullout. Bone screws in the

sacral pedicles are also subjected to dorsally directed pullout forces during flexion, which can lead to screw pullout (Figure 5).

The use of hooks in the sacrum is limited by the fact that the sacral laminae are often thin and do not provide an adequate bone-metal interface. Placing hooks in the more laterally located dorsal sacral neuroforamina often provides a thicker bony surface and results in a better bone-metal interface. The use of sublaminar wire in the sacrum has been reported to result in higher rates of nerve root injury than those observed with wires at other spinal levels, particularly in women. This problem has been minimized with the use of softer multistrand cables in the place of wire. Of note, wires provide less metal-bone contact. Cutting through the bone ("the cheese cutter effect") is occasionally observed.

Angling bone screws away (either medially or laterally) from the sagittal plane increases their pullout strength in bone (the "triangulation ef-

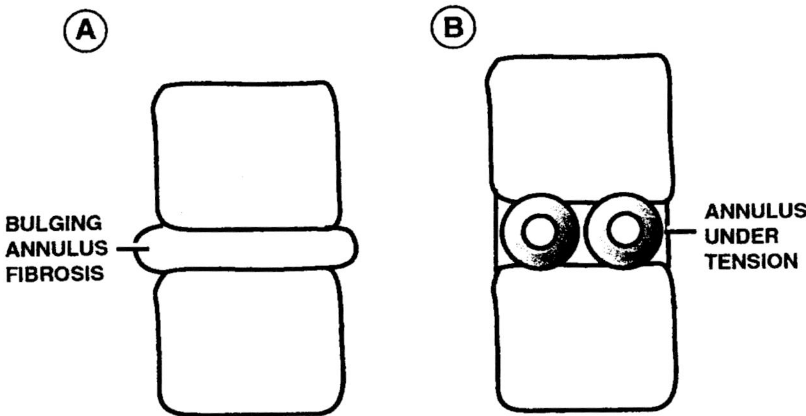

Figure 6: The degenerated disc **(A)** generally has a substantial loss of height and a resulting bulging of the fibers of the annulus fibrosis. The placement of intervertebral body cages **(B)** creates a distraction force between the vertebral bodies. The tension band created by the stretching of the annulus fibers stabilizes the spine.

fect").[37] Directing the screws medially lessens the risk of injury to vital anatomic structures.[31,37] If the longitudinal members (rods or plates) are then linked by crossmembers, a triangulation effect is created. This triangulation effect enhances both the rigidity of the construct and pullout strength.[9,35,37,43] Torsional stability is also enhanced by cross linkage of the longitudinal members.[3,10]

The optimal direction for sacral screw placement, whether medial or lateral, has not been proved. The efficacy of ventromedially placed screws has been tested against that of ventrolaterally placed screws. However, reports regarding which method is superior have been conflicting.[9,37,43] Although conclusions differ regarding the optimal direction for screw placement, there is agreement that directing screws away from the sagittal plane increases pullout resistance. The strength of sacral fixation is enhanced by the placement of additional screws. For example, the use of a screw in the S1 pedicle in combination with a laterally directed screw in the ala or by combining the construct with iliac fixation strengthens the construct.[25,28,30]

The clinical failure rate observed with constructs that include iliac fixation has been reported to be lower than that observed with sacral fixation alone.[8] McCord et al[30] studied mechanism of failure in S1 pedicle screws, S2 pedicle screws, and iliac screws bridging the sacroiliac joint and into the ilium. All constructs failed at the caudal bone-metal interface. In the devices that utilized iliac fixation, the ilium failed first, followed rapidly by the caudal sacral screws, suggesting that the major contribution to stability be from the ilium.

The use of interbody cages has recently gained significant popularity as a technique for lumbosacral stabilization. These devices function as an interbody distractor that pushes firmly against the vertebral bodies to provide tension in the annulus fibrosis and the longitudinal ligaments (Figure 6). It is the ligamentous and annulus tension that actually results in stabilization. The use of interbody cages therefore requires weight-bearing capability in the vertebral bodies and intact ligamentous structures to attain or maintain stability. In the treatment of patients with spine trauma, interbody cages play little role.

The intersection of the middle osteoligamentous column in the sagittal plane and the lumbosacral disc in the transverse plane has been termed the "lumbosacral pivot point." In practical terms, this location is simply the dorsal boundary of the L5-S1 intervertebral disc. It represents the approximate position of the axis of rotation of the L5-S1 motion segment during flexion and extension. Regarding the biomechanical testing of the resistance to flexion, constructs crossing the sacroiliac joint and utilizing the ilium as a fixation site were observed to significantly enhance the rigidity of sacropelvic fixation if they projected ventral to the lumbosacral pivot point.[30]

The optimal depth for screw placement in the sacrum is a controversial issue. In a comparison of screws placed to a depth of 50% of the maximum distance available (the dorsal cortex of the lamina to the ventral cortex of the vertebrae body) with screws placed just up to, but not penetrating, the ventral cortex, Zindrick et al[43] found no significant difference in pullout strength. Other studies, however, have concluded that screw strength is proportional to the depth of penetration.[24]

Cadaveric studies have helped define the optimal directions of sacral screw placement to avoid injury to neural or vascular structures. For screws placed at the S1 pedicle, a "safe zone" exists from the sacral promontory medial to the internal iliac vein laterally.[31] Bicortical purchase of the screw threads increases the pullout strength of the screw but also incurs additional risk of complications.[8,14,24,26,31,43] Overpenetration through the ventral sacral cortex carries the risk of neurological deficit, chronic pain from lumbosacral trunk injury, sympathetic chain injury, peritonitis, sepsis, and hemorrhage.[26,31] Therefore, the surgeon must decide whether the additional biomechanical advantages of bicortical sacral purchase outweigh the risks associated with potential neurovascular and visceral penetration. If these risks are warranted, screws should be oriented toward the safe zone. Additional suggestions to avoid injury include drilling (done slowly and with fluoroscopic guidance, if needed, so that the drill bit barely penetrates the ventral cortex), the use of self-tapping screws, palpation of the ventral aspect of the hole with a depth gauge, the use of a blunted tip screw with tapered distal threads, and the use of a screw length that matches the length measured from the depth gauge.[24]

Perhaps the most important criteria for determining the ability of pedicle screws to bear loads and resist loosening is bone density and quality. Carlson et al[9] found a positive correlation between bone density and maximum load to failure (P <0.05). The ability to resist loosening and the insertion torque required for screw placement is directly proportional to bone mineral density.[9,37,43]

Spinal instrumentation that is extremely rigid can result in load bearing by the instrumentation construct to such a degree that the bony spine carries no significant portion of its normal physiological load. This characteristic, termed "stress shielding," can lead to the progressive loss of bone mineral content and failure of bony arthrodesis. The optimal spinal stiffness that yields the highest fusion rate and the least amount of device-related osteoporosis is not known. McCord et al[30] found that a strain of less than 2% induced device-related osteoporosis, while a strain of greater than 10% yielded excessive instability. Nagel et al[32] demonstrated that a strain of 10% yielded a solid fusion, whereas a strain of 36% would lead to pseudarthrosis 87% of the time.

Another study to evaluate the effects of stress shielding was performed in a dog model by McAfee et al[29] using various instrumentation constructs (and no instrumentation in controls). They found an inverse correlation between the rigidity of instrumentation used and the density of bone in the fusion mass. Systems that are more rigid resulted in fusion masses of lesser density. However, the fusion rates correlated directly with the rigidity of the instrumentation used. The authors concluded that the higher rates of successful arthrodesis more than compensated for the lower bony density; therefore, the use of more rigid instrumentation is justified.

INDICATIONS FOR LUMBOSACRAL OR LUMBOSACROPELVIC INSTRUMENTATION

Instrumentation across the lumbosacral junction or sacroiliac joint serves to maintain stability until bony arthrodesis is complete. The need for instrumentation may arise due to the presence of segmental instability or to the need to maintain deformity correction. Segmental instability at or caudal to the midlumbar (L3) region often requires fixation to the sacrum. This is particularly true in cases where the instability results from trauma. Pelvic obliquity is often present in patients with scoliosis. Since multisegment correction is usually required in such cases, a long lever arm is created by such spinal implants. Rigid fixation to the sacrum and, frequently, instrumentation across the sacroiliac joint are legitimate considerations in these situations.

Spinal fusion is undertaken for reduction of deformity, prevention of deformity progression, or enhancement of stability in any situation where overt instability or segmental dysfunctional motion exists. Although fusion will often alleviate pain, in the absence of radiographic abnormalities that suggest dysfunctional motion, pain alone should seldom be considered an indication of the need for fusion.[15] Indications for fusion to the sacrum are not clearly established. Those most commonly cited are degenerative disc disease, unstable fractures, scoliosis, spondylolysis, spondylolisthesis, pelvic obliquity, and spinal stenosis requiring wide decompression.

Fusion techniques vary, particularly for the lumbosacral spine. In 1911, Hibbs[18] described dorsal fusion in which fusion of the neural arches was induced by overlapping numerous small autologous bone flaps from contiguous spinous processes, laminae, and articular facets. Subsequently, numerous modifications of the Hibbs technique have been described.[38] At present, commonly used fusions include the dorsolateral or intertransverse process, interbody, or combined ventral and dorsal techniques.

The use of rigid instrumentation for enhancing fusion rates has gained popularity. The object of internal fixation is threefold: 1) to immobilize the spine during fusion; 2) to accelerate consolidation; and 3) to reduce pain and disability after surgery. Instrumentation provides temporary fixation and stability while the fusion mass unites, after which the fusion mass itself provides the preponderance of long-term stability. Lorenz et al[27] found a 59% incidence of pseudarthrosis in patients in whom no instrumentation was used; in those with pedicle screw fixation supplementation, no cases of pseudarthrosis formation were observed. In multilevel fusions, Kostuik et al[22] noted a 14% incidence of pseudarthrosis in instrumented patients, compared to a 55% incidence in a historical series.

Although not all reports demonstrate a dramatic discrepancy in fusion rates between instrumented and non-instrumented spines,[39] many clinicians agree that instrumentation does increase fusion rates in humans.[4,21,42] In a prospective randomized comparison of fusion with and without instrumentation, Zdeblick et al[42]

found a 65% rate of successful fusion among non-instrumented patients, while rigid instrumentation was associated with successful fusion in 95% of cases. In most routine fusions of one or two levels that involve the lumbosacral junction, the use of a single bone screw in each S1 pedicle provides adequate sacral fixation. However, in longer fusions and when the case is more complicated, instrumentation to the ilium is often necessary.

Pseudarthrosis rates vary among studies, but do correlate with the extent of fusion. For fusions extending to the sacrum, a one-level fusion (L5-S1) results in a failure rate of approximately 3.5% to 10%, a two-level fusion (L4-S1) results in a pseudarthrosis rate of approximately 15% to 20%, and a three-level fusion (L3-S1) fails in approximately 25% to 33% of cases.[11,23] Pseudarthrosis rates increase in patients with advanced age, tobacco use, non-instrumented constructs, or multisegment constructs.[20,42] Kim et al[20] found that combined ventral and dorsal fusion and rigid postoperative immobilization in a spica pantaloon cast significantly improved fusion rates. Although pseudarthrosis can be very disabling, it has been estimated that 50% of patients with pseudarthrosis have no symptoms.

The time to fusion in the adult population has generally been accepted as 4 months to 1 year. Ogilvie and Bradford[33] reported a mean duration to fusion of 4.9 months, while Kornblatt et al[21] observed a mean time to fusion of 9.2 months. Precise determination of the time to fusion is limited by the difficulty of determining when fusion has occurred via imaging studies.[10] It is further limited by the fact that the findings on surgical exploration (the gold standard for confirming solid arthrodesis) have demonstrated a poor correlation between true arthrodesis and radiographically determined fusion.[6]

Studies analyzing variables that affect outcome in patients treated with fusion are limited. Hanley and Levy[17] investigated patients treated with fusion for isthmic lumbosacral spondylolisthesis and found a negative influence on outcome in patients who are middle aged (30–50 years old), have a smoking habit, have pseudarthrosis on radiography, or have a compensable work situation. Kim et al[20] found a strong correlation between fusion rate and clinical outcome. Among 47 patients with solid fusion, 40 (85%)

had a good or excellent outcome. In contrast, of 18 patients who developed a pseudarthrosis, only seven (38%) had a good or excellent outcome (P = 0.004).

INSTRUMENTATION AND TECHNIQUES

A variety of spinal instrumentations are available for sacral and iliac fixation. Sacral constructs can be divided into three subgroups: screw and plate, screw and rod, and designs using hooks and sublaminar cables or wires. Screw-plate designs may require contouring of the plate to preserve the normal lordosis at the lumbosacral junction. If scoliosis or lateral translation is present, one must also contour the plate in the coronal plane. Contouring of a plate in both the sagittal and coronal planes is difficult, and in such situations, many surgeons choose screw-rod designs. Screw-rod designs provide the ability to attach spinal rods directly to the sacrum with screws. Contouring in the sagittal and coronal planes is a simple matter when rods are used as the longitudinal member.

Iliac fixation can be performed using either rods or screws. The classic Galveston technique, described by Allen and Ferguson,[1,2] provides rigid pelvic fixation through the use of rods inserted into the ilium. A segment of rod (ideally 6 cm) is driven between the cortical bone tables of each ilium from the posterior superior iliac spine ventrally toward the anterior superior iliac spine, passing approximately 1 cm above the sciatic notch. Immediately rostral to the sciatic notch is the area of greatest bone strength in the ilium. Thus, it provides an excellent fixation site.

Screw placement directly into the ilium can provide excellent fixation. One commercially available iliac screw (DePuy-AcroMed, Raynham, MA) can be inserted into the ilium in a direction analogous to the path of the Galveston rod. This method is perhaps simpler to perform than the Galveston rod technique, and connection to the longitudinal member is easily accomplished with a rigid connector device.

Another technique for iliac fixation is the placement of adjustable-angle bone screws into the ilium obliquely from medial to lateral beginning near the posterior superior iliac spine.[5] The oblique direction of passage allows bicortical purchase of the screw threads and positioning of the screw tip ventral to the lumbosacral pivot point. When used in conjunction with sacral pedicle screws and an additional fixation site (such as a screw placed into the ala or the S2 pedicle, or a hook in the S2 dorsal neuroforamen), the construct creates a tripod for load distribution. This splayed geometry of screw placement may also help resist implant pullout. Fluoroscopy is not required since bicortical purchase is confirmed by palpation at the lateral iliac surface. Additionally, the use of variable-angle bone screws allows attachment of the screw to an appropriately contoured rod in nearly any orientation. Therefore, the requirement for preplanning or acquiring special devices and instruments is eliminated, and the degree of rod contouring is minimized. Clinical experience with this method is limited and its use should be confined to situations where conventional methods of sacral screw fixation may be inadequate.

Another technique for lumbosacral fixation involves the use of transpedicular sacral screws combined with rods inserted into the lateral aspect of the sacrum. The screws connect to the rod at oblique angles, thereby allowing the placement of these screws through the pedicle and the rostral aspect of the sacrum for purchase in the dense cortical bone of the endplate. This manner of screw placement provides the biomechanical advantages of bicortical purchase without the dangers posed by screw placement through the ventral sacral cortex. Passage of the rod into the lateral aspect of the sacrum provides a buttressing effect and additional rigidity. Although clinical data regarding this technique are limited, the rationale for its use appears to be sound.[19]

COMPLICATIONS

As with any technically challenging surgical procedure, the complications of lumbosacral and sacropelvic fixation are numerous and can occur even under the most optimal conditions. Intraoperative complications commonly include injury to nerve roots, vascular structures, or the intestine. Avoiding screw overpenetration by the use of a depth gauge and cautious technique, or simply avoiding bicortical purchase altogether, should lessen the incidence of damage to intra-abdominal structures. In the patient with significant scoliosis, it must be remembered that there is coupling of rotation with the lateral curvature. The transverse processes, therefore, are rotated ventrally on the concave side of the curve. This results in the nerve roots being positioned relatively dorsally on the concave side. They can easily be injured during exposure of the transverse processes. The use of blunt dissection, as opposed to sharp or electrocautery techniques, should lessen this risk.

A number of complications related to spinal instrumentation can occur in lumbosacral or sacropelvic fixation construct application. Of course, placement of the hardware must be performed with great caution, but care must also be exercised in optimizing the construct itself. The implants should be as close to the spine as possible to prevent the discomfort caused by high-profile constructs. Caution must also be exercised to avoid the overcorrection of deformities or the elimination of the normal lumbar lordosis, both of which may result in chronic pain and/or neurological deficit.[4,34] If laterally directed implants are placed in the sacrum, avoiding violation of the sacroiliac joint is advisable unless the plan is to fully bridge the joint with the construct. Placing a screw tip in the sacroiliac joint, without truly bridging it, carries the risk of chronic irritation and pain.

As is the case with any instrumentation and arthrodesis procedure, long-term complications can include the loss of correction, implant failure, and pseudarthrosis formation. Every surgeon who performs these procedures will encounter complications. However, through meticulous attention to surgical technique, as well as the use of instrumentation constructs that are matched to the intended type of correction, immobilization, and anticipated load stresses, overall surgical results can be optimized.

REFERENCES

1. Allen BL Jr, Ferguson RL: The Galveston technique for L rod instrumentation of the scoliotic spine. **Spine** 7:276-284, 1982
2. Allen BL Jr, Ferguson RL: The Galveston technique of pelvic fixation with L-rod instrumentation of the spine. **Spine** 9:388-394, 1984
3. Asher M, Carson W, Heinig C, et al: A modular spinal rod linkage system to provide rotational stability. **Spine** 13:272-277, 1988
4. Balderston RA, Winter RB, Moe JH, et al: Fusion to the sacrum for nonparalytic scoliosis in the adult. **Spine** 11:824-829, 1986
5. Baldwin NG, Benzel EC: Sacral fixation using iliac instrumentation and a variable-angle screw device. Technical note. **J Neurosurg** 81:313-316, 1994
6. Brodsky AE, Kovalsky ES, Khalil MA: Correlation of radiological assessment of lumbar spine fusions with surgical exploration. **Spine** 16 (Suppl 6):S261-S265, 1991
7. Brooke R: The sacroiliac joint. **J Anat** 58:297-305, 1924
8. Camp JF, Caudle R, Ashmun RD, et al: Immediate complications of Cotrel-Dubousset instrumentation to the sacro-pelvis: a clinical and biomechanical study. **Spine** 15:932-941, 1990
9. Carlson GD, Abitbol JJ, Anderson DR, et al: Screw fixation in the human sacrum: an in vitro study of the biomechanics of fixation. **Spine** 17 (Suppl 6): S196-S203, 1992
10. Carson WL, Duffield RC, Arendt M, et al: Internal forces and moments in transpedicular spine instrumentation: the effect of pedicle screw angle and transfixation—the 4R-4bar linkage concept. **Spine** 15: 893-901, 1990
11. Cleveland M, Bosworth DM, Thompson FR: Pseudarthrosis in the lumbosacral spine. **J Bone Joint Surg (Am) 30**:302-312, 1948
12. Colombini D, Occhipinti E, Grieco A, et al: Estimation of lumbar disc areas by means of anthropometric parameters. **Spine** 14:51-55, 1989 [erratum appears in **Spine** 14:533, 1989]
13. Dietrich M, Kurowski P: The importance of mechanical factors in the etiology of spondylolysis: a model analysis of loads and stresses in human lumbar spine. **Spine** 10:532-542, 1985
14. Esses SI, Botsford DJ, Huler RJ: Surgical anatomy of the sacrum: a guide for rational screw fixation. **Spine** 16 (Suppl 6):S283-S288, 1991
15. Esses SI, Huler RJ: Indications for lumbar spine fusion in the adult. **Clin Orthop** 279:87-100, 1992
16. Farfan HF, Kirkaldy-Willis WH: The present status of spinal fusion in the treatment of lumbar intervertebral joint disorders. **Clin Orthop** 158:198-214, 1981
17. Hanley EN Jr, Levy JA: Surgical treatment of isthmic lumbosacral spondylolisthesis: analysis of variables influencing results. **Spine** 14:48-50, 1989
18. Hibbs RA: An operation for progressive spinal deformities. **NY J Med 93**:1013-1016, 1911
19. Jackson RP, McManus AC: The iliac buttress: a computed tomographic study of sacral anatomy. **Spine** 18: 1318-1328, 1993
20. Kim SS, Denis F, Lonstein JE, et al: Factors affecting fusion rate in adult spondylolisthesis. **Spine** 15: 979-984, 1990
21. Kornblatt MD, Casey MP, Jacobs RR: Internal fixation in lumbosacral spine fusion: a biomechanical and clinical study. **Clin Orthop** 203:141-150, 1986
22. Kostuik JP, Errico TJ, Gleason TF: Luque instrumentation in degenerative conditions of the lumbar spine. **Spine** 15:318-321, 1990
23. Kostuik JP, Smith TJ: Pitfalls of biomechanical testing. **Spine** 16:1233-1235, 1991
24. Krag MH, Van Hal ME, Beynnon BD: Placement of

transpedicular vertebral screws close to anterior vertebral cortex: description of methods. **Spine 14:**879-883,
1989

25. Leong JCY, Lu WW, Zheng Y, et al: Comparison of the
strengths of lumbosacral fixation achieved with techniques using one and two triangulated sacral screws.
Spine 23:2289-2294, 1998

26. Licht NJ, Rowe DE, Ross LM: Pitfalls of pedicle screw
fixation in the sacrum: a cadaver model. **Spine 17:**
892-896, 1992

27. Lorenz M, Zindrick M, Schwaegler P, et al: A comparison of single-level fusions with and without hardware. **Spine 16 (Suppl):**S455-S458, 1991

28. Louis R: Fusion of the lumbar and sacral spine by
internal fixation with screw plates. **Clin Orthop 203:**
18-33, 1986

29. McAfee PC, Farey ID, Sutterlin CE, et al: 1989 Volvo
Award in basic science: device-related osteoporosis
with spinal instrumentation. **Spine 14:**919-926, 1989

30. McCord DH, Cunningham BW, Shono Y, et al: Biomechanical analysis of lumbosacral fixation. **Spine 17**
(Suppl):S235-S243, 1992

31. Mirkovic S, Abitbol JJ, Stienman J, et al: Anatomic
consideration for sacral screw placement. **Spine 16**
(Suppl 6):S289-S294, 1991

32. Nagel DA, Kramers PC, Rahn BA, et al: A paradigm of
delayed union and nonunion in the lumbosacral
joint: a study of motion and bone grafting of the lumbosacral spine in sheep. **Spine 16:**553-559, 1991

33. Ogilvie JW, Bradford DS: Sublaminar fixation in lumbosacral fusions. **Clin Orthop 269:**157-161, 1991

34. Paonessa KJ, Engler GL: Back pain and disability after
Harrington rod fusion to the lumbar spine for scoliosis. **Spine 17 (Suppl):**S249-S253, 1992

35. Ruland CM, McAfee PC, Warden KE, et al: Triangulation of pedicular instrumentation. A biomechanical
analysis. **Spine 16 (Suppl 6):**S270-S276, 1991

36. Smidt GL, Wei SH, McQuade K, et al: Sacroiliac
motion for extreme hip positions. A fresh cadaver
study. **Spine 22:**2073-2082, 1997

37. Smith SA, Abitbol JJ, Carlson GD, et al: The effects of
depth of penetration, screw orientation, and bone
density on sacral screw fixation. **Spine 18:**1006-1010,
1993

38. Thompson WAL, Gristina AG, Healy WA Jr: Lumbosacral spine fusion: a method of bilateral posterolateral fusion combined with a Hibbs fusion. **J Bone**
Joint Surg (Am) 56:1643-1647, 1974

39. Turner JA, Ersek M, Herron L, et al: Patient outcomes
after lumbar spinal fusions. **JAMA 268:**907-911, 1992

40. White AA III, Panjabi MM: Clinical instability of the
spine, in Evarts CM, Burton RI, Cofield RH, et al (ed):
Surgery of the Musculoskeletal System. 2nd ed. New
York, NY: Churchill Livingstone, 1990, pp 2151-2173

41. White AA III, Panjabi MM: **Clinical Biomechanics of**
the Spine. Philadelphia, Pa: JB Lippincott, 1990

42. Zdeblick TA: A prospective, randomized study of
lumbar fusion: preliminary results. **Spine 18:**983-991,
1993

43. Zindrick MR, Wiltse LL, Widell EH, et al: A biomechanical study of intrapeduncular screw fixation in
the lumbosacral spine. **Clin Orthop 203:**99-112, 1986

CHAPTER 16

PENETRATING INJURIES

HOWARD J. LANDY, MD, FACS, JOSE ARIAS, MD, AND BARTH A. GREEN, MD, FACS

HISTORY

Much of the early literature about spinal missile injuries relates to military experience. During World War I, Cushing and Harvey[14] reported that in the United States Army only patients with incomplete spinal cord injury (SCI) survived; the overall mortality rate was 71.8%. In the British Army, a 65% to 80% mortality rate was reported for patients with SCI;[66,68] urosepsis was believed to be responsible for the majority of deaths.[66]

Controversy surrounded the surgical management of spinal gunshot wounds in the military. Cushing and Harvey[14] reported an operative mortality rate of 62.2%. After World War I, complete injuries were usually treated only with debridement of entrance and exit wounds. Laminectomy was recommended only for patients with incomplete injuries displaying further neurological deterioration.[67]

Progress in resuscitation, urological care, antibiotic agents, and long-term care decreased the incidence of mortality due to SCI during and after World War II. The mortality rate reported in that war ranged from 7.4% to 14.5%.[25,29,43] Matson[43,44] reported that in World War II, SCIs received less uniform treatment than any other injury. The poor prospects for neurological improvement of complete injuries deterred many

surgeons, but some authors maintained that a small fraction of patients with complete lesions benefited from surgical exploration, and laminectomy was recommended for most.[43,46,67] The possibility of surgical improvement in even a small percentage of patients was believed to justify surgical treatment of all patients. Incomplete injuries were generally considered more appropriate for surgical treatment. The operative mortality rate in World War II was reported to range from 4.5% to 11.4%.[29,36,43,53,59,67]

During the Korean War, all patients with penetrating SCIs underwent operative exploration. The operative mortality rate was 1%.[70] In a group of 20 patients operated on for complete cervical cord injury, 13 were reported to show neurological improvement.[70] In the Vietnam Conflict, helicopter evacuation of casualties was efficient and patients received specialized neurosurgical attention quickly.[33,34] In spite of this, no neurological improvement was noted in patients with a complete injury. Compilations of spinal cord missile injuries from armed conflicts continue to be published.[27,58]

The surgical experience of civilians with spinal gunshot wounds has generated even less optimism than military reports.[31,37,62,63,76] In a series of 65 patients, 24 underwent laminectomy for initially complete lesions; none showed significant neurological recovery.[76] In a patient group of 38 civilian cervical cord injuries, recovery of one or two cervical nerve roots occurred after complete injuries, but no long-tract recovery was seen; operative treatment did not improve the outcome for patients with complete or incomplete injuries in that series.[31]

In a report of 185 civilian injuries, Stauffer et al[63] reported that laminectomy had no effect on either complete or incomplete injuries, and surgical treatment led to an increase in morbidity with wound infections, cerebrospinal fluid (CSF) fistulae, and spinal instability. In another group of 59 civilian patients, Six et al[62] reported that no difference in outcome was demonstrated between patients treated surgically and those treated nonsurgically. However, Benzel et al[7] concluded in a study of 42 civilians with spinal gunshot wounds that decompressive surgery was appropriate and beneficial for selected patients with radicular involvement or incomplete myelopathy. In that series, postoperative neurological improvement was believed to be greater than the results would have been without surgery.

Different reports use different criteria for improvement, and not all differentiate between nerve root recovery and long-tract function improvement. In 1980, Feldman and Young[19] pointed out the discrepancy between military and civilian reports, with military reports maintaining that some patients benefit from surgery, while civilian reports generally demonstrate a lack of benefit from operative treatment. An increased incidence of spinal cord concussion from higher velocity military-type missiles might lead to an increased incidence of improvement after uniformly applied surgical exploration in military reports. Such improvement might account for the differences in outcome between the civilian literature and some military reports and might produce misleading data regarding the value of surgical treatment.[75,76]

The literature displays a general consensus that neurological deterioration is an indication for operative exploration, but in patients with stable neurological deficits, the timing of surgery had little bearing on outcome. Priority should be given to associated life-threatening injuries. Plain radiographs, frequently suboptimal, were used to aid in wartime surgical decisions; mod-ern radiographic techniques, particularly computed tomography (CT), have significantly improved anatomic assessment of SCIs.[6,52,54]

In civilian practice, interdisciplinary trauma teams, coupled with helicopter ambulances, have improved the outlook for survival of severe trauma victims, but the prognosis is still poor for significant neurological recovery after a complete SCI. If there is no evidence of long-tract improvement within 24 hours after a complete SCI, the probability of recovery is low.[64]

Civilian spinal gunshot wounds are common in the U.S.[18] due to the prevalence of firearms (Figure 1). In countries where firearms are less readily available, these injuries are rarer. As with other trauma, the most frequent patients are young adult males, and alcohol and drugs are commonly involved. Bystanders, including children, are often victims.[10] The most successful treatment of a disease is to prevent it; many believe that effective gun control is more likely to impact spinal gunshot wounds than advances in therapy.

Spinal injury from stab wounds is more common outside the United States where firearms are not as available. The largest series of stab wounds have been from South Africa,[40,51] although spinal gunshot injuries are becoming increasingly more prominent in South Africa.[69] In the U.S., SCI from a stab wound is much less frequent than from a missile wound (Figure 2). A study of outcomes after spinal stab wounds found no differences in motor recovery compared to other types of spinal injuries.[73]

PATHOPHYSIOLOGY

The term "complete" SCI refers to total loss of motor, sensory, and reflex function below the level of injury. Some authors define complete injury in terms of motor and sensory function only and ignore any preserved reflexes. The physiological transection of complete injury may occur without anatomic transection.

The spinal cord and nerve roots may be injured directly by penetrating projectiles or by bone or disc fragments. Concussive injury to the spinal cord and nerve roots may occur without direct penetration of the spinal canal.

The pathology of injuries from gunshot

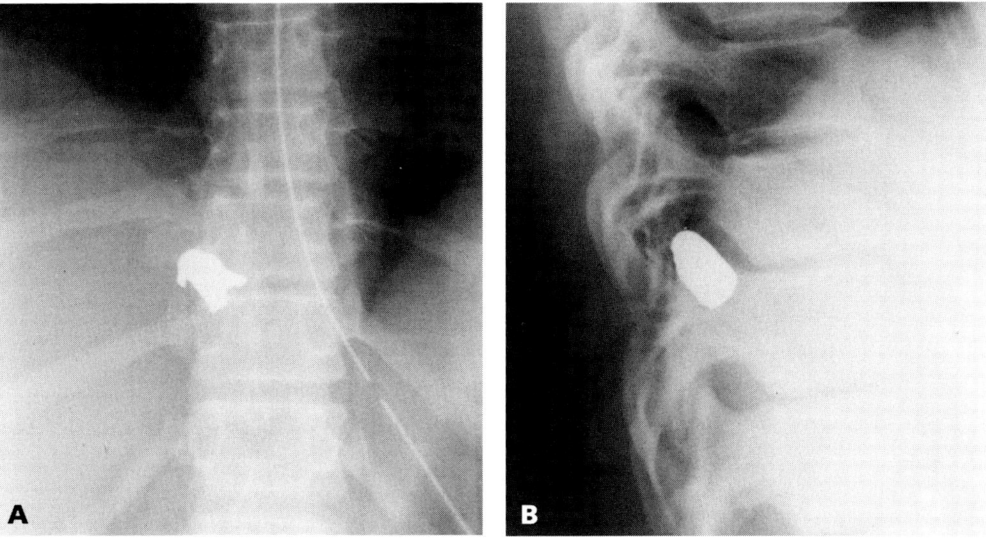

Figure 1: Anteroposterior **(A)** and lateral **(B)** films showing a bullet lodged on the right side of the spinal canal at T9-10.

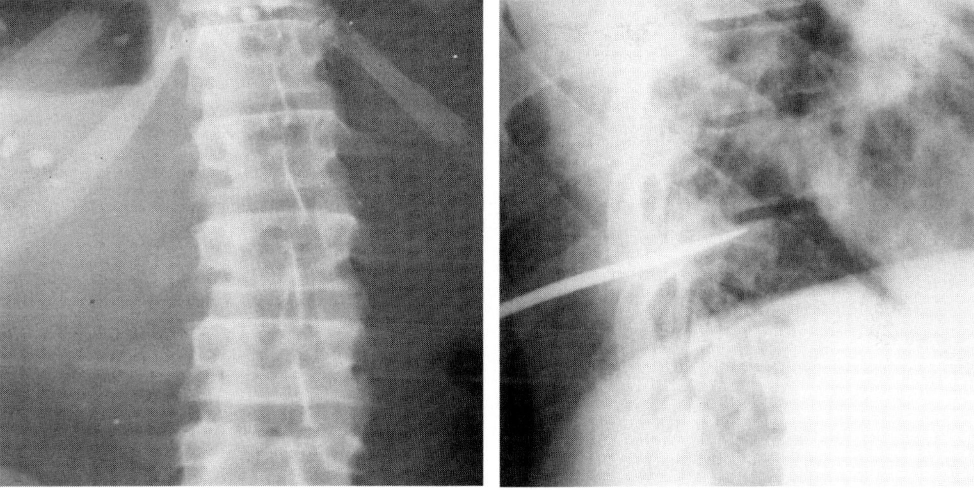

Figure 2: Thoracic spine films demonstrating a broken knife blade entering the spinal canal and resulting in partial injury to the spinal cord.

wounds during World War I was described by Holmes[32] and that of experimental gunshot wounds have been studied.[9] Significant hematoma formation in the epidural or subdural spaces rarely occurs. Intramedullary hemorrhage is frequent, particularly in gray matter, and ranges in amount from small to involving several spinal cord segments. Degenerating axons and myelin may be seen for variable distances on either side of the lesion, and chromatolysis or signs of cell death may be present in neurons. Later, macrophages become prominent and cystic changes occur.

Posttraumatic progressive cystic myelopathy may cause late deterioration of neurological function from progressive syringomyelia. With the advent of improved magnetic resonance imaging (MRI), the syndrome of posttraumatic progressive myelomalacic myelopathy has been suggested as an additional cause of delayed neu-

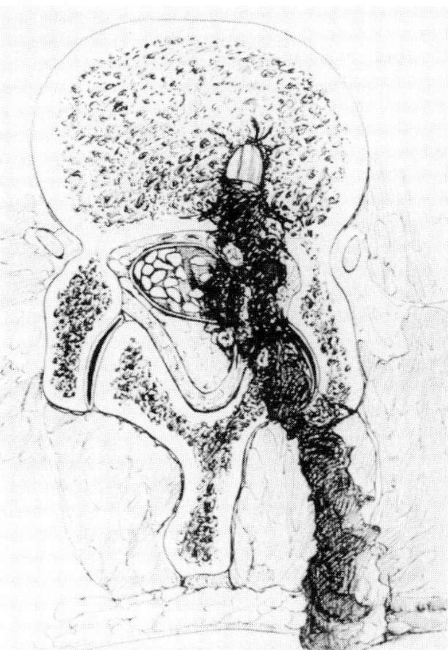

Figure 3: Drawing of a typical missile injury below the conus medullaris affecting the cauda equina and causing nerve root injuries.

rological deterioration. In this instance, microcystic change rather than a confluent syrinx may be the result of spinal cord tethering, usually dorsally and laterally, from scar tissue. Prolonged supine positioning in the immediate postinjury period, when the spinal cord is contused and inflamed, may be an aggravating factor in producing tethering.

Penetrating injuries below the conus medullaris cause injuries to the cauda equina. These are nerve root injuries and are frequently incomplete and asymmetric (Figure 3). It is not unusual for brachial and lumbosacral plexus injuries to be associated with SCIs.

Missile and bone fragments may come to rest in the epidural space, the subdural space, the spinal cord, or among the roots of the cauda equina. Fragments of clothing, skin, or other debris may be carried into the spinal canal with missile fragments. In a study of 245 spinal gunshot wounds, 96 patients had major bullet fragments retained in the spinal canal.[72] Missile fragments may remain mobile within the spinal canal,[3,65] and migration of an intracranial bullet into the spinal canal has also been reported.[77] Intervertebral disc herniation resulting from missile injuries may produce neural compression.[42,55]

Spinal cord concussion[5,41,43] is a partial or complete loss of function that recovers completely within several days after injury. The lesion is related to the shock wave created by a projectile passing through tissue adjacent to the spinal canal without actually penetrating it. The cellular mechanism of this injury is not well understood. High-velocity military-type missiles are more likely to cause spinal cord concussion than the lower velocity wounds often seen in civilian injuries.

Surgical inspection of the cord offers only limited prognostic information, unless complete anatomic transection is observed.[19,31,62,63,75,76] Meningitis, epidural abscess, intramedullary abscess,[53] and osteomyelitis[12,26,56] may occur; the risks of infection increase if the missile passes through the alimentary canal or lung before entering the spinal canal. Although CSF leakage increases the risk of meningitis, it is more likely to occur after surgical intervention.

Spinal instability occurs only rarely after gunshot wounds. High-velocity injuries or gunshot wounds to children are somewhat more likely to result in spinal instability.

Lead projectiles in nervous tissue produce relatively little tissue reaction, whereas copper is much more toxic.[61] Lead intoxication is a risk if bullet fragments are retained in a disc space.[24] Neurological symptoms may initially present at a time remote from the original injury.[2,11,74] Reactive tissue may produce delayed neural compression.[15,49]

Fistula formation may occur between the spine and bowel,[71] bladder,[71] or pleural cavity.[8,16] Headache and chronic subdural hematoma have been reported after prolonged CSF leakage into the epidural space following a stab wound.[4,45] An arteriovenous fistula may result from injuries lacerating the vertebral artery,[38,60] and the carotid artery may also be involved.[57]

In the majority of cases, stab wounds result in incomplete injuries.[73] The description of a classic lesion from a stab wound is similar to that of the Brown-Séquard syndrome, although most injuries do not fit the syndrome definition exactly. The configuration of the spine tends to force the blade to one side of the spinal canal.[51] In some stab injuries, the cord ipsilateral to the penetration may be spared, whereas the contralateral cord is injured from compression against the side of the spinal canal.[25] Epidural hematoma has been reported following a stab wound.[50] Spinal stab wounds may also result in infection,[28] CSF leakage, and delayed neurological deficits. Delayed deficits may occur due to retained weapon fragments.[13,21]

MANAGEMENT

Pre-Hospital and Emergency Room Management

During initial treatment, the fundamentals of resuscitation take precedence over management of the spine. Airway maintenance and respiration may be compromised by penetrating neck injury; if a cervical spine injury is suspected, airway establishment should be performed with as little cervical motion as possible. Respiratory function may be compromised by thoracic injuries, and associated major vascular injuries may result in hypovolemia and shock. Large bore intravenous lines should be established as early as possible.

At the injury scene, the paramedic should maintain spinal immobilization in a neutral position. The spine is usually stable after a gunshot or stab wound; if there is instability, excessive spinal column mobility may increase spinal cord or neural injury when intraspinal bone or missile fragments are present. A brief baseline neurological examination should be performed in the field. When paralysis is present, the involved extremities should be appropriately immobilized and protected.

In the emergency room, further evaluation of associated injuries is performed and decisions relating to treatment priorities are made for possible emergency surgery for vascular or visceral injuries to the neck, thorax, or abdomen. Extremity injuries may be severe enough to require emergency surgical management as well. When paralysis is present, a nasogastric tube should be inserted and placed to suction due to the paralytic ileus usually associated with acute SCI. A urinary catheter is necessary for adequate bladder emptying as well as to aid in the assessment of fluid balance and hemodynamic status.

Careful neurological examination is performed after initial resuscitation. If emergency surgery is necessary for associated injuries, as complete a neurological assessment as possible in the time available should be performed. In an attempt to standardize the nomenclature and quantitate the neurological deficit, the American Spinal Injury Association (ASIA) scoring system[1] was developed and is being increasingly recognized worldwide.

Neurological examination will establish the level and character of the injury. Careful attention should be paid to differentiating between complete and incomplete injuries. Rectal examination should be included, with attention to both volitional contracture of the anal sphincter as well as possible sensory preservation. The presence of lateral column sacral sparing (pain and temperature sensation and volitional sphincter function) improves the prognosis, even in the presence of severe neurological deficit.

Entrance and exit wounds should be carefully inspected with attention to the possible presence of CSF leakage. These wounds may be quite separate from the area of spinal injury, and care should be taken not to miss their presence. Because of significant medicolegal overtones almost always present in these cases, it is recommended that photographs of the entrance and exit wounds be taken in the emergency room. If a camera is not available, the responsible physician should make accurate sketches of these sites once the patient has been clinically stabilized.

The term "spinal shock" refers to the flaccid lower motor neuron status associated with loss of reflexes that occurs acutely below the level of a complete SCI. Reflexes return and commonly become hyperactive at variable times after injury, usually 6 to 16 weeks. In rare cases, rapid resolution of spinal shock occurs with the return of reflexes immediately after injury. The rapid return of reflexes in the setting of a persistent complete deficit carries a poor prognosis for neurological recovery. All patients in spinal shock have complete deficits by definition and, therefore, have a poor outlook for improvement. "Neurogenic shock," differentiated from spinal shock, refers to a combination of bradycardia, hypotension, and hypothermia that accompanies acute SCI. This autonomic paralysis (sympathectomy)[47] is often manageable with fluid resuscitation and warming. Bradycardia usually does not require treatment, but atropine may be used if the pulse rate is less than 40 beats per minute or if associated hypotension does not respond to intravenous fluids. Occasionally, vasopressors are temporarily necessary and, in rare instances, a cardiac pacemaker may be utilized for persistent significant bradycardia.

Initially, the spine is kept immobilized on a board until radiographic determination of stability. Attempts should be made to remove the patient from the spine board or to interpose a gel pad as soon as possible to avoid initiation of a sacral decubitus ulcer. Until spinal stability is documented or fusion performed, the patient may be nursed on a Roto Rest Kinetic Treatment Table.[22,23] The constant rotation of the bed is believed to promote drainage of pulmonary secretions and venous drainage from the lower extremities while maintaining spinal alignment.

Broad-spectrum antibiotics are started in the emergency room and continued for 10 to 14 days after injury. Steroids have not been shown to cure paralysis although they may limit the lesion volume, possibly having important implications as regeneration and transplantation strategies evolve for eventual human treatment trials. Theoretically, high-dose steroids may increase the risk of significant infection after penetrating injury; therefore, our practice is to use these drugs only if the penetrating SCI is not associated with major visceral injury such as penetration of the intestine. The Second National Acute Spinal Cord Injury Study found a statistically significant, although clinically small, benefit from the administration of high-dose methylprednisolone begun within 8 hours after nonpenetrating injury. That study did not include penetrating injuries. Retrospective nonrandomized studies of treatment of penetrating spine injuries with the same high-dose methylprednisolone protocol have shown no neurological benefit.[30,39]

Diagnostic Imaging

Routine spinal radiographs are performed in the emergency room and analyzed for the presence of metal fragments and fractures. Spinal alignment and stability are assessed; instability of the spine is rare after a penetrating injury. CT is very helpful in visualizing the bony injuries and localizing metal and bone fragments and may also visualize significant, although rare, he-

matomas. It is possible for large metal fragments to produce enough CT artifact to obscure details of bony injury at some spinal levels. CT is more useful than MRI in the acute phase after penetrating injury. MRI may theoretically be hazardous if a retained ferrous fragment is present. MRI has been used for imaging patients with spinal gunshot injuries, although some degree of risk must be assumed in MRI when there are retained metallic fragments.[17,20,35]

If delayed neurological deterioration occurs in the chronic phase after injury, plain radiographs, CT, and MRI may be useful in assessment. MRI is the preferred modality for detection of posttraumatic progressive cystic or myelomalacic myelopathy. Occasionally, myelography with immediate and delayed CT may be necessary if retained metal fragments produce too much MRI artifact for adequate imaging.

Surgical Management

If radiographic studies suggest the possibility of cervical instability, MRI-compatible tongs are applied to the skull for traction. The weight required for reduction of a subluxation is approximately 5 lb per interspace and is titrated to the radiographic results.

Complete, penetrating injuries of the spinal cord are usually not subjected to operative exploration. The surgical risks of infection, CSF fistula, and anesthesia complications far outweigh the minimal chances of significant neurological recovery. An incomplete SCI with a significant persistent compressive lesion is usually afforded operative exploration, decompression, and debridement.

A complete cervical injury may be explored if radiographic studies suggest that operative decompression carries significant potential for improvement of function of one or more cervical roots. Recovery of even a single cervical root may enhance rehabilitation potential, whereas recovery of a single thoracic root (below T1) is of no consequence.

In the rare eventuality of persistent CSF fistula or for infection such as epidural abscess or osteomyelitis, a complete or incomplete injury may be treated surgically. A case of persistent CSF fistula will usually respond to 5 to 7 days of continuous lumbar CSF external drainage, obviating the need for surgical repair. When antibiotics are used for 7 to 10 days postinjury, infection is quite rare. In our experience, transoral gunshot wounds carry a higher risk of spinal infection than transabdominal wounds.

If a largely intact bullet or large bone fragments occupy the spinal canal in the setting of a complete or incomplete injury of the cauda equina, the injury is usually explored. Cauda equina injuries are nerve root injuries and have a better prognosis for long-term recovery than SCIs. In addition, large bullet fragments in the cauda equina are more likely to cause chronic pain problems if not removed. Cauda equina injuries with only small intraspinal metal or bone fragments are not usually explored.

The exact timing of surgery depends on associated injuries. Any planned spinal surgery is performed at the first convenient opportunity after systemic stability is achieved. The surgical selection criteria described above are not accepted by all spine surgeons, but if a significant compressive lesion is demonstrated radiographically, there is general agreement that progressive neurological deterioration is an indication for surgical treatment.

Operative exploration is usually performed through laminectomy and should include the removal of significant bone fragments and foreign bodies. At times, anterior cervical, transoral, transthoracic, posterolateral, retroperitoneal or transabdominal approaches may be necessary. Dural repair may require grafts of fascia or lyophilized dura in order to prevent CSF leakage. Intraoperative ultrasonography is useful to aid in localization of bone and metal fragments.[48] Debridement does not require removal of every small fragment; removal of some fragments, especially intramedullary, may be deferred if further spinal cord or neural injury would be risked. Loupe magnification is helpful; the operating microscope is usually not necessary. Somatosensory evoked potentials and electromyography monitoring are performed intraoperatively when appropriate.

After positioning for surgery and prior to incision, intraoperative radiographs should be obtained to check for the position of bullet fragments that may be mobile in the spinal canal. If there is spinal instability, appropriate fusion with bone graft and possible instrumentation is performed at the time of decompression.

Postoperative/Postinjury Management

Early during the postoperative period in the recovery room or the intensive care unit, the ASIA motor/sensory testing score is again documented. Kinetic therapy (Roto Rest Treatment Table) may be employed, and patients with systemic support with vasopressors and mechanical ventilators are weaned as soon as possible. Rapid mobilization of the SCI victim from the bed to a wheelchair is a high priority. The multidisciplinary rehabilitation team becomes involved early to expedite a smooth transition from the acute care setting to the rehabilitation phase. Patients with SCI associated with penetrating wounds often have an increased tendency toward developing chronic problems with pain and spasticity as compared to the closed SCI population. It is not within the scope of this chapter to discuss the treatment of all delayed systemic consequences of SCI, but every SCI patient should be afforded a holistic rehabilitation experience to optimize the chances of their return to being a functional contributing member of society. This requires a strong program stressing not only physical restoration but psychosocial, sexual, vocational, educational, and recreational aspects as well. In cases of penetrating wounds, this can be most challenging since the patient may either be a victim of criminal or accidental injury or the perpetrator. Both come with a significant amount of psychosocial and legal "baggage." A team approach is imperative in rehabilitation of these complex cases.

REFERENCES

1. American Spinal Injury Association, International Medical Society of Paraplegia: **International Standards for Neurological and Functional Classification of Spinal Cord Injury.** Chicago, Ill: ASIA/IMSOP, 1992
2. Amitani K, Tsuyuguchi Y, Hukuda S: Delayed cervical myelopathy caused by bomb shell fragment. Case report. **J Neurosurg** 44:626-627, 1976
3. Arasil E, Tasgioglu AO: Spontaneous migration of an intracranial bullet to the cervical spinal canal causing Lhermitte's sign. Case report. **J Neurosurg** 56: 158-159, 1982

4. Baghal P, Sheptak PE: Penetrating spinal injury by a glass fragment: case report and review. **Neurosurgery** 11:419-422, 1982

5. Baker GS, Daniels F Jr: Concussion of the spinal cord in battle casualties. **J Neurosurg** 3:206-211, 1946

6. Bashir EF, Cybulski GR, Chaudhri K, et al: Magnetic resonance imaging and computed tomography in the evaluation of penetrating gunshot injury of the spine. Case report. **Spine** 18:772-773, 1993

7. Benzel EC, Hadden TA, Coleman JE: Civilian gunshot wounds to the spinal cord and cauda equina. **Neurosurgery** 20:281-285, 1987

8. Beutel EW, Roberts JD, Langston HT, et al: Subarachnoid-pleural fistula. **J Thorac Cardiovasc Surg** 80: 21-24, 1980

9. Brookhart JM, Groat RA, Windie WE: A study of the mechanics of gunshot injury to the spinal cord of the cat. **Milit Surg** 102:386-395, 1948

10. Carrillo EH, Gonzalez JK, Carrillo LE, et al: Spinal cord injuries in adolescents after gunshot wounds: an increasing phenomenon in urban North America. **Injury** 29:503-507, 1998

11. Conway JE, Crofford TW, Terry AF, et al: Cauda equina syndrome occurring nine years after a gunshot injury to the spine. A case report. **J Bone Joint Surg (Am)** 75:760-763, 1993

12. Craig JB: Cervical spine osteomyelitis with delayed onset tetraparesis after penetrating wounds of the neck. A report of 2 cases. **S Afr Med J** 69:197-199, 1986

13. Criado E, Oiler D, Fulghum J: Delayed diagnosis of a foreign body in the spinal canal. **South Med J** 83: 332-334, 1990

14. Cushing H, Harvey SC: **Medical Department of the U.S. Army in the World War. Part I: Report of Senior Consultant in Neurosurgery.** Washington, DC: Government Printing Office, 1927, Vol II, pp 757-758

15. Daniel EF, Smith GW: Foreign-body granuloma of intervertebral disc and spinal canal. **J Neurosurg** 17: 480-482, 1960

16. Diergaian RS, Roberts JD, Ditunno JF Jr, et al: Subarachnoid-pleural fistula in traumatic paraplegia. **Arch Phys Med Rehabil** 63:488-489, 1982

17. Falcone S, Green BA, Finitsis S: Letter. **AJNR** 20:356, 1999

18. Farmer JC, Vaccaro AR, Balderston RA, et al: The changing nature of admissions to a spinal cord injury center: violence on the rise. **J Spinal Disord** 11: 400-403, 1998

19. Feldman RA, Young RE: Management of gunshot wounds of the spine. **Contemp Neurosurg** 2:23, 1980

20. Finitsis S, Falcone S, Green BA: MR of the spine in the presence of metallic bullet fragments: is the benefit worth the risk? **AJNR** 20:354-356, 1999 (Letter)

21. Fung CF, Ng TH: Delayed myelopathy after a stab wound with a retained intraspinal foreign body: case report. **J Trauma** 32:539-541, 1992

22. Green BA, Green KL, Klose KJ: Kinetic nursing for acute spinal cord injury patients. **Paraplegia** 18: 181-186, 1980

23. Green BA, Green KL, Klose KJ: Kinetic therapy for spinal cord injury. **Spine** 8:722-728, 1983

24. Grogan DP, Bucholz RW: Acute lead intoxication from a bullet in an intervertebral disc space. A case report. **J Bone Joint Surg (Am)** 63:1180-1182, 1981

25. Guttmann L: **Spinal Cord Injuries: Comprehensive Management and Research. 2nd ed.** Oxford, Engl: Blackwell Scientific, 1976

26. Hales DD, Duffy K, Dawson EG, et al: Lumbar osteomyelitis and epidural and paraspinous abscesses. Case report of an unusual source of contamination from a gunshot wound to the abdomen. **Spine** 16: 380-383, 1991

27. Hammoud MA, Haddad FS, Moufarrij NA, et al: Spinal cord missile injuries during the Lebanese civil war. **Surg Neurol** 43:432-442, 1995

28. Harries TJ, Lichtman DM, Swafford AR: Pyogenic vertebral osteomyelitis complicating abdominal stab wounds. **J Trauma** 21:75-79, 1981

29. Haynes WG: Acute war wounds of the spinal cord. Analysis of 184 cases. **Am J Surg** 72:424-433, 1946

30. Heary RF, Vaccaro AR, Mesa JJ, et al: Steroids and gunshot wounds to the spine. **Neurosurgery** 41: 576-584, 1997

31. Heiden JS, Weiss MH, Rosenberg AW, et al: Penetrating gunshot wounds of the cervical spine in civilians. Review of 38 cases. **J Neurosurg** 42:575-579, 1975

32. Holmes G: The pathology of acute spinal injuries. **Br Med J** 2:815-821, 1915

33. Jacobs GB, Berg RA: The treatment of acute spinal cord injuries in a war zone. **J Neurosurg** 34:164-167, 1971

34. Jacobson SA, Bors E: Spinal cord injury in Vietnamese combat. **Paraplegia** 7:263-281, 1970

35. Kanal E: Letter. **AJNR** 20:355-356, 1999

36. Klemperer WW: Spinal cord injuries in World War II. I. Examination and operative technic in 201 patients. **US Armed Forces Med J** 10:539-552, 1959

37. Kupcha PC, An HS, Cotler JM: Gunshot wounds to the cervical spine. **Spine** 15:1058-1063, 1990

38. Leape LL, Palacios E: Acute traumatic vertebral arteriovenous fistula. **Ann Surg** 174:908-910, 1971

39. Levy ML, Gans W, Wijesinghe HS, et al: Use of methylprednisolone as an adjunct in the management of patients with penetrating spinal cord injury: outcome analysis. **Neurosurgery** 39:1141-1149, 1996

40. Lipschitz R. Stab wounds of the spinal cord, in Vinken PJ, Bruyn GW (eds): **Handbook of Clinical Neurology, Vol 25(Pt 1).** New York, NY: Elsevier, 1976, pp 197-207

41. Livingston WK, Newman HW: Spinal cord "concussion" in war wounds. **West J Surg** 54:131-139, 1946

42. Mariottini A, Delfini R, Ciappetta P, et al: Lumbar disc hernia secondary to gunshot injury. **Neurosurgery** 15: 73-75, 1984

43. Matson DD: **The Treatment of Acute Compound Injuries of the Spinal Cord Due to Missiles.** Springfield, Ill: Charles C Thomas, 1948

44. Matson DD: Treatment of compound spine injuries in forward army hospitals. **J Neurosurg** 3:114-119, 1946

45. Mayfrank L, Laborde G, Lippitz B, et al: Bilateral chronic subdural haematomas following traumatic cerebrospinal fluid leakage into the thoracic epidural space. **Acta Neurochir** 120:92-94, 1992

46. McCravey A: A plea for exploration of spinal cord and cauda equina injuries. **JAMA** 129:152-154, 1945

47. Meirowsky AM: Penetrating wounds of the spinal canal. Problems of paraplegia and notes on autonomic hyperreflexia and sympathetic blockade. **Clin Orthop** 27:90-110, 1963

48. Montalvo BM, Quencer RM, Green BA, et al: Intraop-

erative sonography in spinal trauma. **Radiology 153:** 125-134, 1984

49. Nino HE, Leppik IE, Lai CW, et al: Progressive sensory loss one year after bullet injury of spinal cord. **JAMA 240:**1173-1174, 1978

50. Olshaker JS, Barish RA: Acute traumatic cervical epidural hematoma from a stab wound. **Ann Emerg Med 20:**662-664, 1991

51. Peacock WJ, Shrosbree RD, Key AG: A review of 450 stab wounds of the spinal cord. **S Afr Med J 51:** 961-964, 1977

52. Plumley TF, Kilcoyne RF, Mack LA: Computed tomography in evaluation of gunshot wounds of the spine. **J Comput Assist Tomogr 7:**310-312, 1983

53. Pool JL: Gunshot wounds of the spine. Observations from an evacuation hospital. **Surg Gynecol Obstet 81:** 617-622, 1945

54. Quencer RM, Green BA, Eismont FJ: Posttraumatic spinal cord cysts: clinical features and characterization with metrizamide computed tomography. **Radiology 146:**415-423, 1983

55. Robertson DP, Simpson RK, Narayah RK: Lumbar disc herniation from a gunshot wound to the spine. A report of two cases. **Spine 16:**994-995, 1991

56. Romanick PC, Smith TK, Kopaniky DR, et al: Infection about the spine associated with low-velocity-missile injury to the abdomen. **J Bone Joint Surg (Am) 67:**1195-1201, 1985

57. Rothman SLG, Pratt AG, Kier EL, et al: Traumatic vertebral-carotid-jugular arteriovenous aneurysm. Case report. **J Neurosurg 41:**92-96, 1974

58. Rukovansjki M: Spinal cord injuries caused by missile weapons in the Croatian War. **J Trauma 40 (Suppl 3):** S189-S192, 1996

59. Schneider RC, Webster JE, Lofstrom JE: A follow-up report of spinal cord injuries in a group of World War II patients. **J Neurosurg 6:**118-126, 1949

60. Sherk HH, Girl N, Nicholson JT: Gunshot wound with fracture of the atlas and arteriovenous fistula of the vertebral artery. Case report. **J Bone Joint Surg (Am) 56:**1738-1740, 1974

61. Sights WP, Bye RJ: The fate of retained intracerebral shotgun pellets. An experimental study. **J Neurosurg 33:**646-653, 1970

62. Six E, Alexander E Jr, Kelly DL Jr, et al: Gunshot wounds to the spinal cord. **South Med J 72:**699-702, 1979

63. Stauffer ES, Wood RW, Kelly EG: Gunshot wounds of the spine: the effects of laminectomy. **J Bone Joint Surg (Am) 61:**389-392, 1979

64. Suwanwela C, Alexander E Jr, Davis CH Jr: Prognosis in spinal cord injury, with special reference to patients with motor paralysis and sensory preservation. **J Neurosurg 19:**220-227, 1962

65. Tanguy A, Chabannes J, Deubelle A, et al: Intraspinal migration of a bullet with subsequent meningitis. A case report. **J Bone Joint Surg (Am):**1244-1245, 1982

66. Thomson-Walker J: The treatment of the bladder in spinal injuries in war. **Proc R Soc Med 30:**1233-1240, 1937

67. Tinsley M: Compound injuries of the spinal cord. **J Neurosurg 3:**306-309, 1946

68. Vellacott PN, Webb-Johnson AE: Spinal injury with retention of urine. The avoidance of catheterisation. **Lancet 1:**733-737, 1919

69. Velmahos GC, Degiannis E, Hart K, et al: Changing profiles in spinal cord injuries and risk factors influencing recovery after penetrating injuries. **J Trauma 38:**334-337, 1995

70. Wannamaker GT: Spinal cord injuries. A review of the early treatment in 300 consecutive cases during the Korean conflict. **J Neurosurg 11:**517-524, 1954

71. Ward WC, Maltby GL: Associated complications in war wounds of the spine. **JAMA 129:**155-157, 1945

72. Waters RL, Adkins RH: The effects of removal of bullet fragments retained in the spinal canal. A collaborative study by the National Spinal Cord Injury Model Systems. **Spine 8:**934-939, 1991

73. Waters RL, Sie I, Adkins RH, et al: Motor recovery following spinal cord injury caused by stab wounds: a multicenter study. **Paraplegia 33:**98-101, 1995

74. Wu WQ: Delayed effects from retained foreign bodies in the spine and spinal cord. **Surg Neurol 25:**214-218, 1986

75. Yashon D: Missile injuries of the spinal cord, in Vinken PJ, Bruyn GW (eds): **Handbook of Clinical Neurology, Vol 25(Pt 1).** New York, NY: Elsevier, 1976, pp 209-220

76. Yashon D, Jane JA, White RJ: Prognosis and management of spinal cord and cauda equina bullet injuries in sixty-five civilians. **J Neurosurg 32:**163-170, 1970

77. Young WF Jr, Katz MR, Rosenwasser RH: Spontaneous migration of an intracranial bullet into the cervical canal. **South Med J 86:**557-559, 1993

CHAPTER 17

PEDIATRIC SPINAL CORD INJURY

PETER J. LENNARSON, MD, AND ARNOLD H. MENEZES, MD

Spinal cord injury (SCI) that results in permanent neurological deficit is a devastating affliction at any age, but especially so in children and adolescents. Fortunately, injury to the spinal cord and vertebral column is relatively uncommon in the pediatric population. Unique anatomic and biomechanical features of the pediatric spine result in injury patterns that differ from those observed in adults. In addition, children have substantial growth potential and, hence, the risk of posttraumatic spinal deformity is much greater than in adults.

This chapter reviews spinal column and cord injury in children and emphasizes the features that distinguish it from traumatic spinal injury in adults.

INCIDENCE AND EPIDEMIOLOGY OF PEDIATRIC SPINAL INJURY

Accurate information regarding the incidence of pediatric SCI is difficult to obtain. Often, clinical series discuss only the incidence of patients who have been hospitalized; this does not take into account the large number of patients who died either at the scene of the accident or prior to admission. Additionally, there is great variation in the ages included as "pediatric" cases. Birth injuries as well as injuries occurring in children with congenital abnormalities of the vertebral column are excluded from some reports.[20,51]

The annual incidence of SCIs in the United States is 30 to 40 per million population, with an additional 20 cases per million dying prior to hospitalization.[59] Each year 230 to 500 children younger than the age of 15 years and 1500 to 2000 individuals less than 20 years of age sustain SCI. The prevalence of SCI based on the 1990 census is estimated at approximately 200,000. There is no estimate of the prevalence of pediatric SCI patients; however, the prevalence in individuals under 25 years of age is estimated to be 26,000.

The anatomy and biomechanics of the spine change from birth through adolescence, producing alterations in the bony and ligamentous relationships. This leads to variations in the etiology and pathophysiology of pediatric SCI. Taken as a whole, motor-vehicle accidents account for approximately 45% of pediatric spinal injuries, diving injuries 23%, falls 12%, gymnastics 7%, and football and other sports 5%; approximately 8% of pediatric SCIs are due to other causes.[23] Up to 25% of patients suffer from multisystem injuries.[1,8,20,34,41] Another analysis points out an increase in the proportion of violence-related SCIs, with estimates approximating 15% in the birth to 8-year-old age group, 27% in the 9- to 15-year-old age group, and 36% in the 16- to 20-year-old age group.[59] The incidence of sports-related SCIs, on the other hand, has been declining, presumably due to education and prevention programs.

While in the adult population, the incidence of SCI is four times higher in males than females, this difference is less marked in the pediatric population. In patients 3 years of age and younger, the incidence in females and males is equal.[59]

Unique Features of the Pediatric Spine

The pediatric spine possesses unique anatomic and biomechanical characteristics that are largely responsible for the variation in injury patterns between children and adults. The spine undergoes dynamic changes beginning at birth and progressing through adolescence that are characterized by the formation of ossification centers and closure of epiphyses. In most individuals, it is estimated that the spine has achieved an adult configuration both anatomically and radiographically by the age of 8 to 10 years. It is not surprising, therefore, that at this age the injury patterns begin to resemble those of adolescents and adults. The biomechanical variations of the pediatric spine are the result of alterations in the geometry of the vertebral bodies, the articulating surfaces, and the physical properties of the developing muscles and ligaments. These variations result in increased physiological mobility of the pediatric spine compared to that of the adult.

The incompletely ossified, wedge-shaped vertebral bodies in children allow excessive motion in the sagittal plane. The facets in the upper three cervical vertebrae have a relatively horizontal orientation in young children and contribute to the instability in this region. The facets eventually achieve their more vertical orientation and ossify in children between the ages of 7 to 10 years.

There is also an incomplete development and flattening of the uncinate processes in children younger than 10 years of age. This makes the spine less able to withstand excessive flexion and rotational forces.[35,62] Because the immature spine is progressively ossifying, injuries in patients under 8 to 10 years of age tend to be avulsions, epiphyseal separations, or fractures of the growth plate rather than true fractures.

Additionally, in children there is a relative laxity of the stabilizing ligaments and joint capsules that have not yet achieved their normal elastic properties. The paraspinous musculature is also underdeveloped and does not become supportive until puberty.[13,41,61] Thus, even minor trauma can result in excessive mobility between vertebral bodies. Finally, the fulcrum of cervical movement is located higher in young children than in adults and adolescents, about C2-3, because the mass of the head is relatively large compared with the body. A pseudosubluxation between the second and third cervical vertebrae is seen in up to 45% of normal children (Figure 1).[14] The above factors make the upper cervical spine particularly vulnerable to injury.

Pathology and Pathophysiology of Spinal Injury

Etiology and Mechanisms of Injury

As mentioned previously, the major etiologies of pediatric SCI include motor-vehicle accidents, violence, sports-related injury sustained in football, diving, gymnastics, etc., falls, and birth injuries.

Despite the varied circumstances associated, pediatric spinal injury can be classified according to the mechanisms of injury as follows: 1) flexion compression; 2) flexion dislocation; 3) axial loading; 4) extension; 5) distraction; 6) rotation; 7) penetrating; and 8) vascular-ischemic.[3,7,24,41,54,58] Each of these mechanisms can occur independently, although more than one mechanism can be implicated in a particular injury. In flexion compression injuries, the most anterior aspect of the vertebral bodies is reduced

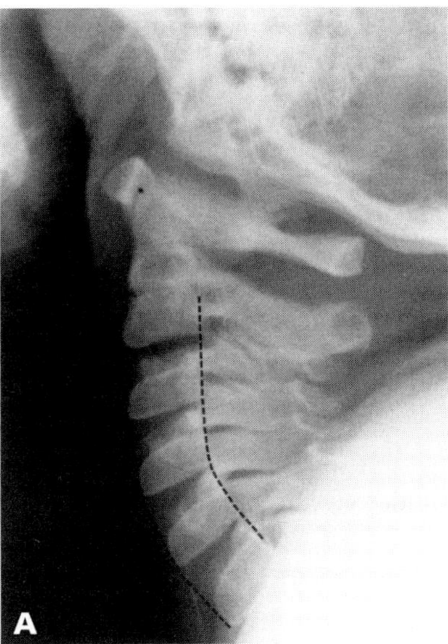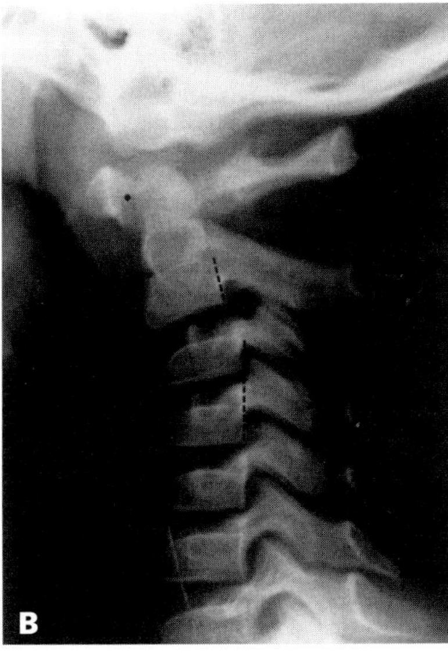

Figure 1: Lateral radiographs demonstrating normal laxity of the cervical spine in a 4-year-old child. **A)** Extension position. Lines drawn tangent to the anterior and posterior margins of the vertebral bodies are smooth *(dotted lines)*. **B)** Flexion position. There is anterior "subluxation" of C2 on C3 with interruption of the tangent lines *(dotted lines)*. The predental space has widened to 5 mm *(dot)*.

in height with associated posterior ligamentous disruptions. Flexion dislocations are associated with maximum ligamentous damage with minimum bone pathology, unilateral or bilateral locked facets, and severe neurological deficits. Compression burst fractures associated with axial loading may shatter vertebral bodies while preserving ligaments. Severe extension injuries may be associated with fractures of the spinous processes, laminae, and facets as well as avulsion fractures of the anterior portions of the vertebral bodies. Distraction injuries are especially prominent at the occipitoatlantal and atlantoaxial joints and can be associated with both cephalic and breech presentations during childbirth. Penetrating spinal injuries, despite causing serious neurological damage, are often associated with a stable spinal column. The penetrating object as well as the resulting shock wave combine to result in the various degrees of neurological deficit. Vascular-ischemic insults may result from damage to the cervical portions of the vertebral arteries and have also been reported with the use of umbilical artery catheters and paradoxical air embolism through transitional cardiovascular shunts in neonates.

Fractures can be simply classified as stable or unstable.[24] Fracture dislocations accompanied by rupture of the ligamentous complex and facet interlock are unstable. Rotational fracture dislocations are the most unstable of all the vertebral fractures and are the result of rotational flexion forces, disruption of the posterior ligament complex, and lateral displacement of the upper vertebral body on the lower. Burst fractures in the cervical spine are frequently associated with severe neurological deficit and instability. Simple wedge fractures of flexion with impaction of fracture fragments and extension fractures localized to the cervical spine are often stable. In these cases the posterior ligaments are intact, maintaining stability in neutral and flexed positions.

In the upper thoracic spine, considerable violence is necessary to produce a fracture or dislocation, and the narrow spinal canal makes it almost inevitable that these children should sustain neurological injury. Despite the severity of the neurological injury, however, the fractures are generally stable as a result of support of the rib cage. The axial loading of wedge compression fractures as well as anterior subluxations are generally stable. Because there is very little rotatory motion of the upper part of the thoracic spine, most injuries occur in flexion with axial loading. The "sagittal slice fracture" occurs when a vertebra above slices into the sagittal plane through the vertebra below, displacing half of the lower vertebra to a lateral position. Spinal dislocation in this instance results from a total disruption of the posterior and anterior ligaments as well as the disc. The resultant instability of this fracture may be compounded by inappropriate laminectomy, during which the posterior supporting elements are removed in the presence of an anterior compression fracture. In this situation, surgical intervention with decompression, internal fixation, and arthrodesis is essential for neurological recovery and prevention of kyphosis. Burst fractures associated with fractures of the neural arch, referred to as "shear" fractures, are limited to the lower thoracic and lumbar regions and frequently occur as a result of seatbelt injuries. These fractures are unstable.

The majority of fractures of the thoracic and lumbar spine occur at the fulcrum of motion, the thoracolumbar junction. All types of fractures may occur at this area, and neurological deficits may result from compression of the conus medullaris or cauda equina. Acute fractures of the thoracolumbar spine should be considered initially unstable and must be immobilized. The most unstable fracture in this region is the rotary fracture dislocation for which early reduction with internal fixation and fusion is the preferred treatment. Vertebral compression fractures with greater than 40% loss of vertebral body height require stabilization.

Location of Spinal Injury

Figures vary regarding the incidence of fractures in specific regions of the spinal column. Although numbers range from 39% to 79%, in all series, a majority of injuries in the pediatric population occur in the cervical spine. Anderson and Schutt[1] reviewed the Mayo Clinic experience encompassing 156 children under the age of 14 years who were admitted with injury of the spinal column or spinal cord between 1950 and 1978. Of these children, 39% had cervical

injuries, 10% had injuries between T1 and T5, 27% between T6 and T12, 17% between L1 and L4, and 6% below L4. The majority of other series report a larger proportion of cervical spine involvement, nearer the 70% range.[20,41]

Multiple levels of injury occur in 13% to 35% of patients and are most common in the thoracic spine as reported by McPhee.[34] In adolescence, the pattern of injury parallels that of the adult population.

Neurological Deficit after Spinal Injury

The majority of SCIs resulting in permanent loss of neurological function do not involve initial physical transection but rather compression and contusion.[38,57] During the first few hours after injury, impulse generation and conduction cease, blood flow to the injured segment decreases, and the consequent ischemia triggers extensive tissue destruction. The predominant pattern is a central to peripheral spread of the pathological condition.

Spinal cord injuries can be classified into the following syndromes: 1) complete lesions with loss of motor, sensory, and autonomic function distal to the injury; 2) central cord syndrome; 3) anterior cord syndrome with preservation of posterior column function; 4) posterior cord syndrome; 5) Brown-Séquard syndrome; and 6) root syndrome with pain and/or loss of neurological function in a radicular distribution.

Regardless of the specific neurological deficit, there is a consistent sequence of events required in the care of a child with SCI. This includes splinting and immobilization, medical stabilization, diagnostic procedures, alignment of the spine, decompression of the compressed neural elements, stabilization of the spine, and rehabilitation. The management of each phase of treatment and the rapidity with which it is effected may influence the final neurological outcome. Management of specific lesions is discussed in the sections that follow.

While the above steps are recommended for all patients with SCI, the administration of methylprednisolone continues to be recommended for those patients with nonpenetrating injury with neurological deficit. Results of the

Third National Acute Spinal Cord Injury Study have recently been published.[9] This study was a randomized double-blind clinical trial comparing the neurological and functional recovery and morbidity and mortality rates 1 year after acute SCI in patients who had received a standard 24-hour methylprednisolone regimen (30 mg/kg bolus followed by 5.4 mg/kg/hour infusion) to patients in whom an identical methylprednisolone regimen had been delivered for 48 hours or who had received 48 hours of a tirilazad mesylate regimen. Benefit from methylprednisolone was again noted in patients initially classified as having complete neurological lesions as well as those with incomplete lesions. However, the recommendation for length of therapy was changed. For patients in whom methylprednisolone therapy can be initiated within 3 hours of injury, a 24-hour course is still recommended. For patients starting therapy within 3 to 8 hours after injury, however, the methylprednisolone infusion should be continued for 48 hours unless there are complicating medical factors.

DIAGNOSIS

Clinical Presentation and Neurological Deficits

The diagnosis of SCI is generally made on the basis of recognized trauma followed by the immediate rapid development of the classic clinical syndrome of paralysis and spinal cord shock. Diagnosis in children is often not straightforward. The unique features of the pediatric spine allow for injuries in the spinal cord at various levels without fracture or dislocation. Additionally, a significant number of patients may have a delayed onset of neurological deficit with the latent period ranging from a few minutes to 3 or 4 days.[15,42,43]

A high index of suspicion is required to diagnose SCI in the acutely injured unconscious child. Injury to the vertebral column or the spinal cord should be suspected in the conscious individual with symptoms of neck pain, back pain, or localized tenderness and in a child in whom an asymmetric response to stimulation is obtained. Frontal or occipital head trauma and limitation of neck movement should alert the clinician to possible hyperextension or hyperflexion injuries to the cervical spine. Bruising across the cervical, thoracic, or lumbar spine often indicates an underlying osseous injury. Abdominal distention with hypotonia in the lower extremities is another clue to SCI. In the awake cooperative child, sensory, motor, and reflex examination allows one to reliably assess the level of cord injury. In spinal shock, there is flaccid paralysis below the level of the lesion and deep tendon reflexes are lost. There is urinary retention and autonomic imbalance resulting in hypotension. If the injury is not too severe, voluntary control is re-established and recovery begins within a few hours of injury. If the injury is severe, however, the spinal cord distal to the injury is isolated and mass reflexes set in, without improvement in voluntary motor activity or sensory perception. Assessment of reflexes is helpful in determining the level of lesion as reflex loss is generally consistent with the degree of motor involvement.

It is important to keep in mind that congenital abnormalities such as os odontoideum, Chiari I malformation, and Down's syndrome as well as underlying pathological conditions such as inflammatory disease of the upper respiratory tract may make the cervical spine prone to atlantoaxial instability with minor trauma.

An additional complicating factor in the evaluation of the child with SCI is that a large percentage of patients with major neurological involvement have normal radiographs. This is more fully discussed in the section on SCI without radiographic abnormality.

On the other hand, spinal fracture or ligamentous injury is frequently incurred without resulting neurological deficit. In a series published by the University of Iowa Hospitals and Clinics, Osenbach and Menezes[41] reviewed 179 children with injuries of the spinal column and cord (Table 1). Fifty-two percent sustained neurological injury. The neurological outcome was dependent on the severity of initial injury. The majority of children with mild to moderate injury regained complete function, while only one patient with complete injury became ambulatory. There was no significant difference between patients managed operatively or conservatively.

TABLE 1

ETIOLOGY, LEVEL, AND CLASSIFICATION OF SPINAL CORD INJURY*

	Group A (0-8 yrs)	Group B (9-16 yrs)
Total cases	62	117
Cause of injury		
Vehicular accidents	28 (45%)	72 (62%)
Falls	15 (24%)	15 (13%)
Athletics	1 (2%)	23 (19%)
Birth trauma	10 (16%)	0 (0%)
Penetrating wounds	3 (5%)	5 (4%)
Miscellaneous	5 (8%)	2 (2%)
Level of injury		
Upper cervical (O-C3)	33 (53%)	31 (26%)
Lower cervical (C4-7)	16 (26%)	32 (27%)
Thoracic	7 (11%)	17 (15%)
Thoracolumbar junction	2 (3%)	15 (13%)
Lumbosacral	4 (7%)	22 (19%)
Pattern of Injury		
Fracture only	23 (37%)	52 (44%)
Fracture-subluxation	9 (15%)	42 (36%)
Subluxation only	9 (15%)	10 (9%)
SCIWORA	21 (33%)	13 (11%)

*Number in parentheses represents percentage of patients within a given age group.

Hadley et al[20] reported a series in which 50% of patients had neurological deficit. The injury was incomplete in 33% and complete in 17%. In 89% of the incomplete injuries, improvement was noted. In a series by Kewalramani et al,[28] 81% of patients with cervical injuries remained quadriplegic and 83% of patients with thoracolumbar injuries remained paraplegic.

Thus, with regard to prognosis for children with traumatic quadriplegia, approximately 85% of patients whose injury was initially "complete" remained complete, while a small percentage regained some motor function in their legs. In severe partial lesions, up to 25% of patients may recover. In central cord lesions with relatively preserved function in the legs, recovery of lost motor power occurs in up to 75% of patients. Data pertaining to thoracic lesions are similar. Prognosis for patients with thoracolumbar junction injuries is better, with as many as 30% of those with initially complete lesions regaining some motor function.[38]

Radiographic Evaluation

When imaging the child with suspected spinal trauma, the aim should be to diagnose the entire extent of the injury. One has to be careful, however, not to worsen the patient's injury in attempting to fully define the extent of trauma. It is essential that the treating physician keep in mind the different modalities of imaging, as well as the order in which they should be implemented. The diagnostic studies should compliment one another and thus each component of the diagnostic process should be undertaken with an appreciation for its limitations and timeliness. The imaging modalities currently employed are plain radiographs, flexion/extension films, fluoroscopy, dynamic motion studies, computed tomography (CT) with or without myelography, and magnetic resonance imaging (MRI). Plain radiographs are utilized for imaging the entire spine. In the cervical region, imaging consists of anteroposterior (AP), lateral, oblique, and open-mouth views. The oblique views are obtained with 30° angulation of the x-ray film unit to the right and left and are useful for visualizing the facets. The open-mouth view, while often difficult to obtain in a child, can reveal fractures of the atlas or axis. Lateral radiographs must clear the C7-T1 interspace, and this frequently requires the patient's shoulders to be pulled down for a "swimmer's" view. The cervical alignment must be checked, and the retropharyngeal soft tissue space appraised. A high suspicion of spinal trauma must be entertained in children who are not awake or who have multiple injuries. With cervical spine injuries in the absence of neurological deficit and obvious fracture, dynamic flexion/extension views should be obtained to assess stability. The patient is instructed to voluntarily flex and extend the spine as far as possible. No attempt is made to increase the patient's range of motion. The extent of subluxation can easily be measured on the radiographs. These motion studies can also be obtained using cine- or fluoroscopic techniques. It must be kept in mind that a painful injury may mask evidence of cervical spine instability due to muscle spasm. If necessary, immobilization should be maintained until the spasm resolves and the radiographs are repeated.

The following criteria have been used to detect instability on plain radiographs at the craniocervical junction in children:[39] 1) predental space of >5 mm in patients younger than 8 years and >3 mm in those older than 10 years; 2) a total overhang of the atlas lateral masses on C2 of >7 mm in the open-mouth view, suggesting a Jefferson (C1) burst fracture with possible disruption of the transverse portion of the cruciate ligament; 3) vertical clivus odontoid translation of >2 mm; 4) "bare" occipital condyles indicating an occipitocervical dislocation; 5) any abnormal relationship between the spinal canal and the foramen magnum, except for widening of the interspace between the occiput and C1 and between C1 and C2 posteriorly; and 6) abnormal cervicocranial motion dynamics.

Pluridirectional tomography and CT have greatly enhanced our understanding of bony pathology. All identified fractures on plain radiographs must be visualized with CT to define the extent of bony injury and rule out potential spinal canal compromise from bony fragments. Any areas poorly visualized on plain radiographs or that are suspicious for injury should also be evaluated with CT. Two-dimensional and, at times, three-dimensional reconstructions are quite helpful.

Despite its usefulness, CT has limitations. This is particularly so when fractures parallel the plane of the scan. In addition, visualization of the spinal cord, ligaments, and other soft tissues is poor. The use of CT myelography has been obviated by MRI. MRI has the advantage of imaging long vertical segments and identifying spinal and spinal cord pathology such as hematomas, ligamentous disruptions, and disc herniations. For patients needing immediate stabilization in traction, MRI-compatible tongs and halo crowns are available.

SPECIAL CONSIDERATIONS IN CHILDREN

Neonatal SCI

Neonatal SCI occurs in approximately one in 60,000 births.[60] The unique structural characteristics of the newborn spine are such that it can be stretched to 5 cm without disruption, while the spinal cord and meninges may rupture with only 5 mm of stretching.[31] Approximately 70% of spinal injuries at birth occur with breech delivery, while 30% are associated with cephalic presentations.[17,26,41,56]

Excessive longitudinal traction, particularly with breech presentation, most commonly results in lower cervical and cervicothoracic junction injuries. Hyperextension of the head increases this risk.

Spinal cord injury occurs in cephalic presentations secondary to torsional forces applied in rotating the head and may be additionally associated with use of forceps. Such injuries typically affect the upper cervical cord. Distortion of the shoulder with traction being transmitted to the spinal cord can also cause SCI. Neonatal SCI in the thoracolumbar region is extremely rare but has been reported in association with breech delivery, prematurity, and vascular accidents.

Spinal cord injuries are easily overlooked at

birth owing to a lack of awareness and understanding of the neonate's susceptibility to injury, as well as the presence of other medical conditions, including lethargy or coma, that can be associated with co-existing hypoxic encephalopathy. A state of shock and difficulty in initiating respiration are common findings with neonatal SCI. Injuries occurring above the C3-4 spinal level are promptly fatal unless the infant is given constant respiratory support. The motor manifestations vary with the site of injury. Damage to the lower cervical and upper thoracic spinal cord, often associated with brachial plexus injuries, produces flaccidity of the arms and hands as well as respiratory embarrassment with paradoxical respiration and, occasionally, a Horner's syndrome. There are varying degrees of flaccidity of the lower extremities. Bladder paralysis is common but often does not require catheterization.

Radiographs of the spine, although usually normal, are useful in excluding congenital anomalies such as spina bifida and may occasionally demonstrate vertebral dislocation. If suspicion of a spinal injury is present, MRI should be performed as soon as possible and include visualization of the spinal canal as well as the posterior fossa.

The state of "spinal shock" subsides generally within the first few weeks, and it becomes possible to establish a reasonably accurate assessment of the infant's neurological status. Repeated examinations are therefore important. The infant is generally alert with few, if any, cranial nerve abnormalities unless the brainstem was injured with traction or by damage to its blood supply. Reflex movements develop in response to noxious stimuli over a wide receptive area in the arms and legs and may be confused with return of function. Spasticity may develop and rarely leads to contracture in the hips and femoral muscles.

Koch and Eng[29] reviewed the long-term prognosis of 14 infants with neonatal SCI. Eight of the 14 patients died: four at <3 months of age, three between 3 months and 1 year of age, and one at 3.5 years of age. Six children survived for more than 2 years. The quality of survival for those with functional levels of C8-T1 and below depended on the presence and severity of medical complications. Another limited study related prognosis according to the early rate of re-

covery.[59] In upper cervical SCI, the presence of breathing movements on Day of Life 1 was associated with only mild or moderate disability, where the absence of breathing movements by Day 2 was associated with severe disability. Persistent absence of breathing movements for the first 3 weeks after birth was associated with permanent total dependency on mechanical ventilation and associated severe spastic quadriplegia.

Trauma in Children Under 8 Years of Age

The majority of spinal canal and spinal cord trauma occurs in the cervical spine. In most children below the age of 8 years, this is referable to a level above C3. The odontoid process is most affected at the neurocentral synchondrosis. The superior segment angulates forward along the atlas vertebra (Figure 2). Radiographs may also reveal fractures of the pars interarticularis with anterior subluxation of the atlas and the body of C2 on C3. This combination of fractures is unstable and reduction is best achieved with the head and neck placed in a hyperextended position over the edge of a mattress.[39] Once adequate reduction of the spinal deformity has been achieved, rigid external immobilization can be obtained with the use of a halo vest. This offers the advantage of prolonged immobilization and active early rehabilitation.

Cervical traction in the toddler can be safely applied provided that factors such as skull thickness, age, and anatomic and biomechanical properties of the pediatric spine are taken into account. In patients under the age of 2 years, a halo ring can be used with eight pins for fixation to evenly distribute the forces at 1 to 2 lb per sq inch. This can be accomplished by tightening the pins using the index finger and thumb. In children between the ages of 2 and 4 years, pins should generally be tightened approximately 2 lb per sq inch. The amount of weight required to achieve reduction of a cervical spine subluxation is considerably less in small children than in teenagers or adults. Therefore, it is imperative that frequent films be obtained to ensure that overdistraction does not occur. Careful attention should be paid to the cleanliness of the halo pin and tong sites. Symptoms of local pain and

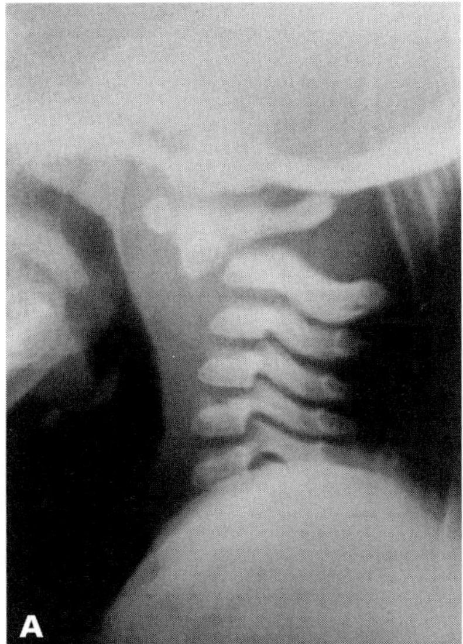
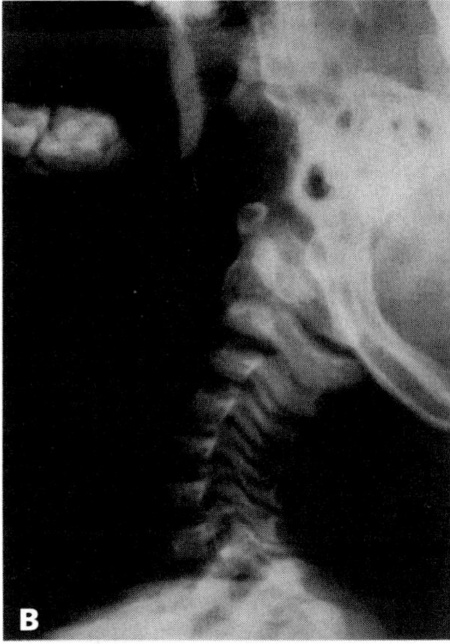

Figure 2: A) Lateral cervical radiograph in a 14-month-old child following a motor-vehicle accident. Note the odontoid fracture through the neurocentral synchondrosis and gross atlantoaxial dislocation. This child had no neurological deficit. **B)** Lateral cervical radiograph of the above patient made 3 months later demonstrating the healed odontoid fracture following traction, reduction, and immobilization.

headache may indicate penetration into the skull, leading to osteomyelitis or even cerebritis.

In up to 5% of children with cervical spine injuries, symptomatic disc herniation may be present.[5,14] Menezes at The University of Iowa has performed anterior cervical discectomies at the C3-4 level in nine patients age 6 to 8 years with good results. Other indications for surgery include the reduction of locked facets, debridement of compound wounds, removal of bone fragments from the spinal canal, and internal fixation of unstable fractures.

When posterior fusion is necessary in the cervical spine, wire fixation alone is inadequate. The wire may cut through the thin poorly ossified lamina or spinous processes. As the child grows, a position of hyperextension may develop or subsequent disruption of the wire with impingement of the spinal cord result.[21,35,41] The optimal fusion construct should be osseous. The optimal treatment is wiring of bone to each individual lamina or facet so that, once incorporation of the bone has taken place, the bone will continue to grow with the child. The bone graft is preferably harvested from a rib; however, the posterior iliac crest and the tibia are viable alter-

natives (Figure 3). In a series of over 200 such cervical fusions in children over the past 15 years, there has been no demonstrable decrease in growth potential or exaggerated lordosis with long-term follow-up.

Trauma in Children Over the Age of 8 Years

In children aged 8 and older, cervical injuries continue to predominate and account for 60% to 70% of injuries.[19,36] Cervical spine fractures are managed with reduction and immobilization. The presence of disc herniation and bone fragments or hematoma impinging on the spinal cord requires decompression and fusion. This may be accomplished via the anterior or posterior approach. Surgery is then followed by external immobilization and early rehabilitation.

Thoracic and thoracolumbar junction injuries are generally related to violent forces that occur with football injuries, crush injury, falls from a height, and motor-vehicle accidents. Unstable thoracic or thoracolumbar spine fractures, whether associated with complete or incomplete

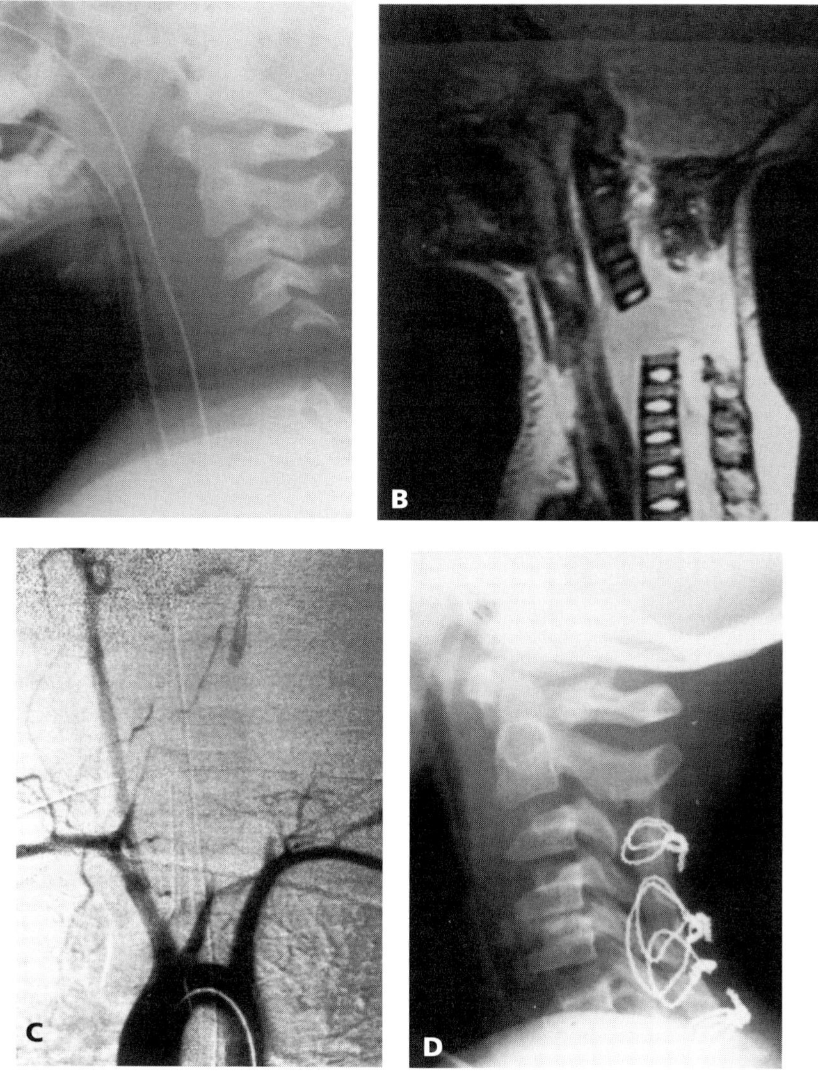

Figure 3: A) Lateral cervical radiograph in a 5-year-old child with acute quadriplegia following a motor-vehicle accident. Note the avulsion injury of the C5 vertebrae with a large gap between C5 and C6 and marked prevertebral swelling. **B)** Midsagittal T2-weighted MRI of the cervical spine reveals avulsion through the C5 vertebral body preserving the disc space with pseudomeningocele formation and nonvisualization of the spinal cord. **C)** Arch aortogram in the same patient revealing patency of the right carotid artery with occlusion of both the vertebrals and the left carotid. **D)** Lateral cervical spine radiograph following bilateral interlaminar rib graft fusion from C3 through C7. The alignment has been restored.

neurological injury, require stabilization. This is accomplished via the anterior route.[7,36,46,54] The transthoracic anterior approach to resect the involved vertebral body and disc allows direct visualization of the ventral dural sac and confirmation of decompression. A rib graft with vascularized pedicle can then be rotated into position and wedged between the vertebrae above and below the level of injury. Removal of the disrupted bony segment prevents kyphosis, and the vascularized rib graft shows incorporation into the recipient site within 6 to 8 weeks.

Thoracic fractures can also be approached via the transpedicular or costotransversectomy posterolateral routes. These approaches allow for satisfactory ventral decompression as well as posterior column instrumentation.

Thoracolumbar junction fractures are best approached via a posterolateral decompressive route, which allows for visualization of the dura and spinal cord.[36,41] A concomitant transpedicular approach to the ventral spinal canal permits the anterolateral bony decompression to be performed. Segmental stabilization is preferred over the use of the long Harrington rod or Luque fixation. As discussed with the cervical spine, bony fusion is mandatory.

Craniovertebral Junction Injuries

The craniovertebral junction encompasses the occipital bone and the atlas and axis vertebrae, along with their stabilizing ligaments. This transition zone between the skull and vertebral joints is unique in that it allows extensive movement and yet its vertebrae are interlocked in an amazingly stable three-dimensional structure. The diagnosis and treatment of trauma to this region require a thorough understanding of the osseous anatomy, ligamentous structures, and their functional properties along with the joint kinematics. This is a particularly important region with regard to pediatric spinal injury because the proportion of injuries involving this complex is extremely high, especially in young children.

Injuries to the craniovertebral junction are divided into the following:[39,61]

- ligamentous injuries (occipitoatlantal dislocation and atlantoaxial dislocation);
- osseous injuries (occipital condyle fracture, Jefferson fracture, and odontoid fractures); and
- complex injuries (transaxial cervicomedullary junction injury, traumatic spondylolisthesis of C2 (hangman's fracture), and combined osseous ligamentous disruptions).

Occipitoatlantal Dislocation

The literature concerning traumatic occipitoatlantal dislocation is limited. Although not uncommon, this diagnosis is not frequently seen clinically because it results in complete disruption of the cervicomedullary junction and immediate death at the scene of the accident. Because the actual incidence is obscured by the devastating nature of the injury itself, occipitoatlantal dislocation had previously been presumed to occur only rarely. Bucholz and Burkhead,[11] in a review of 112 victims of trauma who died at the scene of injury, found that 26 had had cervical spine injury. Of the 26, nine had a traumatic occipitoatlantal dislocation and five had an odontoid fracture. Alker and coworkers in a similar review found 19% to have occipitoatlantal dislocation. In a series of 18 patients with traumatic occipitoatlantal dislocation and four with lesser forms of ligamentous occipitoatlantal disruption, six patients succumbed to their injury.[37] Despite the severity of damage, the number of survivors with this injury has continued to increase owing to improved on-sight resuscitation and transportation by emergency units.

Several mechanisms have been implicated as the cause of occipitoatlantal dislocation, with the most frequent being hyperflexion of the head combined with distraction. Other mechanisms of injury include lateral flexion and extreme hyperextension leading to disruption of the tectorial membrane.[45,48] Forward displacement of the cranium on the atlas is associated with ligamentous disruption of the anterior occipitoatlantal ligament, the tectorial membrane, the alar ligaments, and the posterior elements of the occipitoatlantoaxial complex. Although anterior occipitoatlantal dislocation is most common, lateral occipitoatlantal dislocation, posterior cranial displacement, as well as isolated longitudinal distraction have been reported.

Avulsion of cranial nerves as well as transection of the medulla oblongata and/or upper cervical cord can be found on postmortem examination. Infants and young children who survive frequently have overwhelming neurological dysfunction and are generally comatose with flaccid hemiplegia or quadriplegia and diaphragmatic breathing. In other instances, survivors may have altered levels of consciousness with abnormal lower cranial nerve function and a combination of spinal cord abnormalities.

Several radiographic criteria for the diagnosis of occipitoatlantal dislocation have been proposed to aid in the early diagnosis with plain ra-

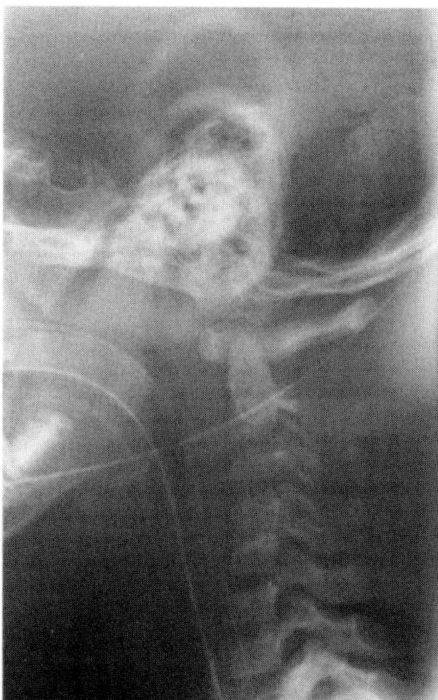

Figure 4: Lateral cervical spine radiograph, including the posterior fossa, in a 6-year-old child following a motor vehicle accident. The patient has no limb extremity movement and is on a ventilator. Note the "bared occipital condyles," an increase in the prevertebral shadow in the retropharyngeal space, and the widened interspace distance between the atlas and the axis vertebra. These findings are suggestive of craniocervical-occipitocervical ligamentous injury.

diography. Separation of the occipital condyles from the atlas with the finding of "bare" occipital condyles and significant displacement of the odontoid from the basion are highly suggestive. The presence of a retropharyngeal hematoma may be the first hint to the diagnosis (Figure 4). Thin-section CT with sagittal and coronal reconstruction is recommended to evaluate all patients with suspicious upper cervical spine radiographs. MRI best identifies the ligamentous disruption as well as spinal cord and brainstem hemorrhagic contusion and the possible presence of epidural hematoma external to the tectorial membrane. Angiography may reveal stenosis or occlusion of the vertebral arteries.

Cervical traction should never be used in patients with known or suspected occipitocervical instability. Occipitocervical dislocation requires immediate immobilization in a halo vest. Operative intervention utilizing a contoured loop for occipitocervical fixation is ideal and should be implemented as soon as the patient's condition allows it. Osseous integration can be achieved by utilizing bone grafts at the same time.

Atlantoaxial Instability and Luxation

The term "luxation" refers to a complete and lasting disruption of the articular facets of synovial joints. Examples of this are the interlocking of interarticular facets or the marked diastasis that occurs with hyperflexion fracture luxation. Atlantoaxial luxations can be divided into anterior, posterior, and rotational subtypes. In the setting of trauma, the frequency of fracture of the odontoid process in children is much greater than atlantoaxial luxation. This is in agreement with the biomechanical study of the atlantoaxial ligament complex by Fielding and Hawkins,[16,22] which showed that the force required to fracture the odontoid process was much less than the force required to cause failure of all the ligaments in the same specimen. The anterior and rare posterior atlantoaxial luxation can be a finding in acute as well as chronic nonunited fractures of the odontoid process. The rotatory luxations require more attention and will be discussed in detail.

Under normal circumstances, rotation of the atlas about the axis is within the range of 35°. If rotation exceeds 40°, facet interlock occurs.[16,35,53] This occurs most frequently in trauma; however, it is not an uncommon finding in children with infections of the upper respiratory system or other inflammatory conditions. In a series of 36 patients with atlantoaxial rotatory luxation, trauma was the causative factor in all patients.[37] Football spearing was present in a significant number of injuries, followed by motor vehicle accidents and wrestling injuries. An associated occipitoatlantal rotatory luxation was not uncommon. This series did not include patients with Down's syndrome, who are also predisposed to abnormalities at the craniovertebral junction.

Children with atlantoaxial rotatory luxation usually present with painful torticollis and a limited range of neck motion. An associated occipitoatlantal rotatory luxation leads to a characteristic "cock-robin" appearance (Figure 5A).[61] Facial flattening is also prominent. The diagnosis may go unrecognized if the symptoms are minor or it may be diagnosed when associated with brainstem dysfunction or cervical myelopathy. Symp-

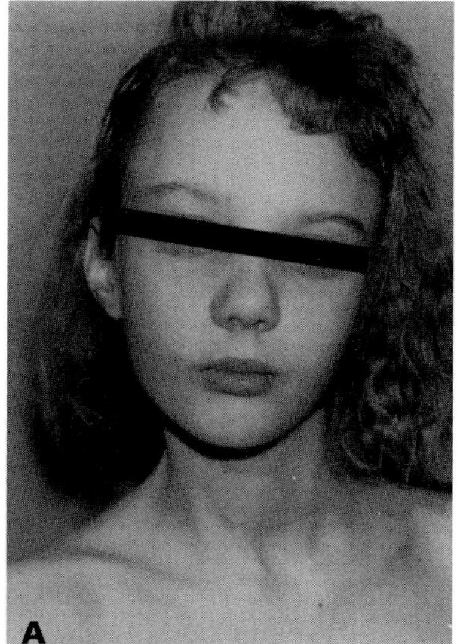
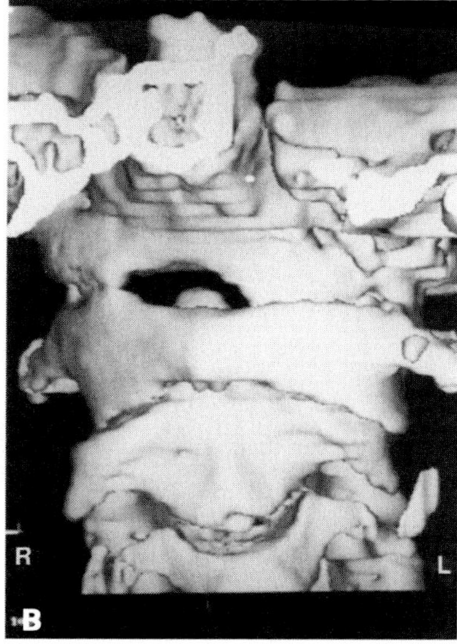
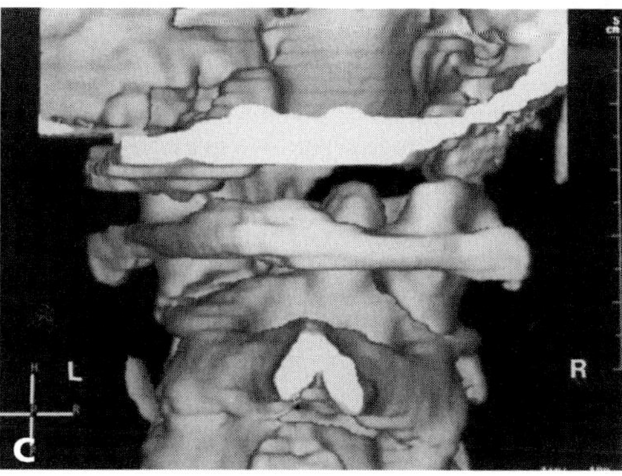

Figure 5: A) Frontal photograph of 9-year-old child with a rotatory occipito-atlantoaxial subluxation following a fall backward while skipping rope. Note the "cock-robin" head position. **B)** Three-dimensional CT of the craniocervical junction, frontal view. Note the perched occipital condyle on the tip of the lateral mass of C1 on the right with a ventral location of the lateral atlantal mass on the left. **C)** The perched right occipitoatlantal articulation is well defined with a tilt of the head. The posterior displacement of the right atlantal mass is better visualized.

toms of neural compression occur when the atlas is separated from the odontoid process by >5 mm, allowing a rotation of the atlas on the axis and thus compromising the spinal canal. Children with rotatory atlantoaxial subluxation have been erroneously diagnosed as having brainstem vascular insults, cerebellar tumor, Chiari malformation, cervical migraine, syringohydromyelia, and ocular palsies (Figure 6B).[35]

The diagnostic procedures utilized are AP and lateral cervical radiographs, pluridirectional tomography, cineradiography, CT, and MRI. The entity may be difficult to diagnose owing to radiographic problems in visualizing the complex anatomy of the area. Overriding of the atlas in relationship to the axis on an AP radiograph is abnormal and a clue to the diagnosis. On a lateral radiograph, there should be normal alignment of the facet joints of the upper cervical spine. Rotation of the atlas is usually seen in relation to the axis, with forward projection of the atlantal lateral masses anterior to the odontoid process. This represents a large bulk of bone in front of the odontoid process, which should also be a clue to the diagnosis (Figure 6A). If the skull and atlas are in a true lateral position, the cervical spine shows a prominence of the facet joints rather than a true lateral picture in the subaxial region. This persistent asymmetry in the atlantoaxial relationship is not corrected by rotation unless it is reduced. This is easily seen on cine CT or cineradiography, which show the subluxed axis and atlas moving as a unit during neck rotation.

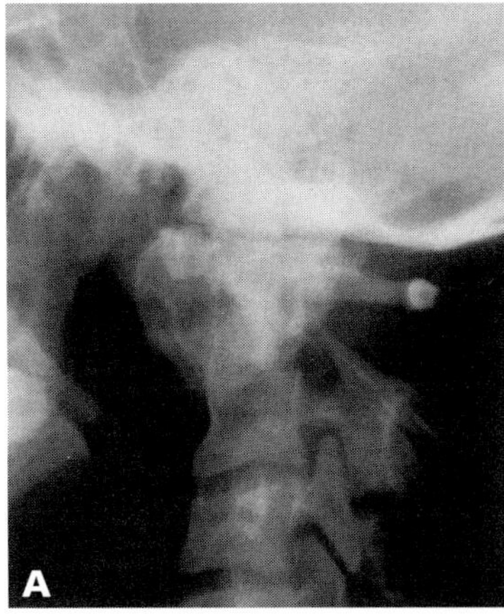
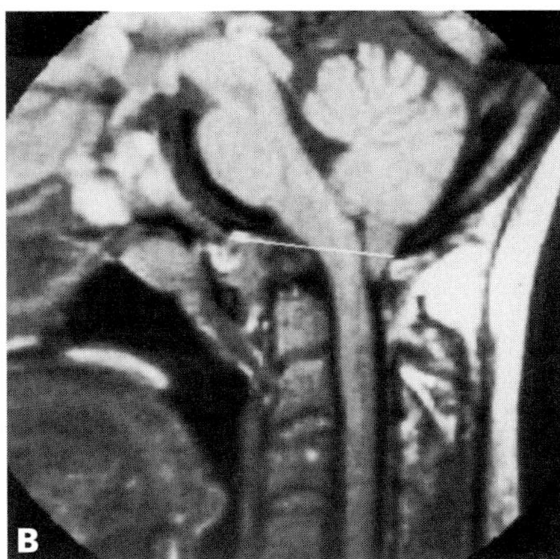
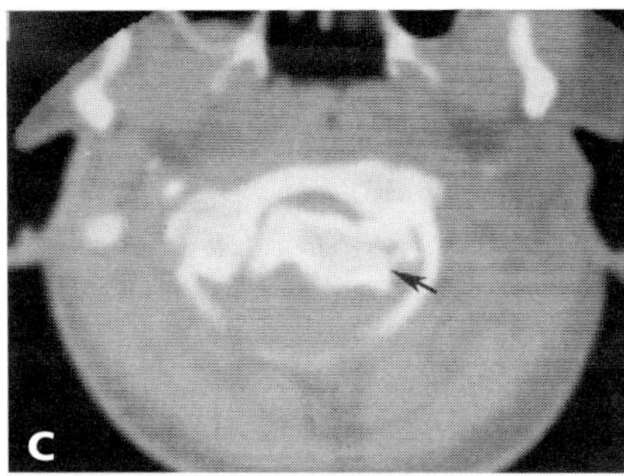

Figure 6: A) Lateral cervical radiograph in a 15-year-old child following neck manipulation for myringotomy and tubes under general anesthesia. There is a large mass to the anterior arch of C1 indicative of an anterior position to the lateral atlantal mass. This finding most likely signifies atlantoaxial rotary subluxation. This diagnosis was missed clinically. **B)** Midsagittal T1-weighted MRI of the posterior fossa and upper cervical spine demonstrating odontoid basilar invagination through the plane of foramen magnum as outlined with ventral compression of the cervicomedullary junction and a downward descent of the cerebellar tonsils. This patient was referred due to a Chiari I malformation. **C)** Axial CT through the plane of the atlas defines atlantoaxial rotary dislocation with a facet interlock on the right.

The best visualization of the abnormality is seen on CT with three-dimensional reconstruction (Figure 5B and C). Alternatively, a dynamic study using CT or MRI can be obtained through the craniovertebral complex.[37,39] No motion is seen at the C1-2 articulation in a fixed luxation, be it unilateral or bilateral. This is easily visualized on CT with the head turned to the extreme right and then turned to the extreme left. MRI provides information regarding the patency of the vascular structures as well as possible neural compromise.

Treatment of this condition depends on the integrity of the transverse ligament and the secondary support ligament complex. If these ligaments are intact, rotation will generally not exceed 40° and, in such cases, reduction and realignment with traction are often successful. The patient is then immobilized in a halo for 3 months or until healing occurs. If the transverse ligament is ruptured, the atlas may be displaced anteriorly, causing compromise of the spinal canal. This situation requires reduction and operative fixation (C1-2 posterior fusion) with postoperative halo immobilization.

Jefferson's Fracture

Jefferson's fracture is caused by excessive axial loading resulting in divergent lines of force passing through the lateral masses of the atlas. The lateral masses are wedged shaped and can be easily displaced in an outward manner with bursting of the C1 ring at the vertebral artery groove, its weakest point. Therefore, posterior arch fractures are the most common; however, the anterior arch of C1 may fracture with axial loading in extreme flexion. In fact, the original fracture described by Jefferson[25] was a four-part burst fracture.

Atlas fractures in children are more common than previously believed.[36,39,61] Neurological deficits are rarely significant in C1 arch fractures, and symptoms are usually limited to localized pain. Jefferson's fracture is considered a stable injury that responds well to conservative management with Philadelphia collar or halo immo-

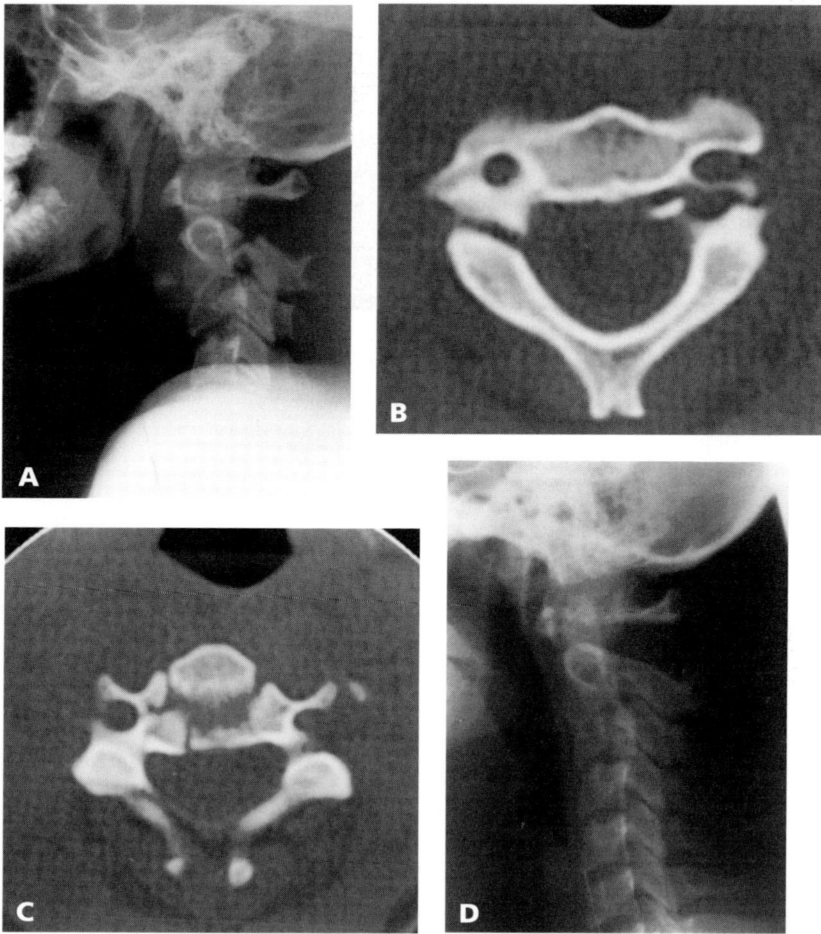

Figure 7: A) Lateral cervical radiograph demonstrating bilateral pars fractures with C2-3 angulation consistent with a "hangman's fracture." **B)** Axial CT through the axis body demonstrating the bilateral pars interarticularis fractures. **C)** Axial CT through the body of C3 defining the comminuted fracture of the body. **D)** Lateral cervical radiograph obtained 1 year following the incident. There is satisfactory upper cervical alignment without canal compromise.

bilization. One must be aware, however, that a significant proportion of patients with C1 fractures have additional associated cervical spine fractures, most commonly of the adjacent axis vertebra.

Axis/Odontoid Fractures

The two most common axis fractures in children are hangman's fracture and fractures of the odontoid process. Most commonly, these injuries occur as a result of major trauma involving either hyperflexion or hyperextension of the head on the cervical spine.

Hangman's fractures are unusual in young children. This injury comprises bilateral fractures of the pars interarticularis of C2, generally resulting from hyperextension and axial loading. The hangman's fracture is usually unstable, although neurological deficit is rare. This injury can be adequately managed with halo immobilization and rarely requires operative fusion in the form of C1-3 posterior arthrodesis (Figure 7).

Odontoid fractures in children present different problems from those seen in the adult. In children up to the age of 10 years, these fractures are avulsion injuries at the neurocentral synchon-

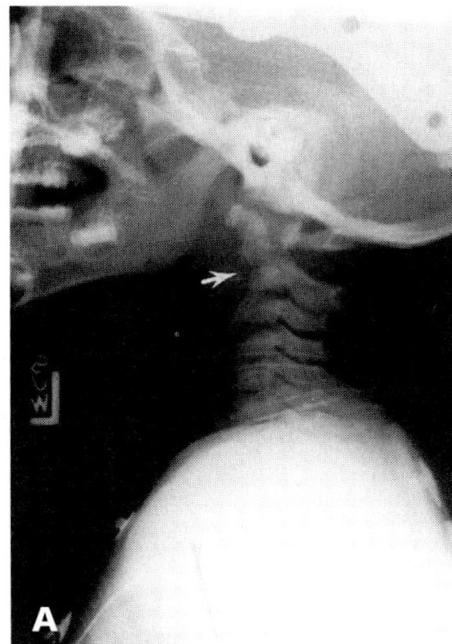

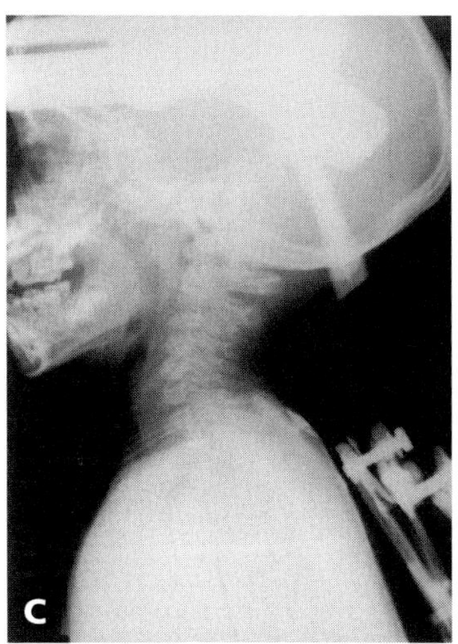

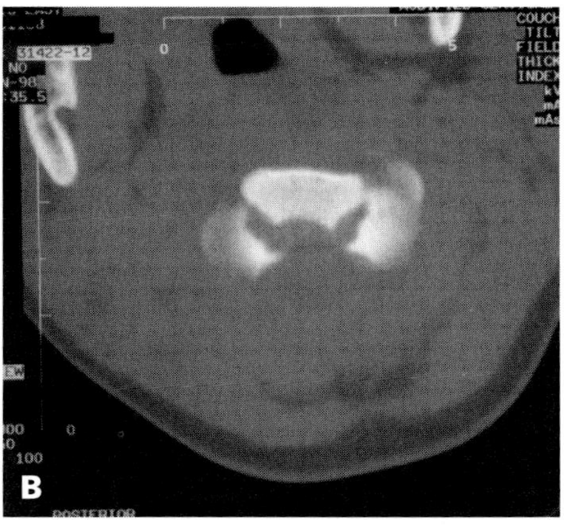

Figure 8: A) Lateral cervical radiograph in a 2-year-old child following neck trauma. Note the avulsion fracture of the odontoid process. **B)** Axial CT through the plane of the axis body demonstrating the avulsion fracture of the body through the neurocentral synchondrosis. **C)** Lateral cervical radiograph in halo with moderate extension at the craniocervical region. This film shows satisfactory reduction of the odontoid onto the axis body with reconstitution of the spinal canal.

drosis. Ligamentous laxity and incomplete ossification in young children make them more susceptible to this type of injury. These fractures can usually be reduced with gentle cervical traction and are managed with complete immobilization in a halo vest or Minerva jacket for 8 to 10 weeks (Figure 8).[20,45] In children older than 8 to 10 years, odontoid fractures can be divided into the adult forms of type I, type II, and type III.

While odontoid fractures in children carry a good prognosis, prompt recognition and treatment are required to prevent later complications. Failure to adequately treat this injury may result in resorption of the base of the dens or os odontoideum with latent atlantoaxial instability (Figure 9).

SCIWORA

SCIWORA (SCI without radiographic abnormality) is the eponym used to describe the occurrence of traumatic myelopathy in the absence of any demonstrable contiguous osseous or ligamentous abnormality. The term "SCIWORA" was coined by Pang and Wilberger[44] in 1982 in their report of a large group of children who sustained traumatic spinal injury despite normal radiographic studies. Earlier, authors reported similar cases of SCI that would fall into this category.[23,30,36,43]

By definition, a SCIWORA has negative radiographic studies. Plain radiographs including flexion/extension views and CT reveal no evidence of abnormality. MRI, however, has made the term SCIWORA inaccurate because it detects injury to the spinal cord and ligaments not previously visualized. Nonetheless, the term is still widely accepted.

The incidence of SCIWORA among all cases of pediatric SCI has been estimated to be as much as 55% to 65%.[44] SCIWORA occurs al-

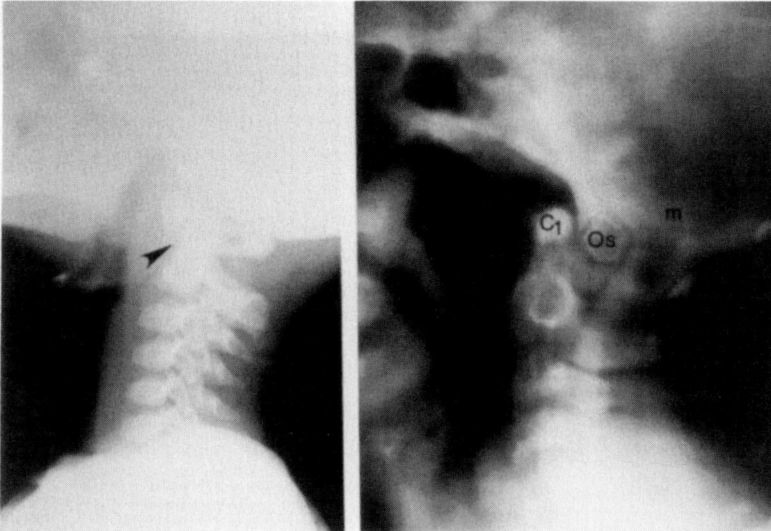

Figure 9: Composite of a lateral cervical radiograph made in a child at age 6 *(left),* and a midline sagittal myelotomogram (Iohexol) of the same patient 7 years later *(right).* The radiograph *(left)* shows a complete odontoid process with atlantoaxial instability present *(arrowhead).* The myelotomogram *(right)* now shows a dystopic os odontoideum (os) causing ventral compression of the medulla (M) and cervicomedullary junction.

most exclusively in the pediatric population, with the majority of cases occurring in children younger than 8 years of age. The high incidence of SCIWORA in this subgroup can be attributed to the previously discussed unique anatomic and biomechanical features of the pediatric spine. Although extremely rare, this injury has been reported in adults.

Multiple mechanisms of injury have been implicated in the pathophysiology of SCIWORA. These include flexion, hyperextension, longitudinal distraction, and ischemia. Flexion forces, which most often result in fracture and/ or dislocation in adolescents, can result in significant translational motion in the pediatric spine with subsequent return of the spinal column to its normal alignment. Flexion injuries tend to occur more commonly in the very young, have been associated with upper cervical injuries, and often result in severe neurological deficit.

Hyperextension may result in inward buckling of the ligamentum flavum with a decrease in the sagittal diameter of the spinal canal by as much as 50%. Hyperextension may also result in

compression and spasm of the vertebral arteries that might lead to spinal cord ischemia and infarction. Hyperextension injuries occur in children of all ages, have been associated with lower cervical injuries, and often result in milder neurological deficit. Excessive distraction has been implicated as an important mechanism of SCIWORA, especially in neonatal injuries, as previously discussed.

Dickman et al[15] reviewed the literature on SCIWORA and were able to find reports of 201 cases, of which 104 had adequate data from which to draw conclusions. They found that cervical and thoracic injuries occurred with about equal frequency (44% and 48%, respectively); however, given the length and number of segments of the cervical spine, a disproportionately large number of injuries seem to involve this region. Osenbach and Menezes[42] reported on 31 children with SCIWORA, of which 26 (84%) were affected in the cervical spine. All upper cervical injuries occurred in children younger than 8 years of age.

Up to 52% of children with SCIWORA pre-

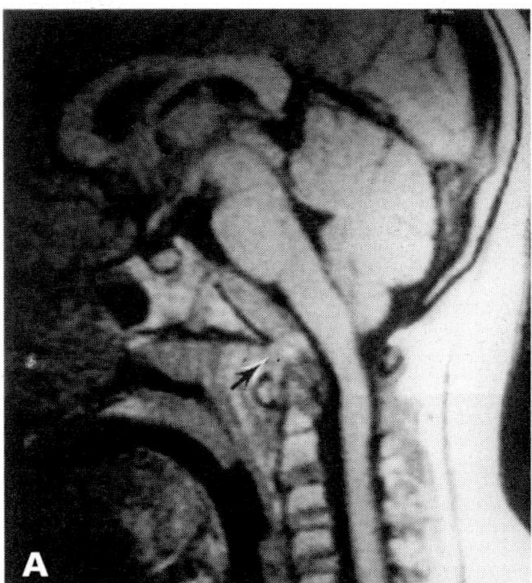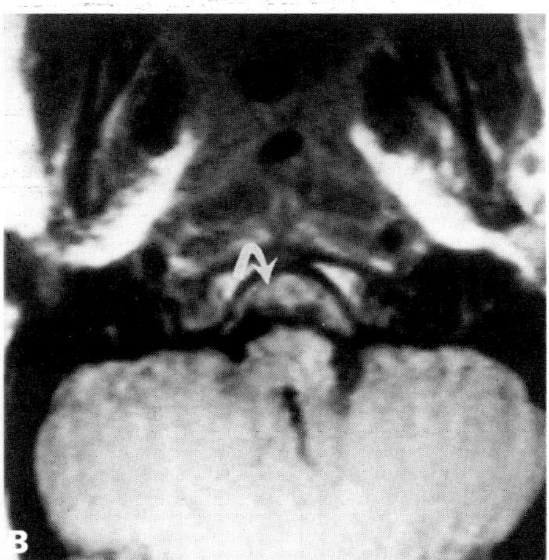

Figure 10: A) Midsagittal T1-weighted MRI of the posterior fossa and upper cervical spine in a 5-year-old child involved in a motor vehicle accident. Note the epidural hematoma behind the clivus and the odontoid process with the cervicomedullary junction being displaced dorsally. **B)** Axial T1-weighted MRI through the middle of the posterior fossa visualizing the epidural hematoma with displacement of the medulla dorsally.

sent with delayed onset of neurological deficit.[42] The delay may range from several hours to 4 days after what may have been considered a trivial injury. Once noted, however, the deficit often progresses rapidly to a severe fixed deficit. In retrospect, many children describe a history of premonitory neurological symptoms such as transient paresthesias, numbness, and/or subjective motor weakness. The neurological examination at the time of initial evaluation may reveal one of four individual syndromes: partial dysfunction of the spinal cord, central cord syndrome, Brown-Séquard syndrome, or complete physiological transection. Given the large proportion of patients who describe a history of premonitory symptoms, even trivial neurological complaints in a child with potential spinal injury must be taken seriously to avoid a potentially preventable disaster.

Diagnosis can be made only after complete evaluation with plain radiographs including flexion/extension views, thin-section CT, and MRI, which is useful for evaluating surgical lesions such as herniated discs and epidural hematoma (Figure 10).

Patients who have minor symptoms and are neurologically intact at presentation should re-frain from physical activity until subsequent clinical follow-up and may benefit from immobilization. At times, follow-up radiographs a week after injury will reveal ligamentous injury and dynamic instability not present on the acute films.

It is not uncommon for children with partial neurological dysfunction to have a recurrent episode a few weeks following the initial insult. To regain ligamentous stability after the initial neurological injury, these children should undergo bracing for 3 months.

Corticosteroids are indicated in SCIWORA with persistent neurological deficit as in other cases of SCI.

SEQUELAE OF PEDIATRIC SCI

Improvements in the acute and chronic care of pediatric SCI patients have resulted in a significant increase in the number who survive into adulthood. Because of the increased life expectancy, complications associated with SCI have become more prevalent. Many problems, including decubitus ulcers, urinary tract infections, pulmonary infections, myositis ossificans, and a variety of psychological problems, are similar to those encountered in the adult. Much literature exists on the diagnosis and treatment of these conditions. Two sequelae have particular relevance to the neurosurgeon: posttraumatic spinal deformity and posttraumatic syringomyelia.

Posttraumatic Spinal Deformity

The incidence of progressive spinal deformity in series of pediatric SCI with long-term follow-up is extremely high, sometimes exceeding 90%.[6,10,32] Posttraumatic spinal deformity is relatively unique to the growing child. It is uncommon in patients who are near the end of their growth cycle. The deformities encountered include scoliosis, kyphosis, and lordosis. Major factors that contribute to progressive spinal curvature are epiphyseal damage (which interferes with normal growth of the spine and leads to the development of scoliosis) and paralysis of the postural muscles of the spine below the level of injury. Lesions caudal to T12-L1 are less likely to result in scoliosis, as most of the postural muscles remain innervated. As the scoliotic curve progresses, additional changes occur in the vertebral bodies. On the concave side of the curve there is deficient growth of the lamina and articular processes, while on the convex side there is excessive growth of the vertebral body and discs.[49] The development of significant spinal deformity leads to pelvic obliquity, difficulty in sitting, and ischial weight bearing, which predisposes to decubitus ulcers. Curves exceeding 60% may compromise cardiopulmonary function as well as result in intestinal and bladder dysfunction.

Age at the time of injury seems to be the most important risk factor for the development of scoliosis. It is generally agreed that in children with unstable thoracolumbar fractures and SCI, early instrumentation and fusion are indicated. In young children with complete SCI, one should consider extending the fusion several segments more than would normally be required for stability alone. External orthoses as a means of delaying spinal fusion are acceptable but should be used as a temporary measure and are inadequate as a definitive treatment. Surgical fusion is ultimately required in the majority of children.

Posttraumatic Syringomyelia

The development of a syrinx following traumatic SCI is a well-documented occurrence. Schurch et al[52] in a prospective study of 449 patients with SCI found MRI-documented syringomyelia in approximately 4%. Experimental studies in animals have documented the presence of myelin microcysts within the vicinity of spinal cord transection.[18,33,55] Kao et al[27] suggested that these microcysts rupture and coalesce to form the syrinx cavity. Tethering of the spinal cord at the site of injury together with elevation of the central venous pressure is believed to ultimately result in transmission of this elevated pressure to the epidural veins. This subsequently alters the tension within the syrinx and leads to dilatation and extension of the cyst.

Posttraumatic syringomyelia may become clinically symptomatic relatively early (within months) following SCI; more commonly, the onset of symptoms is delayed for several years. The average latency from onset of symptoms to diagnosis is approximately 3 years. The clinical onset is usually heralded by pain in the most rostral area of dysfunction. Pain frequently originates in the neck and radiates into the upper extremities; it is typically exacerbated by sneezing, coughing, or other Valsalva maneuvers. There is often upper migration of the lowest area of hypesthesia. As the lesion progresses within the cervical cord, weakness and atrophy involving the arm muscles develop and deep tendon reflexes become hypoactive. Extension of the cavity into the brainstem (syringobulbia) can lead to cranial nerve dysfunction or paroxysmal episodes of unconsciousness. In patients with incomplete spinal cord lesions, the symptoms may consist of increased weakness and spasticity along with progressive loss of bladder, bowel, and sexual function. Hyperhidrosis has also been commonly reported.

Diagnosis is most accurately demonstrated on MRI, which clearly reveals the extent of the syrinx cavity and effectively excludes other pathological processes. The mere presence of a symptomatic posttraumatic syringomyelia, however, is not an indication for treatment. The progression of symptoms should guide the physician in deciding whether an operative procedure is warranted.

The primary procedure of choice for post-traumatic syringomyelia is a syringosubarachnoid shunt. This procedure is facilitated by use of the operating microscope, as meticulous attention to preservation of the arachnoid membrane during dural opening is needed. Intraoperative ultrasonography is useful for locating the syrinx cavity. Median myelotomy is performed, and a small silicone catheter is inserted cephalad for 2-3 cm into the cavity. The catheter is anchored to the arachnoid membrane at the myelotomy site and passed caudally into the subarachnoid space for several centimeters. In a series of 14 patients with posttraumatic syringomyelia treated with syringosubarachnoid shunts, improvement was demonstrated on long-term follow-up in 12 patients.[38] Syringoperitoneal shunting is preferred in cases where there is significant arachnoiditis. A dorsal root entry zone lesion may be considered if pain persists despite demonstration of collapse of the syrinx after shunting.

Conclusions

The anatomic and biomechanical variations of the developing spine result in unique injury patterns in children. An understanding of these variations is essential for the successful management of children with spinal column trauma. The incidence of cord injury is quite high in children who sustain spinal injuries, and the social and economic consequences are devastating. Although the overall management of patients with SCI has advanced, the prognosis for those with severe injuries remains poor. Perhaps the most important contribution that can be made is to educate children of all ages as well as adults in the prevention of these devastating injuries.

References

1. Anderson JM, Schutt AH: Spinal injury in children: a review of 156 cases seen from 1950 through 1980. **Mayo Clin Proc** 55:499-504, 1980
2. Apple DF, Jr, Anson CA, Hunter JD, et al: Spinal cord injury in youth. **Clin Pediatr** 34:90-95, 1995
3. Babcock JL: Cervical spine injuries. Diagnosis and classification. **Arch Surg** 111:646-651, 1976
4. Backe HA, Betz RR, Mesgarzadeh M, et al: Post-traumatic spinal cord cysts evaluation by magnetic resonance imaging. **Paraplegia** 29:607-612, 1991
5. Baily DK: The normal cervical spine in infants and children. **Radiology** 59:712-719, 1952
6. Banniza von Bazan UK, Paeslack V: Scoliotic growth in children with acquired paraplegia. **Paraplegia** 15:65-73, 1977
7. Bohlman HH: Treatment of fractures and dislocations of the thoracic and lumbar spine. **J Bone Joint Surg (Am)** 67:165-169, 1985
8. Bracken MB, Freeman DH Jr, Hellendrand KA: Incidence of acute traumatic hospitalized spinal cord injury in the United States, 1970–1977. **Am J Epidemiol** 113:615-622, 1981
9. Bracken MB, Shepard MJ, Holford TR, et al: Methylprednisolone or tirilazad mesylate administration after acute spinal cord injury: 1-year follow up. Results of the third National Acute Spinal Cord Injury Study randomized. **J Neurosurg** 89:699-706, 1998
10. Bradford DS: Deformities of the thoracic and lumbar spine secondary to spinal injury, in Bradford DS, Lonstein JE, Moe JH, et al (eds): **Moe's Textbook of Scoliosis and Other Spinal Deformities. 2nd ed.** Philadelphia, Pa: WB Saunders, 1987, pp 435-463
11. Bucholz RW, Burkhead WF: The pathological anatomy of fatal atlanto-occipital dislocations. **J Bone Joint Surg (Am)** 61:248-250, 1979
12. Burke DC: Traumatic spinal paralysis in children. **Paraplegia** 11:268-276, 1974
13. Caffey J: The whiplash shaken infant syndrome: manual shaking by the extremities with whiplash-induced intracranial and intraocular bleedings, linked with residual permanent brain damage and mental retardation. **Pediatrics** 54:396-403, 1974
14. Cattell HS, Filtzer DL: Pseudosubluxation and other normal variations in the cervical spine in children. **J Bone Joint Surg** 47:1295-1309, 1965
15. Dickman CA, Rekate HL, Sonntag VKH, et al: Pediatric spinal trauma: vertebral column and spinal cord injuries in children. **Pediatr Neurosci** 15:237-256, 1989
16. Fielding JW, Hawkins RJ: Atlanto-axial rotatory fixation. (Fixed rotatory subluxation of the atlanto-axial joint.) **J Bone Joint Surg (Am)** 59:37-44, 1977
17. Franken EA Jr: Spinal cord injury in the newborn infant. **Pediatr Radiol** 3:101-104, 1975
18. Gabriel KR, Crawford AH: Identification of acute posttraumatic spinal cord cyst by magnetic resonance imaging: a case report and review of the literature. **J Pediatr Orthop** 8:710-714, 1988
19. Garrick JA, Requa RK: Injuries in high school sports. **Pediatrics** 61:465-469, 1978
20. Hadley MN, Zabramski JM, Browner CM, et al: Pediatric spinal trauma: review of 122 cases of spinal cord and vertebral column injuries. **J Neurosurg** 68:18-24, 1988
21. Hasue M, Hoshino R, Omata S, et al: Cervical spine injuries in children. **Fukushima J Med Sci** 20:115-123, 1974
22. Hawkins RJ, Fielding JW, Thompson WJ: Os odontoideum: congenital or acquired. A case report. **J Bone Joint Surg (Am)** 58:413-414,1976
23. Hill SA, Miller CA, Kosnik EJ, et al: Pediatric neck injuries. A clinical study. **J Neurosurg** 60:700-706, 1984
24. Holdsworth F: Fractures, dislocations, and fracture-dislocations of the spine. **J Bone Joint Surg (Am)** 52:

1534-1551, 1970

25. Jefferson G: Fracture of the atlas vertebra. Report of four cases, and a review of those previously records. **Br J Surg 7:**407-422, 1920

26. Jones EL: Birth trauma and the cervical spine. **Arch Dis Child 45:**147, 1970 (Abstract)

27. Kao CC, Chang LW, Bloodworth JMB Jr: The mechanism of spinal cord cavitation following spinal cord transection. Part 2: Electron microscopic observations. **J Neurosurg 46:**745-756, 1977

28. Kewalramani LS, Kraus JF, Sterling HM: Acute spinal-cord lesions in a pediatric population: epidemiological and clinical features. **Paraplegia 18:**206-219, 1980

29. Koch BM, Eng GM: Neonatal spinal cord injury. **Arch Phys Med Rehabil 60:**378-381, 1979

30. Kraus JF: Epidemiological aspects of acute spinal cord injury: a review of incidence, prevalence, causes, and outcome, in Becker DP, Povlishock JT (eds): **Central Nervous System Trauma Status Report.** Bethesda, Md: National Institute of Neurological and Communicative Disorders and Stroke, National Institutes of Health, 1985, pp 313-322

31. Leventhal HR: Birth injuries of the spinal cord. **J Pediatr 56:**447-453, 1960

32. Mayfield JK, Erkkila JC, Winter RB: Spine deformity subsequent to acquired childhood spinal cord injury. **J Bone Joint Surg (Am) 63:**1401-1411, 1981

33. McComas CF, Frost JL, Schochet SS Jr: Posttraumatic syringomyelia with paroxysmal episodes of unconsciousness. **Arch Neurol 40:**322-324, 1983

34. McPhee IB: Spinal fractures and dislocations in children and adolescents. **Spine 6:**533-537, 1981

35. Menezes AH: Traumatic lesions of the craniovertebral junction, in VanGilder JC, Menezes AH, Dolan K (eds): **Textbook of Craniovertebral Junction Abnormalities.** Mt Kisco, NY: Futura, 1987, pp 195-216

36. Menezes AH, Godersky JC, Smoker WRK: Spinal cord injury, in McLaurin RL, Schut L, Venes JL, et al (eds): **Pediatric Neurosurgery: Surgery of the Developing Nervous System. 2nd ed.** Philadelphia, Pa: WB Saunders, 1989, pp 198-317

37. Menezes AH, Muhonen M: Management of occipitocervical instability, in Cooper PR (ed): **Management of Posttraumatic Spinal Instability.** Baltimore, Md: Williams & Wilkins, 1990, pp 65-76

38. Menezes AH, Osenbach RK: Spinal cord injury, in Cheek WR (ed): **Pediatric Neurosurgery. 3rd ed.** Philadelphia, Pa: WB Saunders, 1994, pp 320-343

39. Menezes AH, Piper JG: Anatomy and radiographic pathology of injury to the occipito-atlanto-axial complex, in Wilkins RH (ed): **Disorders of the Spine and Peripheral Nerves Symposia.** Baltimore, Md: Williams & Wilkins, 1993, pp 1-16

40. Menezes AH, Smoker WRK, Dyste GN: Syringomyelia, Chiari malformations and hydromyelia, in Youmans J (ed): **Textbook of Neurological Surgery. 3rd ed.** Philadelphia, Pa: WB Saunders, 1990, pp 1421-1459

41. Osenbach RK, Menezes AH: Pediatric spinal cord and vertebral column injury. **Neurosurgery 30:**385-390, 1992

42. Osenbach RK, Menezes AH: Spinal cord injury without radiographic abnormality in children. **Pediatr Neurosci 15:**168-175, 1989

43. Pang D, Pollack IF: Spinal cord injury without radiographic abnormality in children—the SCIWORA syndrome. **J Trauma 29:**654-664, 1989

44. Pang D, Wilberger JE Jr: Spinal cord injury without radiographic abnormalities in children. **J Neurosurg 57:**114-129, 1982

45. Pang D, Wilberger JE Jr: Traumatic atlanto-occipital dislocation with survival: case report and review. **Neurosurgery 7:**503-508, 1980

46. Paul RL, Michael RH, Dunn JE, et al: Anterior transthoracic surgical decompression of acute spinal cord injuries. **J Neurosurg 43:**299-307, 1975

47. Perlman M: Neonatal spinal cord injury in the infant: etiology, diagnosis, treatment and outcome, in Betz RR, Mulcahey MJ (eds): **The Child with a Spinal Cord Injury.** Rosemont, Ill: American Academy of Orthopaedic Surgeons, 1996, pp 161-167

48. Powers B, Miller MD, Kramer RS, et al: Traumatic anterior atlanto-occipital dislocation. **Neurosurgery 4:** 12-17, 1979

49. Roaf R: Scoliosis secondary to paraplegia. **Paraplegia 8:**42-47, 1970

50. Rossier AB, Foo D, Shillito J, et al: Posttraumatic cervical syringomyelia. Incidence, clinical presentation, electrophysiological studies, syrinx protein and results of conservative and operative treatment. **Brain 108:** 439-461, 1985

51. Ruge JR, Sinson GP, McLone DG, et al: Pediatric spinal injury: the very young. **J Neurosurg 68:**25-30, 1988

52. Schurch B, Wichmann W, Rossier AB: Post-traumatic syringomyelia (cystic myelopathy): a prospective study of 449 patients with spinal cord injury. **J Neurol Neurosurg Psychiatry 60:**61-67, 1996

53. Selecki BR: The effects of rotation of the atlas on the axis. Experimental work. **Med J Aust 1:**1012-1015, 1969

54. Seljeskog EL: Thoracolumbar injuries. **Clin Neurosurg 30:**626-641, 1983

55. Shannon N, Symon L, Logue V, et al: Clinical features, investigation and treatment of post-traumatic syringomyelia. **J Neurol Neurosurg Psychiatry 44:**35-42, 1981

56. Stern WE, Rand RW: Birth injuries to the spinal cord. A report of 2 cases and review of the literature. **Am J Obstet Gynecol 78:**498, 1959

57. Tator CH, Fehlings MG: Review of the secondary injury theory of acute spinal cord trauma with emphasis on vascular mechanisms. **J Neurosurg 75:** 15-26, 1991

58. Venes JL: Spinal cord injury, in McLaurin RL (ed): **Pediatric Neurosurgery.** New York, NY: Grune & Stratton, 1982, pp 333-343

59. Vogel L, DeVivo MJ: Etiology and demographics, in Betz RR, Mulcahey MJ (eds): **The Child with a Spinal Cord Injury.** Rosemont, Ill: American Academy of Orthopaedic Surgeons, 1996, pp 3-12

60. Vogel L, Mulcahy MJ, Betz RR: The child with a spinal cord injury. **Dev Med Child Neurol 39:**202-207, 1997

61. Von Torklus D, Gehle W: The upper cervical spine. Regional anatomy, pathology and traumatology, in Verlag GT (ed): **A Systemic Radiological Atlas and Textbook.** New York, NY: Grune & Stratton, 1972, pp 2-91

62. White AA III, Panjabi MM: The clinical biomechanics of the occipitoatlantoaxial complex. **Orthop Clin North Am 9:**867-878, 1978

CHAPTER 18

SPORTS AND RECREATION AS CAUSES OF SPINAL CORD INJURY: EPIDEMIOLOGY, SCREENING, INJURY MANAGEMENT, AND RETURN TO PLAY

CHARLES H. TATOR, CM, MD, PHD, FRCS(C), FACS

Sports and recreation are common causes of spinal cord injury (SCI). Indeed, depending on the country and region, sports and recreation may comprise 20% or more of the cases of SCI.[9,10,23] In general, the clinical manifestations and principles of management of these injuries are similar to SCI due to other causes. However, there are several unique and special features peculiar to sports and recreation, such as when to remove the helmet on an injured football player and when to return to play. As well, there is the issue of whether an athlete with an SCI, especially an elite athlete, should be treated differently from other patients with SCI. Thus, it is important for all neurosurgeons and orthopedic surgeons to be aware of the principles of management of SCIs occurring in sports and recreation.

EPIDEMIOLOGY

Worldwide, diving is the most common cause of acute SCI in sports and recreation.[7,11,21] The injuries in diving are almost always to the cervical spine, and there is a high incidence of complete SCI. These injuries occur most often in the set-ting of unsupervised recreation at the lakeside, the ocean, or in private pools, and less often in a supervised setting such as a pool at a school. Trained divers seldom sustain SCI. With respect to organized sports, football in the United States and hockey in Canada are the sports with the highest incidence of acute SCI.[14,24] These sports also cause a high incidence of accelerated degenerative spinal changes that can lead to chronic myelopathy and radiculopathy. In the U.S. and in Canada, registries have been developed that provide systematic reporting of the incidence of SCI related to football[14] and hockey.[21] Major prevention programs have been developed to deal with some of the identified causes of these injuries, such as "clotheslining" and "spearing" in football and hitting from behind into the boards in hockey. Other organized sports with a high incidence of spinal injury or SCI are gymnastics (including the trampoline), wrestling, skiing, hang gliding, mountain climbing, rugby, and horseback riding.[2,8] Bicycling and motor sports, including snowmobiles, all-terrain vehicles, dirt bikes, and motorcycle racing, also are involved in large numbers of SCI in specific locations suitable for these recreational activities.

In both organized and unorganized sports and recreation, males comprise approximately 80% of the SCIs, with the exception of horseback riding, which affects males and females in almost equal proportions. In sports and recreation, the SCI victims are usually young. Indeed, SCI in sports such as hockey, football, and rugby often involves teenagers. In sports as well as other activities that cause SCI, children under the age of 11 have a lower incidence of SCI but are prone to ligamentous injuries of the upper cervical spine; older children have injuries in the middle and lower segments of the cervical spine, similar to adults.[13]

LEVEL, SEVERITY, AND TYPE OF NEUROLOGICAL DEFICIT AND VERTEBRAL COLUMN INJURY

Overall, cervical cord injury is much more common in sports and recreation than are thoracic or thoracolumbar injuries.[7] In certain activities such as diving, the SCIs are almost exclusively cervical. Motor sports involving all-terrain vehicles and snowmobiles cause a large number of thoracic and thoracolumbar injuries. Similar to the findings in non-athletic injuries, about 60% of SCIs in sports and recreation are incomplete injuries, with American Spinal Injury Association (ASIA) grades of B, C, and D (see Chapter 4, Table 3, for an explanation of grading); in sports such as diving, complete injuries with an ASIA grade of A predominate. Root injuries may occur in sports and recreation SCIs, especially related to acute disc herniations in the cervical, thoracic, thoracolumbar, and lumbosacral regions.

Many of the sports and recreational injuries of the spine involve axial loading, and this is especially true in football and hockey where burst fractures and compression fractures frequently occur. The combination of flexion and axial loading or extension and axial loading can lead to fracture-dislocations with or without associated disc rupture. Bilateral locked facets in the cervical region with anterior dislocation or fracture-dislocation is common in diving, and gymnasts have a propensity for fractures of the pars interarticularis in the lumbar region.

INJURY PREVENTION

Unfortunately, screening of participants is of limited value in terms of prevention of SCI in sports and recreation. Routine radiological examination of the spine in all athletes is not cost-effective, although there are specific exceptions to this rule. For example, atlanto-axial dislocation is a recognized complication in persons with Down's syndrome[4,19] and in some persons with Klippel-Feil syndrome and other congenital anomalies;[17] all such patients should have flexion-extension views prior to participation. Fortunately, the incidence of SCI in the Special Olympics is very low.[19] The issue of routine radiological screening in high-risk sports such as football and hockey has not been settled. There is no definite evidence that certain presumed radiological risk factors such as the ratio of the diameter of the cervical spinal canal to the cervical body, other measures of spinal stenosis, or the features of the so-called "spear tackler's spine" are proven contraindications to play.[25-27] Lumbar spondylolisthesis has been shown to be present in a high proportion of gymnasts,[3,20] but it has not been shown that this is a proven contraindication to participation, although the continuing pain associated with this condition may limit participation. The same is true of progressive degenerative spondyloarthropathies in sports such as hockey and football. The pain and neurological deficits associated with disc protrusions and osteophytes, which produce radiculopathy and/or myelopathy, may prevent return to play.

The education of players, coaches, trainers, referees, and the administrators of sports leagues and associations is an important aspect of injury prevention. There should be an emphasis on respect for the health and safety of all players, including the opponents. Awareness of the specific risk factors inherent in individual sports is essential. Repeated safety messages can be given via coaching sessions, videos, posters, and other means. Players should be warned about highly dangerous maneuvers such as tackling with the "head into the numbers" in football and checking from behind in hockey. There is mounting evidence that these prevention measures have helped reduce the incidence of SCI in football and hockey.[15,22] There should be screening of the participants in sports such as rugby to exclude small-stature players from vulnerable positions. Proper conditioning also has value, especially neck muscle conditioning in young athletes with poorly developed neck muscles who play contact sports such as hockey and football. Adherence to appropriate return-to-play guidelines as outlined below will also help reduce the incidence of catastrophic spinal injury.

Prevention can also be promoted by attention to the structural and physical aspects of the sports venue and by the use of special equipment that has been developed to enhance sports safety. For example, breakaway goal posts in hockey and padded goal posts in football are strongly advocated, although absolute proof of their effectiveness is lacking. There is a need for improved helmet design in many sports. More research is required to determine the best shape and padding for energy deflection and energy absorption, respectively. It should be noted that there is no definite evidence that helmets have led to an increase in SCI in sports such as hockey or that improved helmets can actually reduce the incidence of SCI. It may be true that "helmets can neither cause nor prevent serious neck injuries."[5] However, it is the view of this author that proper helmet design and use can reduce the incidence and severity of SCI in certain sports such as hockey.

Injury Management

It is important for physicians associated with sports teams or athletic or recreational events to have the necessary equipment and training to safely and effectively provide first aid, and preparation for the management of a catastrophic spinal or head injury is essential.[12] The attending physician or trainer should quickly obtain a thorough history of the injury, inquiring specifically for spinal pain, muscle weakness, and sensory loss followed by a specific examination of the nervous system, including motor power and sensation. Finally, the trainer or physician should perform gentle manual palpation of the entire spine, examining for tenderness and deformity. Effective treatment also includes the prevention of secondary injury by appropriate first aid, the correct diagnosis, and judicious treatment at the injury site. These measures will prevent the worsening of neurological deficits or the initiation of a neurological deficit in persons without an initial deficit who have an unstable spinal injury. It is essential to ensure absolute immobilization of the entire spine during any required transfers and transport. Special attention must be given to careful documentation of all previous injuries, as this information is essential for inclusion in the deliberations regarding return to play.

With few exceptions, the first aid and subsequent hospital management of the athlete with an acute SCI are identical to the management of other patients with these injuries.[12] In football and hockey, one of the specific differences relates to helmet removal in players who are also wearing shoulder pads. When these players are injured, the helmet should not be removed first. If there is a problem with airway management, only the facemask should be removed, and this can be accomplished with heavy wire cutters. Removal of the helmet first in a player wearing shoulder pads may cause extension of the neck because of the thickness of the shoulder pads. Thus, it is recommended that the shoulder pads and helmet be removed simultaneously while maintaining the neck in axial alignment with the trunk.[6,16]

The subsequent in-hospital management of the SCI in athletes is no different from other persons with SCIs, although the issue of return to play presents a specific management challenge in athletes as outlined below. As with other injuries to the spine, athletic injuries require meticulous imaging to detect evidence of present or previous injury to the spine and spinal cord including ligamentous injury, and to detect spinal instability and intracanalicular space-occupying lesions such as herniated discs. Liberal use of magnetic resonance imaging is recommended to detect ligamentous injury and subtle evidence of previous or current cord injury, sometimes evident only on high-resolution T2-weighted images.

Return-to-Play Guidelines

In general, the neurosurgeon or orthopedic surgeon should use the same guidelines when treating athletes as used when treating the general population of patients. However, the practi-

TABLE 1

CRITERIA FOR DETERMINING RETURN TO
SPORTS OR RECREATION FOLLOWING A SPINAL INJURY

Safe Criteria for Allowing Return to Play Following a Spinal Injury
- No residual neurological symptoms or signs of neurological deficit
- No residual symptoms of vertebral column disorder, including a painless full range of motion of the spine
- No radiological or imaging lesion of the cord or nerve roots
- No radiological or imaging lesion of the cord or nerve roots including absence of instability on flexion-extension views

Absolute Indications for Advising No Return to Play Following a Spinal Injury
- Residual neurological deficit related to cord injury
- Unstable spinal column
- Major spinal stenosis
- Congenital or operative fusion of two or more motion segments
- Evidence on MRI of spinal cord lesion such as T2-weighted signal change, syrinx, etc.

Possible Indications for Advising No Return to Play Following a Spinal Injury
- Residual neurological deficit related to root injury
- Congenital or operative fusion of one or more motion segments
- Cervical spondylosis of advanced degree
- Repeated transient spinal cord injury or spinal cord concussion

tioner should anticipate that athletes may treat themselves differently from the general population. The practitioner should be prepared to resist intimidation by relatives, coaches, trainers, league officials, and players' agents.

Many factors need to be considered when advising athletes about return to play after sports and recreational injuries of the spine. Although there have been very good attempts to develop guidelines about return to play after a spinal injury,[1,18,25] there is still a great deal of uncertainty. The decision about return to play depends primarily on the nature of the injury and the nature of the activity in which the athlete is engaged (Table 1).

The Nature of the Injury

Athletes with both neurological and spinal column injuries pose special problems compared to those with spinal column injuries alone. After a permanent SCI, it is best to advise the patient to not return to contact sports. However, if the cord injury has been transient, or if the injury involves only a root injury and there is no significant spinal column injury, the athlete may be eligible for return to play. The nature of the spinal column injury is the next most important variable to consider. If the spinal column injury is stable, such as a spinous process or transverse process fracture, or a mild compression fracture, then the athlete can probably be allowed to return to play, with or without surgical treatment. In the case of an unstable injury, the athlete should not be permitted to return to play unless stability can be restored either by conservative or operative means. Athletes who have had an operative fusion involving one spinal motion segment or who have undergone a single corpectomy for burst fracture may be eligible for return to play 6-12 months later. Most athletes who have had a radiculopathy due to a herniated disc can be allowed to return to play following conservative or operative treatment.

The Nature of the Sports or Recreational Activity

With contact sports such as hockey, football, or rugby, the potential for recurrent injury is much greater, and athletes with significant neurological or spinal column injuries can seldom return to play. Caution must also extend to sports with potential contact such as skiing, horseback riding, and baseball. Less caution is required for non-contact activities such as tennis.

Athletes who require surgery such as cervical or lumbar fusion are permitted a gradual return to activity beginning with walking only in the first month, and progressing to floor exercises and bicycling. In the second month postoperative, weight training can begin and swimming is encouraged. In the third month, treadmill workouts can be allowed, with return to aerobic exercises in the fourth month. With respect to contact sports, athletes should not participate until next season after a cervical or lumbar fusion or after disc removal.

In summary, players should not return to play if there is persisting neurological deficit and/or spinal column instability. In patients with a neurological deficit, return to play may be permitted when there has been full recovery of the neurological deficit and if the spinal column is stable. In those without a neurological deficit, return to play may be permitted if the spinal column is stable. All of these possibilities are tempered by the nature of the activities involved.

REFERENCES

1. Bailes JE, Hadley MN, Quigley MR, et al: Management of athletic injuries of the cervical spine and spinal cord. **Neurosurgery 29:**491-497, 1991
2. Bruce DA, Schut L, Sutton LN: Brain and cervical spine injuries occurring during organized sports activities in children and adolescents. **Primary Care 11:**175-194, 1984
3. Caine DJ, Lindner KJ, Mandelbaum BR, et al: Gymnastics, in Caine DJ, Caine CG, Lindner KJ (eds): **Epidemiology of Sports Injuries.** Champaign, Ill: Human Kinetics, 1996, pp 213-246
4. Chang FM: The disabled athlete, in Stanitski CL, DeLee JC, Drez D (eds): **Pediatric and Adolescent Sports Medicine.** Philadelphia, Pa: WB Saunders 1994, Vol. 3, pp 48-76
5. Clarke KS, Jordan BD: Sports neuroepidemiology, in Jordon BD, Tsairis P, Warren RF (eds): **Sports Neurology. 2nd ed.** Philadelphia, Pa: Lippincott Raven, 1998, pp 3-13
6. Ford M: Neck, spinal cord and back, in Bull RC (ed): **Handbook of Sports Injuries.** New York, NY: McGraw-Hill, 1999, pp 55-71
7. Katoh S, Shingu H, Ikata T, et al: Sports-related spinal cord injury in Japan (from the nationwide spinal cord registry between 1990 and 1992). **Spinal Cord 34:**416-421, 1996
8. Keene JS, Albert MJ, Springer SL, et al: Back injuries in college athletes. **J Spinal Disord 2:**190-195, 1989
9. Kraus JF: Epidemiologic features of injuries to the central nervous system, in Anderson DW (ed): **Neuroepidemiology, a Tribute to Bruce Schoenberg.** Boca Raton, FL: CRC Press, 1991 pp 333-357
10. Kraus JF, Franti CE, Riggins RS, et al: Incidence of traumatic spinal cord lesions. **J Chron Dis 28:**471-492, 1975
11. Kurtzke JF: Epidemiology of spinal cord injury. **Exp Neurol 48(3 Pt 2):**163-236, 1975
12. Leidholt JD: Spinal injuries in athletes: be prepared. **Orthop Clin North Am 4:**691-707, 1973
13. McGrory BJ, Klassen RA, Chao EY, et al: Acute fractures and dislocations of the cervical spine in children and adolescents. **J Bone Joint Surg (Am) 75:**988-995, 1993
14. Mueller FO, Blyth CS: An update on football deaths and catastrophic injuries. **Phys Sportsmed 14:**139-142, 1986
15. Mueller FO, Zemper ED, Peters A: American football, in Caine DJ, Caine CG, Lindner KJ (eds): **Epidemiology of Sports Injuries.** Champaign, Ill: Human Kinetics, 1996, pp 41-62
16. Palumbo MA, Hulstyn MJ, Fadale PD, et al: The effect of protective football equipment on alignment of the injured cervical spine: radiographic analysis in a cadaveric model. **Am J Sports Med 24:**446-453, 1996
17. Pizzutillo PD: Klippel-Feil syndrome, in **The Cervical Spine Research Society Editorial Committee: The Cervical Spine, 2nd ed.** Philadelphia, Pa: JB Lippincott, 1987, pp 258-271
18. Rappoport LH, Cammisa FP Jr, O'Leary PF: Fractures and dislocations of the cervical spine, in Jordan BD, Tsairis P, Warren RF (eds): **Sports Neurology. 2nd ed.** Philadelphia, Pa: Lippincott-Raven Press, 1998, pp 157-179
19. Robson HE: The Special Olympic games for the mentally handicapped—United Kingdom 1989. **Br J Sports Med 24:**225-230, 1990
20. Sward L: The thoracolumbar spine in young elite athletes. Current concepts on the effects of physical training. **Sports Med 13:**357-362, 1992
21. Tator CH: Diving, in Jordan BD, Tsairis P, Warren RF (eds): **Sports Neurology. 2nd ed.** Philadelphia, Pa: Lippincott-Raven Press, 1998, pp 375-380
22. Tator CH, Carson JD, Cushman C: Spinal injuries in Canadian ice hockey players, 1966-1996, in Cantu RC (ed): **Neurologic Athletic Head and Spine Injuries.** Orlando, Fla: WB Saunders, 2000 (In press)
23. Tator CH, Duncan EG, Edmonds VE, et al: Changes in epidemiology of acute spinal cord injury from 1947 to 1981. **Surg Neurol 40:**207-215, 1993
24. Tator CH, Edmonds VE, Lapczak L, et al: Spinal injuries in ice hockey players, 1966–1987. **Can J Surg 34:**63-69, 1991
25. Torg JS, Glasgow SG: Criteria for return to contact activities following cervical spine injury. **Clin J Sport Med 1:**12-26, 1991
26. Torg JS, Pavlov H: Cervical spinal stenosis with neuropraxia and transient quadriplegia. **Clin Sports Med 6:**115-133, 1987
27. Torg JS, Sennett B, Pavlov H, et al: Spear tackler's spine: an entity precluding participation in tackle football and collision activities that expose the cervical spine to axial energy inputs. **Am J Sports Med 21:**640-649, 1993

CHAPTER 19

NUTRITION ASSESSMENT AND MANAGEMENT IN SPINAL CORD INJURY PATIENTS

DONNA J. RODRIGUEZ, MS, RD, CNSD

Close attention to the metabolic alterations and nutritional status of patients with spinal cord injury (SCI) is necessary to optimize medical and neurological outcomes. Following injury, well-documented hypermetabolic and hypercatabolic responses can result in the detrimental consequences of malnutrition, loss of lean body mass, increased susceptibility to infections, and impaired wound healing. Paralysis and functional losses that commonly occur after SCI produce additional metabolic and nutritional derangements.

Optimal nutritional assessment and management of SCI patients can potentially minimize complications associated with acute traumatic injury and long-term rehabilitation. This chapter describes postinjury metabolic responses, nutritional assessment methods, specific nutrient considerations, and nutrition support techniques for SCI patients.

METABOLIC RESPONSES TO SCI

Two unique metabolic responses to SCI, distinguished by acute and chronic time frames, impose several confounding variables onto this complex pathophysiological process.

Acute Stage

Major injury has been described as a "sudden stimuli to which the organism is not quantitatively or qualitatively adapted."[28] Increased circulating levels of glucagon, cortisol, catecholamines, and cytokines are primarily responsible for the initial metabolic alterations after traumatic injury.

Energy Expenditure

Following injury, remarkable increases have been observed in energy expenditure, endogenous protein catabolism, and nitrogen excretion.[15,34,36,42,43,77] Extensive multisystem trauma, soft tissue injury, and long bone fractures commonly associated with SCI can further augment the hypermetabolic response.[53] Body temperature and energy expenditure also increase after SCI due to pulmonary or urinary tract infections and pancreatitis.[9,16] The metabolic rate does not appear to be influenced by the small decreases in plasma thyroxine levels that are observed after injury.[23]

In addition to postinjury hypermetabolism, decreased energy expenditure related to paralysis and immobility contribute to the acute metabolic state. The loss of sympathetic innervation and the inability of muscles to shiver also lead to wide ranges in basal metabolic rates.[10,22,66] The degree of impaired temperature regulation is proportional to the extent and spinal level of paralysis.

To determine more accurately the initial energy expenditures after SCI, studies have compared actual resting energy expenditure (REE) measurements to the Harris-Benedict equation (basal energy expenditure (BEE)).[37]

$$BEE_m \text{ (men)} = 66 + (13.7 \times \text{weight [kg]}) + (5 \times \text{height [cm]}) - (6.8 \times \text{age [yrs]})$$

$$BEE_w \text{ (women)} = 655 + (9.6 \times \text{weight [kg]}) + (1.7 \times \text{height [cm]}) - (4.7 \times \text{age [yrs]})$$

During the first and second weeks after SCI, actual REE measurements are similar to estimated calorie needs when the BEE is used in conjunction with the stress/injury factor of 1.6.[61,62] Elimination of the activity factor of 1.2 (bed rest) was suggested to avoid overestimation of caloric needs. Kearns and associates[41] reported that the mean REE following acute SCI in 10 patients was only 67% of the predicted Harris-Benedict BEE. They hypothesized that nonspecific changes in neurogenic stimuli and decreased oxygen consumption by flaccid muscles contributed to their findings. Of interest, they also observed that the REE increased by 5% as muscle tone returned.[41]

Obligatory Negative Nitrogen Balance

Acute postinjury nitrogen requirements are much higher than maintenance levels. Accelerated catabolism of lean body mass results in a supply of amino acids for acute-phase protein synthesis, for gluconeogenesis, and for wound repair. Glucocorticoid administration after SCI can also exacerbate protein catabolism. In some traumatized patients, the administration of growth hormone has reduced nitrogen losses and could prove to prevent muscle wasting after SCI.[51]

Urinary nitrogen losses, due primarily to muscle atrophy from paralysis, increase in proportion to the severity of the SCI.[27,28] Cooper and Hoen[27] reported that urinary nitrogen excretion of >25 gm/day during the first two postinjury weeks is a poor prognostic sign for the functional recovery of paralyzed muscles. Nitrogen losses following SCI are obligatory and persist for at least 7 weeks.[27,28,43,62] Despite the delivery of adequate calories and protein, a negative nitrogen balance (NB) commonly occurs in acute SCI patients, peaking during the third week after injury.[62] This same phenomenon has been observed with severe cases of botulism poisoning that have resulted in muscle paralysis.[17]

The obligatory negative NB that follows SCI has been associated with additional findings. During the first week following injury, many SCI patients have a transiently positive NB, possibly due to an initial delay in nitrogen losses.[62] Dietrick et al[31] evaluated four conscientious objectors who were immobilized in pelvic girdles and leg casts for 6 to 7 weeks on a metabolism ward. All four subjects showed an increase in nitrogen excretion and a negative NB. This, however, also took 4 to 5 days to develop. In conclusion, acute immobilization of paralyzed patients contributes to the increased nitrogen excretion that begins about 1 week after injury.

Impaired Glucose and Lipid Metabolism

Glucose and lipid metabolism are impaired in the acute postinjury stage. Hyperglycemia results from increased hepatic gluconeogenesis and peripheral insulin resistance. Derangements in glucose metabolism in relation to acute neural injury have been extensively studied, especially as they relate to ischemia.[32,47,50,59,60] These studies suggest that hyperglycemia immediately following head trauma or SCI may worsen outcome. High serum glucose levels increase substrate availability for anaerobic glycolysis, and thus for the production of lactic acid,[52] which may have an adverse effect on the neurological recovery from injury.[7] Prevention of hyperglycemia, especially during the first 2 to 8 hours postinjury, appears to be crucial for optimal recovery. After 2 to 8 hours postinjury, increased glucose levels may be advantageous, allowing for enteral or parenteral feedings to begin soon after injury.[7] Elevated serum triglyceride levels may also occur due to accelerated lipogenesis, decreased lipoprotein lipase activity, and an impaired triglyceride clearance.

Negative Calcium Balance

After acute SCI, decreased osteoblastic activity and bone collagen losses lead to dramatic increases in bone degradation.[20,74] This rapid and intense bone resorption begins within 10 days and lasts for at least 6 months postinjury, resulting in hypercalciuria and, possibly, hypercalcemia. A low calcium intake is not effective in decreasing high urine or serum calcium levels and is not advisable.[74]

Hyponatremia

Hyponatremia (<135 mM/L after correction for hyperglycemia) is much more prevalent in acute SCI patients than in other surgical or medical populations.[21,57] Low serum sodium levels are commonly observed within the first week, but have also been noted in the chronic stages following SCI. Patients with motor and sensory complete SCI are at the highest risk for development of hyponatremia. This metabolic abnormality is related to impaired intrarenal and arginine vasopressin-dependent osmoregulatory mechanisms, which lead to decreased free water excretion and increased urinary sodium losses.[46]

Chronic Stage

Energy Expenditure

The metabolic response to long-standing SCI is marked by reduced energy expenditures in comparison to predicted energy needs. When Agarwal et al[1] studied 15 quadriplegic patients with a mean duration of injury of 9.2 ± 6.5 years, the average measured energy expenditures were 25% lower than the predicted BEE calculations. Kearns et al[40] demonstrated that when standard formulas were used for five critically ill quadriplegic patients, calculated calorie needs exceeded measured energy expenditures by as much as 70%. Although the duration of injury was not specified in the Kearns study, they suggested reducing the estimated number of calories by 20%. Clarke[19] concluded that REE equations used to calculate the recommended dietary allowance for able-bodied subjects overestimated caloric expenditures by 25% to 47% in active paraplegics, even when allowances are made for body weight. The loss of metabolically active lean body mass due to paralysis and immobilization could account for these REEs.[65]

The calorie needs of SCI patients appear to be inversely correlated to the spinal level of injury and the corresponding muscle atrophy (Table 1). In a study of 22 SCI patients at more than 2 months postinjury, Cox et al[29] demonstrated that quadriplegics required 22.7 kcal/kg/day, whereas paraplegics required 27.9 kcal/kg/day. Mollinger et al[54] confirmed a significant inverse association between energy expenditure and the level of SCI, and lower energy expenditures than predicted by BEE. Studies by Alexander et al[2] and Liu et al[49] also reported lower measured energy expenditures in quadriplegics compared to paraplegics. However, SCI patients with pressure ulcers had higher energy needs than their SCI counterparts (quadriplegia or paraplegia) without pressure ulcers.

Impaired Glucose and Lipid Metabolism

Long-standing SCI predisposes individuals to abnormalities in glucose and lipid metabolism. This was demonstrated in a study including 100 veterans with SCI (equally divided between those with paraplegia and those with quadriplegia) and 50 able-bodied veteran controls matched for age and body mass index.[5] Diabetes mellitus and impaired glucose tolerance was diagnosed in 22% and 34% of those with SCI, but in only 6% and 12% of the control group, respectively. Subjects with SCI also showed decreased high-density lipoprotein cholesterol levels (38.1 ± 1 mg/dL), direct correlation between peak serum insulin and triglyceride levels, and a strong inverse correlation between serum triglycerides and high-density lipoprotein cholesterol. These carbohydrate and lipid abnormalities possibly resulted from insulin resistance as a consequence of extreme physical inactivity.[5]

Alterations in Body Composition

A loss of muscle and body cell mass following SCI are progressive processes that occur over a prolonged period of time.[21,35,65,67] Body composition studies by Sedlock and Laventure[65] indicate that, although their SCI subjects were not overweight, they had an increased proportion of

TABLE 1

PREDICTED ENERGY EXPENDITURES OF SCI PATIENTS

Predicted Energy Expenditure	Condition
BEE × 1.6 (injury/stress factor)[61]	Acute traumatic stage; no pressure ulcers
BEE ×1.2 (injury/stress factor)[18]	Chronic stage; with grade II pressure ulcers
BEE ×1.5 (injury/stress factor)[18]	Chronic stage; with grade III and IV pressure ulcers
30-40 kcal/kg/day[11]	With pressure ulcers
Paraplegic	
34.4 ± 7.9 kcal/kg/day[54]	Postacute stage; high paraplegia (T1-10)
35.8 ± 6.5 kcal/kg/day[54]	Postacute stage; low paraplegia (<T10)
27.9 kcal/kg/day[29]	Chronic stage; no pressure ulcers
2200-2300 kcal/day[19]	Chronic stage; healthy, active; ages 19 to 26 years
21.4 ± 0.6 kcal/kg/day[2]	Chronic stage; no pressure ulcers
25.9 ± 1.2 kcal/kg/day[2]	Chronic stage; with pressure ulcers
Quadriplegic	
19.0 ± 2.9 kcal/kg/day[54]	Postacute stage; high quadriplegia (>C6)
31.0 ± 7.4 kcal/kg/day[54]	Postacute stage; low quadriplegia (C6-T1)
22.7 kcal/kg/day[29]	Chronic stage; no pressure ulcers
20.9 ± 0.8 kcal/kg/day[49]	Chronic SCI; no pressure ulcers
24.3 ± 1.1 kcal/kg/day[49]	Chronic SCI; with pressure ulcers

body fat, with decreased lean body mass. Claus-Walker and Halstead[21] demonstrated that the atrophied muscle is replaced by connective tissue, lipids, and water. Shizgal et al[67] stated that in well-nourished quadriplegics, the loss of body cell mass is accompanied by a similar loss of extracellular mass as the body size decreases. On the contrary, Greenway and associates[35] noted no consistent trends in body composition changes in long-term SCI patients. They suggested that caloric restriction compensates for reduced muscle activity, which prevents increases in body fat.

Impaired Bone Metabolism

Excessive calcium and bone collagen losses eventually lead to osteoporosis in paralyzed skeletal structures. Major bone loss occurs during the first 6 months after SCI and stabilizes between 12 to 16 months at two thirds of the original bone mass.[74] In a study of bone metabolism, results demonstrated that bone mineral density of the proximal femur decreased and reached fracture threshold at 1 to 5 years after SCI.[71] A retrospective study by Ragnarsson and Sell[58] showed a greater incidence of lower-extremity fractures in paraplegic than in quadriplegic patients, probably due to greater levels of activity in the paraplegic patients. Most fractures occurred in osteoporotic bones following trivial injuries, not traumatic ones.[58]

Pressure Ulcers

All SCI patients are at increased risk for the development of pressure ulcers due to immobility, prolonged focal pressure, and collagen degradation. After SCI, increased degradation of skin collagen results in increased urinary excretion of hydroxyproline, hydroxylysine, and glucosyl-galactosyl hydroxylysine.[24,25,63] This results in decreased amino acid content per unit weight of skin and may account for its decreased tensile strength and increased sensitivity to mechanical insults. The lack of weight-bearing contributes to collagen degradation in SCI patients.[19] Defective wound healing has also been reported in non-decubitus wounds below the level of the spinal lesion.[4]

Major nutritional factors associated with pressure ulcer development and impaired wound healing are weight loss, anemia, hypoproteinemia, and micronutrient deficiencies.[64,70] Weight loss reduces fat and muscle tissue, resulting in increased pressure over bony prominences and damage to microcirculation. Anemia, assessed by low hemoglobin (<14 mg/dL) and low hematocrit (<36%) levels, reduces the oxygen supply in the blood and interferes with wound healing.[63] Low levels of serum total protein (<6.4 gm/dL) and albumin (<3.5 gm/dL) precipitate edema, which causes the skin to become less elastic and interferes with oxygen and nutrient transport from the blood to the skin.[70] Edema could also increase local tissue pressure, causing a regional loss of blood flow and tissue damage. Losses of albumin and protein into the pressure ulcer exudate further augment protein deficiencies. Deficiencies of zinc and vitamin C have been associated with poor wound healing. Supplementing these micronutrients in SCI patients who do not have deficiencies does not enhance the healing of pressure ulcers.[8,12]

NUTRITION ASSESSMENT

Nutritional status impacts the morbidity and mortality of critically ill SCI patients. As might be expected, quadriplegics are at a higher risk for malnutrition than are paraplegics. In addition, two thirds of SCI patients admitted to a rehabilitation unit are reportedly malnourished.[55] Therefore, the goal for the SCI patient should be either maintenance of optimal nutritional status or repletion of nutrient deficiencies.

No single parameter consistently assesses nutritional status or predicts the effects of nutrition on prevention and treatment of complications. Serial measurements to evaluate trends over time may be useful for first estimating baseline nutritional status and then monitoring the response to a nutrition intervention. Recommended evaluations should be interpreted collectively, with consideration of possible contributing factors such as age, gender, over- or underhydration, drug-nutrient interactions, metabolic stress, infection, and concurrent illnesses.

Dietary History

A dietary history can determine the adequacy of an individual's usual food intake. In SCI pa-

tients, adequate nutrient intake is hindered by many factors including food intolerances and allergies, difficulty with chewing and swallowing, difficulty with food acquisition and preparation, immobility, neglect, lack of knowledge, poverty, depression, and anorexia. In a study of 51 acute SCI patients, anorexia was present in 57% of patients 2 weeks after injury; in 33%, anorexia continued until 8 weeks postinjury.[45]

Successful dietary management often includes meal patterns with six small meals daily; modification of food textures; increased amount of foods high in protein, complex carbohydrates, vitamins, and minerals; and decreased amount of dietary fat.[48] If SCI patients are not physically able to feed themselves, assistance at mealtimes may be necessary. The use of adaptive eating devices can help SCI patients to become more independent.

Compromised gastrointestinal function can impair intake in SCI patients. Gastric dilatation and paralytic ileus occur acutely, although bowel activity commonly returns within the first postinjury week.[53] For SCI patients who experience dysphagia or esophageal stricture, pureed or mechanical soft diets often improve nutritional intakes. Constipation can be prevented by adequate dietary intake of fiber and fluids, and appropriate bowel regimens. Although early satiety is a common complaint, normal rates for gastric emptying of both liquids and solids have been demonstrated, regardless of the level or completeness of SCI.[78]

Anthropometric Measurements

Although ideal body weight, triceps skinfold thickness, midarm circumference, and midarm muscle circumference are common nutrition assessment measures, they may not be valid following SCI.[18,54,55] Due to water shifts, muscle atrophy from disuse, an increased percentage of body fat, and unavoidable weight loss that normally occur in SCI patients, anthropometric standards may not apply. In SCI patients, early weight loss primarily consists of muscle rather than fat.[45]

For long-term paraplegics, the ideal body weight has been estimated to be 10 to 15 lb below the Metropolitan Life Insurance guidelines for a given height and frame size. For quadriplegics, it is estimated to be 15 to 20 lb below the recommended guidelines.[10] In malnourished SCI patients, the body weight may actually increase due to an expansion in extracellular mass, even in the presence of a corresponding loss of body cell mass. Severe muscle wasting can be masked by water retention. For these reasons, body weight may not be a valid predictor of nutritional status.

Biochemical Parameters

Urinary Nitrogen Excretion and Nitrogen Balance

The breakdown of muscle mass results in urinary excretion of nitrogenous by-products, urea, creatinine, and 3-methyl-histidine.[41] When inadequate calories and protein are provided, endogenous protein stores are used as an amino acid supply. Net protein losses, therefore, can usually be minimized by increasing calorie and protein deliveries.

To calculate the nutrition balance, the daily protein intake (grams) from all sources is divided by 6.25 for conversion to nitrogen intake (grams). Nitrogen output consists primarily as urine urea nitrogen. An aliquot of a 24-hour urine collection is assayed for its urea nitrogen content using a standard enzymatic laboratory technique (Beckman Astra, Beckman Instruments, Fullerton, California). This value, plus 4 (the constant used for nitrogen losses from the skin and feces), is subtracted from the grams of nitrogen intake during the same 24-hour period to calculate the NB. The formula to calculate the nitrogen balance is: NB = protein intake/6.25 − (24-hour urine urea nitrogen + 4).

Nitrogen equilibrium is reached when the nitrogen intake equals the nitrogen output (NB = 0). A positive NB, or anabolic, state exists when nitrogen intake exceeds nitrogen output. A net 24-hour positive NB of 2 to 4 gm is optimal for anabolism. A negative NB, or catabolic, state exists when nitrogen excretion is greater than nitrogen intake.

Creatinine-Height Index

Creatinine-height index is based on the amount of creatinine excreted in the urine over a 24-hour period. Usually, this index is compared with standard values to assess nutritional status. However, muscle atrophy due to paralysis and inactivity decreases urine creatinine excretion to 85% of normal, regardless of nutritional intake adequacy. Thus, the creatinine-height index may not truly reflect the SCI patient's nutritional status.[10] Nevertheless, a value of <60% of the standard index has been established as an indicator of nutritional risk in SCI patients.[55]

Serum Protein Levels

Serum total protein and albumin levels are often distorted by fluid shifts and acute blood loss. Hepatic transport proteins such as albumin respond as acute-phase proteins, causing serum levels to decline with physiological stress.[28] Patients with an SCI have an extremely high elimination rate of serum albumin.[18,55] With a long half-life of 18 to 21 days, serum albumin is an insensitive marker of the adequacy of nutritional support and may be a better indicator of severity of illness. Serum prealbumin may be a more appropriate nutrition assessment parameter with a half-life of 1 to 2 days.[34]

Hemoglobin and Hematocrit

Anemia is a common complication of acute SCI, even in the absence of significant blood loss.[18,38] In a study of 28 acute SCI patients, Huang and colleagues[38] found 71% of patients with normochromic normocytic anemia and 14% with normochromic microcytic anemia. Decreased serum levels of iron-binding capacity, transferrin, iron, and iron saturation were found in 86%, 79%, 50%, and 50% of the 28 SCI patients, respectively. Folate and iron deficiencies, alterations in bone marrow maturation, and the effects of physiological stress were believed to be causative factors. Impairment in erythropoiesis has not been found in SCI patients.[38]

In long-term SCI patients, the most common type of anemia is associated with chronic disorders, such as urinary tract infections and pressure ulcers.[56] However, malnutrition is also a contributing factor. Anemia is related to an increased length of stay by SCI patients in rehabilitation centers.[13] Recognition and treatment of the causes of anemia might speed up the rehabilitation process.

Nutritional Requirements

Predicting energy and nutrient requirements is a major component of the management of SCI patients (see Appendix). Underfeeding can result in muscle wasting, intestinal mucosal atrophy, decreased immunocompetence, and poor wound healing. On the other hand, overfeeding is associated with fluid overload, hyperglycemia, elevated blood urea nitrogen, elevated triglyceride levels, increased hepatic enzyme levels, respiratory distress due to increased CO_2 production, and ventilator weaning difficulties.[14,34,44] Accurate, individualized nutrient delivery is certainly desirable.

The estimation of nutritional requirements involves more than a few simple calculations. The professional expertise of a registered dietitian or clinician is necessary to evaluate clinical and morphometric data prior to the application of equations that predict energy and protein requirements.

Prediction of Calorie Requirements

Several methods have been reported for prediction of energy expenditures (PEE) (Table 1). However, predictive equations can be complicated and invalidated by several confounding factors including infection and sepsis; hypercaloric nutrition support regimens; clinical procedures; surgical operations; medications; and alterations in body weight, such as anasarca, obesity, amputations, and significant weight loss. The sicker a patient is, the poorer is the ability to predict metabolic rates. This could be due to the following reasons:[76]

- varying degrees of severity of illness are difficult to assess objectively;
- greater fluid retention and subsequent increased body weight lead to falsely elevated predictions;
- ventilated patients are not spontaneously breathing;
- critically ill patients are in a sedated and relatively motionless state; and
- substrate utilization is in an unstable, nonsteady state.

Therefore, actual energy expenditure measurements are often necessary.

Calorimetry: Measurement of Energy Expenditures

Calorimetry is a more sophisticated and expensive technique requiring equipment and technical skills that are not needed for predictive methods. Direct or indirect calorimetry can be used to determine energy expenditures.

Direct calorimetry measures heat production by or heat loss from the body.[30] An individual is placed in a sealed chamber with a supply of oxygen. Because the chamber is well insulated, the heat produced by the body is absorbed by a known volume of water that circulates through pipes located in the chamber. The change in water temperature reflects the heat loss or expended metabolic energy. Obviously, this method cannot be used for acutely traumatized or critically ill patients.

Indirect calorimetry is a valid and accurate alternative for measuring the REE. Heat production, or REE, is determined using a metabolic cart (Critical Care Monitor, Medical Graphics Corp., St. Paul, MN) by measuring the respiratory gas exchange between the inspired and expired samples.[30] This is based on the assumption that oxygen consumption (VO_2) and carbon dioxide production (VCO_2) accurately reflect a significant portion of intracellular metabolism. With the data obtained from a metabolic cart study, the Weir equation is used to determine the REE[75] (REE = $[3.9 \times VO_2 + 1.1 \times VCO_2] \times 1.44$).

The metabolic cart is also used to determine the respiratory quotient (RQ) (the ratio of VCO_2/VO_2) which is an indicator of substrate utilization.[30] Each energy source is oxidized at a known RQ (carbohydrate at 1.00, protein at 0.82, and fat at 0.71). Mixed substrate oxidation has an RQ of 0.85. When the RQ is >1.0, lipogenesis is assumed to occur from overfeeding of either carbohydrate or calories. The amount of metabolized protein can be quantified and the remaining caloric expenditure can be differentiated into carbohydrate and fat components. Based on the REE and RQ, amounts of substrate can be adjusted in the nutritional support regimen.

TABLE 2

PROTEIN RECOMMENDATIONS FOR
SCI PATIENTS

Condition & Amount of Protein*

Acute stage; septic
2 gm/kg[61,62]

With pressure ulcers
1.2-1.5 gm/kg[73]
1.5-2.0 gm/kg[11]

Chronic stage; with grade II pressure ulcers
1.2-1.5 gm/kg[12]

Chronic stage; with grade III and IV pressure ulcers
1.5-2.0 gm/kg[12]

---

*Gm protein/kg of Ideal Body Weight. For Ideal Body
Weight calculations, see Appendix.

Protein

Protein is necessary for tissue growth, maintenance, and repair, and for the synthesis of hormones, enzymes, antibodies, and transport molecules. When excess protein is ingested, it is either metabolized to energy or stored as fat. Recommendations for protein intake in SCI patients vary according to the acute or chronic stage after injury, and the presence or absence of pressure ulcers (Table 2).

Carbohydrate

Glucose is the preferred energy substrate by central nervous system tissue, blood cells, granulation tissue, testis, and renal medulla. A minimum of 100 to 150 gm of glucose per day is required for these functions and for the prevention of endogenous protein breakdown.[68] The normal rate at which the body oxidizes carbohydrate or glucose is about 2 to 4 mg/kg/min. During periods of severe stress, the oxidation rate of glucose is increased to 3 to 5 mg/kg/min. In most patients, the provision of more than 400 to 500 gm of glucose per day exceeds the body's ability to oxidize and use it for energy. Sources of glucose include not only nutrition support fluids, but also intravenously administered dextrose and peritoneal dialysis fluid. The excess glucose is converted to fat (lipogenesis) and results in an increased ratio of VCO_2/VO_2 (or RQ).[15]

Lipids

The provision of lipid as a concentrated source of calories can facilitate protein sparing, decrease the risk of carbohydrate overfeeding, and limit total fluid volume. Lipids should generally comprise about 30% of the total calorie delivery. In the acute postinjury stage, large amounts of fat, especially as linoleic or omega-6 fatty acids, can have an immunosuppressive effect by stimulating the release of arachidonic acid.[68] This leads to prostaglandin formation, and, subsequently, depresses delayed cell-mediated hypersensitivity, lymphocyte proliferation, and natural killer cell function. In the presence of sepsis, high serum triglyceride levels (>250 gm/dL) also indicate lipid intolerance and the need for reduced delivery of intravenous lipid emulsions. A minimum of 4% of total energy needs as essential fatty acids is necessary to avoid deficiencies.[68]

Patients with long-term SCI are at an increased risk for cardiovascular disease and cardiopulmonary morbidity and mortality due to excessive intake of fats and nominal activity levels. Decreased intakes of saturated fat and cholesterol are advised to decrease these risks.

Micronutrients

Adequate amounts of minerals and vitamins are usually provided in a well-balanced diet. Supplementation of micronutrients may be necessary if deficiencies are suspected due to prolonged inadequate intake or increased needs due to specific disease conditions. Deficiencies of zinc, vitamin C, and vitamin D have been especially associated with SCI patients.

Zinc

Zinc, often given to enhance healing of pressure ulcers, is known to be involved in the structural integrity of collagen. However, serum zinc levels are reportedly similar in patients who do and do not develop pressure ulcers.[8] Oral zinc sulfate supplements (220 mg daily) do not affect healing rates of pressure ulcers within a 2- to 3-month time period.[12] Adverse physiological effects, such as impaired copper metabolism, copper deficiencies, and anemia, may result from long-term supplementation of high amounts of zinc.[33]

Vitamin C

Vitamin C has a well-established role in the formation of collagen. However, dietary intake of vitamin C has not been correlated to the development of pressure ulcers.[8] In addition, supplementation of vitamin C does not accelerate healing of pressure ulcers in patients who are not deficient in vitamin C.[72] Because a subclinical deficiency state is difficult to detect, the minimum intake of the recommended dietary allowance of 60 mg has been suggested.

Vitamin D

Patients with an SCI have a predisposition to the development of vitamin D deficiency. Contributing factors include lack of exposure to sunlight due to hospitalizations and limited mobility and avoidance of calcium-containing foods that are often fortified with vitamin D. In a study of 100 veterans with chronic SCI (equally divided between those with paraplegia and quadriplegia) and 50 healthy controls, low serum 25-hydroxy-vitamin D (25-OH D) levels were detected in 30 (30%) of the SCI individuals compared to eight (16%) of the controls.[6] In the SCI group, a negative correlation existed between the serum 25-OH D levels and parathyroid hormone. With secondary hyperparathyroidism, bone losses increase, further compounding the complication of osteoporosis. Active measures should therefore be taken to detect and correct vitamin D deficiency in SCI individuals.

NUTRITION SUPPORT

In 1950, Cooper and associates stated "It is not a rare occurrence to see a patient who is paraplegic . . . literally die of starvation, despite vigorous attempts to supply adequate nutrients."[28] The effectiveness of early, aggressive nutrition support has not been established in terms of improved outcome and decreased incidence of complications in SCI patients.[45] However, nutrition support measures are indicated for maintenance or repletion of optimal nutritional status in SCI patients.

Oral Supplements

A variety of specialized commercial formulas are available for both oral and tube feeding supplementation (Table 3). These supplements differ by calorie and protein densities, fiber contents, osmolalities, form of nutrients, amounts of micronutrients, and the presence or absence of flavorings.[39] Most commercial formulas provide the recommended dietary allowance for vitamins and minerals in approximately 1000 to 1500 mL. Selection of the appropriate formula is based on the individual's digestive and absorptive capacity as well as the specific characteristics of and indications for each product.

Enteral Nutrition (Tube Feeding)

Indications

If the gastrointestinal tract is functional, enteral tube feeding is the preferred method for nutritional support. Use of the enteral route for nutrient administration is always preferable to parenteral feedings. The benefits of enteral feedings include increased physiological metabolism and utilization of nutrients, maintenance of gut integrity, decreased risk of bacterial translocation, decreased expense of nutrient delivery, and decreased risk of catheter-related infections.[39]

Administration

Decisions regarding the most appropriate enteral access route depend on the anticipated duration of tube feeding and the risk of pulmonary aspiration of gastric contents (Figure 1).[26] Short-term (<6 weeks) enteral access is possible via the nasogastric, nasoduodenal, or nasojejunal routes. Surgical or percutaneous endoscopic gastrostomy and jejunostomy tubes can be inserted for long-term (>6 weeks) nutrition support. However, gastric feedings should not be instituted in patients without an intact gag reflex, with gastroesophageal reflux, with gastro-

TABLE 3

COMMERCIAL FORMULAS FOR ORAL SUPPLEMENTS AND TUBE FEEDINGS*

	Kcal/mL	Protein (gm/L)	MOsm/ kg Water
Standard (for noncatabolic states, anorexia, and the inability to eat solid foods)			
Ensure[a]	1.0	37	555
Isocal[b]	1.0	34	270
Isosource[e]	1.2	43	360
Nutren 1.0[c]	1.0	40	300
Osmolite[a]	1.0	37	300
Fiber-containing (for regulation of bowel function)			
Compleat[e]	1.0	43	300
Ensure/Fiber[a]	1.1	40	480
Fibersource HN[e]	1.2	53	390
Jevity[a]	1.0	44	300
Promote/Fiber[a]	1.0	63	370
Sustacal/Fiber[b]	1.0	43	480
Ultracal[b]	1.0	44	310
Vitaneed[d]	1.0	40	300
High protein (for catabolic states, pressure ulcers, and wound healing)			
Ensure/High Protein[a]	1.0	48	610
Isocal HN[b]	1.0	44	270
Osmolite HN[a]	1.0	44	300
Promote[a]	1.0	63	340
Protain XL[d]	1.0	57	340
Replete[c]	1.0	63	300
Sustacal[b]	1.0	61	650
High-caloric density (for hypermetabolic and catabolic states, and volume restriction)			
Isosource HN[e]	1.2	53	390
Jevity Plus[a]	1.2	56	450
Osmolite HN Plus[a]	1.2	56	360
Comply[d]	1.5	60	410
Ensure Plus[a]	1.5	55	690
Ensure Plus HN[a]	1.5	63	650
Nutren 1.5[c]	1.5	60	430
Resource Plus[e]	1.5	55	600
Sustacal Plus[b]	1.5	61	670
Traumacal[b]	1.5	83	560
Deliver 2.0[b]	2.0	75	640
Magnacal[d]	2.0	70	590
Nutren 2.0[c]	2.0	80	720
TwoCal HN[a]	2.0	84	690
Elemental or peptide-based (for acute or chronic maldigestion, malabsorption)			
Accupep HPF[d]	1.0	40	490
Criticare HN[b]	1.0	38	650
Peptamen[c]	1.0	40	270
Reabilan[c]	1.0	32	350
Tolerex[e]	1.0	21	550
Travasorb STD[c]	1.0	30	560
Vital HN[a]	1.0	42	460
Vivonex Plus[e]	1.0	38	630
Special Disease States			
Metabolic stress; Acute trauma; Sepsis			
Alitraq[a]	1.0	53	575
Crucial[c]	1.5	94	490
Peptamen VHP[c]	1.0	63	300
Perative[a]	1.3	67	385
Reabilan HN[c]	1.3	58	490

TABLE 3 (cont'd)
COMMERCIAL FORMULAS FOR ORAL SUPPLEMENTS AND TUBE FEEDINGS

	Kcal/mL	Protein (gm/L)	MOsm/kg	
Compromised respiratory function; Ventilator-dependent				
Nutrivent[c]	1.5	68	450	
Pulmocare[a]	1.5	63	475	
Respalor[b]	1.5	76	580	
Abnormal glucose tolerance due to stress; Diabetes mellitus				
Choice dm[b]	1.0	45	440	
Glucerna[a]	1.0	42	355	
Glytrol[c]	1.0	45	380	
Acute or chronic renal failure				
Amin-Aid[f]	2.0	19	700	(predialysis)
Renalcal[c]	1.35	23	600	(predialysis)
Suplena[a]	2.0	30	600	(predialysis)
Magnacal Renal[d]	2.0	75	570	(hemodialysis)
Nepro[a]	2.0	70	635	(hemodialysis)
Hepatic failure				
NutriHep[c]	1.5	40	690	
Hepatic-Aid[g]	1.2	44	560	
Fat malabsorption				
Lipisorb[b]	1.35	57	630	
Travasorb MCT[c]	1.0	50	250	
Compromised immune function				
Immun-Aid[g]	1.0	37	460	
Impact[e]	1.0	56	375	
HIV Infection; AIDS				
Advera[a]	1.28	60	680	
Pediatric (for children aged 1 to 10 years)				
Pediasure[a]	1.0	30	345	
Pediasure/Fiber[a]	1.0	30	345	
Peptamen Jr[c]	1.0	30	260	
Kindercal[b]	1.0	34	300	
Modular supplements (for modifying commercial formulas to meet unique patient requirements)				
Glucose polymers				
Polycose[a]	2.0	–	900	
Polycose Powder[a]	32 kcal/T	–	–	
Protein powder				
Casec[b]	17.0 kcal/T	4.7g/T	–	
Elementra[c]	12.5 kcal/T	2.6g/T	–	
Promod Powder[a]	12.0 kcal/T	3g/T	–	
Fat emulsion and medium chain triglycerides (MCT)				
Microlipid[d]	4.5	–	80	
MCT Oil[b]	7.7	–	–	

*This table is for reference only and is not all-inclusive. Some of the formulas listed in the table may be appropriate in more than one of the above categories. For detailed information, contact the product's manufacturer.

[a] = Ross Products Division, Abbott Laboratories, Columbus, Ohio
[b] = Mead Johnson Nutritionals, Evansville, Indiana
[c] = Nestle Clinical Nutrition, Deerfield, Illinois
[d] = Sherwood Medical, St. Louis, Missouri
[e] = Novartis Nutrition, Minneapolis, Minnesota
[f] = R & D Laboratories, Marina del Rey, California
[g] = Braun-McGaw, Inc., Irvine, California

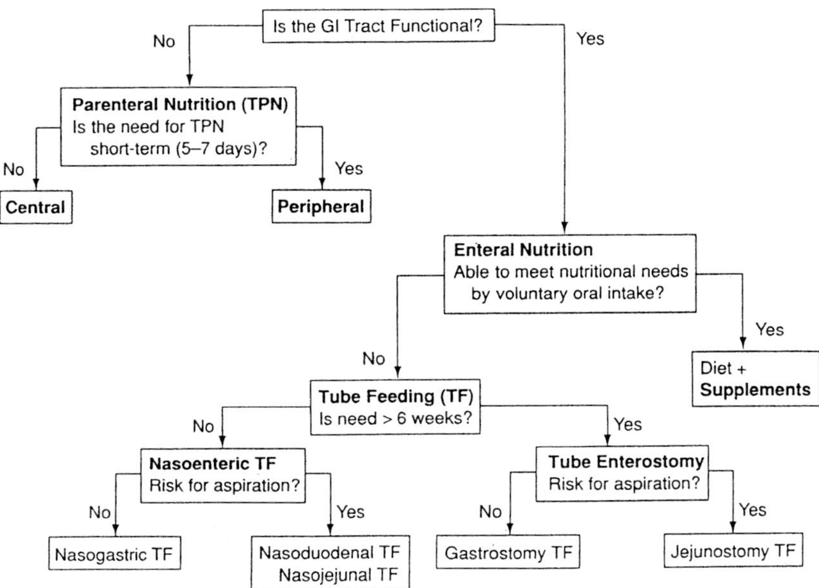

Figure 1: Decision-making process for nutritional support. (Reproduced from Rodriguez DJ, Benzel EC: Nutritional support, in Benzel EC (ed): *Spine Surgery: Techniques, Complication Avoidance, and Management.* Philadelphia, Pa: Churchill-Livingstone, 1999, p 1325, with permission.)

paresis, with gastric outlet obstruction, or with gastric atony.[39] Jejunal feedings, which can usually be initiated immediately after injury, potentially reduce the risk of aspiration.

Enteral formulas (Table 3) can be administered by bolus, intermittent, or continuous methods. Bolus feedings involve rapid delivery of 300 to 400 mL of formula over 10 minutes several times daily. Intermittent feedings are also given several times daily, but over at least 30 minutes. The bolus and intermittent methods are especially suited for gastric feedings. Small-volume (<125 mL/hour) continuous-drip feedings over 10 to 24 hours are recommended for intestinal delivery of nutrients. Continuous feedings are usually better tolerated than bolus feedings in critically ill patients.[39] The delivery of tube feedings only during the night can supplement dietary intake without interfering with appetite.

The final goal amount of delivered formula depends on the product's nutrient density (Table 3) and the individual's estimated daily calorie and protein requirements. Bolus and intermittent feedings can be initiated with 100 mL of formula. The bolus volume can be advanced by 50 mL every 4 hours to the goal amount if gastric residuals are not significant (<100 mL or

one half the volume previously delivered) when aspirated before each feeding.[26] The initiation of continuous tube feeding can range from rates of 20 to 50 mL/hr. Rates are advanced by 10 to 25 mL/hr every 6 hours to the goal amount as the patient tolerates.

Complications

Complications of enteral feedings can prevent adequate nutrient deliveries. Diarrhea and tube obstruction are the most common problems that interfere with tube feeding delivery. Possible causes of diarrhea are:

- formula hyperosmolality;
- low residue formula;
- lactose-containing formula;
- rapid delivery of a large volume (bolus) of formula;
- bacterial contamination of formula;
- bacterial overgrowth of the gastrointestinal tract;
- gut atrophy due to prolonged NPO status; and
- concurrent drug therapy, such as antibiotics and magnesium-containing antacids.

Tube feeding obstruction often results from

delivery of medications through the feeding tube and irregular irrigation of the tube. Prevention or treatment of these complications can improve formula tolerance and increase nutrient intakes.[39]

Parenteral Nutrition

Indications

Total parenteral nutrition (TPN) may be needed if optimal nutritional status cannot be achieved through enteral feedings. Indications for TPN include the mechanical obstruction of the gastrointestinal tract, prolonged ileus, severe gastrointestinal hemorrhage, severe diarrhea, intractable vomiting, and high-output gastrointestinal tract fistula. Combinations of TPN and small amounts of enteral feedings as tolerated can together provide nutritional needs and maintain gut integrity.

Administration

Specialized techniques for TPN delivery are available to prevent malnutrition (Figure 1). Central or peripheral veins can be used for delivering TPN solutions. However, concentrated TPN formulas should only be infused through a central venous catheter to prevent thrombophlebitis of smaller peripheral veins.[69] Central vein access is appropriate for delivery of TPN for more than 5 to 7 days, because peripheral vein access is difficult to maintain for this length of time. Parenteral solutions with <900 mOsm can be administered via peripheral venous access.

Standard TPN solutions, which can be ordered from stock TPN order forms, are available in most institutions. The institution's pharmacy can provide information regarding standard TPN formulas and how to order them. If standard formulas are unavailable or inappropriate, patient-specific formulas can be designed to meet calorie, protein, and fluid requirements. Energy substrates included in TPN are 5% to 70% initial concentrations of dextrose, and 10% (1.1 kcal/mL) to 20% (2 kcal/mL) lipid emulsions.[69] Protein can be provided as 3% to 15% initial concentrations of crystalline L-amino acid solutions. Electrolyte additives, multivitamins, trace minerals, and medications can also be administered in TPN solutions.

Complications

Complications of TPN include mineral and electrolyte imbalances, acid-base disorders, substrate intolerance (hyperglycemia, hypertriglyceridemia, and elevated blood urea nitrogen levels), and catheter-related infections.[69] In the acute postinjury stage, the daily monitoring of serum electrolytes, glucose, blood urea nitrogen, and creatinine is necessary to detect and minimize excesses or deficiencies. Changes in sodium, potassium, magnesium, and phosphorus deliveries are frequently needed in critically ill patients. The careful evaluation of fluid balance by daily weights and intake and output records is necessary to prevent volume depletion or overload. Meticulous line care is essential for the prevention of catheter-related infections.

CONCLUSION

Unique metabolic alterations are present in both the acute and chronic stages following SCI. The achievement of optimal nutritional status is necessary whether the SCI patient is critically ill or undergoing rehabilitation. Estimates of energy needs can provide the framework for initial nutritional management, and actual REE measurements can facilitate fine-tuning of subsequent nutrition support. Adjustments can also be made based on the patient's clinical condition, available feeding routes, substrate tolerance, and changes in requirements as the hospital course progresses. The use of available assessment techniques and a variety of nutritional supplements can optimize nutritional management of SCI patients.

REFERENCES

1. Agarwal N, Lee BY, Corcoran L, et al: Energy expenditure in quadriplegic patients. JPEN 8:98, 1984 (Abstract)
2. Alexander LR, Spungen AM, Liu MH, et al: Resting metabolic rate in subjects with paraplegia: the effect of pressure sores. Arch Phys Med Rehabil 76:819-822, 1995
3. American Diabetes Association and American Dietetic Association: A Guide for Professionals: The Effective Application of Exchange Lists for Meal Planning. New York, NY, 1977, p 17
4. Basson MD, Burney RE: Defective wound healing in paraplegic patients. Surg Forum 32:78-80, 1981
5. Bauman WA, Spungen AM: Disorders of carbohy-

drate and lipid metabolism in veterans with paraplegia or quadriplegia: a model of premature aging. **Metabolism** 43:749-756, 1994

6. Bauman WA, Zhong YG, Schwartz E: Vitamin D deficiency in veterans with chronic spinal cord injury. **Metabolism** 44:1612-1616, 1995
7. Benzel EC, Wild GC: Biochemical mechanisms of posttraumatic neural injury, in Barrow DL (ed): **Perspectives in Neurological Surgery.** St Louis, Mo: Quarterly Medical, 1991, Vol 2, pp 95-126
8. Bergstrom N, Braden B: A prospective study of pressure sore risk among institutionalized elderly. **J Am Geriatr Soc** 40:747-758,1992
9. Berlly MH, Wilmot CB: Acute abdominal emergencies during the first four weeks after spinal cord injury. **Arch Phys Med Rehabil** 65:687-690, 1984
10. Blissitt PA: Nutrition in acute spinal cord injury. **Crit Care Nurs Clin North Am** 2:375-384, 1990
11. Breslow RA, Hallfrisch J, Guy DG, et al: The importance of dietary protein in healing pressure ulcers. **J Am Geriatr Soc** 41:357-362, 1993
12. Brewer RD, Mihaldzic N, Dietz A: The effect of oral zinc sulfate on the healing of decubitus ulcers in spinal cord injured patients. **Proc Annu Clin Spinal Cord Inj Conf** 16:70-72, 1967
13. Burr RG, Clift-Peace L, Nuseibeh I: Haemoglobin and albumin as predictors of length of stay of spinal injured patients in a rehabilitation centre. **Paraplegia** 31:473-478, 1993
14. Bursztein S, Elwyn DH, Askanazi J: Energy metabolism and indirect calorimetry in critically ill and injured patients. **Acute Care** 14/15: 91-110, 1988/1989
15. Bynoe RP, Kudsk KA, Fabian TC, et al: Nutrition support in trauma patients. **Nutr Clin Pract** 3:137-144, 1988
16. Carey ME, Nance FC, Kirgis HD, et al: Pancreatitis following spinal cord injury. **J Neurosurg** 47:917-922, 1977
17. Cashman MD, Wightkin WT, Madden JE, et al: Massive azoturia and failure to achieve positive nitrogen balance in a botulism patient. **JPEN** 10:316-318, 1986
18. Chin DE, Kearns P: Nutrition in the spinal-injured patient. **Nutr Clin Pract** 6:213-222, 1991
19. Clarke KS: Caloric costs of activity in paraplegic persons. **Arch Phys Med Rehabil** 47:427-435, 1966
20. Claus-Walker J: Clinical implications of the disturbance in calcium and collagen metabolism in quadriplegia. **Int J Rehabil Res** 3:540-541, 1980
21. Claus-Walker J, Halstead LS: Metabolic and endocrine changes in spinal cord injury: I. The nervous system before and after transection of the spinal cord. **Arch Phys Med Rehabil** 62:595-601, 1981
22. Claus-Walker J, Halstead LS: Metabolic and endocrine changes in spinal cord injury: II (Section 1). Consequences of partial decentralization of the autonomic nervous system. **Arch Phys Med Rehabil** 63:569-575, 1982
23. Claus-Walker J, Halstead LS: Metabolic and endocrine changes in spinal cord injury: III. Less quanta of sensory input plus bedrest and illness. **Arch Phys Med Rehabil** 63:628-631, 1982
24. Claus-Walker J, Halstead LS: Metabolic and endocrine changes in spinal cord injury: IV. Compounded neurologic dysfunctions. **Arch Phys Med Rehabil** 63: 632-638, 1982
25. Claus-Walker J, Singh J, Leach CS, et al: The urinary excretion of collagen degradation products by quadriplegic patients and during weightlessness. **J Bone Joint Surg (Am)** 59:209-212, 1977
26. Clevenger FW, Rodriguez DJ: Decision-making for enteral feeding administration: the why behind where and how. **Nutr Clin Pract** 10:104-113, 1995
27. Cooper IS, Hoen TI: Metabolic disorders in paraplegics. **Neurology** 2:332-340, 1952
28. Cooper IS, Rynearson EH, MacCarty CS, et al: Metabolic consequences of spinal cord injury. **J Clin Endocrinol** 10:858-870, 1950
29. Cox SAR, Weiss SM, Posuniak EA, et al: Energy expenditure after spinal cord injury: an evaluation on stable rehabilitating patients. **J Trauma** 25:419-423, 1985
30. Damask MC, Schwarz Y, Weissman C: Energy measurements and requirements of critically ill patients. **Crit Care Clin** 3:71-96, 1987
31. Dietrick JE, Whedon GD, Shorr E: Effects of immobilization upon various metabolic and physiologic functions of normal men. **Ann J Med** 4:3-36, 1948
32. Duckrow RB, Beard DC, Brennan RW: Regional cerebral blood flow decreases during hyperglycemia. **Ann Neurol** 17:267-272, 1985
33. Eleazer GP, Bird L, Egbert J, et al: Appropriate protocol for zinc therapy in long term care facilities. **J Nutr Elderly** 14:31-38, 1995
34. Fry DE, Borzotta AP: Options in nutritional support of the surgical patient. **Probl Gen Surg** 4:427-440, 1987
35. Greenway RM, Houser HB, Lindan O, et al: Long-term changes in gross body composition of paraplegic and quadriplegic patients. **Paraplegia** 7:301-318, 1970
36. Hadley MM: Hypermetabolism after CNS trauma: arresting the "injury cascade." **Nutrition** 5:143, 1989 (Editorial)
37. Harris JA, Benedict FG: **A Biometric Study of Basal Metabolism in Man. Carnegie Institute of Washington, Publication #279.** Philadelphia, Pa: JB Lippincott, 1919, pp 190-227
38. Huang CT, DeVivo MJ, Stover SL: Anemia in acute phase of spinal cord injury. **Arch Phys Med Rehabil** 71:3-7, 1990
39. Ideno KT: Enteral nutrition in Gottschlich MM, Matarese LE, Shronts EP (eds): **Nutrition Support Dietetics Core Curriculum.** Silver Spring, Md: American Society of Parenteral and Enteral Nutrition, 1992, pp 71-104
40. Kearns PJ, Pipp TL, Quirk M, et al: Nutritional requirements in quadriplegics. **JPEN** 6:577, 1982 (Abstract)
41. Kearns PJ, Thompson JD, Werner PC, et al: Nutritional and metabolic response to acute spinal-cord injury. **JPEN** 16:11-15, 1992
42. Kinney JM, Duke JH Jr, Long CL, et al: Tissue fuel and weight loss after injury. **J Clin Pathol** 4 (Suppl):65-72, 1970
43. Kolpek JH, Ott LG, Record KE, et al: Comparison of urinary urea nitrogen excretion and measured energy expenditure in spinal cord injury and nonsteroid-treated severe head trauma patients. **JPEN** 13:277-280, 1989
44. Lanschot JJB, Feenstra BWA, Vermeij CG, et al: Calculation versus measurement of total energy expenditure. **Crit Care Med** 14:981-985, 1986

45. Laven GT, Huang CT, DeVivo MJ, et al: Nutritional status during the acute stage of spinal cord injury. **Arch Phys Med Rehabil 70**:277-282, 1989

46. Leehey DJ, Picache AA, Robertson GL: Hyponatremia in quadriplegic patients. **Clin Sci 75**:441-444, 1988

47. LeMay DR, Gehua L, Zelenock GB: Insulin administration protects neurologic function in cerebral ischemia in rats. **Stroke 19**:1411-1419, 1988

48. Levine AM, Nash MS, Green BA, et al: An examination of dietary intakes and nutritional status of chronic healthy spinal cord injured individuals. **Paraplegia 30**:880-889, 1992

49. Liu MH, Spungen AM, Fink L, et al: Increased energy needs in patients with quadriplegia and pressure ulcers. **Adv Wound Care 9**:41-45, 1996

50. Longstreth WT Jr, Inui TS: High blood glucose level on hospital admission and poor neurologic recovery after cardiac arrest. **Ann Neurol 15**:59-63, 1984

51. Manson JM, Wilmore DW: Positive nitrogen balance with human growth hormone and hypocaloric intravenous feeding. **Surgery 100**:188-197, 1986

52. Marsh WR, Anderson RE, Sundt TM Jr: Effect of hyperglycemia on brain pH levels in areas of focal incomplete cerebral ischemia in monkeys. **J Neurosurg 65**:693-696, 1986

53. McCagg C: Postoperative management and acute rehabilitation of patients with spinal cord injuries. **Orthop Clin North Am 17**:171-182, 1986

54. Mollinger LA, Spurr GB, El Ghatit AZ, et al: Daily energy expenditure and basal metabolic rates of patients with spinal cord injury. **Arch Phys Med Rehabil 66**:420-426, 1985

55. Peiffer SC, Blust P, Leyson JFJ: Nutritional assessment of the spinal cord injured patient. **J Am Diet Assoc 78**:501-505, 1981

56. Perkash A, Brown M: Anaemia in patients with traumatic spinal cord injury. **J Am Paraplegia Soc 20**:235-236, 1982

57. Peruzzi WT, Shapiro BA, Meyer PR Jr, et al: Hyponatremia in acute spinal cord injured patients. **Crit Care Med 22**:252-258, 1994

58. Ragnarsson KT, Sell GH: Lower extremity fractures after spinal cord injury: a retrospective study. **Arch Phys Med Rehabil 62**:418-423, 1981

59. Rawe SE, Lee WA, Perot PL: Spinal cord glucose utilization after experimental spinal cord injury. **Neurosurgery 9**:40-47, 1981

60. Robertson CS, Grossman RG: Protection against spinal cord ischemia with insulin-induced hypoglycemia. **J Neurosurg 67**:739-744, 1987

61. Rodriguez DJ, Benzel EC, Clevenger FW: The metabolic response to spinal cord injury. **Spinal Cord 35**:599-604, 1997

62. Rodriguez DJ, Clevenger FW, Osler TM, et al: Obligatory negative nitrogen balance following spinal cord injury. **JPEN 15**:319-322, 1991

63. Rodriguez GP, Claus-Walker J: Biochemical changes in skin composition in spinal cord injury: a possible contribution to decubitus ulcers. **Paraplegia 26**:302-309, 1988

64. Salzberg CA, Byrne DW, Cayten CG, et al: A new pressure ulcer risk assessment scale for individuals with spinal cord injury. **Am J Phys Med Rehabil 75**:96-104, 1996

65. Sedlock DA, Laventure SJ: Body composition and resting energy expenditure in long term spinal cord injury. **Paraplegia 28**:448-454, 1990

66. Sherrington CS: Notes on temperature after spinal transection, with some observations on shivering. **J Physiol (Lond) 58**:405-424, 1924

67. Shizgal HM, Roza A, Leduc B, et al: Body composition in quadriplegic patients. **JPEN 10**:364-368, 1986

68. Shronts EP, Lacy JA: Metabolic support, in Gottschlich MM, Matarese LE, Shronts EP (eds): **Nutrition Support Dietetics Core Curriculum.** Silver Spring, Md: American Society of Parenteral and Enteral Nutrition, 1992, pp 361-365

69. Skipper A, Marian MJ: Parenteral nutrition, in Gottschlich MM, Matarese LE, Shronts EP (eds): **Nutrition Support Dietetics Core Curriculum.** Silver Spring, Md: American Society of Parenteral and Enteral Nutrition, 1992, pp 105-123

70. Strauss EA, Margolis DJ: Malnutrition in patients with pressure ulcers: morbidity, mortality, and clinically practical assessments. **Adv Wound Care 9**:37-40, 1996

71. Szollar SM, Martin EME, Sartoris DJ, et al: Bone mineral density and indexes of bone metabolism in spinal cord injury. **Am J Phys Med Rehabil 77**:28-35, 1998

72. ter Riet G, Kessels AGH, Knipschild PG: Randomized clinical trial of ascorbic acid in the treatment of pressure ulcers. **J Clin Epidemiol 48**:1453-1460, 1995

73. Thomas DR: Specific nutritional factors in wound healing. **Adv Wound Care 10**:40-43, 1997

74. Uebelhart D, Demiaux-Domenech B, Roth M, et al: Bone metabolism in spinal cord injured individuals and in others who have prolonged immobilisation. A review. **Paraplegia 33**:669-673, 1995

75. Weir JB: New methods for calculating metabolic rate with special reference to protein metabolism. **J Physiol 109**:1-9, 1949

76. Williams RR, Fuenning CR: Circulatory indirect calorimetry in the critically ill patient. **JPEN 15**:509-512, 1991

77. Young B, Ott L, Phillips R, et al: Metabolic management of the patient with head injury. **Neurosurg Clin North Am 2**:301-320, 1991

78. Zhang RL, Chayes Z, Korsten MA, et al: Gastric emptying rates to liquid or solid meals appear to be unaffected by spinal cord injury. **Am J Gastroenterol 89**:1856-1858, 1994

Appendix
Steps For Planning Nutrition Support Regimens

Step 1: Determine the Ideal Body Weight (IBW) and calculate the percent of IBW as actual body weight.

Ideal Body Weight:[3]
    Men (5' tall) = 106 lbs + 6 lbs for every inch taller
    Women (5' tall) = 100 lbs + 5 lbs for every inch taller
If patient's Actual Weight is 20% greater than the IBW, calculate the adjusted IBW
Adjusted IBW = [(Actual Weight – Ideal Weight) × 0.25] + Ideal Weight.

Step 2: Calculate the predicted energy expenditure (Table 1). If actual weight is 20% greater than the IBW, use the adjusted IBW to calculate the basal energy expenditure.

Step 3: Estimate the protein requirements (Table 2).

Step 4: Determine the nutrition support regimen:
- Select the appropriate nutrition support access route (Figure 1).
- Select the enteral tube feeding formula (Table 3) according to the patient's clinical condition, access route, and tolerance.
- Select the TPN formula according to the patient's nutritional requirements and via regional or institutional standards. Obtain information on standard TPN formulas from the institution's pharmacy.
- Base initial goal rates of tube feedings, TPN, or intravenously administered lipids on the amount of formula needed to meet assessed needs for calorie, protein, and fluid.

Step 5: Monitor the clinical and nutritional parameters in the acute stage and whenever the patient is receiving enteral feedings and/or TPN.

Daily
- Weight
- Fluid intake and output
- Tolerance to nutritional support regimen
- Strict calorie counts (when on oral diet)
- Serum electrolytes, glucose, blood urea nitrogen, creatinine, and complete blood count with differential

Weekly
- Prealbumin
- Liver function profile, triglycerides (if receiving TPN)

Biweekly
- Indirect calorimetry or metabolic cart studies (ideally when tube feeding or TPN and intravenously administered lipids are at goal rates)

Step 6: Adjust the calorie and substrate deliveries according to indirect calorimetry (metabolic cart) measurements.

Step 7: Taper the tube feeding as oral diet intake improves (documented by calorie counts); taper the TPN as the patient tolerates enteral feedings or as oral intake improves.

CHAPTER 20

PREVENTION AND TREATMENT OF MEDICAL COMPLICATIONS

RAN VIJAI P. SINGH, MD, SONIA SUYS, MD, AND PHILIP A. VILLANUEVA, MD

The rapid identification of neurological impairment and protection of the spinal cord from further primary or secondary damage are major factors that determine the eventual outcome of patients with a spinal cord injury (SCI). A top priority should be early treatment of associated injuries to other parts of the body and focus should be on prevention of complications. When the patient is stable, early comprehensive rehabilitation should be started to enable the patient to return to a social and vocational life.

It has long been proven that early treatment at SCI centers decreases the number of complications and is cost-effective. Therefore, an attempt should be made to transport these patients to an SCI center if the patient is stable and less than 1 hour is needed to get to the center. However, nothing is gained from transferring unstable patients who may have received better care in the SCI center if only they had reached the center while alive.[14,30]

PRE-HOSPITAL AND EMERGENCY ROOM CARE

During the prehospital care phase and while in the emergency room, it is important to look for and deal with any pathology of other systems due to associated injuries or secondary to the SCI. To assess the patient appropriately, all cloth-ing should be cut away and removed and vital signs monitored (body temperature, blood pressure, heart rate, and respiratory rate). Immobilization of the whole spine must be continued using a rigid straight board.[1,30]

Systematic Assessment

A primary survey should be initiated according to the advanced trauma life support priorities. The first concern is provision of an adequate airway; therefore, all debris, blood, dentures, and vomit must be removed from the patient's mouth. In an unresponsive patient, an oral airway may be needed. A chin-lift or jaw thrust can also increase the patency of the airway.[30] The patient is then given supplemental oxygen. This is mandatory in all trauma patients and particularly critical in SCI patients because better oxygenation improves the neurological recovery of the spinal cord. If ventilation remains inadequate, respiratory causes should be sought. One problem may be associated chest trauma. Chest examination may reveal bruises, flail segments, decreased respiratory excursion, a displaced trachea, decreased breath sounds, subcutaneous emphysema, etc. Pneumothorax, hemothorax, or less frequently hemopneumothorax are common injuries (occurring in approximately 15%) and may require a chest drain insertion.[27,30] Pulmonary contusion is present in about 1% of SCIs but is more difficult to detect without arterial blood gas (ABG) measurement or a chest x-ray. Other causes are usually directly related to the SCI. In injuries above C5, the abdominal and intercostal muscles are nonfunctional and the diaphragm (C3-5) and accessory muscles (C2-8) are affected to a variable extent depending upon the exact level of SCI. Therefore, breathing and ventilation will be inadequate and most patients will need artificial ventilation. Aspiration is another cause for concern because it decreases the available area for gas exchange and later may be the cause of aspiration pneumonitis, further deteriorating oxygenation. Because many of these patients are unconscious or intoxicated with alcohol, aspiration is common in SCI. Any kind of trauma, and especially SCI, delays gastric emptying and makes aspiration more likely. For this reason, every SCI patient should have a nasogastric tube inserted while in the emergency room.[30]

Often during these initial stages of care, a decision about artificial ventilation will be necessary. Artificial ventilation is started if PO_2 <70 mm Hg, PCO_2 >45 mm Hg, respiration rate >30/min, or vital capacity (VC) <500 ml. Aspiration of vomitus, abnormal breathing patterns, or increased work of breathing due to the level of SCI may be relative indications for artificial ventilation. It is vital to keep the cervical spine immobilized, and intubation of SCI patients presents a challenge. Several options are available. Physicians can either perform a blind nasotracheal intubation or use a fiberoptic bronchoscope. A tracheostomy may be the method of choice in a high cervical injury when more prolonged ventilation is anticipated. In emergency situations, a cricothyroidotomy may be necessary.[9,19]

Attention is then focused on the circulatory system. Shock is common and is due to neurogenic shock in 80% of cases and hypovolemia in the remaining 20%. Loss of sympathetic tone in lesions above T6 that results in loss of vasomotor tone and loss of sympathetic innervation to the heart is responsible for the hypotension and bradycardia of neurogenic shock. Unopposed vagal activity accentuates the bradycardia.[32] Hypovolemic shock is related to injuries of the chest or abdomen or to fractures of the pelvis or limbs, accounting for considerable overt or concealed blood loss. If the cardiovascular regulatory mechanisms are intact, hypovolemic shock is accompanied by tachycardia in most cases. In young patients, tachycardia may be the only sign. Differential diagnosis is important because hypovolemic shock may hide an emergency situation without obvious symptoms or signs. A distinguishing feature is tachycardia in pure hypovolemia, in contrast to the bradycardia present in SCI or in mixed hypovolemic-neurogenic shock. Usually, a diagnosis of neurogenic shock is made by exclusion. This means that one must seek associated injuries that may be the cause of hypovolemia. Pelvic and chest x-rays may assist in this, and a peritoneal lavage may be needed if it is impossible to assess the abdomen in the patient with sensory loss. Fluid replacement and treatment of the underlying pathology are necessary in hypovolemic shock. Initial treatment of neurogenic shock is volume expansion, but extreme care is needed to prevent overhydration because this may lead to pulmonary edema. Insertion of a central line to monitor the central venous pressure, or better still, a pulmonary arterial catheter to maintain a pulmonary capillary wedge pressure of 18 mm Hg can help prevent overhydration.[28] Military antishock trousers are occasionally useful as a short-term measure because they evoke a volume shift by compressing the lower limbs. The inotropic agents dopamine and dobutamine are used if hypotension is not corrected by volume expansion. Intravenous atropine may be needed in SCI with severe bradycardia. Blood samples should be obtained for routine hematologic and biochemical investigations, for typing and cross-match, and for ABG analysis. Two large-bore intravenous cannulas should be inserted and Ringer's lactate solution infused or blood replaced. This is also the time to insert a urinary catheter to monitor urinary output and to drain the atonic bladder, because a volume of more than 500 ml will stretch the detrusor and delay the return of bladder function.[1,30]

A neurological examination should be performed, noting the level of consciousness and the function of the brain stem. Cranial nerve function and the peripheral nervous system are evaluated to establish the exact extent of the sensory and motor damage caused by the SCI.[9,32]

Missed Injuries

Missed injuries are a particular problem in SCI and are very costly for the patient and society. They are often the cause of a preventable death and, in a less critical situation, may make additional surgery necessary and prolong the hospital stay considerably. In a study by Ryan et al,[27] 42% of patients with SCI had an injury that was missed during the initial assessment; of these, 45% were spinal and 55% nonspinal. There are many reasons for missed injuries. Multiple physiological changes due to the SCI focus the initial attention on the SCI and its complications. Patients may be more difficult to assess due to an altered level of consciousness secondary to a head injury or alcohol or drug ingestion. Some patients are intubated and may be hemodynamically unstable. The differential diagnosis between hemorrhagic shock and neurogenic shock is almost always an exclusion diagnosis, and causes of hypovolemic shock are much less easily detectable. When present, quadriplegia makes the diagnosis of multiple injuries more difficult due to the loss of skin sensation and visceral pain perception. When there is loss of abdominal muscle tone, a valuable sign of intra-abdominal pathology (i.e., abdominal guarding) is absent.

Associated injuries more likely to be diagnosed at the time of presentation include head injuries, soft-tissue thoracic injuries, fractures of the long bones, and vascular injuries. Spinal fractures at a different level and intra-abdominal pathology are among the most frequently missed injuries. These are followed closely by pneumothorax, hemothorax, hemopneumothorax, paralyzed diaphragm, and renal contusion.

A low index of suspicion and inadequate x-rays are among the most easily remedied causes of missed injury.[9,27] It is a mistake to believe that missed injuries only occur in patients with a low Glasgow Coma Scale score or low Revised Trauma Score. Therefore, the physician should scrutinize all patients with SCI very carefully for associated injuries. The incidence of associated injury correlates well with the level and the mechanism of injury. Of patients with a cervical SCI, 12% have an associated injury. These include skull fractures, facial fractures, and closed head injuries. The possibility of a vertebral artery injury or esophageal disruption, although much less common, should be borne in mind.

Thoracic SCIs carry the highest risk of a missed injury (46%), consisting of intra-thoracic trauma, abdominal pathology, and limb fractures. Injuries of the lumbar region and lesions of the cauda equina are associated with intra-abdominal pathology such as liver or splenic trauma in 22% of patients.[7,27] Penetrating cervical SCIs are often accompanied by injury to the airway, the esophagus, or the blood vessels, and retroperitoneal damage is common in penetrating injuries of the lumbar spinal cord. High-speed deceleration injuries can cause tears of the mesentery and laceration of intra-abdominal organs, mainly the liver and spleen. Whiplash injuries (acceleration-deceleration injuries) occasionally coexist with vertebral artery spasm presenting with blurred vision, tinnitus, nystagmus, and vertigo. Inadequate radiographs are another cause of missed injury, especially thoracic, because chest x-rays taken in the supine position may be inadequate. The missed injury may be remote from the SCI and progressive neurological deterioration may be the first indication.[27]

CARE IN THE CRITICAL CARE UNIT

When the patient is transferred to the critical care unit, evaluation and therapy of all systems continues.

Cardiovascular Complications

Autonomic Complications

Medical cardiovascular complications occur either as a result of sympathetic disruption in SCI above T6 or as a result of immobility.

Hypovolemia. The nursing staff should scrutinize for hypovolemia. This can be due to hemorrhage secondary to a missed injury, previous surgery, or newly arising complications such as gastrointestinal (GI) bleeding. Most frequently, hypovolemia is relative as a consequence of venous pooling. The aim is to maintain blood pressure between 80 and 100 mm Hg systolic[32] and pulmonary capillary wedge pressure at 18 mm Hg.[28] Adequacy of perfusion can be evaluated quickly by assessment of mental status and a urine output of 0.5 cc/kg/hr. Treatment of hypovolemia consists of elevation of the legs or placing the patient in the Trendelenburg position. Intravenous fluid replacement may be necessary. Crystalloids are the fluids of choice and colloids are occasionally necessary. Blood products should only be used in case of obvious blood loss. If the blood pressure remains low despite adequate fluid resuscitation, dobutamine and dopamine can be used as pressure agents.[28]

Quite often, hypovolemia becomes symptomatic when the patient is first placed upright and venous pooling in the legs increases. Therefore, it is important to monitor the blood pressure closely at this time. Measures that can help prevent syncope are elastic stockings, an abdominal binder, and slow changes in position. In some patients, ephedrine may be given before mobilization. It is usual practice to begin mobilization by gradually elevating the head of the bed. Once this is tolerated, the patient can be placed in a reclining wheelchair or on a tilt table. Eventually the patient is able to maintain stable blood pressure while in the upright position.

Hypothermia. Hypothermia is another concern in SCI patients because the loss of sympathetic control causes vasodilatation below the level of injury. Therefore, patients with an SCI are dependent on the environmental temperature for control of their body temperature. Prevention and treatment consist of warming the intravenous fluids, using a warming blanket, and assuring a comfortable room temperature.[14,28,30]

Bradycardia. Another result of the loss of sympathetic control is bradycardia, which may be associated with sinus pauses that increase the risk of cardiac arrest. Bradycardia is often exacerbated by changing body position, endotracheal suctioning, hypoxia, or hypothermia. If bradycardia occurs due to a change in body position, returning the patient to the original position may be necessary. If a certain position is critical, prophylactic atropine may be used. Artificial ventilation or oxygen therapy can correct hypoxia and only suctioning to clear airway secretions may be enough to improve oxygenation and reverse bradycardia. One must be aware, however, that suctioning in itself can produce bradycardia. Hypoxia and tracheal suction both increase vagal activity and therefore may result in bradycardia. It is wise to pre-oxygenate patients and to occasionally give prophylactic atropine before attempting endotracheal suctioning.[30] Measures to combat hypothermia have been described previously.

Autonomic Dysreflexia. After the period of spinal shock, approximately 50% of patients with lesions above T6 display autonomic dysreflexia. This consists of an uncontrolled sympathetic reflex response to a variety of innocuous or mildly noxious stimuli such as a distended bladder or bowel, passive movement of the hip, etc. It causes sudden headache, flushing, sweating, anxiety, and hypertension (200-240/100-170 mm Hg) usually associated with bradycardia. The most important treatment is removal of the stimulus and elevation of the head of the bed. If the blood pressure does not return rapidly to normal, antihypertensive medication may be needed. In the acute stages, intravenous hydralazine or diazoxide, or oral chlorpromazine or nifedipine is used. In the more chronic treatment, alleviation of the cause is the main concern: propantheline is used to decrease detrusor activity, phenoxybenzamine or prazosin to decrease sphincter tone, and Xylocaine can be used before inserting suppositories.[14,30]

Deep Venous Thrombosis and Pulmonary Embolism

Pathogenesis. Deep venous thrombosis (DVT) occurs in up to 80% of SCI patients, depending on the level of injury (thoracic > cervical or lumbar), the extent of the injury (motor complete > motor incomplete), and the detection methods used.[11,12,19,25,33] In about 20% of patients, calf DVT will extend into the popliteal, femoral, or iliac vein where it can cause obstruction of venous return or from where thrombi may dislodge and cause fatal pulmonary embolism (PE) in 2% to 16% of patients.[11] DVT is most common during the first 2 weeks after injury, with a peak incidence between Days 7 and 10. The occurrence of DVT is higher in SCI patients with a high lesion, associated long-bone fractures, extensive soft-tissue trauma, persistent infection, and obesity. Immobilization in SCI causes stasis due to loss of pump action of the calf muscles and dilatation of the calf veins. External pressure on immobile limbs may cause indirect damage to the blood vessels. Several studies have shown abnormal coagulation in patients with SCI. These abnormalities consist of a raised platelet count, factor VIII, fibrinogen and von Willebrand factor, and increased platelet aggregation. Blood viscosity may be raised secondary to dehydration. Loss of sympathetic tone may account for loss of vasoconstriction, which results in stasis causing capillary leakage and endothelial changes.[11,12,14] DVT is more likely to occur in patients with heart disease, previous DVT, or varicose veins due to increased stasis. Advanced age (especially over 50 years) is another risk factor, as is obesity, which is associated with decreased fibrinolytic activity and possibly with stasis. Hormonal alterations such as estrogen-containing oral contraceptives also increase risk. DVT is less likely to occur in patients with blood group O compared with patients with other blood groups, especially A.

Diagnosis of Deep Vein Thrombosis. The diagnosis of DVT is somewhat difficult as often there will be very few symptoms and signs, and any symptoms tend to be nonspecific inflammatory changes: redness, swelling, warmth, pain, decreased function, or fever of unknown origin. Therefore, it is important to maintain a high level of suspicion and use objective investigations to establish the diagnosis. The gold standard against which all other diagnostic methods are compared is still venography. Impedance plethysmography is based on the finding that changes in blood volume cause alterations in electrical resistance in the calf. These changes in electrical resistance are reduced in patients with popliteal or proximal vein thrombosis. Plethysmography should not be used for screening because the specificity and sensitivity are not very high. False-positive results are common in conditions interfering with venous return (e.g., chronic cardiac failure, constrictive pericarditis, and external compression of the veins by tumors). False-negative results are present in nonocclusive thrombi or in proximal vein thrombosis with a high number of collaterals. Plethysmography is a good diagnostic test for patients with suspected DVT of the proximal veins.

[125]I-labeled fibrinogen leg scanning may be used in screening, because it has a sensitivity of 95% for picking up calf DVT, but it is relatively insensitive (70%) as a diagnostic procedure. After a single injection of ^{125}I, the test is repeated daily for 7 to 10 days. Increased radioactivity of more than 20% for 24 hours is considered a positive test. This test is not reliable for the detection of thrombosis in the upper thigh or pelvic veins. Sensitivity to ^{125}I is seldom serious. Despite its usefulness as a screening test, it is seldom used in a clinical setting because it is not very cost effective and effective DVT prophylaxis is available.

Doppler ultrasound is based on detection of a change in blood flow velocity. The flow sound is absent in stasis; it varies with respiration and is increased by calf compression or by ankle movement. DVT modifies the quality of the sound and the changes during manipulation. Doppler ultrasound is highly sensitive to detect popliteal and more-proximal DVT (85%) and has a low rate of false-positive results in these situations. Its use is limited by its subjectivity and the need for expert interpretation. It is not reliable for the diagnosis of calf DVT or as a screening test. Overall, a high degree of suspicion is needed and a suspected diagnosis of DVT should be confirmed with additional tests: venography in calf DVT and Doppler ultrasound in more proximal DVT. At present there does not seem to be a reliable, cost-effective screening method for routine use in asymptomatic patients.[11]

Diagnosis of Pulmonary Embolism. PE presents another diagnostic challenge. The symptoms are often atypical or PE may be clinically silent. The presentation depends on pre-existing heart and lung conditions and on the size of the embolus. Massive PE can present with sudden severe dyspnea, cardiovascular collapse, and apprehension, but it has also been diagnosed in patients with only minimal dyspnea. Symptoms of pulmonary infarct such as pleuritic chest pain, cough, and hemoptysis together with dyspnea may accompany a submassive PE. Unexplained pyrexia, tachycardia, tachypnea, or a change in cardiac rhythm may be the only symptoms of PE. As with DVT, it is important to have a high index of suspicion and to investigate further to confirm the diagnosis.

Pulmonary angiography is the only specific diagnostic test that shows an intraluminal filling defect or an abrupt cutoff in the artery in cases of PE. However, it is highly invasive and may not always be available. When PE is suspected, a chest x-ray is essential. It will show only nonspecific changes, but is important to exclude other causes of dyspnea and is needed for proper interpretation of the ventilation-perfusion scan. The chest x-ray in PE may be normal or show pulmonary infiltrates, atelectasis, elevation of the diaphragm, pleural effusion, or altered vascular markings. The electrocardiogram in PE will also be nonspecific and, even in massive PE, only 50% of patients show abnormalities. There may be T wave inversion, right axis deviation, or right bundle branch block denoting right ventricular strain. At times, only supraventricular arrhythmias are present.

An isotope lung scan, also called ventilation-perfusion (V/Q) scan, with a minimum of four and preferably six views can be very helpful in the diagnosis of PE. The ventilation scan is performed using ^{133}Xe and is usually normal in PE, whereas the perfusion scan will show a defect. This V/Q mismatch may signify that a PE is present, but false-positive results due to altered perfusion are possible in patients with chronic obstructive airway disease, asthma, chronic cardiac failure, or pleural effusion. A V/Q mismatch accompanied by a large perfusion defect makes the diagnosis of PE highly probable. A V/Q match, however, does not rule out PE. If both the chest x-ray and the V/Q scan are normal, the patient is unlikely to have a PE. In V/Q scans of low or intermediate probability, further investigation may be warranted.

If clinical suspicion is high, the patient should undergo pulmonary angiography; if suspicion is low, only a Doppler ultrasound is needed to look for the presence of a DVT.[12] Other ancillary tests include ABG measurements, tests that detect intravascular fibrin formation, and fibrin degradation products. Ascending venography can be used to detect the presence of a DVT that may be the cause of PE; however, a DVT is not present in all cases of PE.

Prevention. Because DVT is such a common complication in SCI and the risk of a fatal PE is high, it is important to use every method available for the prevention of these complications in SCI patients with motor paralysis.[5] Simple measures such as elastic graduated-pressure stockings, intensive physiotherapy consisting of passive and active exercises, and massage can decrease the incidence of DVT by one-third. Early treatment of vertebral fracture(s) with open reduction and internal fixation may reduce DVT as it allows for much earlier mobilization.

Electrical calf stimulation is another option but can only be used in anesthetized patients (i.e., during the operation) or in patients with complete sensory loss and is unlikely to be of benefit in the prolonged immobilization of SCI. Intermittent pneumatic calf compression diminishes stasis by acting as a muscle pump; it also seems to

increase fibrinolytic enzyme activity[11,17] and decrease the affinity of platelets for collagen.[12]

The main pharmacological agents used to prevent DVT are heparin and coumarin derivatives such as warfarin. Warfarin is a competitive inhibitor of vitamin K and causes dysfunction of factors II, VII, IX, and X. Heparin inhibits factors IX, X, XI, and XII as well as thrombin by increasing the effect of antithrombin III. Low doses are needed for inactivation of factor X, and large doses for the inhibitory effect on thrombin. For prophylaxis, low-dose subcutaneous heparin, 5000 U given twice a day is used in our center. Recently, low-molecular-weight heparin is being advocated as a better method of prevention. It consists of a single daily injection because it has a longer half life. It is better absorbed from subcutaneous depots and there is less variability in the anticoagulation response. For the same antithrombotic effect, it causes less bleeding.[11,12,17] Adjusted-dose heparin reduces the risk of DVT more than low-dose heparin but has an unacceptable risk of bleeding.

A combination of intermittent pneumatic compression, graduated elastic stockings, and low-dose heparin (5000 U given twice a day) as used at the Jackson Memorial Medical Center reduces the risk of DVT from between 49% and 72% to 5% and decreases the size of the clot if one forms.[25] Primary prophylaxis should be started as soon as possible. In the early postinjury period, intermittent pneumatic compression may be difficult to maintain due to frequent transport and surgery, but every attempt should be made to continue it. Anticoagulants may be contraindicated due to the increased risk of bleeding. DVT does not usually occur in the first 3 days. Therefore it is common practice to begin heparin on Day 3.[11] If surgery is performed after the start of prophylaxis, heparin should be stopped 24 hours before the operation and resumed 6 hours postoperatively.[11] Intermittent pneumatic compression should continue during the operation and the patient must continue to wear graduated-compression stockings. Because DVT is most common in SCI during the first 2 weeks postinjury (but the risk remains increased during the period of immobilization and flaccidity), anticoagulation should be continued until ambulation or for 3 months in persistent paralysis.[11,12,24,25] There also seems to be a late-onset thrombosis in about

10% of patients, but further studies are pending.

Treatment. Treatment in established DVT is aimed at preventing propagation of the clot and occurrence of PE in the acute stages, whereas in the chronic phase the focus is on prevention of recurrence of DVT or PE. As soon as s diagnosis of DVT or PE is made, a bolus injection of 5000 U of heparin is given. This is followed by continuous infusion at a rate of 1000 to 1500 U/hr. The activated partial thromboplastin time needs to be checked every 6 hours until 1.5 to 2.5 times the patient's baseline value is reached, and the infusion rate is changed accordingly. Warfarin is started on the same night or by the third night (10-10-5 mg or 9-6-3 mg regimen), and both drugs are continued until the international normalized ratio is between 2 and 3, at which time heparin can be discontinued. Warfarin should be continued for 3 months in DVT and 6 months in PE.[5,24]

Thrombolytic treatment (intravenous plasmin, urokinase, or streptokinase) may be used in some SCI patients. On the whole, there are few studies of the effect of this treatment in SCI patients. The aim is to reduce the burden of the clot, to restore patency, and to prevent postphlebitic syndrome. It is associated with a considerable risk of bleeding especially in patients with recent trauma or major surgery less than 10 days ago. It should only be used in extensive DVT with compromised limb viability or in PE with severe hypotension, hypoxia, tachypnea, and tachycardia.[11,15-24]

Caval filters are useful to prevent PE in certain patients with proven DVT. Indications for the use of caval filters are recurrent PE while undergoing treatment, bleeding during therapeutic anticoagulant treatment, failure of the previous filter, and postembolectomy status, and contraindication to anticoagulant treatment. Caval filters may be used prophylactically in very high-risk patients without DVT or PE in whom there is a contraindication for routine prophylaxis. Preoperatively, those patients need inferior vena cava studies to determine the presence, extent, and location of the clot, to determine the size, contour, and anomalies of the inferior vena cava, and to identify the renal veins. This study is critical for the selection of the type of filter and for correct placement. Commonly used filters are the Greenfield filter and Bird's Nest filter. Caval filters have a low rate of complications, such as thrombosis of the filter with bilateral leg edema, incorrect placement of the filter, migration of the device, extrusion of the prongs, and retroperitoneal hematoma.[24]

Recurrent DVT and PE should receive the same initial therapy as when acute, but treatment should be continued for 1 year. In the event of several episodes of recurrent DVT or PE, a caval filter and long-term anticoagulation are necessary.

The main side effect of warfarin therapy is bleeding, occurring in 2% to 5% of patients, and it is frequently associated with the use of other medications.[16] The risk of bleeding is also increased in certain medical conditions (e.g., atrial fibrillation, stroke, chronic renal failure, anemia, and a previous history of GI bleeding). Patients aged over 65 years are also more likely to suffer this complication. Some SCI patients are at increased risk due to recent surgery or invasive procedures, closed head injuries, and multiple fractures. With a therapeutic international normalized ratio of 2 to 3, the risk of bleeding is minimal. If bleeding occurs, it may be related to excessive anticoagulation, vigorous range of motion exercises, or a triad of low hemoglobin, low hematocrit, and leg swelling.[23] Treatment of clinically symptomatic bleeding complications is via fresh frozen plasma infusion and 10 mg of parenteral vitamin K1.

Heparin is known to cause bleeding in 5% to 20% of patients.[5] The treatment of bleeding consists of local measures and decreasing the dose of heparin. Protamine sulfate can be given in a dose of 1 mg/100 U of heparin with a maximum of 50 mg over 10 minutes. Extreme care is needed when using protamine because it can cause severe hypotension, anaphylactic shock, and hypersensitivity reactions. Heparin can also cause thrombocytopenia (occurring in approximately 2% of patients), usually in the first week, with a relative drop in thrombocytes of more than 50% or an absolute level of <70,000. Thrombocyte counts should therefore be checked regularly while on heparin. Despite the low thrombocyte count, thrombotic complications are still possible. Rarely, osteoporosis may occur in cases of long-term heparin use. Skin necrosis is not a recognized complication of heparin therapy. Low-molecular-weight heparin has a lower incidence of both bleeding complications and thrombocytopenia.[18]

Respiratory Complications

Of the 10,000 new SCIs each year, about 50% are quadriplegic with a complete or partial loss of respiratory muscle function. Upper thoracic SCI patients also have involvement of respiratory muscles. This means that 65% of SCI patients are at risk for developing respiratory problems. About 35% develop respiratory complications, mainly pneumonia or atelectasis, during their first month postinjury. Of these, 30% patients die as a result of their respiratory pathology.[18]

Respiratory Changes in SCI

Pathophysiology. According to the level and completeness of SCI, the respiratory musculature is paralyzed to a varying degree. In lesions above C3, there is no diaphragmatic or intercostal function and the accessory muscles are also affected. The accessory muscles are primarily postural and there is no cyclical activity during sleep; in most cases, these patients die during the night. All of these patients need artificial ventilation. Lesions at C3-5 cause varying degrees of diaphragmatic dysfunction. Under normal circumstances, the diaphragm generates 75% of the normal tidal volume (V_T) by increasing the vertical and lateral diameters of the thorax. Patients with midcervical lesions are at risk from respiratory complications during the early stages and may need some respiratory assistance. Once recovered, they can usually be weaned from the ventilator. Lesions of the lower cervical and thoracic spine do not interfere with diaphragmatic function. The intercostal muscles, however, either have no or impaired function. In normal circumstances, the external intercostal muscles increase the anteroposterior chest diameter. Impairment of the external intercostal muscles decreases chest mobility and the ability to breath deeply. Contraction of the diaphragm in these patients creates negative intrapleural pressure and, due to the paralysis of the intercostal muscles, causes depression of the rib cage, known as paradoxical breathing. The internal intercostal muscles are affected to the same extent. They are normally responsible for a decrease in the anteroposterior diameter in forced expiration, hence forced expiration is impaired in low cervical and thoracic SCI. In these patients, abdominal muscle function is absent or impaired. Abdominal tone assists normal expiration by supporting the viscera and pushing the diaphragm back to its resting position. With the loss of abdominal tone, the diaphragm has a lower resting position and a reduced inspiratory capacity on contraction. Abdominal contraction is also needed for forceful expiration, as in coughing. In thoracic injuries, inspiration is almost normal but expiration is impaired. Lumbar lesions do not cause paralysis of any of the respiratory muscles and, therefore, have little effect on ventilation.[4,18]

The position of the patient also affects breathing. The vital capacity decreases and the residual volume and functional residual capacity both increase in the upright position. In the supine quadriplegic patient, there is paradoxical movement of the upper rib cage in early inspiration due to the negative intrapleural pressure. The weight of the abdominal organs pushes the diaphragm up where it can generate more force. Contraction of the diaphragm also produces outward excursion of the abdomen and flattening of the diaphragm. During the late inspiratory stages, the already flattened diaphragm pulls in the lower rib cage and causes paradoxical movement. Changes in both the anterior and posterior diameter are abnormal in the supine position. In the upright position in SCI, the effect of gravity cannot be offset by an increase in abdominal muscle tone and the diaphragm assumes a lower resting position. There is less compliance of the abdomen as it has reached its elastic limit. Hence, contraction of the diaphragm causes less abdominal wall movement and more lifting of the rib cage. It can be concluded that, although the inspiratory force of the diaphragm is greater in the supine position, it is mainly wasted in distorting the rib cage (paradoxical movement). Respiratory performance is better in the upright position if the abdominal sag is prevented with a corset or abdominal binder.[4]

Ventilatory capacity is poor in the acute stages because flaccid muscle, mobile rib cage joints, and the supine position are responsible for considerable distortion of the rib cage during respiration. In midcervical lesions, the VC usually drops to 30% immediately after an SCI but improves quickly between 3 and 5 weeks postinjury.[4] As edema of the spinal cord decreases, there may be partial recovery of neurological function, in particular of respiratory muscles. The rib cage also becomes stiffer over time and, as a percentage of diaphragmatic energy is used to distort the rib cage, the diaphragm is under some tension, which constitutes a form of training. As the period of spinal shock subsides, there is also some return of tone or even spasticity, which is usually beneficial, as it increases the stability of the rib cage.

Respiratory Failure. Respiratory failure may be due to a failure in gas exchange, pump failure from impairment in central drive (intoxication), abnormalities in the chest wall (scoliosis), or muscle failure (muscle fatigue). Muscle fatigue is an important cause of respiratory failure in SCI. It can either be caused by a decrease in energy supply or by an increase in energy demand of the muscle. The catabolic state immediately postinjury causes a lack of substrate. Sympathetic loss is responsible for cardiovascular compromise and results in decreased O_2 and nutrient delivery. These and competing metabolic demands due to fever or sepsis can interfere with energy supply to the respiratory muscles. In an acute SCI, the energy demand is greatly raised secondary to an increased work of breathing with an increased respiratory rate and a reduced V_T above optimal and a low respiratory reserve. Respiratory load is also often increased as a result of pneumonia or atelectasis. Normal adaptive mechanisms, such as dysrhythmic breathing and rotation of the respiratory muscles under stress, are absent in SCI. Very few muscles are available for recruitment. Treatment is based on early detection of fatigue. Its presence can be marked by rapid, shallow breathing with signs of hypercarbia and passive indrawing of the abdominal wall. More sophisticated lung function tests measuring serial VC or maximum inspiratory and expiratory pressures can confirm the diagnosis. Impaired contractility can be shown by means of flow/frequency curves or inspiratory muscle electromyography having more low- and less high-frequency components. Treatment consists of eliminating the underlying cause whenever possible and resorting to early mechanical ventilation and rest if needed.[4]

Accumulation of Secretions. Bronchial secretions are increased in SCI patients because there is loss of sympathetic control and unopposed vagus activity. This, together with an impaired cough reflex, accounts for the reduced airway clearance in SCI.[18] A normal cough reflex is initiated by mechanochemical irritation of the larynx and the first two divisions of the bronchial tree. For an efficient cough, the patient must be able to rapidly inspire a large volume of air and to generate a large pressure once the glottis closes. As soon as the glottis opens, a large expiratory flow results, expelling mucus or foreign particles. In quadriplegics, the expiratory force is produced by the elastic recoil of the lung and depends grossly on the depth of the previous inspiration. The maximum expiratory flow rate is 65% of normal at the usual lung volumes and slightly greater at lower lung volumes. At 25% of lung volume, the maximum expiratory flow is 80% of normal.[4] The maximum pleural pressure that quadriplegic patients can generate is also considerably reduced. The pleural pressure causes a dynamic compression of the airways downstream of the equal pressure point, and the increasing linear velocity of the gas flow removes the foreign bodies. Patients with a high SCI are unable to increase the linear velocity to a great extent. The cascade of coughs can also not include the maximum lung volumes so that the equal pressure point will never reach the largest airways. Quadriplegics can only clear their smaller airways, and secretions become lodged in their main airways and trachea.

Loss of Fine Control of Breathing. Fine control of breathing is dependent on sensory receptors in the lung, the diaphragm, and the intercostal muscles. In lesions below T1, a considerable amount of sensory afferents are preserved and the patient has a normal sensation of load and normal breath-holding capabilities. Midcervical lesions are associated with the loss of most of these sensations. Most afferent pathways from the rib cage and the diaphragm are interrupted. Only reflexes mediated by the vagus are intact. These remaining reflexes only respond to large changes in lung volume and, consequently, an abnormal respiratory rhythm ensues and may result in apnea. The perception of elastic load is absent as it is transmitted via the phrenic nerve, but the perception of resistive loads transmitted via the vagus nerve is intact. The reflex that induces sighing is lost and micro-atelectasis is consequently very common. Because chest wall reflexes are lost, the breath-holding time is greatly increased because only hypoxia will end it. Sudden death is a common complication in SCI as the drive to breathe may be considerably decreased.[4]

Assessment of Respiratory Function

The SCI patient should be continuously assessed to detect any deterioration in respiratory function. Hemorrhage or edema of the spinal cord can cause the level of injury to ascend and may increase the neurological deficit within the first 48 to 72 hours. Direct or indirect injury to the lung such as pneumothorax, hemothorax, flail chest, pulmonary contusion or aspiration, pneumonia, and adult respiratory distress syndrome can worsen respiration. Aside from being potentially fatal, PE can impair a patient's breathing considerably. Paralytic ileus and acute gastric dilatation are frequently the bases for vomiting and aspiration. Increased metabolic demands may further worsen borderline respiratory function.[18]

It is important to establish the patient's respiratory status on admission to the intensive care unit (ICU). It is highly relevant to note the existence of previous chest disease, associated chest injuries, and the level of neurological injury. Respiratory rate, rhythm, and depth together with the quantity and quality of secretions are used to assess respiration. The symmetry of respiration, the use of accessory muscles, the efficiency of the diaphragm (abdominal extrusion), and the strength of the abdominal muscles (assessed during a cough) are good indices of muscle function. A chest x-ray may show associated injuries or other complications. Occasionally, fluoroscopic screening of the diaphragm may be useful. Negative inspiratory force, V_T, and serial VC are objective indicators of respiratory muscle function and reserve, but are position-related. A low VC is associated with an increase in complications. A VC of <1000 ml together with an inability to clear secretions is an indication for intubation and ventilation. Serial ABG measurements evaluate the efficiency of gas exchange. Hypoxia with a rise in CO_2 occurs in hypoventilation and may be a sign of muscle fatigue. A pulse oximeter enables noninvasive assessment of the adequacy of gas exchange.[18]

Sources of hypoxemia in SCI are diffusion defects due to increased bronchial secretions, V/Q inequalities due to the effect of gravity, PE, or shunt (atelectasis, pneumonia, aspiration, near-drowning, lung contusion, adult respiratory distress syndrome, etc.), and most importantly hypoventilation. Although shunts are not responsive to oxygen treatment, all other causes of hypoxemia are. Pre-existing lung diseases can fall within these categories and should be treated in the standard way. The physician should consider the medication that the patient was taking prior to injury because it may affect an already compromised autonomic nervous system.

Treatment of Respiratory Complications Due to Paralysis

Treatment of respiratory problems due to paralysis consists of artificial ventilation and physiotherapy.

Artificial Ventilation. Hypoventilation is most frequently the result of impaired muscle function mainly in cervical SCI. The muscles are unable to move sufficient air, V_T and VC are reduced, and $PaCO_2$ is raised. Positive-pressure ventilation is necessary in 20% to 30% of SCI patients in cases of ventilatory failure, hypoxemia that is not corrected by other means, and impending fatigue.[18] Certain problems with mechanical ventilation should be anticipated. Intubation must be performed with extreme care by a knowledgeable physician because of possible neurological deterioration by moving the cervical spine. Sympathetic vascular tone is absent in these SCI patients, and they are therefore subject to high swings in blood pressure when put on the ventilator. Easy access for suction is present after intubation, but care must be taken because any instrumentation in the airway can stimulate the unopposed vagus and cause extreme bradycardia and cardiac arrest. In that case, atropine and oxygen may be necessary. Only humidified gases should be used with an endotracheal tube in situ or with a tracheostomy; otherwise, secretions will be very viscous and the risk of atelectasis and pneumonia will be very high.

If the SCI is ≥C4, it may be expected that permanent ventilatory support will be needed. In these cases, tracheostomy should be performed as early as possible and the use of a portable ventilator considered. Tracheostomy should be performed within 7 days if prolonged (>14 days) intubation is expected. Low-pressure, high-volume cuffed tubes are utilized to minimize tracheal injury. If the injury is <C4, and the pulmonary

problem has stabilized, consideration may be given to weaning. There is no single "best" means for weaning a patient with SCI. The experience in our institution shows that a reduction of positive end-expiratory pressure levels by 2- to 3-cm decrements to a baseline of 5 cm H_2O is a reasonable first stage. If a pulmonary artery catheter is in place, shunt fractions of 15% to 20% may be used as a guideline for this reduction. Another parameter is the maintenance of a PaO_2:FiO_2 (fraction of inspired oxygen) ratio of approximately 300:1. The FiO_2 is then reduced to 21% (room air FiO_2). The use of an oxygen saturation monitor previously described is very helpful and eliminates the need for frequent ABG sampling. The last stage in weaning is reduction of the ventilatory rate. The goal is reduction to zero. It is during this period that the greatest degree of anxiety on the patient's part develops as the work of breathing is progressively increased, occasionally beyond the patient's capacity. Several monitoring systems are available to monitor work of breathing and assist in the prediction of successful weaning. When such systems are not available, more traditional parameters, such as negative inspiratory force and spontaneous V_T, are helpful.

The advent of the current generation of volume ventilators has introduced several new modalities to the weaning process. Both pressure support (PS) and flow-by help ease the transition to the "no mandatory breath" state. The use of a weaning schedule which combines a minimum tolerable intermittent mandatory ventilation (IMV) (usually 2 to 4 breaths/minute) with continuous positive airway pressure (CPAP +5 cm) and PS ($+10 \pm 15$ cm) may help. Initially, 4-hour blocks divided into a 3:1 ratio of IMV:CPAP/PS are used. The ratio is gradually adjusted to provide continuous CPAP/PS. The PS is then decreased by 3- to 5-cm decrements until a ventilator setting of CPAP +5 cm, FiO_2 21%, and PS +5 cm is reached. Extubation is considered if at that point the spontaneous respiratory rate is <30/min, FiO_2:PaO_2 ratio is approximately 300:1, PaO_2 ≥70 mm Hg, and $PaCO_2$ <50 mm Hg, there is no evidence of respiratory distress, and no obvious airway impairment. After extubation, helpful adjuncts are continued: vigorous chest physiotherapy, incentive spirometry, and mobilization (if the spine is stable). Occasionally, intermittent positive-pressure breathing may be used to treat small areas of atelectasis.

When the injury is >C4, phrenic pacing is an option if the lower motor neurons (phrenic nerve) are intact and if there is a good response of the diaphragm to electrical stimulation and a normal cerebral function. Continuous pacing results in fatigue and, therefore, alternate pacing of one hemidiaphragm every 12 hours is performed in adults. In children under 10 years old or in patients with a subnormal diaphragmatic function, pacing needs to be alternated with mechanical ventilation. If diaphragmatic pacing is impossible, the best option is long-term intermittent positive-pressure ventilation usually with a portable ventilator.[4]

Physiotherapy. In SCI patients in a halo vest, a respiratory restriction of 10% of the VC may occur due to the vest.[18] In a patient with borderline ventilation, this can be important. Hence, it is advisable to measure the VC before and after application of the halo vest and to maintain a rigorous pattern of pulmonary hygiene.

As noted before, SCI patients need intensive physiotherapy directed at clearing secretions and preventing atelectasis and pneumonia. Atelectasis and pneumonia are most common during the first month postinjury (mean Day 8) in motor complete SCI. The occurrence does not seem to be related to the date of any surgical intervention. Because it determines the degree of compromise of the respiratory muscles, the level of injury is a significant determinant of the incidence of atelectasis and pneumonia. During the first month, approximately 74% of patients with high-level quadriplegia, 27% with low-level quadriplegia, and 10% with paraplegia suffer an episode of atelectasis or pneumonia. The predominant anatomic location for these respiratory complications is the left lower lobe (76% of SCI patients).[10] The dependent position of the lower lobes makes them more prone to the accumulation of secretions. It is also more difficult to clear secretions from the lower lobes because the cough is impaired and available treatment does not clear secretions from the lower lobes. Chest physiotherapy and fiberoptic bronchoscopy clear only the proximal airways. Postural drainage can shift secretions from the periphery more centrally where they are better accessible to other treatment modalities. Clearance of the lower lobes requires the patient to be in a 15° to 20° Trendelenburg semiprone position in right decubitus for clearance of the left lower lobe and in left decubitus for the right lower lobe.

A nurse or physiotherapist should change the position of the patient with SCI every 2 hours. Patients should perform deep-breathing exercises and incentive spirometry every 4 hours. Chest physiotherapy includes assisted coughing, tracheal suctioning, chest percussion, and postural drainage. Patients can also be placed on a Kinetic bed that rotates sideways through 124° and provides continuous postural drainage. The rotation may have to be unilateral in the case of unilateral lung disease. When patients are moved to a regular bed, even with a variable air mattress overlay, they will need more vigorous pulmonary hygiene. In case of a lobar collapse despite adequate prevention, fiberoptic bronchoscopy combined with suction and lavage may be able to clear the mucus plug. Should pneumonia ensue, sputum is collected for culture and sensitivity and antibiotics are started empirically according to prevalent organisms in the ICU and adjusted once the microbiology results are available.

Treatment of Respiratory Complications Not Due to Paralysis

Certain respiratory complications are a result of the injury but are not directly related to paralysis. PE is a major cause of mortality in the early SCI, and prevention and treatment have been outlined earlier in this chapter.

Neurogenic Pulmonary Edema. Neurogenic pulmonary edema is due to the mechanical trauma to the spinal cord causing a short-lived increase in autonomic discharge with bradycardia, hypertension, and a high number of bizarre arrhythmias. The autonomic discharge is responsible for an increase in total peripheral resistance, with a shift of blood into the more compliant pulmonary circulation. A rise in pulmonary pressure accompanied by some loss of capillary integrity results in pulmonary edema. Systemic and pulmonary hypertension return to normal early on, but pulmonary edema persists. Attempts to raise the blood pressure in SCI patients with crystalloids may be another cause of pulmonary edema by producing dilution and a reduction in oncotic

pressure ending in more leakage of fluids. Central venous pressure monitoring is of some use, but quite often there is a disproportionate rise in pulmonary capillary wedge pressure long before the rise in central venous pressure. Therefore, monitoring pulmonary capillary wedge pressure is suggested. Therapy with oxygen or intermittent positive-pressure ventilation is usually sufficient for the patient because the episode is short-lived and reversible. Diuretics only impair the circulatory volume and should be used carefully. Occasionally, this type of pulmonary edema is intractable and may progress into full-blown adult respiratory distress syndrome.[4]

Associated Pulmonary Trauma. Several respiratory complications result from associated trauma. Pulmonary trauma (aspiration, rib fractures, flail segments, pneumothorax, hemothorax, pulmonary contusion, and ruptured diaphragm) usually causes hypoventilation and increases the risk of pneumonia. In unilateral lung pathology, the effect of gravity can be offset by placing the patient with the healthy lung down. The dependent lung gets the most perfusion; hence, an optimum V/Q ratio and, therefore improved gas exchange, is obtained. Trauma at more distant sites can also interfere with respiration. Loss of consciousness in head injuries is responsible for aspiration. In some head injuries, the respiratory drive is lost and neurogenic edema tends to be more common. Long-bone fractures are a major cause of fat emboli.

Gastrointestinal Complications

GI complications such as acute dilatation of the stomach and paralytic ileus make the excursion of the diaphragm more difficult. Patients with these injuries may need mechanical ventilation. Specific therapy of these complications is needed but is beyond the scope of this chapter.

Patients with SCI are prone to certain GI complications. They can be a result of the neuroendocrine response to stress or can be due to the abrupt changes in nervous control of the GI tract or to direct injury to the GI tract. Assessment of the abdomen is difficult in patients with SCI due to the loss of traditional clinical signs. Anorexia, nausea, or vomiting may be the only symptoms. Occasionally, there is a dull, poorly localized pain.

Referred pain to the interscapular region or to the testis or the thigh may be present. Abdominal percussion does not usually accentuate pain but may cause increased spasticity. Abdominal distention is only significant if it occurs suddenly, is progressive, or is accompanied by air-fluid levels on radiographs. Nonspecific indicators of abdominal pathology are low-grade fever, elevated serum and urine amylase levels, incontinence of bowel or bladder, and spinal reflex sweating.[4]

Acute Changes in Gastrointestinal Motility

The earliest GI complications are acute gastric dilatation and paralytic ileus. They occur as a direct response to trauma. Paralytic ileus occurs immediately in thoracolumbar lesions, within 24 hours in midthoracic SCI, and at approximately 48 hours in cervical injuries. The ileus resolves usually within the first 3 or 4 days, but may last somewhat longer (about 1 week) in cervical injuries.[16] The diagnosis is made by the abdominal distention, the absence of bowel sounds in ileus, the presence of a gastric splash in gastric dilatation, and gaseous distention on an abdominal x-ray. Loss of large volumes of fluid and electrolytes in the GI tract can produce hypovolemia, shock, and electrolyte disturbances. Hypotension can be accentuated by the decreased venous return due to pressure of the distended gut on the inferior vena cava. Severe hypokalemia predisposes to cardiac arrhythmias in a patient who often already has cardiovascular compromise. Hyponatremia may cause lethargy and, if severe enough, can cause convulsions. The large amount of fluids sequestrated in the gut induces vomiting with a high risk for aspiration especially in cervical SCI patients who have lost their protective reflexes. The sheer volume of fluid within the GI tract pushes the abdominal wall outward and the diaphragm upward and makes breathing considerably more difficult. Patients with SCI need a nasogastric tube and no oral intake until the ileus and the acute gastric dilatation are resolved. Hydration is maintained with intravenous fluids. If the period of ileus continues beyond a few days, then total parenteral nutrition needs to be instituted.[20] Cholinergic agents are sometimes used in these conditions, but their role in stasis after SCI has not been established.

Stress Ulceration

Stress ulceration in the stomach or the duodenum occurs in up to 22% of patients with SCI during the first month, with the main incidence between Days 6 and 14.[4] In 85% of patients, hyperemia of the stomach can be found.[16] A much smaller percentage suffers ulceration, bleeding, or perforation. The exact pathogenesis remains a mystery. Several factors have been implicated, including breakdown of the mucosal barrier, decreased mucosal blood flow, raised intraluminal acid concentration, low intramural pH, and diminished epithelial regeneration. Shock, catecholamines, and steroids have been implicated, but no conclusive evidence has been found. Cushing ulcers are found in serious central nervous system (CNS) injury and are due to adrenocorticotropic hormone release and an increased parasympathetic discharge producing a rise in serum gastrin and an increase in the secretion of gastric hydrochloric acid and pepsin. These deep erosions are typically multiple and can be located in the esophagus, stomach, and duodenum. In SCI, they are most frequently situated on the anterior gastric wall and along the lesser curve.

The main problem in diagnosing ulcers is the lack of symptoms and signs. The presence of an ulcer often remains silent until a complication such as perforation or bleeding arises. Bleeding occurs in about 5% of patients and is more prevalent in complete lesions and in cervical SCI. Bleeding is most likely from Day 4 to 10 but may be seen up to 6 weeks after the injury. Most patients do not have a previous history of GI dysfunction. The loss of normal sympathetic compensatory mechanisms accounts for the rapid deterioration and a mortality rate of 80%.[16] Ulcers can be prevented by the placement of a nasogastric tube that continuously removes the acidic contents. Early nutritional support also protects against GI bleeding. The underlying mechanism is uncertain but may be a reduced hydrochloric acid secretion due to the presence of amino acids modifying the response of parietal cells to neural and humoral stimulation. The incidence of bleeding drops from 7.5% in patients who are fed enterally when clinically ready to 2% in the group where total parenteral nutrition is started if the patient is still nil per os (NPO) on Day 5.[20]

All patients with SCI should be given magnesium- or aluminum-containing antacids. Sucralfate is a nonsystemic agent that, in the presence of an acid pH, coats the ulcer bed and promotes healing. It has no significant side effects. H_2 antagonists are the mainstay of treatment because of sustained acid reduction and increased ulcer healing rates. They can be used in prevention and treatment. The two main H_2 antagonists are cimetidine and ranitidine. Cimetidine has been available longer and the side effects are considerable including CNS depression, deterioration of pre-existing hepatic and renal impairment, and alteration of the metabolism of warfarin, diazepam, anticonvulsants, etc. Ranitidine was introduced more recently and does not affect the CNS nor does it alter drug metabolism.[6,16] However, both have been implicated in aspiration pneumonitis. Presumptively, both reduce gastric acidity, which in turn may allow an increase in bacterial content of the stomach. If aspiration occurs, this elevation may lead to an increased number of bacteria aspirated.

Associated Abdominal Trauma

Abdominal trauma accompanies the SCI in about 6.8% of cases.[16] As mentioned earlier, it is often missed due to the lack of symptoms or signs. Abdominal trauma may present with an increasing abdominal girth (ileus) although this is not diagnostic. Hypotension may be the first indication of a problem. A drop in hemoglobin and/or hematocrit is a late sign of bleeding, and bleeding may not be in the abdomen. For the multi-injured patient with paraplegia, a peritoneal lavage should be performed since the abdominal examination is unreliable. This is useful to detect free intraperitoneal blood. False-positive results are possible in pelvic fractures where blood may have leaked into the free peritoneal cavity. False-negative results are more serious and present in 2% of patients. They are due to isolated injuries of the pancreas and the duodenum, which are retroperitoneal. False-negative results are also possible in injuries to the diaphragm, the small bowel, or the bladder, which do not bleed enough to produce >100,000 red blood cells/cu mm. A computed tomography scan should be performed despite the negative peritoneal lavage if there is clinical suspicion of an abdominal injury.[1,16]

Esophageal injury is rare but can occur with either penetrating cervical trauma or with nonpenetrating injury to the larynx and trachea. The only sign may be subcutaneous emphysema.

Surgical Gastrointestinal Emergencies

Surgical GI emergencies such as appendicitis, cholecystitis, a perforated viscus, infarcted bowel, and pancreatitis are possible in the SCI patient at the same or slightly higher rate as in the general population but carry a much greater risk of death. They are difficult to diagnose because of the limited sensory input from the parietal peritoneum. A high level of suspicion and early investigation are of utmost importance. Ultrasound scanning is less useful in SCI patients because of the increased amount of gas present in the bowel. Pancreatitis is particularly important in SCI and can be a direct result of the abdominal trauma. The incidence is also increased in this patient group in the later stages because of the predominant activity of the parasympathetic nervous system causing overdistention of the sphincter of Oddi and more viscous secretions. Direct activation of trypsinogen by hypercalcemia is possible.[16] Gallstones also occur slightly more frequently due to gallbladder hypomotility and hypercalcemia.[14]

Long-Term Alterations in Gastrointestinal Motility

GI motility is grossly altered in SCI patients. Extrinsic sympathetic control is lost in all injuries above T6. Parasympathetic control up to the left colon is through the vagus nerve and is therefore intact. The more distal parasympathetic outflow is via the sacral nerves (S2-4) and is altered in a variable way in SCI. In the esophagus, the altered nervous control is responsible for gastroesophageal reflux and possible hiatus hernia. SCI patients with a high injury have delayed emptying of the stomach, which can be responsible for nausea and a feeling of fullness. Colonic motility is also altered. The gastrocolic reflex is lost and, for a given distention, there is a much higher pressure; also, motility is decreased, especially in the left side of the colon. Continence is usually maintained by the internal and external anal sphincter. Normal evacuation requires relaxation of the internal sphincter upon rectal distention.

This anorectal reflex is dependent upon the enteric intrinsic plexus and is preserved in SCI. The external sphincter increases its tonic activity upon rectal distention via a spinal reflex contraction; this soon decreases but voluntary control of the external sphincter allows the CNS to suppress defecation. This voluntary control is lost in patients with SCI. Patients with an upper motor neuron lesion (anal wink and cremasteric reflex present) have automatic defecation upon rectal distention. They can initiate defecation with suppositories and digital stimulation after relaxation of the internal sphincter. Evacuation ensues in about 30 minutes. In lower motor neuron lesions, there is damage to the parasympathetic system and to the nervi erigentes to the external sphincter; the defecation reflex is absent, resulting in severe constipation and fecal incontinence. The intrinsic defecation reflex is present but very weak. Manual evacuation is necessary because digital stimulation is ineffective. In incomplete lesions, bowel emptying after abdominal massage or a Valsalva maneuver may be possible. Suprasacral SCI is associated with impaction proximal to the splenic flexure at the boundary of vagus and parasympathetic innervation. Patients with a sacral injury may suffer from distal impaction due to loss of the defecation reflex.[2-14]

Bowel Management

Bowel management is very important in all patients with SCI and should include a high-fiber diet, maintaining an upright position early after injury, and a healthy level of activity. Regular timing of meals and adequate fluid intake are easy to maintain. In the acute period, suppositories every other day and saline enemas are used to establish a regular bowel pattern.[2,14-16] Prevention of impaction is very important but, if present, impaction should be treated with laxatives, enemas, or manual disimpaction. Saline enemas are preferable as they are mild irritants of the colon and break up stool particles. Sodium absorption may be a problem in concomitant renal failure. We recommend bulk laxatives, mainly a high-fiber diet or bran, because they hold water in the stool and cause an expanded and softened stool that reduces intracolonic pressure and transit time. The osmotic laxatives, mainly lactulose, are effective and relatively safe and should be given in a dose of 2 to 7 gm once or twice a day. Stool softeners have a detergent action and cause accumulation of water in the gut lumen. They disrupt the gastric and intestinal mucosa and therefore increase the absorption of other drugs. Stimulant laxatives such as bisacodyl, senna, cascara, and danthron act by increasing fluid secretion and peristalsis. They cause a dilated, atonic bowel and should be avoided. Enemas and colonic cleansing preparations induce anal leakage and incontinence in the long term and should also be avoided.

Nutrition

Adequate nutrition is an important and difficult issue because the normal response to trauma is complicated by some problems specific to the SCI. Nutrition management is discussed in detail in Chapter 19.

Metabolic Response to Trauma in SCI

The normal neuroendocrine response to stress consists of an ebb phase lasting 24 to 48 hours followed by a flow phase. The ebb phase is characterized by a decrease in metabolic rate. The decreased release of insulin and the raised levels of catecholamines, corticosteroids, antidiuretic hormone, renin-angiotensin, and aldosterone are responsible for hyperglycemia, hypokalemia, and retention of sodium and water. The flow phase is an acute catabolic state. Corticosteroids and catecholamines cause the breakdown of proteins to amino acids to be used for gluconeogenesis and repair. The raised concentration of catecholamines and corticosteroids, together with insulin resistance, are responsible for a state of hyperglycemia. Urinary nitrogen excretion is high, and the catabolic state normally peaks after 4 to 8 days in patients with uncomplicated SCI.[16] In multisystem injuries or after surgery there is a much greater and prolonged response. Fever, infection, and sepsis also cause an exaggerated response. The basal metabolic rate raises 13% per degree Celsius above 37°C and an extra 10% in case of sepsis.[3] Some initial weight loss is expected in these patients. Eventually, paraplegics have a weight 10 to 15 pounds below the ideal weight as established by Metropolitan Life Insurance, and the weight of quadriplegics drops to 15 to 20 pounds below the ideal weight.

Nutritional Problems in SCI

Several factors complicate the estimation of energy needs in the SCI patient.[3] Denervation atrophy and paralysis cause muscle atrophy; this provides amino acids for gluconeogenesis and less energy is needed to move the decreased muscle mass. However, even simple activities take up much energy in patients with SCI. Some have glucose intolerance due to insulin resistance or due to the increased supply of glucose. The latter is produced by the hypercatabolic state (raised levels of corticosteroids and catecholamines) and by the use of total parenteral nutrition containing high levels of glucose. Postacute obesity can occur due to limited mobility and a caloric intake far above the caloric needs.

In estimating the nutritional needs of SCI patients, attention should be paid to the provision of adequate amounts of vitamin C, zinc, fluids, and proteins as patients with SCI are prone to skin and wound breakdown due to impaired mobility, preinjury obesity, anemia, and malnutrition. These patients also have increased caloric needs as a consequence of their poikilothermy, especially in hyperthermia. Anemia may be present as a result of associated trauma or GI bleeding. Anemia may have been pre-existing or may be due to an increased red blood cell breakdown secondary to the stress response. This causes oxygen transport to be low at a time of increased energy demand for tissue repair and synthesis. Nutritional management is also complicated by respiratory paralysis and by atelectasis or pneumonia. Protein-energy malnutrition can cause a decrease in diaphragmatic mass and hamper respiration. Overfeeding increases glucose oxidation and CO_2 production; the hypoventilating patient cannot eliminate CO_2, which may prolong the ventilator or oxygen dependency. Overhydration causes pulmonary edema, and dehydration makes secretions more viscous putting the patient at risk for atelectasis and pneumonia. The chances of aspiration are higher in abdominal distention associated with early feeding, unabsorbed food, and a high-fiber diet begun too early. If the paralytic ileus lasts for more than 5 days, total parenteral nutrition should be started. Gastric ulceration is more common in prolonged fasting and may also occur as a result of irritation by a nasogastric tube. For bowel training to be successful, the correct amount of food, fiber, and fluids is necessary. Hyperosmolar tube feeding, lactose intolerance, and pseudomembranous colitis following antibiotic treatment can complicate matters by causing diarrhea.

To prevent nutritional deterioration as well as fluid and electrolyte abnormalities associated with diarrhea, the patient may revert to the NPO state and receive parenteral nutrition with supplements to correct fluid and electrolyte imbalances. Bladder training with eventual intermittent catheterization in most patients will require a limitation of fluid intake to avoid overdistention. A maximum urine output of 400 to 500 cc every 4 to 6 hours is acceptable. Hypercalcemia and hypercalciuria are common in SCI and due to mobilization of bone that begins at Day 10 and continues for 6 months or more. Decreasing the calcium intake does not seem to affect the level of calcium in the blood or urine.

Appetite in patients with SCI is often decreased as a result of sensory loss or immobilization. Patients may have difficulty swallowing, and the tracheostomy tube can interfere with the relaxation of the gastroesophageal sphincter. Narcotics can prolong the ileus or cause constipation. Poor dentition, maxillofacial injuries, and a reduced level of consciousness as in head injury may also interfere with normal feeding.[3,16]

Estimation of Energy Requirements

Daily weighing and biochemical estimations may give some idea of the patient's nutritional state. Pre-albumin and transferrin reflect nutritional changes relatively well and better than albumin, which has a longer half life. Low levels of total body iron, lymphocyte count, hematocrit, and hemoglobin are all associated with malnutrition. Total energy requirements (TER) are arrived at by multiplying the basal energy expenditure (BEE) by a stress factor. Maintenance protein requirements are 0.8 gm/kg body-weight. Protein needs in stress such as SCI are raised to 1 to 1.5 gm protein/kg body-weight. A better way to estimate protein requirements is from urinary nitrogen excretion. The amount of calories per nitrogen is 150/1 in minimal protein depletion, but in SCI it should be much nearer to 100/1.[3,20]

TER = BEE × stress factor [1.5-1.75 in acute SCI and 1.75-2.0 in acute SCI with multiple trauma]

BEE (men) = 66.0 + (13.7 × weight (in kg)) + (5 × height (in cm)) − (6.8 × age (in years))

BEE (women) = 655 + (9.6 × weight (in kg)) + (1.7 × height (in cm)) − (4.7 × age in years)

Estimated total nitrogen excretion = (total urinary nitrogen excretion in gm/24 hrs) + 2 gm extra-urinary loss/24 hrs [Note: more than 2 gm nitrogen is lost extra-urinary in large wounds, decubitus, or diarrhea]

Urea nitrogen in urine in gm/24 hrs = urinary volume in liters/24 hrs × urea nitrogen in urine in gm/liter

Anabolic protein requirements = [(urea nitrogen in urine in gm/24 hrs + 2 gm/24 hrs) × 6.25] + (10 to 30 gm)

Total parenteral nutrition should be started if the patient is NPO on Day 5. The total energy requirements are then reached within 48 hours of caloric supplementation. If the patient is still NPO by Day 17, a feeding jejunostomy should be considered.[20]

Urological Management

Changes in urological management in the SCI patient have had some of the greatest impact on patient survival. During the early part of the 20th century, mortality associated with urological problems was close to 80%. Late mortality was due to renal failure in 40% of patients.[29,34] Dramatic improvement in survival has been due to the introduction of sterile intermittent catheterization in the hospital by Guttmann and Frankel[15] and by the introduction of clean, intermittent catheterization at home by Lapides et al.[21] A better understanding of the urodynamics of the lower urinary tract, selective use of sphincterotomy, and the advent of antibiotics have further decreased the mortality rate. The main goals of urological treatment are a functional lower urinary tract and an infection-free urinary system.[26,31]

In the acute period, an indwelling catheter size 16 to 18 French gauge is used to monitor urinary output and to prevent detrusor overdistention following SCI or operation. Baseline urea, creatinine, and urine culture should be obtained. The evaluation of pre-existing problems such as in-continence, prostate enlargement, or renal pathology is important for decisions regarding long-term management. The aim is for the patient to have a functioning bladder that stores well and empties easily with a minimum of urinary tract infections and with absence of urinary incontinence and autonomic dysreflexia.[16,34] The principles of management of the urinary tract in SCI are given in Chapter 21.

Pressure Sores

Pressure ulcers are another highly prevalent complication of SCI carrying high morbidity and mortality rates. They occur in 28% to 85% of patients with SCI. According to the National SCI Statistical Center, the incidence of pressure sores during the initial hospital stay is 32%; another study reported a pressure sore rate of 59% during the first month after injury.[22]

Definition and Pathogenesis

A pressure sore is a localized area of cellular necrosis of the skin and the subcutaneous tissues due to occlusion of the blood supply. They are located over areas of high pressure such as the sacrum, the greater trochanter, the ischial tuberosities, the occiput, the scapulae, the malleoli, and the calcaneus. Pressure sores have been described by Enis and Sarmiento (Table 1).[8] Different grades need different types of treatment and have a different complication rate.

Several factors contribute to the origin of pressure sores.[8-14,16-20,22] The main external factor is increased pressure for extended periods of time. This increase in local pressure impairs the capillary circulation and at the same time occludes the lymphatic vessels causing extravascular accumulation of tissue fluid and metabolites and further impairs an already precarious blood supply. Intrinsic host factors are more numerous. Different degrees of loss of sympathetic supply and unopposed vagus activity that produce cardiovascular changes occur in all patients with SCI. Loss of vasomotor tone produces vasodilatation, bradycardia, an increased cardiac index that results in an increased stroke volume and a decreased venous return. The reduction in venous return is further accentuated by the low muscle tone and the absence of the muscle pump. Gravity, mainly

TABLE 1

GRADING SYSTEM OF PRESSURE SORES*

Grade I	Ulceration of epidermis and superficial dermis
	Inflammation of all layers
	Nonblanching erythema
Grade II	Ulceration up to junction with subcutaneous fat
	Adinoxal structures destroyed
Grade III	Ulceration into the subcutaneous fat
	Extensive undermining of the skin
Grade IV	Invasion of the deep fascia, muscle onto bone, and joint
	Osteomyelitis is common and a source of septicemia

*Reproduced with permission from Enis and Samiento.[8]

with the patient in the sitting position, and decreased negative inspiratory force due to pulmonary insufficiency may also diminish venous return. These cardiovascular alterations are responsible for vascular stasis and tissue hypoxia. Pulmonary insufficiency can cause hypoxemia, further impairing tissue oxygenation. The decreased host resistance to pressure ulcers in SCI is an important factor in the pathogenesis. The sensory loss in SCI accounts for patient lack of awareness of any numbness, pain, or sensation of ischemia. Adaptive mechanisms present in normal persons such as shifting the body weight and changing position are therefore not employed by patients with SCI, at least not as an automatic reflex.[14] Due to atrophy of tissues in SCI, the thickness of the protective layers of skin, fat, and muscle over bone is greatly diminished. Fecal and urinary incontinence result in a moist, macerated skin much more prone to damage. Shearing stresses in SCI are increased threefold partly as a result of lower-limb spasticity (especially of the adductor muscles) and partly as a result of paralysis that causes the patient to slide down when sitting upright in bed. In SCI, blood flow below the level of injury is reduced to one-third of its normal value. One study has also shown a decrease in transcutaneous oxygen tension even in the absence of pressure.[22]

Prevention and Treatment

The basis of treatment is prevention because pressure sores take a long time to heal when they occur. The loss of fluid and proteins from the pressure sore and the presence of infection also put a high strain on the patient's nutritional status. In the worst scenario, decubitus ulcers can proceed to osteomyelitis and life-threatening sepsis. Absence of pressure sores is an exquisite example of good nursing. Patients need repositioning at least every 2 hours. The positions need to be changed between supine, prone, and on the side in a 20° to 30° angle supported by soft pillows. Not all of these positions may be possible to achieve during the early stages of SCI due to intubation, traction, etc. The head of the bed should be elevated only for short periods since this position greatly increases shearing forces. Control of flexor spasm with muscle relaxants will decrease shearing. Friction can be minimized by using sheepskin and an egg-crate mattress; several special beds are available on the market.[14] Some have inflatable mattresses, others are oscillatory, still others are flotation beds filled with air, water, or silicone beads and air.

In the authors' experience, the Kinetic bed has proved to be extremely beneficial. Patients should be lifted across the bed rather than dragged across it when their position is manually changed. When the patient advances to wheelchair use, the chair must be fitted with suitable pressure-relieving cushions. The patient needs to adhere to a strict pattern of "push ups" or side shifts every 20 to 30 minutes.[14] Sympathetic tone improves slightly in time and consequently there is minor improvement in host resistance.

Electrical stimulation has been used to improve cutaneous blood flow, thereby preventing the development of ulcers and promoting the healing of ulcers already present. Transcutaneous electric nerve stimulation increases the skin temperature and improves the cutaneous microcirculation beginning after 15 to 30 minutes and lasting several hours. Functional electrical stimulation also increases the blood flow to the skin. Subcutaneous stimulation with microelectric medical stimulation can relieve pain, improve the cutaneous blood flow, increase the skin temperature, and promote ulcer healing. High-voltage pulsed galvanic stimulation increases the healing rate of cutaneous wounds and decreases their contamination. Fibroblasts located at the negative electrode have a maximum protein and DNA synthesis at voltages of 50 and 75 mV supplied at a frequency of 100 Hz.[22] Despite its apparent usefulness, electrical stimulation is seldom used for this purpose in SCI.

Conservative treatment is based on removal of pressure and regular debridement of necrotic tissue. Infection control may necessitate oral antibiotics. Epithelialization in Grade I and II pressure sores can be promoted by keeping them clean, dry, and protected. Grade III ulcers can be treated by using wet-to-dry packing with gauze soaked in dakin's solution, sterile saline, H_2O_2, or silver nitrate. Currently, hydroactive dressings and granules or calcium alginate have become the treatment of choice for these pressure sores. Superficial well-granulated wounds can be covered with a split-thickness skin graft. Grade IV ulcers need extensive excision of all infected bone and necrotic tissue. Myocutaneous flaps may be used in these ulcers because of their good blood supply and mobility. Moreover, they may not require optimal sterile conditions and have a great cavity-filling capacity often needed to cover the large defects left by these ulcers.[14,23]

Pain

In the past, the catastrophic consequences of SCI took priority in the SCI treatment. Most patients now have a normal life span and pain becomes a much more important issue. Several studies indicate that in 10% to 25% of patients, there is sufficient pain to interfere with normal functioning. The first occurrence of pain is highly variable. One-third of patients have pain dating from the time of injury, but in some, pain appears more than a decade after the injury.[4] Pain early after the injury is usually directly related to the injury itself. It can be due to soft-tissue trauma or to fractures. This type of pain can be treated with acetaminophen or acetylsalicylic acid with or without codeine. If the pain is mainly inflammatory then naproxen can be of use. Painful spasms are treated with benzodiazepines. Opiate analgesia may be necessary in certain conditions; for example, after orthopedic procedures. Caution is needed because the most painful syndromes in SCI do not respond well and the tendency is to increase the dosage with increasing tolerance as a result. Opiates have several unwanted side effects such as apathy, loss of appetite, and constipation.

They have a central action and therefore more easily mask other pathology. Their short-lasting anxiolytic and antidepressant effect can be beneficial. Opiates should be given only for short periods of time. Morphine, superior to meperidine due to its shorter action, must be reduced as soon as possible and an analgesic with codeine substituted. As pain subsides, simple analgesia will be sufficiently strong.

Some patients may have pain of neurological origin in the acute period; for example, radicular pain, hyperalgesic border reactions (painful hyperesthesia in the area adjoining the damaged dermatome), and central pain syndromes. Psychotropic drugs are effective to relieve pain due to neurological injury, but there are no substantial reports of their effectiveness after SCI.

Pain due to spasm can be prevented by antispasticity medication such as benzodiazepines, dantrolene, and baclofen. Neuralgias and dysesthesias (especially stabbing pain) respond to anticonvulsant therapy such as carbamazepine, valproate, and phenytoin.

For chronic pain, several other treatment modalities are available: electroanalgesia, several forms of surgery, and psychotherapy.[4]

CONCLUSION

Spinal cord injury remains a devastating disease because often there is either minimal or no reversal of the damage. The outcome in SCI, however, has greatly improved since the beginning of the century. The advent of specialized, multidisciplinary centers has assured optimum patient care. Improved early management has prevented deterioration of the neurological lesion and has significantly decreased the complication rate. Advances in the treatment of complications such as urosepsis, PE, and pneumonia have greatly increased quality of life and longevity. The emphasis in current treatment focuses on rehabilitation and adaptation to the disability. Continuing efforts should be made to ensure that these patients live a meaningful and productive life.

REFERENCES

1. American College of Surgeons Committee on Trauma. **Advanced Trauma Life Support Student Manual.** Chicago, Ill: American College of Surgeons, 1993

2. Banwell JG, Creasey GH, Aggarwal AM, et al: Management of the neurogenic bowel in patients with spinal cord injury. **Urol Clin North Am 20:**517-525, 1993

3. Blissitt PA: Nutrition in acute spinal cord injury. **Crit Care Nurs Clin North Am 2:**375-383, 1990

4. Bloch RF, Basbaum M: **Management of Spinal Cord Injuries.** Baltimore, Md: Williams & Wilkins, 1986

5. Dhami MS, Bona RD: Using anticoagulants safely. Guidelines for the therapeutic and prophylactic regimens. **Postgrad Med 90:**121-130, 1991

6. DiMarino AJ Jr, Daberies MA: Gastrointestinal diseases, in Myers AR (ed): **Medicine (NMS Series).** Baltimore, Md: Williams & Wilkins, 1986, pp 147-149

7. Ducker TB, Saul TG: The poly-trauma and spinal cord injury, in Tator CH (ed): **Early Management of Acute Spinal Cord Injury.** New York, NY: Raven Press, 1982, pp 53-58

8. Enis JE, Sarmiento A: The pathophysiology and management of pressure sores. **Orthop Rev 2:**25-34, 1973

9. Fenstermaker RA: Acute neurological management of the patient with spinal cord injury. **Urol Clin North Am 20:**413-420, 1993

10. Fishburn MJ, Marino RJ, Ditunno JF Jr: Atelectasis and pneumonia in acute spinal cord injury. **Arch Phys Med Rehabil 71:**197-200, 1990

11. Green D: Deep vein thrombosis in spinal cord injury—summary and recommendation. **Chest 102 (Suppl):**633S-635S, 1992

12. Green D: Prevention of thromboembolism after spinal cord injury. **Semin Thromb Hemost 17:** 347-350, 1991

13. Green D: Prophylaxis of thromboembolism in spinal cord injured patients. **Chest 102 (Suppl):**649S-651S, 1992

14. Gutierrez PA, Young RR, Vulpe M: Spinal cord injury—an overview. **Urol Clin North Am 20:**373-382, 1993

15. Guttmann L, Frankel H: The value of intermittent catheterization in the early management of traumatic paraplegia and tetraplegia. **Paraplegia 4:**63-83, 1966

16. Halm MA: Elimination concerns with acute spinal cord trauma. **Crit Care Nurs Clin North Am 2:** 385-398, 1990

17. Hull RD: Venous thromboembolism in spinal cord injury patients. **Chest 102 (Suppl):**658S-661S, 1992

18. Kocan MJ: Pulmonary considerations in the critical care phase. **Crit Care Nurs Clin North Am 2:**369-374, 1990

19. Kulkarni JR, Burt AA, Trumans AJ: Prophylactic low dose heparin anticoagulant therapy in patients with spinal cord injuries: a retrospective study. **Paraplegia 30:** 169-172, 1992

20. Kuric J, Lucas CE, Ledgerwood AM: Nutritional support: a prophylaxis against stress bleeding after spinal cord injury. **Paraplegia 27:**140-145, 1989

21. Lapides J, Diokno AC, Silber SJ, et al: Clean intermittent self-catheterization in the treatment of urinary tract disease. **J Urol 107:**458, 1972

22. Mawson AR, Siddiqui FH, Biundo JJ Jr: Enhancing host resistance to pressure ulcers: a new approach to prevention. **Prevent Med 22:**433-450, 1993

23. McGregor JC: Pressure sores: a personal comment. **Paraplegia 30:**116-117, 1992

24. Merli GJ: Management of deep vein thrombosis in spinal cord injury. **Chest 102 (Suppl):**652S-657S, 1992

25. Merli GJ, Crabbe S, Doyle L: Mechanical plus pharmacological prophylaxis for deep vein thrombosis in acute spinal cord injury. **Paraplegia 30:**558-562, 1992

26. National Institute on Disability and Rehabilitation Research Consensus Statement: The prevention and management of urinary tract infections among people with spinal cord injuries. **J Am Paraplegia Soc 15:** 194-204, 1992

27. Ryan M, Klein S, Bongard F: Missed injuries associated with spinal cord trauma. **Am Surg 59:**371-374, 1993

28. Schwenker D: Cardiovascular considerations in the critical care phase. **Crit Care Nurs Clin North Am 2:** 363-367, 1990

29. Selzman AA, Hampel N: Urologic complications of spinal cord injury. **Urol Clin North Am 20:**453-461,

30. Stinson Kidd S: Emergency management of spinal cord injuries. **Crit Care Nurs Clin North Am 2:** 349-356, 1990

31. Tuel SM, Meythaler JM, Cross LL, et al: Cost-effective screening by nursing staff for urinary tract infection in the spinal cord injured patient. **Am J Phys Med Rehabil 69:**128-130, 1990

32. Walleck CA: Neurological considerations in the critical care phase. **Crit Care Nurs Clin North Am 2:** 357-360, 1990

33. Weingarden SI: Deep venous thrombosis in spinal cord injury—overview of the problem. **Chest 102 (Suppl):**636S-639S, 1992

34. Wheeler JS Jr, Walter JW: Acute urological management of the patient with spinal cord injury. **Urol Clin North Am 20:**403-410, 1993

CHAPTER 21

UROLOGICAL MANAGEMENT OF THE SPINAL CORD INJURY PATIENT

SENDER HERSCHORN, BSC, MDCM, FRCSC, AND RAUL C. ORDORICA, MD

Normally, the bladder acts as a storage vessel and as an organ of expulsion. The bladder stores increasing volumes of urine and is an organ of expulsion by which coordinated detrusor muscle contraction and sphincter relaxation completely and efficiently empties its contents at a socially acceptable time. The human's ability to exercise complete volitional control over lower urinary tract function is taken for granted until an injury to the nervous system, such as a spinal cord injury (SCI), alters lower urinary tract control. Proper functioning of the lower urinary tract is required not only for continence, which has both social and health implications, but also for long-term preservation of renal function. Underlying this ability are the interactions of a complex neurological framework responsible for urinary storage and voiding. SCI can result in the disruption of this delicate balance, with both acute and chronic effects on the urinary tract.

This chapter discusses and outlines the urological management of spinal cord trauma within the first month following injury.

ANATOMY AND PHYSIOLOGY OF THE NORMAL LOWER URINARY TRACT

The lower urinary tract, made up of the bladder and the urethra, is responsible for both low-pressure storage and the efficient emptying of its contents. The bladder muscle is the detrusor, a meshwork of interlacing smooth muscle fibers coalescing at the bladder neck, which in the relaxed state allows the accommodation of increasing volumes of urine.[24] Continence is maintained by the two sphincteric mechanisms located at the bladder neck and in the urethra, which are identified as the proximal and distal sphincters.

The proximal sphincter is formed by a continuation of inner longitudinal detrusor fibers through the bladder neck into the urethra, along with outer detrusor fibers that spiral around the bladder neck with an abundance of elastic connective tissue.[24,61] While the proximal sphincter in both sexes is capable of maintaining continence in the isolated setting, it is unable to achieve pressures as high as that of the distal sphincter. The distal sphincter is formed by intrinsic and extrinsic components.[24] The intrinsic portion is made up of slow-twitch striated muscle fibers that surround the membranous urethra as it pierces the pelvic floor. These slow-twitch fibers allow for the continued tonic contraction of the external sphincter without fatigue. The extrinsic portion is formed by the pelvic floor musculature in the form of fast-twitch striated muscle fibers that envelop the intrinsic portion of the external sphincter. The extrinsic portion rapidly fatigues, offering brief additional support with voluntary contraction during stress maneuvers to counteract increases in intra-abdominal pressure. The male distal sphincter is capable of higher physiological pressures than the female, although both are deficient in intrinsic fibers along their dorsal aspect.[23] The female urethra is supplied with a hormonally responsive vascular plexus that forms a pliant cushion, believed to contribute an additional seal against urinary leakage.

The autonomic nerves supplying the bladder and urethra consist of parasympathetic and sympathetic components.[60] The parasympathetic preganglionic motor fibers to the detrusor arise in the intermediolateral column in the second, third, and fourth sacral cord segments (the conus medullaris). These myelinated fibers run into the pelvic plexus as the pelvic nerves.[43]

The sympathetic preganglionic motor fibers to the bladder and urethra are believed to originate in the intermediolateral nuclei of cord segments T10 to L2. They traverse the paravertebral ganglia and the superior hypogastric plexus over the aorta, and divide into right and left hypogastric nerves. The hypogastric and pelvic nerves of each side meet and branch repeatedly to form the pelvic plexus. Branches of the pelvic plexus innervate both ipsilateral and contralateral portions of pelvic organs.[60]

Postganglionic nerve fibers to the bladder and urethra are mainly short segments that arise close to or within the structures that they innervate. Their ganglia, which contain cholinergic, adrenergic, and small intensely fluorescent cells, may further mediate synaptic interactions between sympathetic and parasympathetic pathways.[15,19]

Innervation of the urethral striated sphincter, along with the surrounding pelvic floor muscles, is generally believed to be somatic from the sacral cord pudendal (Onuf's) nucleus via the pudendal nerve.[60] Controversy exists with reports of pelvic nerve innervation to the intrinsic external sphincter.[17,24] Afferent nerve fibers from the bladder and urethra have been demonstrated in the pelvic, pudendal, and hypogastric nerves, conducting various stimuli to the spinal cord.

While the exact neurological pathways involved with micturition have not been completely elucidated, several concepts are supported by both experimental animal and clinical human data.[6,16] The sacral spinal cord, the brainstem, and the cerebral cortex contain centers for the integration and control of micturition. Upon voiding, coordinated contraction of the detrusor occurs to form the expulsive force for emptying. While the proximal sphincter relaxes with bladder contraction, in part due to the inherent configuration of the detrusor fibers at the bladder neck, there also exists sympathetic control in the form of (alpha) receptors. The synchronous relaxation of the distal sphincter requires neurological coordination. The brainstem center is responsible for sustaining detrusor contraction and synergic external sphincter relaxation until the bladder is completely emptied. This is continued even after proprioceptive afferent impulses from the bladder have fallen below the threshold necessary to maintain the micturition reflex with partial emptying. The cerebral cortex can inhibit, initiate, or interrupt voiding at any time.

The lower urinary tract, therefore, has two phases, filling and voiding. During the filling phase, the sympathetic innervation is activated, the striated sphincters are contracted, and the parasympathetic is quiescent. During the voiding phase, the parasympathetic innervation is activated, the sympathetic is quiescent, and the striated sphincters relax. Through learned behavior, higher centers co-ordinate and control the interactions.

Initial Urological Management of the SCI Patient

Immediate urological management of the patient with SCI involves treating any associated trauma to the urinary tract and assuring proper drainage. Upper lumbar vertebral fractures should raise the suspicion of renal injuries, with significant trauma to the parenchyma, collecting system, or vascular pedicle. Sacral injuries and pelvic fractures may be associated with bladder and urethral injuries. Hematuria has typically been used as a guide for the detection of urological trauma, but may be notably absent if the patient is hypotensive or if there is a renal vascular pedicle disruption.[42] Intravenous pyelography (IVP) (and computed tomography) are utilized to evaluate upper tract injury, with the latter demonstrating more accuracy in staging the extent of renal damage.[10] Surgical exploration and intervention are advocated for uncontrolled renal hemorrhage, interruption of renal blood supply, or marked disruption of the collecting system.[11,38,50] Bladder disruption may be demonstrated by cystography, and urethral injuries are initially identified by retrograde urethrography. Bladder ruptures may be surgically repaired upon initial presentation, depending on their continuity with the peritoneal cavity.[14,49] Dorsal urethral injuries can be treated with suprapubic catheters or stented with a catheter, either acutely or within the first few weeks after injury.[29] Following the appropriate management of lower urinary tract trauma, urinary drainage is immediately established with a Foley catheter.

EFFECT OF SCI ON LOWER URINARY TRACT FUNCTION

A determination is made regarding the level of the SCI and its relationship to the sacral reflex arc, located at S2-4 (corresponding to the T11-12 vertebrae). Although of less significance during the initial phase of spinal shock, the level of injury in part determines the subsequent bladder behavior. Except for cases of complete cauda equina injury, the presence of the bulbocavernosus reflex is of lesser value when predicting the level of injury as it is typically present despite the occurrence of spinal shock.[1,36,52]

Initial bladder function following SCI is characterized by the presence of spinal shock, which most often lasts 6 to 8 weeks, but can range from 1 week to 1 year.[48] During this period, the bladder is completely areflexic; however, the precise causes of detrusor areflexia remain unclear.[21,61] It has been suggested that there is a loss of the facilitatory influences of suprasacral micturition centers, leading to bladder acontractility.[39,65] With the loss of parasympathetic efferent activity, the bladder accommodates increasing volumes of urine without reflex detrusor contractions.

Although detrusor tone is minimal, outlet resistance of the sphincter mechanisms may not actually be decreased. The resting sympathetic tone of various portions of the external sphincter has been demonstrated by urodynamic investigations of patients in spinal shock who had injuries above the sacral reflex arc.[4,40,44,52] Electromyographic activity has been recorded in the striated sphincter of patients in spinal shock. The measured maximum pressure is lower than normal. The normal guarding reflex is absent, and there is no voluntary control.[22] With this continued elevation in outlet pressure, urinary incontinence occurs only with significant elevations in bladder pressure. Bladder emptying is not effectively accomplished with the Valsalva maneuver or the Credé method due to the poor relaxation of the outlet at this stage.[51] If the bladder is not drained, it may become overstretched, and/or overflow incontinence may result. Appropriate methods of urinary drainage can best assure an outcome designed to minimize urological morbidity with preservation of bladder anatomy upper tract function.

INITIAL BLADDER MANAGEMENT

In the presence of spinal shock, with the patient unable to void or express urine, bladder drainage is initially managed with an indwelling catheter. Following stabilization of the patient, continued use of an indwelling catheter may appear to be more convenient for the nursing staff and the patient. However, indwelling catheters allow the continued colonization of the urinary tract with bacteria despite aseptic techniques, closed drainage systems, and the use of antimicrobials.[7,32,58] The incidence of colonization and infection with resistant organisms increases over time, with rates for developing bacteriuria consisting of 5% to 10% per day during the first week, until the patient has become infected by the end of the first month. In addition, poor drainage of prostatic and urethral secretions caused by indwelling catheters, along with local mucosal inflammatory reactions, can result in further infection and eventual stricture formation in male patients. Furthermore, attempts to treat infections in the presence of an indwelling catheter lead to the emergence of resistant organisms.

Patients who require large amounts of intravenous fluids, constant output monitoring, or who have large urine outputs are probably best managed with indwelling catheters until the output decreases. Patients with associated lower urinary tract injuries also required indwelling tubes in the early phase. Most other patients may be started on intermittent catheterization after the immediate post-injury period, usually within 3 days (range 1 to 7 days).[5,54]

INTERMITTENT CATHETERIZATION

Since its introduction in 1947 by Guttman and Frankel, intermittent catheterization has become the mainstay of early bladder management in most centers.[5,26,27] Lapides et al[34] in 1972 modified the procedure by advocating a clean rather than sterile technique. Intermittent catheterization is easily learned and applied in a sterile manner in the institutional setting, and with a clean technique in the non-institutional setting. The nonsterile technique improves patient compliance by making it easier for their training. While the clean technique may allow for greater introduction of bacteria into the bladder compared with the sterile method, it is safe with normal host resistance. This is better assured if the catheterization is performed gently, if the bladder is not permitted to become overdistended, and if the bladder is completely drained. Lapides et al[33] suggested that the increased susceptibility to bacterial invasion observed with bladder overdistention is caused by decreased blood flow in the bladder muscle and mucosa. To prevent this, bladder volumes should be maintained at 500 ml or below. Patients usually tolerate catheterization at 4- to 6-hourly intervals, with a 24-hour urine output of less than 2.5 liters. Fluid restriction may help decrease the frequency of catheterization.

Either a No. 14 or a No. 16 French straight catheter is well suited for intermittent catheterization. Patients with benign prostatic hypertrophy may require the use of a coudé, or curve-tipped, catheter to allow passage over an enlarged median lobe of the prostate. Marked difficulty with catheter passage should alert the clinician to the possible presence of a urethral stricture, false passage, or undiagnosed urethral injury, warrant-

ing urological investigation. For patients who prove unsuitable for early intermittent catheterization, placement of a trocar suprapubic catheter may be justified in the preliminary management.[13,20,53] For patients in whom intermittent catheterization is feasible, the urological complication rates with infection, stones, and detrimental changes in the bladder and/or urethral walls associated with chronic indwelling catheters, even those introduced suprapubically, have been markedly reduced.[12,18,28,31,34,63] Urinary tract infection that develops with intermittent catheterization management may be eradicated with appropriate antibiotic therapy without the similar fear of development of resistant organisms associated with indwelling catheters.

Although generally agreed that intermittent catheterization is an excellent form of management, it may not be feasible in some settings. In those instances, the short-term use of a small-bore Foley catheter or suprapubic tube has been shown to be a reasonable option.[35]

LOWER URINARY TRACT RECOVERY FOLLOWING SPINAL SHOCK

Following spinal shock, there is a gradual return of the reflex activity of the centers of undamaged spinal cord segments below the level of injury. During this recovery phase, the detrusor develops reflex contractions that initially are not sustained or of significant pressure. These inadequate contractions, along with poor relaxation of the bladder neck and external sphincter, result in inadequate emptying of the bladder. Gradually, the detrusor contractions may become more sustained and powerful. The reflex bladder activity may result in voiding between catheterizations. Varying degrees of bladder emptying can develop depending upon the bladder contraction along with the degree of proximal and/or distal sphincter dyssynergia or incoordination.[45,47,64,66] The patterns ultimately observed are combinations of interactions between the bladder and the sphincters. With higher lesions, the bladder may be hyperactive (hyperreflexic) with various patterns and degrees of proximal and/or distal sphincter dyssynergia. With lower

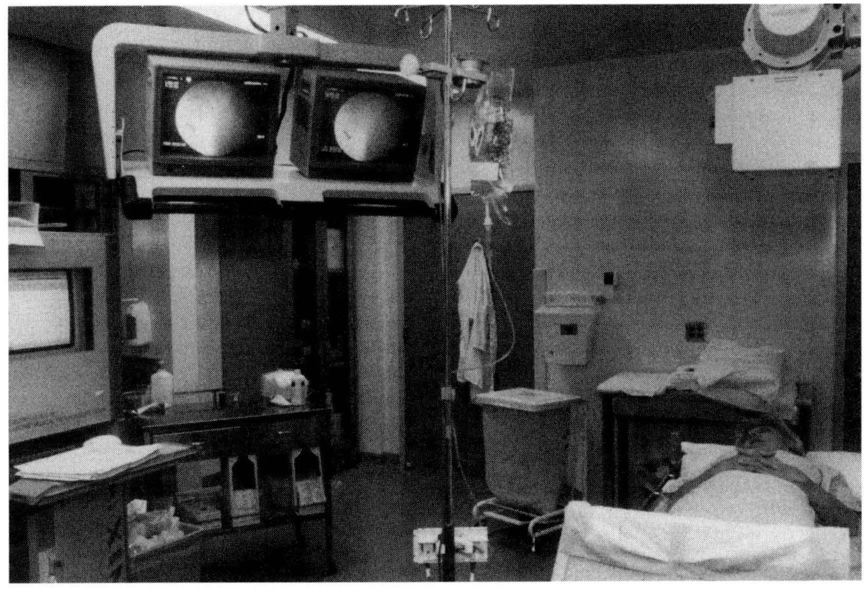

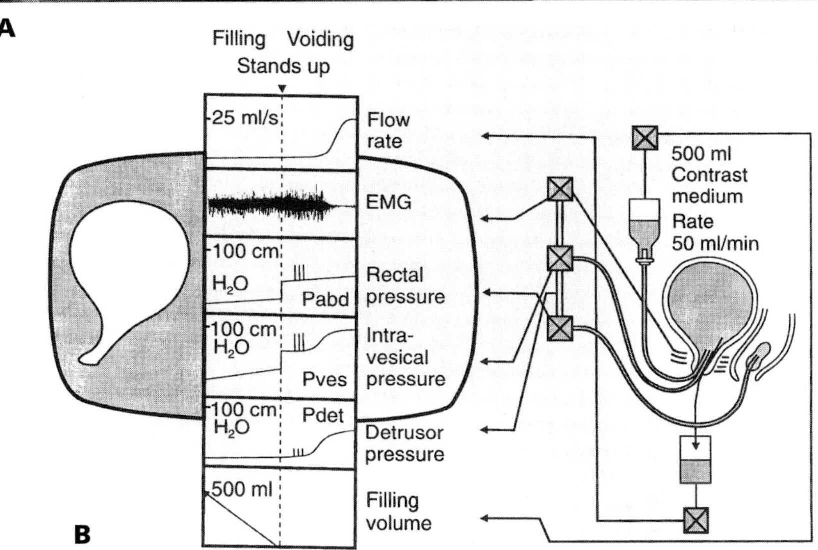

Figure 1: A) Photograph of the video-urodynamics laboratory. The patient is lying on the table under the fluoroscopy tube. The urodynamics recorder and the simultaneous imaging on the screens are to the right. **B)** Schematic diagram of a urodynamic study. The patient's bladder is catheterized with the filling and measuring catheters. A rectal pressure line measures intra-abdominal pressure to obtain detrusor pressure. The study is recorded on the urodynamics machine along with a fluoroscopic picture of the lower urinary tract. The urodynamic study is displayed on the screen in the centre. EMG = electromyography.

suprasacral lesions, bladder hyperreflexia with distal sphincter dyssynergia may be present. With sacral lesions, there may be bladder areflexia with failure of relaxation of the sphincters. This last combination may eventually result in a bladder that complies very poorly with filling and becomes a high-pressure storage system.

A video-urodynamics laboratory and a diagram of a urodynamic study are seen in Figure 1. Urodynamic studies of patients with SCI are demonstrated in Figure 2.

The bladder behavior of an SCI patient con-

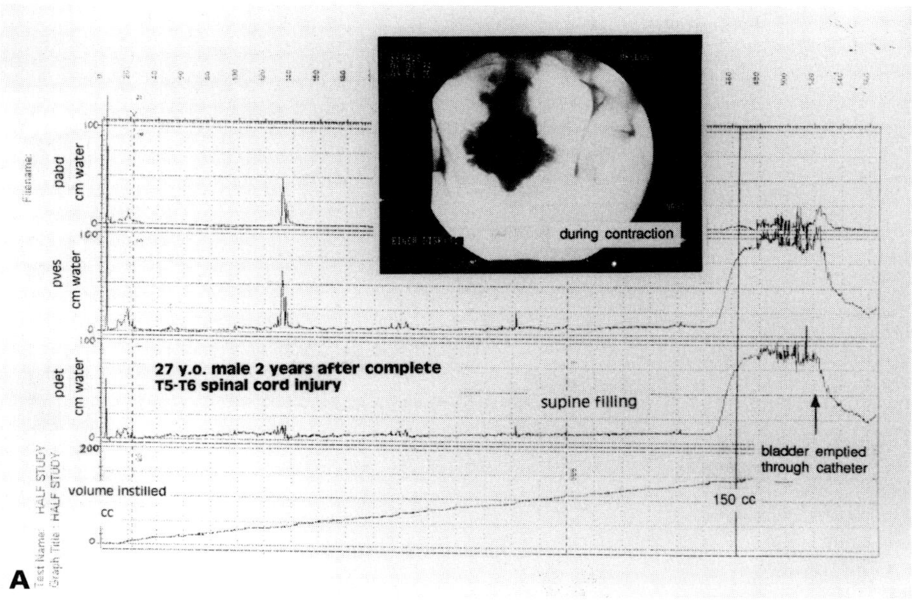

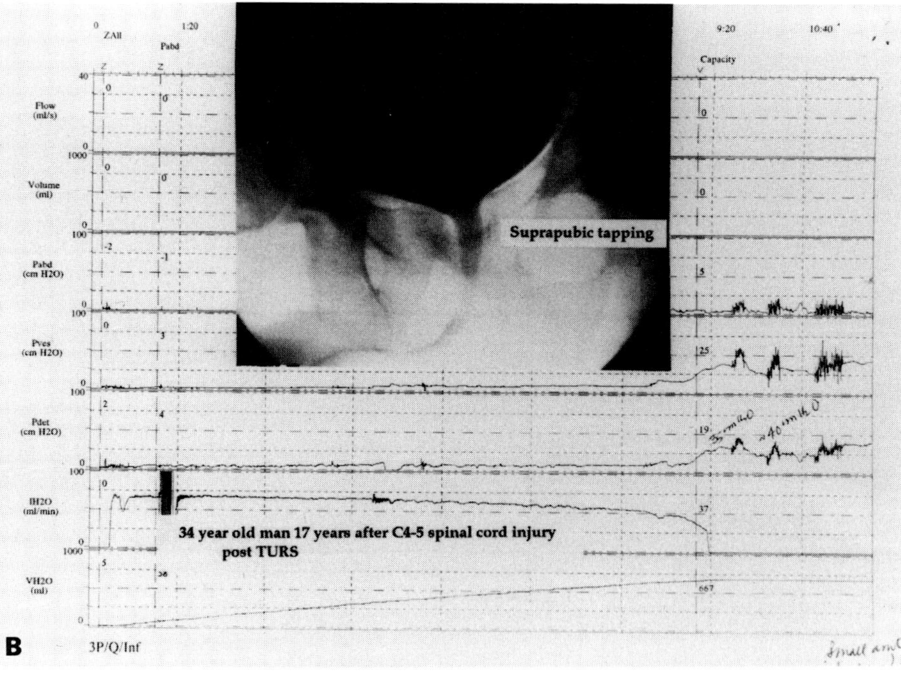

Figure 2: Urodynamic studies in two patients with spinal cord injury. **A)** This 27-year-old male was found to have bilateral hydronephrosis on kidney ultrasound. His video-urodynamic study demonstrated a heavily trabeculated bladder. The bladder holds only 150 cc and exhibits high-pressure contractions (hyperreflexia). During the contractions, the sphincter remained closed indicating detrusor sphincter dyssynergia. The patient subsequently had a transurethral sphincterotomy to lower the voiding pressure and relieve the hydronephrosis. **B)** This 34-year-old male is being followed after a transurethral sphincterotomy. He is managing well on condom drainage. The video-urodynamic study demonstrates a smooth-walled bladder. He has low-pressure contractions after bladder filling with approximately 650 cc. During the voiding phase, the bladder neck opens and there is flow throughout the urethra at a low pressure, indicating a good result.

TABLE 1

GOALS OF UROLOGICAL MANAGEMENT AFTER SPINAL CORD INJURY*

- Upper tract preservation
- Absence or control of infection
- Adequate storage at low intravesical pressure
- Adequate emptying at low intravesical pressure
- Adequate control
- No catheter or stoma
- Social acceptability and adaptability
- Vocational acceptability and adaptability

*Table reproduced from Walsh PC, Retik AB, Vaughan ED Jr, et al (eds): *Campbell's Urology, 7th ed.* Philadelphia, PA: WB Saunders, 1998, with permission.

trasts from normal bladders in which contraction of the detrusor occurs with a sustained relaxation of the urethral sphincter mechanisms. While this is not achieved to the same degree in the SCI patient, where there is by definition interruption between the brainstem region (responsible for such coordination) and the remainder of the cord, the goal in bladder rehabilitation is the development of a "balanced" bladder. Criteria for a balanced bladder are that the patient voids no more frequently than every 2 hours and that the residual urine is less than 100 ml.[25] Goals of management are found in Table 1.[59] This balanced bladder must be a safe bladder that preserves the upper urinary tract. The main requirements in the lower urinary tract to prevent renal deterioration are a low-pressure reservoir during the filling phase and that the voiding phase does not have prolonged and/or excessively high pressures.[41] The clinical criteria are easily determined by history and measurement of post-void residual volumes. However, the urodynamic requirements in the lower urinary tract may not be readily evident in the continent patient who appears to empty sufficiently, since a strong detrusor can overcome an obstructive sphincter and give a false sense that there is "balance" in the system. Even though the function of the lower urinary tract is somewhat predictable from the level of the lesion, urodynamic studies should be obtained for accurate definition, identification of high pressures that may lead to upper tract deterioration, and identification of pathology such as

bladder trabeculation or vesicoureteral reflux that may portend upper tract problems.

According to Graham,[25] 57% to 70% of patients can achieve a balanced bladder with no specific urological intervention. Perlow and Diokno[48] concluded that patients with lesions above T7 generally develop reflex neurogenic bladders, those with lesions below T11 have lower motor neuron bladders, and that those with lesions in the T8-10 range are in a clinically unpredictable gray area. To further characterize bladder behavior, our own results in 136 SCI patients demonstrated that, while high-pressure voiding predominated in patients with lesions above T7, 35% of patients with lesions below T7 exhibited this finding. In one retrospective analysis of 489 patients with various levels of SCI, urodynamic evaluation demonstrated that there was no absolute or specific correlation between the neurological level of injury and the expected bladder function.[30] Of 117 patients with cervical spinal cord lesions, 20 had detrusor areflexia, a finding more typical of lower motor neuron lesions involving the sacral cord or below. Additionally, 26 of 84 patients with sacral cord lesions had bladder function typically characteristic of upper motor neuron lesions. The authors concluded that the accurate assessment of bladder function is dependent upon urodynamic investigations due to the poor predictive value of the level of injury alone.

The initial urodynamic investigation with filling- and voiding-pressure studies can be performed following the period of spinal shock. In our patients, this usually occurs within the first 2 to 3 months.[53] The purpose of such assessment is to define the bladder behavior and to gain information not provided with static studies such as IVP, ultrasound, and post-void residual volume measurement. Anderson[3] studied 80 male acute SCI patients with reflex bladder voiding by serial pressure/flow measurements and correlated these findings with subsequent radiographic evidence of bladder deterioration. While post-void residual volume measurements were not clinically helpful in identifying patients with subsequent bladder deterioration, urodynamic study performed as early as 1 to 3 months following injury did reveal high-risk patient groups. Upper tract imaging with ultrasound or IVP is also done to establish a post-injury baseline.

ENHANCING LOWER URINARY TRACT RECOVERY

The aim of early bladder management is not only to prevent complications but to also influence the development of "balanced" bladder function. It has been suggested that the central nervous system develops supersensitivity to neurotransmitters that accounts for the return of reflex activity, along with the development of neural sprouting.[38] Furthermore, long routing of the ascending and descending tracts of motor neurons of the pontine detrusor nucleus has been found in experimental animals.[8,9] The neurophysiology of the recovering spinal cord suggests that eventual bladder function is not predetermined by merely the level and degree of injury; it is an active process in which one might be able to influence the outcome in terms of bladder function.

Various bladder management strategies have been investigated to improve the chances of developing a balanced bladder. Guttman and Frankel[27] initially promoted intermittent catheterization as a method used to retrain the bladder. Some authors believe that periodic distention of the bladder wall between catheterization promotes the early return of a reflex bladder.[12,28] Wyndaele et al[63] reviewed 115 patients who had various methods of bladder drainage following SCI and noted that patients who underwent intermittent catheterization had the shortest time from injury to established micturition. Thus, intermittent catheterization may assist in the development of favorable bladder behavior as well as prevent local complications.

Other strategies to influence bladder function have included pharmacological management. Investigations in an animal model documented various effects of alpha and beta adrenergic stimulation and blockade on urethral and bladder function during spinal shock.[2] Alpha blockade and beta stimulation resulted in a marked decrease in urethral pressure to allow bladder emptying with the Credé maneuver, but carried with it marked hypotension. Perkash[46] studied 111 SCI patients who underwent bladder rehabilitation. While not randomized, those patients who received bethanechol chloride, a cholinergic agonist, required less time to recover reflex bladder activity. Bethanechol, however, is not recognized to improve bladder emptying as it also results in a marked increase in urethral pressure due to its nicotinic action.[2,66] The use of naloxone, an opioid antagonist, during spinal shock resulted in an increased detrusor pressure and a decrease in the activity of the external sphincter in eight men with traumatic paraplegia.[56] Despite this, voiding occurred only transiently in one patient. Thyrotropin-releasing hormone, another endorphin antagonist, has also been shown to result in an increase in detrusor pressure and a decrease in bladder compliance.[57] The perceived benefit of this drug over naloxone is the lack of interference with narcotic analgesics that may be required. Bladder activity has also been reported to reappear following the administration of phenoxybenzamine, an alpha sympathetic blocker, in patients within 2 weeks following SCI.[37] While these investigations are encouraging, at present there is no clearly demonstrated efficacy in pharmacological management during spinal shock to influence the development of efficient voiding.

AUTONOMIC DYSREFLEXIA

Autonomic dysreflexia is a potentially life-threatening emergency that is unique to the SCI population. It is defined as an acute syndrome of a massive disordered autonomic response to a specific stimulus seen in patients with injuries above the level of the splanchnic outflow, generally above T6 but as low as T8.[55] It is seen more frequently in cervical (60%) than in thoracic (20%) lesions. The spinal cord distal to the segment must be viable in order for the patient to have the condition.

Many terms have been used to name the syndrome including autonomic hyperreflexia, spinal poikilopiesis, paroxysmal neurogenic hypertension, autonomic spasticity, paroxysmal hypertension, autonomic reflex, sympathetic hyperreflexia, mass reflex, and the neurovegetative syndrome.

The syndrome characteristically includes excessive sweating, flushing of the face and body above the lesion, nasal congestion, pounding headache and hypertension, piloerection, and bradycardia or tachycardia. Varying degrees of hypertension may be seen including that causing a mild headache to life-threatening cerebral hemorrhage or seizure. The stimulus for this exaggerated response arises most commonly from a full bladder or from rectal distention. It may be precipitated by detrusor sphincter dyssynergia simple instrumentation of the urethra, a catheter change, fecal impaction, long bone fracture, pressure sores, and other skin lesions. Other precipitants can be urinary tract infection, epididymitis, radiological procedures with distention of viscera, biliary or renal colic, gastrointestinal tract inflammatory conditions, ejaculation in males, and sexual intercourse in both males and females.

The differential diagnosis includes pheochromocytoma, migraine or cluster headaches, posterior fossa neoplasms, toxemia of pregnancy, and essential hypertension.

Pathophysiology

Nociceptive stimuli below the level of the injury, whether somatic or visceral, result in uninhibited reflex sympathetic motor outflow that causes spasm in pelvic viscera, arteriolar spasm and hypertension, pilomotor spasm, and sweating. It also causes an increase in cardiac output and rate. The increase in blood pressure activates the baroreceptors in the carotid sinus and aortic arch. The signal then travels to the medulla where the vasoconstrictor center is inhibited and the vagal center is activated. This subsequently decreases peripheral resistance, heart rate and cardiac output, and blood pressure. In the SCI patient with a lesion above the splanchnic outflow, the inhibitory effect of vagal stimulation cannot reach the effector organs. Vasodilatation above the cord lesion occurs with bradycardia. The patient may present with complaints of a pounding headache, but may have all of the other hallmarks of the syndrome mentioned above.

Treatment and Prevention

A diagnostic cystometrogram in a controlled setting following the return of reflex activity has been recommended to evaluate the propensity of the patient for the condition.[62] Generally, the goal of management is to prevent its occurrence with the use of appropriate bowel and bladder programs and fastidious skin care. When necessary,

treatment is aimed at eliminating the noxious stimulus and lowering the elevated blood pressure with various pharmacological agents.[40] Prophylaxis with various agents can also be used.

When the condition is noticed as an acute symptomatic occurrence, the patient should be placed in the upright position. Tight clothing should be removed and bladder distention relieved, if necessary. Other causes such as rectal impaction or abdominal pathology should be sought and treated as required. If hypertension persists after relieving bladder distention or removing another noxious stimulus, pharmacological treatment should be instituted. Hypertension can be lowered acutely with parenteral ganglionic blockers, alpha blockers, or peripheral vasodilators. Oral nifedipine, a calcium channel blocker, can be given either sublingually (10 to 20 mg) to treat the episode or orally (10 mg) prior to a procedure for prophylaxis. The daily administration of 5 mg of terazosin (an alpha-1 blocker) has also been used for long-term management and prevention.[59]

Autonomic dysreflexia may be seen with various interventional procedures. Topical anesthetics may not prevent the sympathetic response to a noxious stimulus, so nifedipine prophylaxis may be necessary. Autonomic dysreflexia may also occur during a general anesthetic. It is important to know that spinal anesthetic may prevent autonomic dysreflexia by blocking the visceral afferent sacral reflex.

For patients with severe and continual symptoms who fail to respond to management, a number of ablative procedures have been reported including sympathectomy, rhizotomy, cordectomy, and dorsal root ganglionectomy. Furthermore, transurethral sphincterotomy is occasionally done for persistent autonomic dysreflexia in patients with detrusor sphincter dyssynergia.

UROLOGICAL MANAGEMENT IN THE EARLY REHABILITATION PHASE

The management of the patient with SCI in the early rehabilitation phase primarily includes intermittent catheterization for those reasons outlined above. If possible, the patient is taught how to perform intermittent catheterization in the early stages. An initial evaluation of the upper urinary tract with IVP or ultrasound in the early rehabilitation phase documents the baseline condition. Early recovery of bladder function, while encouraging for the patient, should be within acceptable urodynamic parameters (i.e., low residual urine, low filling pressure (<40 cm H_2O), and low voiding pressure (<60 cm H_2O)). Urodynamic studies are carried out after the spinal shock phase to provide a baseline. Early follow-up studies are performed when changes in voiding or complications occur such as febrile infection or autonomic dysreflexia. When selecting the early form of management for the lower urinary tract after voiding, a review must be made of the sex of the patient, the level of injury, manual dexterity, and urodynamic parameters. Pharmacological agents, such as anticholinergics, may improve incontinence resulting from bladder hyperactivity. Females are usually managed with intermittent catheterization with or without anticholinergic agents; if intermittent catheterization is not feasible, an indwelling Foley catheter may be used. Males are managed with intermittent catheterization with or without condom drainage and anticholinergic agents. Interventional maneuvers such as sphincterotomy to relieve outflow obstruction are rarely performed in patients in the early rehabilitative phase unless conservative measures have failed to eliminate the resultant autonomic dysreflexia or upper tract changes.

In treating 101 patients at the Sunnybrook Regional Spinal Cord Injuries Unit managed according to the principles outlined above (i.e., early intermittent catheterization in the acute setting with continuation into the rehabilitative setting, and achievement of a low-pressure system guided by urodynamic studies), the results of the authors[5] have been excellent. After a follow-up period of 25 months, clean intermittent catheterization was used by 17 patients, 43 were voiding with no appliance and were continent, and 29 with or without a sphincterotomy had reflex or spontaneous voiding into a condom. The 12 patients with indwelling catheters included five incontinent females, three quadriplegic males who did not respond to sphincterotomy, and four patients who chose to have an indwelling catheter. When compared to a matched control group treated simultaneously at other institutions, mainly with indwelling catheters, these patients displayed significantly better outcomes. The patients were able to be transferred to the rehabilitation center in one half the time, had one tenth the incidence of urological complications, and one seventh the incidence of clinical urinary infection. In the control group, three patients had supravesical diversions and two died of urosepsis; whereas, no patient in the Sunnybrook study had similar experiences. Although the initial costs in establishing the unit with its team of catheter technicians to carry out the intermittent catheterizations were high, the costs were more than offset by the attendant savings in urological morbidity and the cost of treating the complications that were observed in the control group.

SUMMARY

The normal function of the lower urinary tract may be significantly disrupted by SCI. The acute management of the bladder, while the patient is being resuscitated, is by indwelling catheter. Following stabilization of the patient, intermittent catheterization is the preferred method of lower urinary tract drainage. Pharmacological manipulation to achieve voiding during the spinal shock phase has not been shown to be effective. Many patients void after the spinal shock phase and develop a seemingly "balanced" bladder. The actual bladder behavior cannot be completely predicted by the level and extent of the spinal cord lesion; urodynamic assessment, beginning after 2 to 3 months, is important in the management and for the prevention of bladder and renal deterioration. The goal of management is the achievement of a low-pressure system, with or without intermittent catheterization, and the use of anticholinergic agents. The choice of bladder management is determined by the patient's gender, the level of the lesion, and the functional capacity of the patient.

REFERENCES

1. Abdel-Azim M, Sullivan M, Yalla SV: Disorders of bladder function in spinal cord disease. **Neurol Clin 9:**

727-740, 1991

2. Alastair GS, Tulloch AG, Rossier AB: The autonomic nervous system and the bladder during spinal shock—an experimental study. **Paraplegia 13**:42-48, 1975

3. Anderson RU: Urodynamic patterns after acute spinal cord injury: association with bladder trabeculation in male patients. **J Urol 129**:777-779, 1983

4. Awad SA, Bryniak SR, Downie JW, et al: Urethral pressure profile during the spinal shock stage in man: a preliminary report. **J Urol 117**:91-93, 1977

5. Barkin M, Dolfin D, Herschorn S, et al: The urologic care of the spinal cord injured patient. **J Urol 129**:335-339, 1983

6. Blaivas JG: The neurophysiology of micturition: a clinical study of 550 patients. **J Urol 127**:958-963, 1982

7. Blenkharn JJ: Prevention of bacteriuria during urinary catheterization of patient in an intensive care unit: evaluation of the "Ureofic 500" closed drainage system. **J Hosp Infect 6**:187-193, 1985

8. Bradley WE, Rockswald GL, Timm GW, et al: Neurology of micturition. **J Urol 115**:481-496, 1976

9. Bradley WE, Timm GW, Scott FB: Innervation of the detrusor muscle and urethra. **Urol Clin North Am 1**:3-27, 1974

10. Carroll PR, McAninch JW: Staging of renal trauma. **Urol Clin North Am 16**:193-201, 1989

11. Cass AS: Renovascular injuries from external trauma: diagnoses, treatment, and outcome. **Urol Clin North Am 16**:213-220, 1989

12. Comarr AE: Intermittent catheterization for the traumatic cord bladder patient. **J Urol 108**:79-81, 1972

13. Cook JB, Smith PH: Percutaneous suprapubic cystotomy after spinal cord injury. **Br J Urol 48**:119-121, 1976

14. Corriere JN Jr, Sandler CM: Management of extraperitoneal bladder rupture. **Urol Clin North Am 16**:275-277, 1989

15. de Groat WC: Anatomy and physiology of the lower urinary tract. **Urol Clin North Am 20**:383-401, 1993

16. de Groat WC, Booth AM: Physiology of the urinary bladder and urethra. **Ann Intern Med 92**:312-315, 1980

17. Donker PJ, Droes JTPM, Van Ulder BM: Anatomy of the musculature and innervation of the bladder and the urethra, in Chisholm GD, WIlliams DI (eds): **Scientific Foundations of Urology.** Chicago, Ill: Year Book Medical, 1982, pp 404-411

18. Donnelly J, Hackler RH, Bunts RC: Present urologic status of the World War II paraplegic: 25 year followup: comparison with the status of the 20 year Korean War paraplegic and the 5 year Vietnam paraplegic. **J Urol 108**:558-562, 1972

19. Elbadawi A: Ultrastructure of vesicourethral innervation, II: postganglionic axoaxonal synapses in intrinsic innervation of the vesicourethral lissosphincter: a new structural and functional concept in micturition. **J Urol 131**:781-790, 1984

20. Fam BA, Rossier AB, Blunt K, et al: Experience in the urologic management of 120 early spinal cord injury patients. **J Urol 119**:485-487, 1978

21. Fam BA, Sarkarati M, Yalla SV: Spinal cord injury, in Krane RJ, Siroky MD (eds): **Clinical Neurourology. 2nd ed.** Boston, Mass: Little, Brown & Co, 1979, pp 237

22. Fam BA, Yalla SV: Vesicourethral dysfunction in spinal cord injury and its management. **Semin Neurol 8**:150-155, 1988

23. Gosling J: The structure of the bladder and urethra in relation to function. **Urol Clin North Am 6**:31-38, 1979

24. Gosling JA, Chilton CP: The anatomy of the bladder, urethra and pelvic floor, in Mundy AR, Stephenson TP, Wein AJ (eds): **Urodynamics: Principles, Practice and Application.** New York, NY: Churchill Livingstone, 1984, pp 3-13

25. Graham SD: Present urological treatment of spinal cord injury patients. **J Urol 126**:1-4, 1981

26. Guttman L: Management of paralysis, intermittent catheterization. **Br Surg Pract 6**:445, 1949

27. Guttman L, Frankel H: The value of intermittent catheterization in the early management of traumatic paraplegia and tetraplegia. **Paraplegia 4**:63-84, 1966

28. Herr HW: Intermittent catheterization in neurogenic bladder dysfunction. **J Urol 113**:477-479, 1975

29. Herschorn S, Thijssen A, Radomski SB: The value of immediate or early catheterization of the traumatized posterior urethra. **J Urol 148**:1428-1431, 1992

30. Kaplan SA, Chancellor MB, Blaivas JG: Bladder and sphincter behavior in patients with spinal cord lesions. **J Urol 146**:113-117, 1991

31. Kuhn W, Rist M, Zaech GA: Intermittent urethral self-catheterization: long term results. **Paraplegia 29**:222-232, 1991

32. Kunin CM, McCormack RC: Prevention of catheter-induced urinary-tract infections by sterile closed drainage. **N Engl J Med 274**:1155-1161, 1966

33. Lapides J, Diokno AC, Gould FR, et al: Further observations on self-catheterization. **J Urol 116**:169-171, 1979

34. Lapides J, Diokno AC, Silber SJ, et al: Clean intermittent self-catheterization in the treatment of urinary tract disease. **J Urol 107**:458-461, 1972

35. Lloyd LK, Kuhlemeier KV, Fine PR, et al: Initial bladder management in spinal cord injury: does it make a difference? **J Urol 135**:523-527, 1986

36. Lucas MG, Thomas DG: Lack of relationship of conus reflexes to bladder function after spinal cord injury. **Br J Urol 63**:24-27, 1989

37. Mathe JF, Labat JJ, Lanoiselee JM, et al: Detrusor inhibition in suprasacral spinal cord injuries: is it due to sympathetic overactivity? **Paraplegia 23**:201-206, 1985

38. McAninch JW, Carroll PR: Renal exploration after trauma: indications and reconstructive techniques. **Urol Clin North Am 16**:203-212, 1989

39. McCouch GP, Austin GM, Liu CN, et al: Sprouting as a cause of spasticity. **J Neurophysiol 21**:205-216, 1958

40. McGuire EJ, Wagner FM, Weiss RM: Treatment of autonomic dysreflexia with phenoxybenzamine. **J Urol 115**:53-55, 1976

41. McGuire EJ, Woodside JR, Borden TA: Upper urinary tract deterioration in patients with myelodysplasia and detrusor hypertonia: a follow-up study. **J Urol 129**:823-826, 1983

42. Mee SL, McAninch JW: Indications for radiographic assessment in suspected renal trauma. **Urol Clin N Am 16**:187-192, 1989

43. Mundy AR: Clinical physiology of the bladder, urethra and pelvic floor, in Mundy AR, Stephenson TP, Wein AJ (eds): **Urodynamics: Principles, Practice and Applications.** New York, NY: Churchill Livingstone, 1984, pp 14-25

44. Nanninga JB, Meyer P: Urethral sphincter activity fol-

lowing acute spinal cord injury. **J Urol 123:**528-530, 1980

45. Perkash I: Detrusor-sphincter dyssynergia responses. **J Urol 120:**469-474, 1978

46. Perkash I: Intermittent catheterization and bladder rehabilitation in spinal cord injury patients. **J Urol 114:**230-233, 1975

47. Perkash I: Problems of catheterization in long-term spinal cord injury patient. **J Urol 124:**249-253, 1980

48. Perlow DL, Diokno AC: Predicting lower urinary tract dysfunction in patients with spinal cord injury. **Urology 18:**531-535, 1981

49. Peters PC: Intraperitoneal rupture of the bladder. **Urol Clin North Am 16:**279-282, 1989

50. Peterson NE: Complications of renal trauma. **Urol Clin North Am 16:**221-236, 1989

51. Rossier AB, Fam BA: From intermittent catheterization to catheter freedom via urodynamics: a tribute to Sir Ludwig Guttman. **Paraplegia 17:**73-85, 1979

52. Rossier AB, Fam BA, Dibenedetto M, et al: Urodynamics in spinal shock patients. **J Urol 122:**783-787, 1979

53. Smith PH, Cook JB, Burt AA: Percutaneous cystotomy in paraplegia: a follow-up of 41 patients. **Paraplegia 14:**135-137, 1976

54. Tator, CH, Rowed, DW, Schwartz, ML, et al: Management of acute spinal cord injuries. **Can J Surg 27:**289-294, 1984

55. Trop CS, Bennett CJ: Autonomic dysreflexia and its urological implications: a review. **J Urol 146:**1461-1469, 1991

56. Vaidyanathan S, Rao MS, Chary KSN, et al: A modulation of vesicourethral function with naloxone in traumatic paraplegics during the spinal shock phase: preliminary report. **Ann Clin Res 14:**98-102, 1982

57. Vaidyanathan S, Rao MS, Sharma PL, et al: Modulation of urinary bladder function with thyrotropin-releasing hormone in patients with spinal cord injuries during the spinal shock phase. **Ann Clin Res 15:**66-70, 1983

58. Warren JW, Platt R, Thomas RJ, et al: Antibiotic irrigation and catheter associated urinary tract infections. **N Engl J Med 299:**570-573, 1978

59. Wein AJ: Neuromuscular dysfunction of the lower urinary tract and its treatment, in Walsh PC, Retik AB, Vaughan ED Jr, et al (eds): **Campbell's Urology. 7th ed.** Philadelphia, Pa: WB Saunders, 1998, pp 953-1006

60. Wein AJ, Barrett, DM: Peripheral innervation of the lower urinary tract, in Wein AJ, Barrett DM (eds): **Voiding Function and Dysfunction.** Chicago, Ill: Year Book Medical, 1988, pp 45-52

61. Wein AJ, Barrett DM: Relevant anatomy, in Wein AJ, Barrett DM (eds): **Voiding Function and Dysfunction.** Chicago, Ill: Year Book Medical, 1988, pp 6-21

62. Wheeler JS, Walter JW: Acute urologic management of the patient with spinal cord injury: initial hospitalization. **Urol Clin North Am 20:**403-411, 1993

63. Wyndaele JJ, De Sy WA, Claessens H: Evaluation of different methods of bladder drainage used in the early care of spinal cord injury patients. **Paraplegia 23:**18-26, 1985

64. Yalla SV, Blunt KJ, Fam BA, et al: Detrusor-urethral sphincter dyssynergia. **J Urol 118:**1026-1029, 1977

65. Yalla SV, Fam BA: Spinal cord injury, in Krane RJ, Siroky MD (eds): **Clinical Neurourology, 2nd ed.** Boston, Mass: Little, Brown & Co, 1991, pp 319

66. Yalla SV, Rossier AB, Fam BA: Dyssynergic vesicourethral responses during bladder rehabilitation in spinal cord injury patients: effects of suprapubic percussion, Crede method and bethanechol chloride. **J Urol 115:**575, 1976

CHAPTER 22

SPINAL ORTHOTICS

EDWARD C. BENZEL, MD, FACS

GOALS OF SPINE BRACING

The goals of bracing the spine include: 1) restriction of movement; 2) realignment of the spine; and 3) trunk support. An understanding of these goals when the patient is undergoing bracing and an ability to appraise within reason the properties of individual orthoses that allow the achievement of these goals is imperative.[5]

LIMITATIONS OF SPINE BRACING

Several problems are associated with spine bracing, the most significant of which is the relative lack of effectiveness in achieving its stated goal, which is to minimize "excessive" spinal movement. The amount of soft tissue separating the spine and the brace itself minimizes the effectiveness of the brace. In fact, an inverse relationship exists between the thickness of the soft tissue between the spine and the inner surface of the brace and the effectiveness of the brace. Furthermore, for spinal stability, a longer brace is usually more efficacious than a shorter brace. Therefore, the length/width ratio of the brace plays a significant role in the efficacy of spinal stabilization (Figure 1).

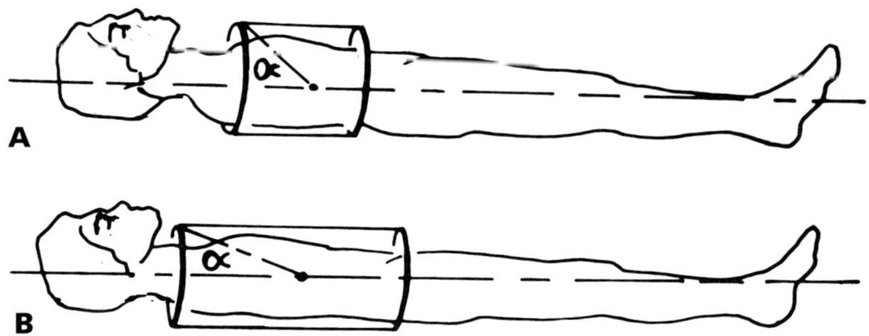

Figure 1: An inverse relationship exists concerning the axial distance between the spine and the inner surface of the brace. This is theoretically defined by following: Efficacy of bracing is proportional to the cosine of the angle as depicted. Alpha is the angle defined by the edge of the brace, the instantaneous axis of rotation at the unstable segment, and the long axis of the spine. This angle is dictated by both the length of the brace and the thickness of tissue between the spine and the inner surface of the brace. A short **(A)** and long **(B)** brace are depicted. A significant reduction of efficacy ensues with the utilization of a shorter, wider brace (i.e., the length/width ratio of the brace is too small).

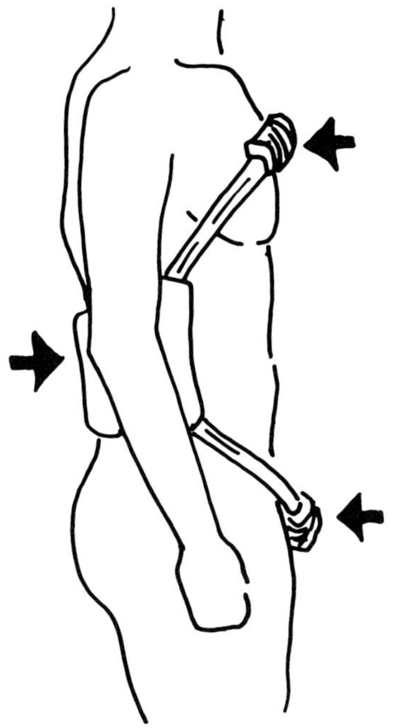

Figure 2: The design of the Jewett brace does not utilize the intrinsic advantage of the body shell and minimizes the surface area contact with the torso. It does allow for the application of three-point bending forces *(arrows)*. These forces are similar to those applied by spinal implants (e.g., the Harrington distraction rod).

CONFORMATION OF THE ORTHOSES TO THE TORSO

Splinting devices that do not closely conform to the torso (including the halo and the Jewett brace) have several disadvantages. The Jewett brace, for example, applies a dorsally directed force at the sternum and the pubic region. Because the pressure applied may be significant, discomfort may result. In the case of lumbar instability, the Jewett brace does not place the ventrally directed force in an appropriate location (i.e., in the low lumbar or lumbosacral spine). Furthermore, the Jewett brace and similar techniques do not promote the maintenance of the cylindrical body shell (i.e., contact with the torso is made over a relatively small surface area). The concept of the body shell has been previously addressed from several viewpoints.[26,27,30,41]

The Jewett brace, however, does provide a three-point bending biomechanical advantage (Figure 2).[30,38] This has been shown to be of significant value with regard to the stability achieved with external splinting. Maintenance of the body shell also increases the stability of the ventral and dorsal spinal elements (columns). Morris et al[27] demonstrated and illustrated the significant role of the trunk as a stabilizer of the spine. Lastly, the Jewett braces and those similar to it do not significantly restrict lateral bending.

The conformation and close "fit" between the ventral and dorsal halves of a brace are critical when assessing the ability of the brace to stabilize the spine. In addition to having the halves of the brace secured so that one half does not slide past the other half, the halves should be rigidly attached to each other (Figure 3).

ORTHOTIC MATERIALS

Spinal orthotics are constructed of a variety of materials, supplying both rigidity and comfort. Rigidity is provided by such materials as metals and plastics, and comfort is provided by cushioning effects such as cloth and foam. Thermoplastics are commonly used for spinal orthotic construction.

The thermoplastic use for spinal orthotics is divided into low temperature and high temperature. Low-temperature thermoplastics require no greater than 180°F to become workable and they may be molded directly to the body. They are not effective in applications where high stress is anticipated. High-temperature thermoplastics require temperatures no lower than 350°F and must be formed over a plastic model. They are more resistant than low-temperature thermoplastics to change in shape with continued stress and body heat and are ideal for long-term use in limb and body orthotics. Kydex, polypropylene, low-density polyethylene, and Vitrathene are the most commonly used high-temperature thermoplastics. Kydex and polypropylene are the most preferred thermoplastics for spinal orthotics due to their light weight, rigidity, and durability. These thermoplastics are applied to customized molds and lined with a closed cell thermofoam for added patient comfort.

Lightweight metals such as aluminum are often used as spacers, stabilizers, or reinforcers.

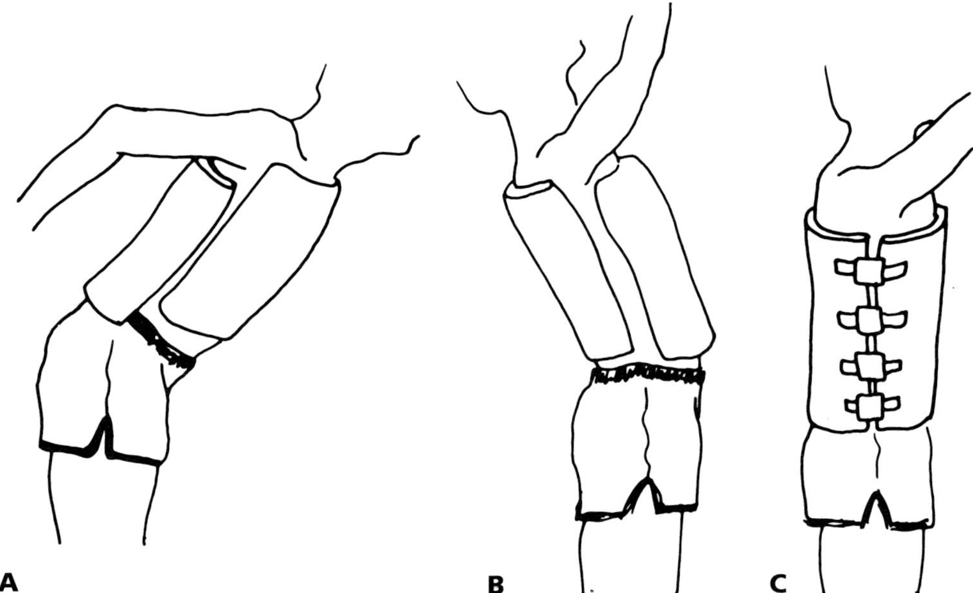

Figure 3: A poorly fitted brace where the anterior and posterior halves are allowed to slide past each other is depicted, and flexion **(A)** and extension **(B)** movements are significantly restricted. The elimination of this sliding motion and an accompanying tight security between the halves (the brace functions as a single solid unit) minimize this occurrence **(C).**

An aluminum strut that connects two portions of a brace (i.e., the cervical and thoracic portions of a Minerva jacket) can also be used for brace fit adjustment (via bending).

CERVICAL SPINE BRACING

The cervical spine is perhaps the region of the spine that is most effectively stabilized by external splinting techniques. This is, in part, related to the lesser amount of soft tissue separating the brace and the spine itself. However, it is also related to the substantial points of fixation available at its extreme (i.e., the cranium and the thoracic cage).

The difficulty associated with preventing rotation and bending in all directions is present in various amounts with each technique.[6,13,14,16-18] The extent of lateral bending is difficult to assess. One has to rely on anteroposterior radiographs for assessment, which are inherently more difficult to assess than equivalent lateral radiographs.

Rotation is even more difficult to assess. Maiman et al[24] and Johnson et al[17] utilized a goniometer scheme to assess rotation following cervical bracing. With regard to concerns of clinical stability, lateral and rotatory movement is usually of lesser significance than sagittal plane movement.

It is often very desirable to prevent sagittal plane movement and, thus, it is the most useful to measure. Sagittal plane movement allows for assessment of flexion-extension movement at each cervical motion segment, while simultaneously allowing one to assess (and to quantitate) unwanted responses to external splinting (i.e., the parallelogram-like bracing effect and snaking, see below).

The parallelogram-like bracing effect is a characteristic unique to cervical spine bracing. It is related both to the significant mobility of the cervical spine and to the lack of adequate fixation points in the mid to lower cervical region. The extensive mobility of the upper cervical (atlanto-occipital) and mid and lower cervical spine combines the unique characteristics of both capital and true neck flexion-extension

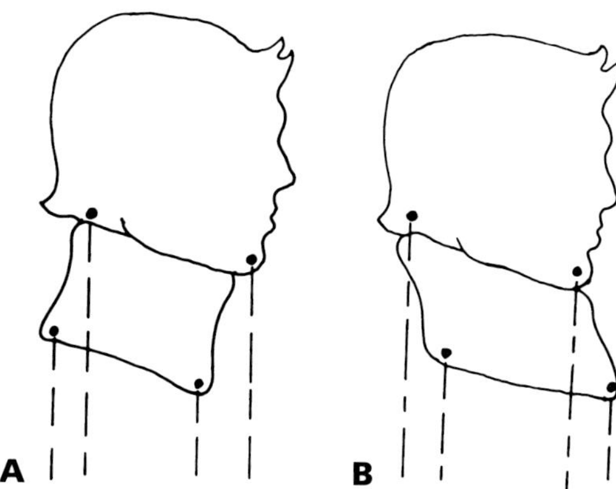

Figure 4: The parallelogram-like bracing effect is a unique aspect of cervical spine bracing that is associated with the combination of capital and true neck movements and the unique points of fixation available. When there is inadequate low cervical/thoracic fixation, true neck flexion and extension is relatively unimpeded. The compensatory relationship between capital and true neck movement is not significantly thwarted. In this example, low cervical flexion is accompanied by compensatory capital extension. This may be encouraged somewhat by the brace itself **(A)**; the converse is also true **(B)**. The *vertical dashed lines* highlight the parallelogram movements.

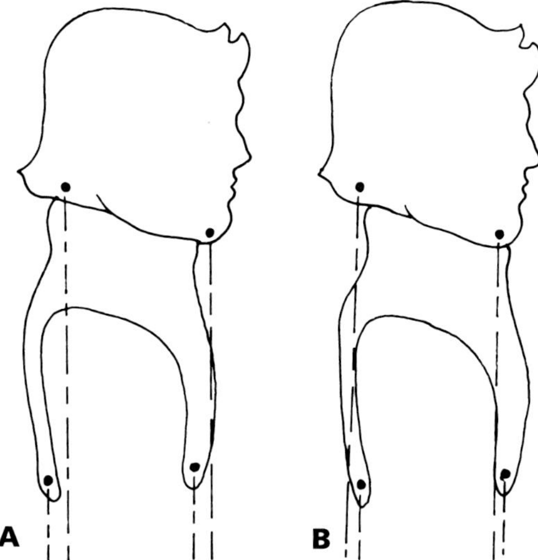

Figure 5: The parallelogram-like bracing effect depicted in Figure 4 can be significantly diminished by minimizing movement in the low cervical and cervicothoracic regions; via a three-bending mechanism. This maneuver restricts true neck flexion **(A)** and extension **(B)**.

movements to exaggerate the parallelogram-like bracing effect (Figure 4).[5] Braces that attempt fixation from the mandibular region to the base of the neck and shoulder often do not effectively prevent parallelogram-like movement and, in fact, may encourage it. A review of published data regarding cervical orthotic effectiveness illustrates this point (Tables 1 and 2).[17] The devices that utilize the mandible without chest fixation points allow excessive movement at each motion segment. The prevention of lower cervical spine movement via the attainment of solid points of chest fixation appears to provide significant reduction of segmental movement at all cervical spine levels. This may pertain to upper thoracic spine segmental movement, as well.[21] The combination of capital and compensatory true neck movement (or vice versa) can be controlled by limiting one type of movement or the other, as they are compensatory. Since capital (upper) cervical movement is difficult to restrict, the most effective alternative is the minimizing of true (mid-low) cervical neck movement. This

is attained by utilizing solid points of chest fixation (Figure 5).

Another challenge associated with cervical spine fixation is "snaking." This phenomenon is defined as "a serpentine movement of the spine, whereby a simple overall movement (such as flexion or extension) is accompanied by an unexpected combination of flexion and extension movements at each intervertebral level."[6,17] Although overall movement from the head to the chest may be minimal, the accumulative segmental movement between these points may be substantial. Therefore, snaking can be quantitatively defined as the difference between the sum of all segmental movements between the head and the chest and the overall movement between the head and the chest.[6] Although one cannot objectively assess segmental movement of the spine due to inconsistent responses of the patient (see below), the difference between the observed overall movement and the sum of segmental movements can be measured. This measurement becomes more of a subjective assess-

TABLE 1

FLEXION AND EXTENSION ALLOWED AT EACH SEGMENT LEVEL[*]

Test Situation	Motion	Occiput-C1	C1-2	C2-3	C3-4	C4-5	C5-6	C6-7	C7-T1
Normal unrestricted	Flexion	0.7±0.5	7.7±1.2	7.2±0.9	9.8±1.0	10.3±1.0	11.4±1.0	12.5±1.0	9.0±1.1
	Extension	18.1±2.1	6.0±1.2	4.8±0.8	7.8±1.1	9.8±1.2	10.5±1.3	8.2±1.2	2.7±0.7
Soft collar	Flexion	1.3±1.3	5.1±1.9	4.5±1.2	7.4±1.5	8.4±2.4	9.9±1.7	9.7±0.9	7.7±2.5
	Extension	13.7±3.5	1.9±1.4	3.9±1.0	5.8±1.7	6.8±1.6	7.8±1.2	7.4±1.4	2.8±1.9
Philadelphia collar	Flexion	0.9±1.0	4.0±1.8	1.6±1.0	3.1±1.1	4.6±1.8	6.2±1.9	6.2±1.6	5.5±1.8
	Extension	6.8±2.2	4.5±1.5	1.8±0.9	3.4±1.0	5.8±1.2	5.9±1.2	5.8±2.0	1.3±0.9
SOMI brace	Flexion	3.6±1.8	2.7±1.8	0.9±0.7	1.6±1.1	1.9±0.8	2.8±1.2	2.9±1.6	3.1±1.8
	Extension	9.1±2.6	5.4±1.9	4.4±1.1	6.3±1.4	6.0±1.8	6.0±2.0	5.6±1.8	2.1±1.1
Four-poster brace	Flexion	2.9±2.0	4.4±2.1	1.6±1.0	2.1±1.1	1.8±0.9	3.0±1.2	3.9±1.6	2.8±1.4
	Extension	9.3±2.2	3.2±1.4	2.0±0.7	3.2±1.2	3.4±1.3	2.9±0.9	3.1±1.5	1.6±0.8
Cervicothoracic brace	Flexion	1.3±0.9	5.0±1.9	1.8±0.8	2.9±1.2	2.8±0.7	1.6±0.8	0.7±0.6	2.4±1.0
	Extension	8.4±2.1	2.5±0.8	2.1±0.7	1.6±0.7	2.2±0.9	2.8±0.9	3.4±1.1	1.7±0.8

[*]Data from Johnson et al.[17] Flexion and extension movements are separately depicted. Data are expressed as mean degrees and 95% confidence limits of the mean.

TABLE 2

AVERAGE MOVEMENT OF EACH INTERVERTEBRAL LEVEL FROM MAXIMUM FLEXION TO MAXIMUM EXTENSION[*]

Stabilization Device	O-C1	C1-2	C2-3	C3-4	C4-5	C5-6	C6-7	Sum of Angles	Movement at Each Level	Sum of Angles O to C6 or C7	Measured Movement
Halo jacket	4.5±2.7	1.3±1.1	4.1±2.6	4.1±3.2	3.1±2.6	3.0±1.9	6.3±5.7	23.4±13.7	3.7±3.1†	23.4±13.7	5.2
Minerva jacket	3.5±2.1	2.1±1.1	1.7±1.7	1.9±1.2	2.0±2.1	2.5±1.6	2.3±1.8	14.8±4.4	2.3±1.7†	14.8±4.4	5.2

[*]Data from Benzel et al.[6] Data are expressed in degrees as means ± standard deviations. O = occiput. † = statistically significant difference ($P<.025$).

ment that relies on each subject as his/her own control.[6]

Finally, it must be noted that the means used to assess the efficacy of cervical bracing techniques are somewhat artificial. Therefore, a heavy reliance on the published data is not suggested. The movement measured in most studies is elicited by neck movement, the extent of which depends on the cooperation of the braced individual. Furthermore, and of much greater significance, the movement depends on a consistent submaximal attempt at flexion, extension, rotation, or lateral bending. This consistency is nearly impossible to attain and, more importantly, to quantitate. These factors are of importance in the cervical spine and also play a role in the thoracic and lumbar spine.

Individual external cervical spine splinting techniques are discussed in relation to data known regarding their attributes and faults. The techniques are grouped to facilitate the objective assessment of each, with this assessment being emphasized. These groupings are: 1) limited cervical bracing techniques; 2) cervical-shoulder bracing techniques; 3) cervical-thoracic bracing techniques; and 4) cranial-thoracic bracing techniques.

Limited Cervical Bracing Techniques

Limited cervical braces have no neck base or shoulder fixation points. These points of fixation

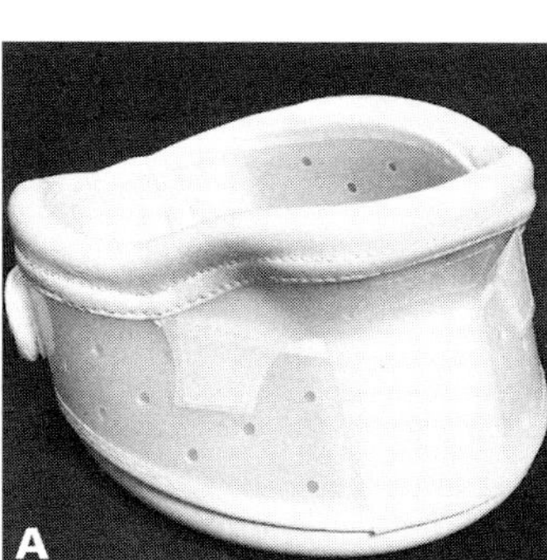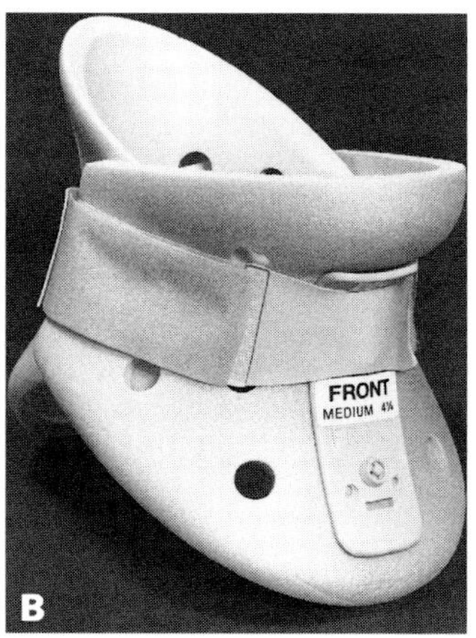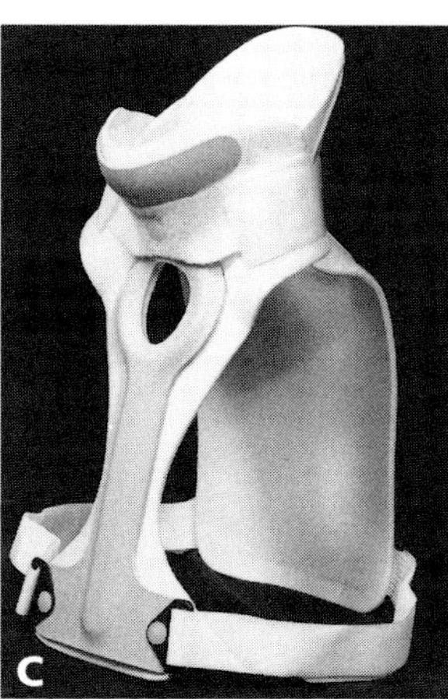

Figure 6: A) Limited cervical bracing techniques provide little stabilization of the cervical spine. The length/width ratio is insufficient and their points of contact with the torso are not solid. **B)** Cervical-shoulder bracing techniques provide a slight advantage over limited cervical bracing techniques by extending the brace to include the neck base-shoulder region. This has a minimal influence on movement in the low cervical region. This, in turn, has significant impact on upper cervical segmental movement (see Figure 4). **C)** Cervical-thoracic bracing techniques provide a biomechanical advantage by limiting low cervical and cervical-thoracic motion and, hence, compensatory higher cervical segmental movements. They are typified by the SOMI, four-poster, and cervical-thoracic braces.

are of considerable importance with regard to their ability to restrict cervical motion. All provide, to one degree or another, a mandibular point of fixation. Their ability to affix to the base of the neck, shoulder, or chest region is variable. Collars that do not affix to the base of the neck, shoulder, or chest regions, including the soft cervical semi-rigid collars, are the least effective (Figure 6A). Flexion-extension movement is essentially unrestricted by these cervical collars (Table 1). Since movement is not restricted in any direction, these devices do not enhance the parallelogram-like bracing effect. However, their overall ineffectiveness regarding the restriction of cervical movement makes this a moot point.

Cervical-Shoulder Bracing Techniques

The extension of a limited cervical brace to include the mandible rostrally and the neck, base, or shoulder caudally provides some restriction of movement (e.g., the Philadelphia collar) (Figure 6B). However, it simultaneously causes an exaggeration of parallelogram-line spinal movements (i.e., the parallelogram-like bracing

effect) (Figure 4). These two points are obviously a tradeoff. The parallelogram-like bracing effect cannot be quantitated. The relative extent of its presence, however, can be assessed (admittedly subjectively) by observing flexion- and extension-induced motion in the upper cervical region (capital flexion and extension). Note that in Table 1 capital and true cervical flexion-extension movements are relatively unimpeded by cervical-shoulder bracing techniques (e.g., the Philadelphia collar).

The advantage of the cervical-shoulder bracing technique is that it provides some degree of restriction of movement (Table 1). The significance of movement restriction is difficult to assess. Recent studies have demonstrated efficacy and significant differences between braces.[2,15,19,22,31,33] Clinical series have shown that cervical-shoulder braces may be effective for indications previously believed to require more extensive bracing strategies.[12]

Cervical-Thoracic Bracing Techniques

The extension of a cervical brace caudally to include the chest region provides a three-point bending biomechanical advantage, whereas the previously discussed devices provide less restriction of movement or they exaggerate the parallelogram-like bracing effect. These splinting techniques (the SOMI, four-poster, and cervicothoracic braces) (Figure 6C) provide substantial restriction of movement in the mid to low cervical region (Table 1).

Cranial-Thoracic Fixation Techniques

For several years, the halo device has been the "gold standard" for cervical bracing.[9,29] However, other orthoses have been used. The rigid (halo) and the semi-rigid (Minerva) fixation of the cranium to the chest provide the greatest degree of segmental cervical spine movement restriction. As mentioned, this maybe largely due to the ability of both devices to limit mid to low cervical movement. This type of fixation provides a significant limitation of segmental movement while simultaneously minimizing the parallelogram-like effect (as is evidenced by the diminished segmental movement observed in the upper cervical region; Table 2).

It has been observed that a significant difference exists between the overall movement between the head and the chest from flexion to extension and the summation of segmental movement between both regions.[6,17] This difference can be quantitatively derived from radiographs (Figure 7), which provide an objective measure of snaking.[6] Obviously, of much greater importance than overall movement between the head and the chest is the movement allowed at each segmental level, since instability is most often a segmental and not a global phenomenon.

The rigid cranial fixation afforded by the halo provides significant restriction of capital flexion and extension movements; hence the parallelogram-like bracing effect is minimized.[37] However, this occurs at the expense of exaggeration of the snaking of the mid to low cervical spine (Table 2).[6] This correlates with clinical data regarding an unexpected deficiency in halo efficacy in patients with unstable cervical spine injuries.[1,20,42]

The Minerva jacket provides a similar advantage regarding the minimization of the parallelo-

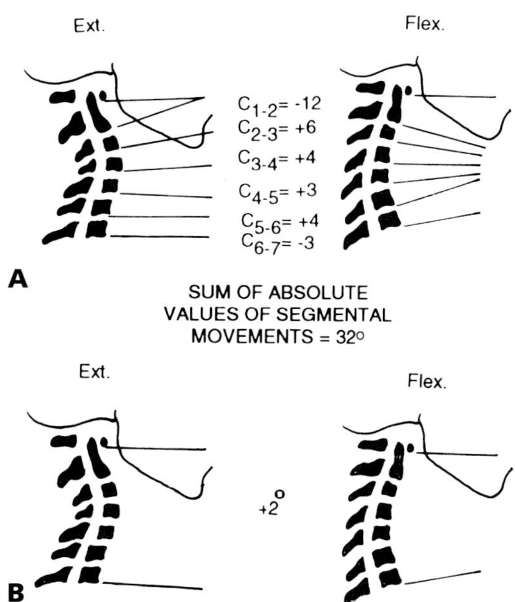

Figure 7: The assessment of segmental movement at each level (in degrees) can be measured and calculated from flexion and extension radiographs. The total of their absolute numbers is the sum of angles. The overall movement between the cranium and the low cervical region (lowest segment assessed) is the measured movement. The differences in segmental levels are depicted by this hypothetical example **(A)**. The overall movement between the cranium and the lowest segment assessed is much less than the sum of the individual angles **(B)**.

gram-like bracing effect. The advantage of the Minerva jacket in this regard is due predominately to the extent of chest fixation, which provides a three-point bending biomechanical advantage (Figure 5). The Minerva jacket, however, does not have the ability to control capital flexion and extension movement[35] and cannot effectively provide these force applications. The major advantage of the Minerva jacket is its minimal effect on snaking.[6,17,24]

If one compares data on the halo and Minerva jacket, it is apparent that the Minerva jacket is more effective at controlling sagittal plane segmental motion. However, the halo has a greater ability to control capital flexion and extension movement.[6,17,24] The degree of control of capital flexion and extension (via manipulation of the degree of tilt of the halo ring with the halo), com-

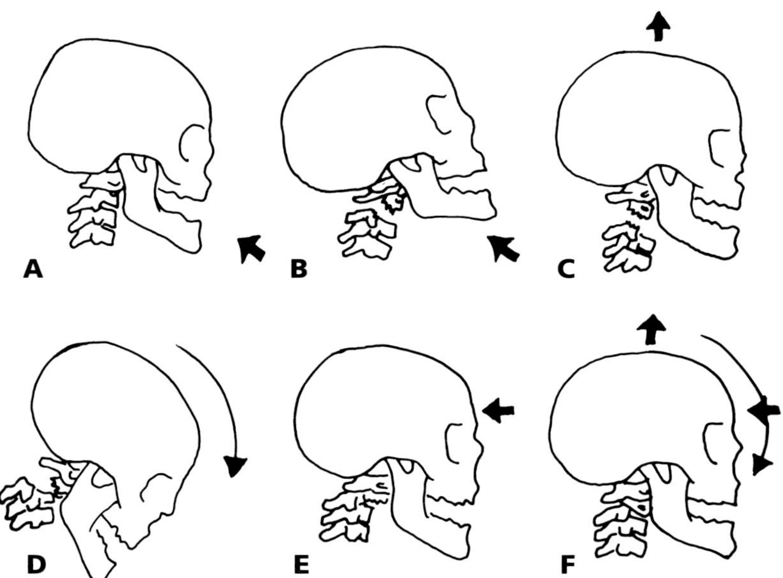

Figure 8: An unstable hangman's fracture can be managed by applying a complex set of forces to the unstable segment. The fracture itself is a result of a hyperextension loading to failure **(A)**. This usually results in a subluxation of C2 and C3 and on disruption of the pars interarticularis of C2 **(B)**. Neither simple distraction **(C)**, capital flexion **(D)**, nor true neck extension **(E)** by itself can provide adequate reduction. However, a combination of slight simple distraction, moderate capital flexion, and moderate true neck extension provides an optimum force complex application for reduction **(F)**. *Arrows* depict the forces and moments applied.

bined with its ability to manipulate true neck flexion and extension movement (by moving the ring ventrally or dorsally) places the halo in the unique position of being the only technique with the ability to manipulate craniocervical translational and flexion and extension movement. The three-point bending biomechanical advantage provided by chest fixation assists in this regard (Figure 5). These points are of particular importance when dealing with situations such as a hangman's fracture, which is very unstable or difficult to reduce (Figure 8).

The cranial extension of the Minerva jacket (occiput and forehead) appears to be of minimal significance (unpublished data). Therefore, a significant portion of the efficacy of the Minerva jacket is provided by the mandible and chest points of attachment. This is not unexpected (Figure 5). The significance of the cervical points of attachment, however, should not be underestimated. They minimize spinal snaking by maintaining the cervical shell. The halo jacket does not offer this advantage. Therefore, the greater seg-

mental movement restriction provided by the Minerva jacket may in part be related to this phenomenon. The relatively minimal amount of soft tissue separating the external splint (Minerva jacket) and the spine allows a particular advantage regarding the maintenance of the body shell (Figure 1).

The extension of a Minerva or the halo brace to a lower chest or lumbar attachment increases the lever arm available for three-point bending force application. The length of the construct is, at least theoretically, proportional to its efficacy, as assessed by its ability to resist bending moments at the unstable segment.

Most splinting techniques cause little compression or distraction of the cervical spine. Furthermore, axially oriented force application is generally difficult to quantitate. However, Koch and Nickel[21] assessed distraction and compression forces with the halo by inserting a transducer into the stabilizing bars of the halo. A surprising variation of axial forces (a variation of nearly 22 lb total) was observed during the assumption of several positions of normal daily activity.[21] These data were corroborated by Lind et al,[23] with their conclusions as follows:

- Significant flexion and extension motion occurs in each motion segment of the cervical spine in spite of the halo-vest fixation.
- The motion pattern of the cervical spine stabilized with a halo vest is similar to a curling snake.
- The motion is greatest in the upper portion of the cervical spine and decreases further down.
- The halo vest provides distraction across the neck during the entire treatment period (3 months).
- There are large variations of force across the neck depending upon the type of exercise performed or the position of the body (mean maximal variation: 175 N).
- A tightly fitted vest exaggerates the variations of force across the neck.
- Large distraction force across the neck of the patient in the supine position results in a large variation of force and great motion in the motion segments of the cervical spine (r=0.8).

These factors could adversely affect stability. For example, an interbody fusion or a dense fracture would heal less well if repetitively subjected to distractive forces. Conversely, a wedge-compression fracture-related deformity could be exaggerated by compression axial force application (Figure 9). Others have also noted factors that affect halo efficacy, including increasing vest tightness, decreasing the deformability of the vest, and ensuring a good fit can reduce motion.[25]

Finally, pin site complications with the halo are not infrequent. These include dislodgment, calvarial penetration, and cosmetic problems. Many cannot be eliminated. However, it behooves the surgeon to most effectively affix the device to the calvarium. Appropriate torque and technique are obviously imperative. In this regard, the perpendicular insertion of halo pins into the skull maximizes the structural properties of the interface.[39] The application of this alone may reduce the incidence of pin site complications.

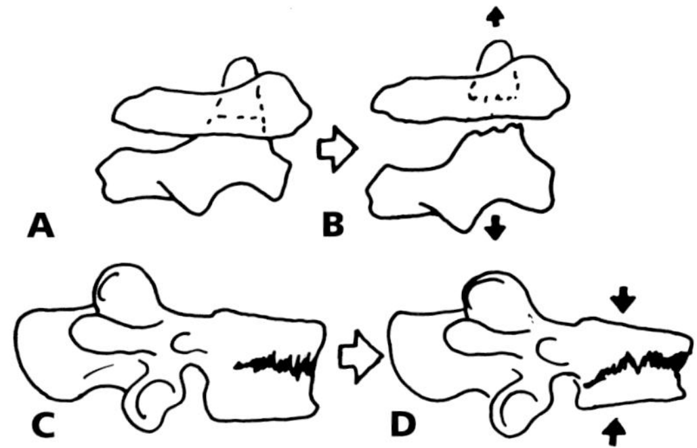

Figure 9: The distraction and compression force transmission to the cervical spine may be problematic in the face of a dens fracture **(A)**, where overdistraction may decrease the chance of union **(B)** or a subaxial wedge compression fracture **(C)**, and where further compression could exaggerate the deformity **(D)**.

CERVICOTHORACIC SPINE BRACING

The external splinting of the cervicothoracic region can be accomplished as a result of extending a thoracic brace to include the cervical region (by attaining a mandible point of fixation) or by utilizing the halo technique with a caudal extension of the brace to include the thoracolumbar or lumbar region. Of interest in this regard are the data from Koch and Nickel[21] that demonstrate the gradual increased efficacy of the halo technique in limiting flexion and extension movement as the cervical spine is descended into the cervicothoracic region (Figure 10). If this information is extrapolated into the upper thoracic spine with a caudally extended halo technique, a substantial splinting advantage provided by the halo technique in this region might be expected.

THORACIC SPINE BRACING

The thoracic spine is unique in that it is the only segment of the spine to which traditional external splinting principles can be applied. Because it has two axial segments above (cranial and cervical) and two axial segments below (lumbar and sacro-pelvic), adequate points of fixation can be attained. The thickness of soft tissue separating the spine and the external splint is relatively unimportant in this region because of the relatively firm rib cage.

Data for the segmental external splint restriction of movement for the thoracic spine are lacking. Bracing, nevertheless, can be assumed to be at least somewhat effective. In fact, the resurgence of interest in the "nonoperative" management of spine trauma patients is partially related to the use of effective bracing strategies.[10,11,28]

LUMBAR AND LUMBOSACRAL SPINE BRACING

The lumbar, and particularly the low lumbar, region is difficult to externally splint because of the limitations created by an inadequate caudal fixation point.[43] In order to qualify as an adequate fixation point, it is necessary that there be two points that are at least four or five vertebral levels proximal and distal to the unstable segment and that are amenable to immobilization by an external splint. The pelvic region does not provide this because the distance from the unstable segment to the pelvic points of fixation is inadequate. In addition, hip flexion, even with hip spica application, allows unacceptable movement that may result in inadequate protection. Partial compensation for this can be achieved by lengthening the brace. This is accomplished either by adding an extension to a single lower extremity in the form of a hip spica or by extending the brace downward to the inguinal region over the iliac crests. To effectively stabilize this region, sitting must be virtually eliminated. These braces are, in general, not well tolerated. In addition, their efficacy is suspect.[4]

Objective data regarding the efficacy of external lumbar and lumbosacral splints are lacking. The available data, however, suggest that the comments of Sypert are rational and objective.[3] Sypert[36] cogently states "the effectiveness of the various lumbosacral orthoses in lumbosacral immobilization (excluding the spica type devices) is related more to their discomfort than to the actual magnitudes of the forces (abdominal compression, three-point fixation) transmitted from the appliance to the body. Thus, the function of most lumbosacral orthoses are to remind and

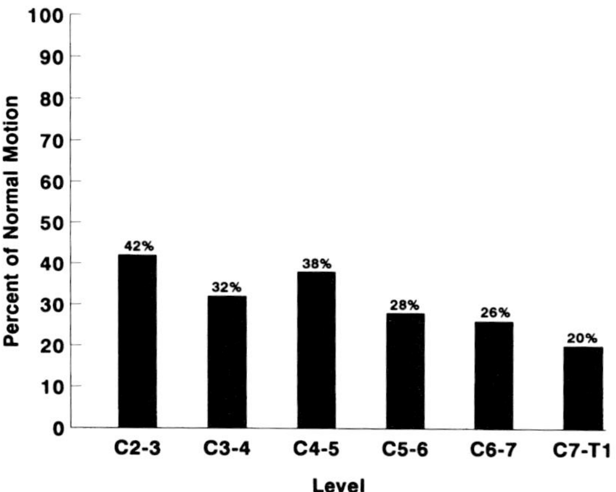

Figure 10: Koch and Nickel[21] determined the percent of normal cervical spine motion allowed in a halo device. The average was 31%, ranging from 42% in the upper cervical spine to 20% in the low cervical spine. The percent loss of segmental motion declined as the spine level descended.

to irritate the patient so that he restricts movements, to support the abdomen to alleviate some of the load on the lumbosacral spine, to provide some movement restriction of the upper lumbar and the thoracolumbar spine by three-point fixation, and to reduce excessive lumbar lordosis to provide a straighter and more comfortable low back." An understanding of these principles is of utmost importance so that the spine surgeon does not expect unattainable results from external spinal splinting techniques.[7,32,40]

COMPLICATIONS

Among the complications of orthoses are the following: 1) pain; 2) pressure; 3) psychological dependence; 4) poor hygiene; 5) axial muscle weakness and disuse atrophy; 6) restriction of activity; 7) aggravation of spinal symptoms; 8) vascular (venous) compromise; and 9) ineffective stabilization. In addition to these complications, halo bracing is associated with pin site complications that include cosmetic problems, osteomyelitis, brain abscess, and other soft-tissue and wound-healing problems. Therefore, spinal orthoses should be judiciously employed and employed only as long as there is a therapeutic advantage.

A rarely seen but potentially fatal complication of spinal bracing is the body cast syndrome. It is a manifestation of duodenum obstruction following the application of a body cast. Acute gastric dilatation with vomiting may be followed by aspiration, airway compromise, cardiac arrest, or gastric perforation and peritonitis. Removal of the brace as well as additional symptomatic therapy may be urgently required.[8,34] Its incidence is related to the excessively tight application of lumbar braces and the infrequent use of casts that are not removed or loosened.

REFERENCES

1. Anderson PA, Budorick TE, Easton KB, et al: Failure of halo vest to prevent *in vivo* motion in patients with injured cervical spines. **Spine 16 (Suppl 10):** S501-S505, 1991
2. Askins V, Eismont FJ: Efficacy of five cervical orthoses in restricting cervical motion. A comparison study. **Spine 22:**1193-1198, 1997
3. Axelsson P, Johnsson R, Stromqvist B: Effect of lumbar orthosis on intervertebral mobility. A roentgen stereophotogrammetric analysis. **Spine 17:**678-681, 1992
4. Axelsson P, Johnsson R, Stromqvist B: Lumbar orthosis with unilateral hip immobilization. Effect of intervertebral immobility determined by roentgen stereophotogrammetric analysis. **Spine 18:**876-879, 1993
5. Benzel EC: **Biomechanics of Spine Stabilization: Principles and Clinical Practice.** New York, NY: McGraw-Hill, 1994
6. Benzel EC, Hadden TA, Saulsbury CM: A comparison of the Minerva and halo jackets for stabilization of the cervical spine. **J Neurosurg 70:**411-414, 1989
7. Benzel EC, Larson SJ: Postoperative stabilization of the posttraumatic thoracic and lumbar spine: a review of concepts and orthotic techniques. **J Spinal Disord 2:**47-51, 1989
8. Berk RN, Coulson DB: The body cast syndrome. **Radiology 94:**303-305, 1970
9. Bucholz RD, Cheung KC: Halo vest versus spinal fusion for cervical injury: evidence from an outcome study. **J Neurosurg 70:**884-892, 1989
10. Cantor JB, Lebwohl NH, Garvey T, et al: Nonoperative management of stable thoracolumbar burst fractures with early ambulation and bracing. **Spine 18:** 971-976, 1993
11. Chow GH, Nelson BJ, Gebhard JS, et al: Functional outcome of thoracolumbar burst fractures managed with hyperextension casting or bracing and early mobilization. **Spine 21:**2170-2175, 1996
12. Coric D, Wilson JA, Kelly DL Jr: Treatment of traumatic spondylolisthesis of the axis with nonrigid immobilization: a review of 64 cases. **J Neurosurg 85:** 550-554, 1996
13. Hart DL, Johnson RM, Simmons EF, et al: Review of cervical orthoses. **Phys Ther 58:**857-860, 1978
14. Hartman JT, Palumbo F, Hill BJ: Cineradiography of the braced normal cervical spine: a comparative study of five commonly used cervical orthoses. **Clin Orthop 109:**97-102, 1975
15. Hughes SJ: How effective is the Newport/Aspen collar? A prospective radiographic evaluation in healthy adult volunteers. **J Trauma 45:**374-378, 1998
16. Johnson RM, Hart DL, Owen JR, et al: The Yale cervical orthosis. **Spine 58:**865-871, 1968
17. Johnson RM, Owen JR, Hart DL, et al: Cervical orthoses. A guide to their selection and use. **Clin Orthop 154:**34-45, 1981
18. Jones MD: Cineradiographic studies of the collar-immobilized cervical spine. **J Neurosurg 17:**633-637, 1960
19. Kauppi M, Neva MH, Kautiainen H: Headmaster collar restricts rheumatoid atlantoaxial subluxation. **Spine 24:**526-528, 1999
20. Kelly EG: Frequent lateral films key to control cervical displacement in halo cast. **Surg Practice News 10:**21, 1981
21. Koch RA, Nickel VL: The halo vest: an evaluation of motion and forces across the neck. **Spine 3:**103-107, 1978
22. Lau YC, Chang RK, Cheng YC, et al: Study of low-temperature thermoplastic modified custom-molded cervical orthosis for cervical spine fixation. **J Spinal Disord 7:**504-509, 1994
23. Lind B, Sihlbom H, Nordwall A: Forces and motions across the neck in patients treated with halo-vest. **Spine 13:**162-167, 1988
24. Maiman D, Millington P, Novak S, et al: The effect of the thermoplastic Minerva body jacket on cervical spine motion. **Neurosurgery 25:**363-368, 1989
25. Mirza SK, Moquin RR, Anderson PA, et al: Stabilizing properties of the halo apparatus. **Spine 22:**727-733, 1997
26. Morris JM: Spinal bracing, in Wilkins RH, Rengachary SS (eds): **Neurosurgery.** New York, NY: McGraw-Hill, 1985, pp 2300-2305
27. Morris JM, Lucas DB, Bresler B: Role of the trunk in stability of the spine. **J Bone Joint Surg (Am) 43:** 327-351, 1961
28. Mumford J, Weinstein JN, Spratt KF, et al: Thoracolumbar burst fractures. The clinical efficacy and outcome of nonoperative management. **Spine 18:** 955-970, 1993
29. Nickel VL, Perry J, Garrett A, et al: The halo. A spinal skeletal traction fixation. **J Bone Joint Surg (Am) 50:** 1400-1409, 1968
30. Norton PL, Brown T: The immobilizing efficiency of back braces. The effect on the posture and motion of the lumbosacral spine. **J Bone Joint Surg (Am) 39:** 111-138, 1957
31. Rae GL: Spine Section Newsletter. American Association of Neurological Surgeons, July 1994
32. Redford JB: **Orthotics Etcetera. 3rd ed.** Baltimore, Md: Williams & Wilkins, 1986
33. Sandler AJ, Dvorak J, Humke T, et al: The effectiveness of various cervical orthoses. An in vivo comparison of the mechanical stability provided by several widely used models. **Spine 21:**1624-1629, 1996
34. Schwartz DR, Wirka HW: The cast syndrome. A case report and discussion of the literature. **J Bone Joint Surg (Am) 46:**1549-1552, 1964

35. Sharpe KP, Rao S, Ziogas A: Evaluation of the effectiveness of the Minerva cervicothoracic orthosis. **Spine 20:**1475-1479, 1995
36. Sypert GW: External spinal orthotics. **Neurosurgery 20:**642-649, 1987
37. Tomonaga T, Krag MH, Novotny JE: Clinical, radiographic, and kinematic results from an adjustable four-pad halovest. **Spine 22:**1199-1208, 1997
38. Triggs KJ, Ballock T, Byrne T, et al: Length dependence of a halo orthosis on cervical immobilization. **J Spinal Disord 6:**34-37, 1993
39. Triggs KJ, Ballock T, Lee TQ, et al: The effect of angled insertion on halo pin fixation. **Spine 14:**781-783, 1989
40. van Poppel MNM, Koes BW, van der Ploeg T, et al: Lumbar supports and education for the prevention of low back pain in industry. A randomized controlled trial. **JAMA 279:**1789-1794, 1998
41. Waters RL, Morris JM: Effects of spinal supports on the electrical activity of muscles of the trunk. **J Bone Joint Surg (Am) 52:**51-60, 1970
42. Whitehill R, Richman JA, Glaser JA: Failure of immobilization of the cervical spine by the halo vest. A report of five cases. **J Bone Joint Surg (Am) 68:**326-332, 1986
43. Willems PC, Nienhuis B, Sietsma M, et al: The effect of a plaster cast on lumbosacral joint motion. An *in vivo* assessment with precision motion analysis system. **Spine 22:**1229-1234, 1997

CHAPTER 23

FUNDAMENTALS, TECHNIQUES, AND EXPECTATIONS OF THE REHABILITATION PROCESS

CHRISTOPHER S. FORMAL, MD, JOHN F. DITUNNO, JR., MD, AND EDWARD C. BENZEL, MD, FACS

Spinal cord injury (SCI) rehabilitation is a complex field that addresses the medical, functional, and psychosocial needs of persons with SCI. Spinal Cord Medicine has become a subspecialty of Physical Medicine and Rehabilitation.

Annually in the United States, approximately 30 to 40 persons per million population survive a traumatic SCI until hospitalization, a total of 183,000 to 230,000 persons.[28] The median age at the time of injury is 26 years, and 82% of injuries are sustained by males. The most common cause is a motor-vehicle accident, followed by a fall, and an act of violence. Life expectancy, while less than that for the general population, has improved over the past decades, and an improved outcome after SCI can be expected, particularly when specialized centers are utilized. It is in this vein that early, aggressive care of the person with SCI is deemed important and, thus, is addressed in this chapter.

PROGNOSIS

Neurological Recovery

The initial severity of injury can be used to predict outcome.[32] Physical examination is the primary method for evaluating severity, while other diagnostic tests, such as imaging studies, somatosensory evoked potentials, and transcra-

nial magnetic stimulation also provide information. Severity is measured using the American Spinal Injury Association (ASIA) impairment scale[1] (see Table 3 in Chapter 4, p 23). The prognosis for those with an initial grade of A (complete injury) is poor, with the majority demonstrating no change in grade and very few gaining functional strength in muscles innervated below the injury[19] (Table 1). The prognosis for those with an initial grade of D (incomplete injury) or E (normal) is good, and for those with an initial grade of B or C (incomplete injury) is less certain; 28% with an initial grade of B and 55% with an initial grade of C, improve to D or E. The prognosis for those with an initial grade of B may be more favorable in those sparing of pin sensation.[15] The prognosis for ambulation in those

TABLE 1

CORRELATION OF INITIAL AND DISCHARGE ASIA IMPAIRMENT SCALE GRADES*

Admit Grade	Discharge Grade				
	A	B	C	D	E
A	89%	5%	3%	3%	0%
B	5%	49%	16%	28%	1.7%
C	2%	1%	41%	53%	1.3%
D	1%	1%	1%	90%	6.5%

* Data from Ditunno et al.[19]

with an initial grade of C is good if there is a quadriceps muscle grade of >3/5 at 2 months.[14] While those with an initial grade of A do not usually improve in terms of the ASIA Impairment Scale grade, improvement in motor function at the level of injury is common, most likely due to the peripheral sprouting of nerves.[34]

Late or delayed neurological changes often occur in patients with an incomplete SCI. While changes can continue for more than a year after injury, most improvement occurs within the first 6 months.

A minority of patients deteriorate neurologically in the acute postinjury period. This is sometimes related to surgery or the method of immobilization. Deterioration in a person with a chronic injury is not expected and its occurrence should prompt a search for spinal instability or a second process, such as posttraumatic cystic myelopathy.

A brief discussion of "complete myelopathy" is warranted. A complete injury corresponds to a grade of A in the ASIA impairment scale, with absence of sensation and motor function in the sacral segments S4-5. The term implies the absence of long-tract neural transmission past the injured segments of the cord; the neurological prognosis is poor.[41]

Survival after Spinal Cord Injury

During World War II, survival after SCI was unlikely, with most patients succumbing in the initial weeks to sepsis from the urinary tract or pressure ulcers.[20] The recent decades have brought considerable improvement. For example, a 20-year-old person who survives at least 24 hours after sustaining tetraplegia, with an injury level of C5-8, and, at most, nonfunctional lower-extremity strength, has a life expectancy of 34 years from the time of injury.[16] Lung infection (pneumonia and influenza), non-ischemic heart disease, and sepsis (often from urinary tract infection, pneumonia, or pressure ulcers) are the most frequent causes of death.

Tetraplegia with Ventilator Dependence

Ventilator dependence after SCI is compatible with a prolonged life expectancy. A majority of ventilator-assisted tetraplegic individuals are alive 9 years after injury.[8] Patients often perceive a good quality of life, comparable to or better than that perceived by autonomously breathing individuals with tetraplegia.[5] Modern ventilators are compact and can be easily accommodated by an appropriate powered wheelchair. Management most frequently is with a cuffless tracheotomy tube, allowing phonation. Those with intact phrenic nerve function can be considered for placement of a phrenic nerve pacemaker.[45] Noninvasive technology can be used to replace conventional management by tracheotomy.[3]

GOALS OF REHABILITATION

SCI rehabilitation addresses a patient's physical status, functional ability, and psychosocial integration. This corresponds to treating their impairment, disability, and handicap. Physical rehabilitation involves minimizing the ultimate neurological deficit, developing the full potential of spared segments, and preventing and treating complications that occur in both the acute and chronic phases. Functional restoration includes maximizing mobility, developing self-care abilities (such as feeding, dressing, and bathing), and the management of the bowel and bladder. Psychosocial integration includes eventual discharge, whenever possible to a community setting, and the return to an educational or work setting.

A fundamental principle of SCI rehabilitation is that the process of rehabilitation does not cause neurological recovery. Rather, rehabilitation can take advantage of existing function or recovered function by strengthening non-paralyzed muscles. It can also utilize non-paralyzed muscles in novel manners to substitute for lost functions. Adaptive equipment can be used to provide function that would otherwise be lost. When an activity cannot be performed, despite appropriate retraining and provision of equipment, family members or other care providers can be instructed regarding assistance.

Realistic Expectations

Following complete and incomplete injuries, what can the patient's outcome be expected to be? Functional gains and life expectancy vary so much that each patient must be considered individually. Some predictions can be made and utilized to guide treatment plans. For example, patients with a complete SCI can expect little recovery of distal long-tract function. Potential levels of functioning based upon the neurological level are noted below.

Changing Expectations

Today, the quality of life for patients with an SCI can be expected to be higher than that achieved several decades ago by a patient with similar injuries. In addition to better physical and functional outcomes, legislation such as the Americans with Disabilities Act has improved psychosocial integration. Social issues may have a greater effect upon a patient's perceived quality of life than the severity of the neurological deficit.[25,26]

CURRENT SCI REHABILITATION TECHNIQUES

Rehabilitation after SCI should begin as soon as possible during the acute admission. New potentials may develop after hospital discharge, while new deficits may appear as the patient becomes older. The prevention and treatment of complications are always of concern. Thus, rehabilitation is a life-long process.

Acute Treatment Strategies

Surgery to stabilize the spine can facilitate early mobilization from the bed. This decreases the hospital length of stay and costs as well as the deleterious effects of bed rest.[21]

Orthostatic hypotension may develop during initial mobilization due to the lack of sympathetic tone, as well as the deconditioning effects of bed rest. An abdominal binder, elastic stockings, and gradual adaptation to erect positioning can be helpful. Recalcitrant cases can respond to treatment with oral salt supplementation, fludrocortisone, and possibly midodrine.[35] Asymptomatic "low blood pressure" is common in patients with tetraplegia and need not be treated.

Prophylaxis for deep vein thrombophlebitis can minimize but not eliminate potentially catastrophic complications of immobilization. The use of mechanical calf-compression devices for 2 weeks after injury, combined with low-dose subcutaneous heparin for 8 to 12 weeks, is a reasonable regimen.[13]

Turning regimens for the prevention of integument-pressure injury were introduced during World War II. Specialized frames and beds simplify the task of intermittently relieving pressure while maintaining alignment of the injured spine. Acutely, sacral pressure ulceration is most common; later, the ischii, trochanters, and heels are at risk.[44]

The physiology of acute spinal shock, in which a spinal upper motor neuron injury results in areflexia, is obscure.[2] After a period of days or weeks, the gradual picture of an upper motor neuron injury, with hyperreflexia and spasticity, emerges.

Pulmonary complications are common in the acute and chronic phases of SCI.[30] Physical measures such as turning, chest physical therapy, "quad coughing," and suctioning are critical in preventing atelectasis, mucous plugging, and pneumonia. A deficiency of suctioning is its inability to clear the left lung due to the acute angle of the left main bronchus.[24] The use of a mechanized insufflation-exsufflation device may address this problem and avoid the trauma of suctioning.[4]

The economic cost of SCI is high. Charges incurred in the first year after injury, including emergency services, acute hospital care, and rehabilitation, exceed $350,000 for a patient with high tetraplegia.[17]

Functional Restoration

Functional retraining is a team endeavor, with occupational and physical therapists working in concert with the physiatrist, nurse, social worker, and other professionals. The initial training is in an inpatient setting; after discharge, home and outpatient therapy are continued.

The neurological level (the most caudal spinal segment with normal motor and sensory function above the spinal lesion) can be used to predict the functional level after rehabilitation in patients with complete lesions.[38] If in an accessible environment, a person with a level of neurological injury above C4 may require the use of a ventilator but may still be entirely independent in mobility (and weight-shifting to prevent pressure ulcers) in a powered wheelchair. Those with a level of injury above C7 require some physical assistance for transfer from bed to chair, and for dressing and bathing. A person with a level of injury at C7 can achieve complete independence in self-care and mobility with the assistance of a wheelchair. A person with paraplegia can ambulate with long leg braces and a walker, but this is exhausting and wheelchair locomotion is often preferable. A person with intact function through the L3 myotome has functional quadriceps strength and, thus, can stabilize the knees, obviating the need for long-leg braces. However, short leg braces are still needed to stabilize the ankles, while the hips remain unstable due to the lack of strength for hip abduction and extension. This necessitates the use of canes, crutches, or a walker.

Standard rehabilitation measures can be augmented by the selective use of biofeedback training, electrical stimulation, and functional reconstructive surgery. Biofeedback utilizes surface electrodes to detect muscle contraction. The signal is then amplified and converted to a modality, such as sound, that can be utilized by the patient to guide exercise.[7,40] Functional electrical stimulation involves the programmed delivery of a stimulus to peripheral nerves in a pattern that can be used for exercise (e.g., bicycle ergometry) or function (e.g., walking).[31,33] Functional reconstructive surgery can be applied to the upper extremity, with the use of intact muscles to perform movements that have been lost. For example, a person with a C6 injury could achieve active elbow extension by transfer of the dorsal deltoid muscle to the triceps tendon.[42] Reconstructive surgery can also reverse deformities caused by spasticity, such as a foot held in equinovarus.

Psychosocial Adaptation

Depression is not the rule after SCI, although the risk of suicide is increased.[23] Most with SCI are grateful to have survived the trauma. The perceived quality of life appears less dependent upon the severity of the neurological injury than upon the level of social integration.[25,26]

Most persons with an SCI reside within the community. Compared to comparable healthy individuals, the rate of marriage is decreased following SCI. For those married at the time of SCI, the rate of divorce is increased, although a majority of those married at the time of injury remain married after 5 years postinjury. The level of education achieved by those with SCI eventually exceeds that of the general population. The rate of employment 10 years after injury is approximately 30%.[18]

Medical Management & Follow-Up

Medical management and follow-up of the person with an SCI is a specialty-oriented endeavor. Physiatrists, orthopedic surgeons, plastic surgeons, neurosurgeons, urologists, internists, and family physicians can play a role in this process. However, a single physician should direct the primary care of these patients. This physician should maintain a high index of suspicion for a multitude of potential complications and play an active role in their prevention. Several of the more common challenges are discussed below.

Pain perceived at or caudal to the spinal lesion is common.[6,22] Management includes patient education, maintenance of a high level of physical and social activity, and treatment of other morbidities. Antidepressant medications (e.g., nortriptyline) and anticonvulsants (e.g., gabapentin) are useful; nortriptyline may be more effective for constant and diffuse discomfort, while gabapentin may help with lancinating, "electric shock" pain. The possible contribution of a directly treatable lesion, such as posttraumatic cystic myelopathy, or an unstable spine, should be considered.

Autonomic hyperreflexia presents as an excruciating headache and hypertension in a person with a spinal injury level of T8 or higher.[10,11] It is triggered by a noxious stimulus, such as a distended bladder, that elicits a sympathetic response from the isolated spinal cord, resulting in constriction of the visceral vascular beds and hypertension. Management involves placing the person in a sitting position, loosening clothing, and searching for the triggering stimulus, such as a blocked urethral catheter. Acute medicinal treatment includes sublingual or topical nitroglycerin. If it is believed that the patient is at a low risk for a cardiovascular complication, bite-and-swallow nifedipine can be used.

Pressure ulcer prevention is affected by patient education and motivation. Appropriate bed and wheelchair cushions, with frequent weight shifts to relieve pressure, are integral to prevention.[37]

Initially, the bladder is drained by an indwelling catheter. For long-term use, intermittent catheterization is preferred. Here, urine output is controlled by fluid restriction. Reflex bladder contractions may necessitate the use of medications such as oxybutynin or tolterodine. A tetraplegic man may be unable to perform intermittent catheterization, but can sometimes void, by reflex, into an external catheter. In this circumstance, dyssynergic contraction of the external bladder sphincter, which then leads to high bladder pressures during voiding, can eventuate in urinary reflux, hydronephrosis, and renal deterioration. Voiding pressures can occasionally be decreased by medications such as terazosin or tamsulosin or by surgery that defeats the external sphincter. A tetraplegic female may also void by reflex, but an effective external catheter is lacking.[20]

The goal of bowel management is to achieve predictable emptying, without accident or impaction. Proper stool consistency is achieved by a diet including adequate fiber and water. Reflex bowel emptying can be achieved by a daily bowel routine, triggered by digital stimulation or a bisacodyl suppository or enema.[12]

Although spasticity usually develops after SCI, it need not be problematic. When it interferes with comfort or function, spasticity may respond to a program of regular stretching and medications (e.g., baclofen, tizanidine, diazepam, and dantrolene). When a limited number of muscles are responsible for the problems of spasticity, phenol motor point block or botulinum toxin injection can be helpful. Spasticity unresponsive to other measures usually responds to intrathecal baclofen.[39]

The most common causes of morbidity after SCI are urinary tract infection and pressure ulceration.[43] As noted, common causes of mortality in chronic SCI include pneumonia, cardiac disease, and sepsis (often from urinary tract infection, pressure ulceration, and pneumonia).[16]

The Comprehensive Program

The neurosurgeon or orthopedic surgeon often asks, "Where should I send my patient for SCI rehabilitation?" An adequate program must comply with surgical instructions, particularly with regard to the use of immobilization devices. The program must obtain routine surgical follow-up, as well as more urgent evaluation when a problem is detected. SCI rehabilitation is a lifelong process, and an outpatient program for the provision of life-long follow-up is a necessity.

THE FUTURE

What can the patient of the future expect? Are there reasonable expectations regarding reduc-

tion of the incidence of SCI and improvements in the quality of life for those with an SCI? Safety education and advances in motor vehicle engineering may decrease the incidence of SCI. Current investigations are approaching the problem of acute intervention to reduce the resulting neurological deficit; other investigations examine the potential for improving a chronic deficit. Reports from large-scale human trials involving the use of GM-1 ganglioside and 4-aminopyridine are pending.[27,29] Animal research has demonstrated some restoration of function after surgical spinal cord repair.[9] Other research examines the possibility of improving function given a static neurological deficit. A large-scale human trial, involving the use of a body weight support system for the purpose of achieving functional ambulation, is planned.[36] Such intervention may exploit the use of a spinal pattern generator for gait. Finally, the quality of life for those with SCI may be considerably improved by a more physically assessable environment and a more enlightened societal attitude.

Can we meet the challenge of SCI prevention and management in a cost-effective manner? In the future, we will be required to demonstrate efficacy in both cost and medical care. Therefore, we should turn our attention in this direction.

REFERENCES

1. American Spinal Injury Association, International Medical Society of Paraplegia: **International Standards for Neurological and Functional Classification of Spinal Cord Injury, Revised 1996.** Chicago, Ill: ASIA/IMSOP, 1996
2. Atkinson PP, Atkinson JLD: Spinal shock. **Mayo Clin Proc 71:**384-389, 1996
3. Bach JR: Alternative methods of ventilatory support for the patient with ventilatory failure due to spinal cord injury. **J Am Paraplegia Soc 14:**158-174, 1991
4. Bach JR: Mechanical insufflation-exsufflation. Comparison of peak expiratory flows with manually assisted and unassisted coughing techniques. **Chest 104:**1553-1562, 1993
5. Bach JR, Tilton MC: Life satisfaction and well-being measures in ventilator assisted individuals with traumatic tetraplegia. **Arch Phys Med Rehabil 75:**626-632, 1994
6. Bowsher D: Central pain of spinal origin. **Spinal Cord 34:**707-710, 1996
7. Brucker BS, Bulaeva NV: Biofeedback effect on electromyography responses in patients with spinal cord injury. **Arch Phys Med Rehabil 77:**133-137, 1996
8. Carter RE: Respiratory aspects of spinal cord injury management. **Parplegia 25:**262-266, 1987
9. Cheng H, Cao Y, Olson L: Spinal cord repair in adult paraplegic rats: partial restoration of hind limb func-

tion. **Science 273:**510-513, 1996

10. Colachis SC III: Autonomic hyperreflexia with spinal cord injury. **Topics Spinal Cord Inj Rehabil 3**(1):71-81, 1997

11. Consortium for Spinal Cord Medicine: **Acute Management of Autonomic Dysreflexia: Adults with Spinal Cord Injury Presenting to Health-Care Facilities.** Washington, DC: Paralyzed Veterans of America, 1997

12. Consortium for Spinal Cord Medicine: **Neurogenic Bowel Management in Adults with Spinal Cord Injury.** Washington, DC: Paralyzed Veterans of America, 1998

13. Consortium for Spinal Cord Medicine: **Prevention of Thromboembolism in Spinal Cord Injury.** Washington, DC: Paralyzed Veterans of America, 1997

14. Crozier KS, Cheng LL, Graziani V, et al: Spinal cord injury: prognosis for ambulation based on quadriceps recovery. **Paraplegia 30:**762-767, 1992

15. Crozier KS, Graziani V, Ditunno JF Jr, et al: Spinal cord injury: prognosis for ambulation based on sensory examination in patients who are initially motor complete. **Arch Phys Med Rehabil 72:**119-121, 1991

16. DeVivo MJ, Stover SL: Long-term survival and causes of death, in Stover SL, DeLisa JA, Whiteneck GG (eds): **Spinal Cord Injury. Clinical Outcomes from the Model Systems.** Gaithersburg, Md: Aspen, 1995, pp 289-316

17. DeVivo MJ, Whiteneck GG, Charles ED Jr: The economic impact of spinal cord injury, in Stover SL, DeLisa JA, Whiteneck GG (eds): **Spinal Cord Injury. Clinical Outcomes from the Model Systems.** Gaithersburg, Md: Aspen, 1995, pp 234-271

18. Dijkers MP, Abela MB, Gans BM, et al: The aftermath of spinal cord injury, in Stover SL, DeLisa JA, Whiteneck GG (eds): **Spinal Cord Injury. Clinical Outcomes from the Model Systems.** Gaithersburg, Md: Aspen, 1995, pp 185-212

19. Ditunno JF Jr, Cohen ME, Formal C, et al: Functional outcomes, in Stover SL, DeLisa JA, Whiteneck GG (eds): **Spinal Cord Injury. Clinical Outcomes from the Model Systems.** Gaithersburg, Md: Aspen, 1995, pp 170-184

20. Ditunno JF Jr, Formal CS: Chronic spinal cord injury. **N Engl J Med 330:**550-556, 1994

21. Donovan WH: Operative and nonoperative management of spinal cord injury. A review. **Paraplegia 32:** 375-388, 1994

22. Eide PK: Pathophysiological mechanisms of central neuropathic pain after spinal cord injury. **Spinal Cord 36:**601-612, 1998

23. Elliott TR, Frank RG: Depression following spinal cord injury. **Arch Phys Med Rehabil 77:**816-823, 1996

24. Fishburn MJ, Marino RJ, Ditunno JF Jr: Atelectasis and pneumonia in acute spinal cord injury. **Arch Phys Med Rehabil 71:**197-200, 1991

25. Fuhrer MJ, Rintala DH, Hart KA, et al: Depressive symptomatology in persons with spinal cord injury who reside in the community. **Arch Phys Med Rehabil 74:**255-260, 1993

26. Fuhrer MJ, Rintala DH, Hart KA, et al: Relationship of life satisfaction to impairment, disability, and handicap among persons with spinal cord injury living in the community. **Arch Phys Med Rehabil 73:**552-557, 1992

27. Geisler FH, Dorsey FC, Coleman WP: Recovery of motor function after spinal-cord injury—a randomized, placebo-controlled trial with GM-1 ganglioside. **N Engl J Med 324:**1829-1838, 1991

28. Go BK, DeVivo MJ, Richards JS: The epidemiology of spinal cord injury, in Stover SL, DeLisa JA, Whiteneck GG (eds): **Spinal Cord Injury. Clinical Outcomes from the Model Systems.** Gaithersburg, Md: Aspen, 1995, pp 21-55

29. Hayes KC, Blight AR, Potter PJ, et al: Preclinical trial of 4-aminopyridine in patients with chronic spinal cord injury. **Paraplegia 31:**216-224, 1993

30. Jackson AB, Groomes TE: Incidence of respiratory complications following spinal cord injury. **Arch Phys Med Rehabil 75:**270-275, 1994

31. Jacobs PL, Nash MS, Klose J, et al: Evaluation of a training program for persons with SCI paraplegia using the Parastep1 Ambulation System: Part 2. Effects on physiological responses to peak arm ergometry. **Arch Phys Med Rehabil 78:**794-798, 1997

32. Kirshblum SC, O'Connor KC: Predicting neurologic recovery in traumatic cervical spinal cord injury. **Arch Phys Med Rehabil 79:**1456-1466, 1998

33. Klose KJ, Jacobs PL, Broton JG, et al: Evaluation of a training program for persons with SCI paraplegia using the Parastep1 Ambulation System: Part 1. Ambulation performance and anthropometric measures. **Arch Phys Med Rehabil 78:**789-793, 1997

34. Marino RJ, Herbison GJ, Ditunno JF Jr: Peripheral sprouting as a mechanism for recovery in the zone of injury in acute quadriplegia: a single-fiber EMG study. **Muscle Nerve 17:**1466-1468, 1994

35. Nobunaga AI: Orthostatic hypotension in spinal cord injury. **Topics Spinal Cord Inj Rehabil 4**(1):73-80, 1997

36. Norman KE, Pepin A, Ladouceur M, et al: A treadmill apparatus and harness support for evaluation and rehabilitation of gait. **Arch Phys Med Rehabil 76:**772-778, 1995

37. Panel for the Prediction and Prevention of Pressure Ulcers in Adults: **Pressure Ulcers in Adults: Prediction and Prevention. Clinical Practice Guideline, Number 3.** Rockville, Md: Agency for Health Care Policy and Research, Public Health Service, U.S. Department of Health and Human Services, 1992

38. Staas WE Jr, Formal CS, Freedman MK, et al: Spinal cord injury and spinal cord injury medicine, in DeLisa JA, Gans BM (eds): **Rehabilitation Medicine: Principles and Practice. 3rd ed.** Philadelphia, Pa: Lippincott-Raven, 1998, pp 1259-1291

39. Stein AB, Pomerantz F, Schechtman J: Evaluation and management of spasticity in spinal cord injury. **Top Spinal Cord Inj Rehabil 2**(4):70-83, 1997

40. Stein RB, Brucker BS, Ayyar DR: Motor units in incomplete spinal cord injury: electrical activity, contractile properties and the effects of biofeedback. **J Neurol Neurosurg Psychiatry 53:**880-885, 1990

41. Waters RL, Adkins RH, Yakura JS: Definition of complete spinal cord injury. **Paraplegia 29:**573-581, 1991

42. Waters RL, Sie IH, Gellman H, et al: Functional hand surgery following tetraplegia. **Arch Phys Med Rehabil 77:**86-94, 1996

43. Whiteneck GG, Charlifue SW, Frankel HL, et al: Mortality, morbidity, and psychosocial outcomes of persons spinal cord injured more than 20 years ago. **Paraplegia 30:**617-630, 1992

44. Yarkony GM, Heinemann AW: Pressure ulcers, in Stover SL, DeLisa JA, Whiteneck GG (eds): **Spinal Cord Injury. Clinical Outcomes from the Model Systems.** Gaithersburg, Md: Aspen, 1995, pp 100-119

45. Yarkony GM, Jaeger RJ: Phrenic nerve pacemakers for tetraplegia. **Topics Spinal Cord Inj Rehabil 1**(1): 77-82, 1995

CHAPTER 24

THE SPINAL CORD INJURY UNIT IN THE NEW MILLENNIUM: A PARADIGM SHIFT

W. P. WARING, III, MS, MD, AND DENNIS J. MAIMAN, MD, PHD

Between 8000 and 10,000 traumatic spinal cord injuries (SCIs) are reported annually in the United States. Although this number pales in comparison to the incidence of other disabilities (stroke: 500,000 or congenital disabilities: 100,000), several factors make SCIs unique: 1) medically, SCIs are very expensive, with a mean cost of $200,000 during the first year following injury and $25,000 annually thereafter; 2) societal costs are very high within this group due to the increasing life expectancy, with annual direct costs of $2.7 billion and indirect costs of $3.7 billion; and 3) the complex nature of SCIs requires a host of specialists who are often found only in larger medical centers, which has led to the development of SCI programs.[8]

Over the last 50 years, enormous strides have been made in the care of individuals with SCIs, including emergency medical care, acute care after injury, acute rehabilitation, and community integration. The apex of progress for SCIs was the evolution of regional SCI centers that integrate emergency care, acute care, rehabilitation, and post-acute care. Within this concept of SCI centers, SCI units have been established in which acute care and initial rehabilitation can be effectively and efficiently combined. These improve-ments are evidenced by the fact that more than 90% of patients discharged from model systems SCI centers return to the community, and survival, although not normal, can often be measured by decades (Table 1).

The 1990s saw several changes that challenged the concepts and goals of SCI centers and units. These changes include: 1) limiting the access of patients to hospitals by health maintenance organizations (HMOs), which can undermines the volume of cases needed to maintain expertise and makes it financially unfeasible to operate distinct SCI units; 2) third-party payors targeting SCI care for cost containment, resulting in progressively shorter lengths of stays in SCI units and a shift from rehabilitation discharge outcomes to more of a medical model; 3) third-party payors limiting access to SCI outpatient clinics and the long-term care that outpatient clinics offer; 4) decreasing reimbursement on a "per diem" basis, which impacts the amount of care and rehabilitation services that can be delivered per day; and 5) a shift in epidemiology that is resulting in more SCIs caused by violence, especially gunshot wounds and falls, and fewer patients injured in motor-vehicle and sport accidents. These shifts also resulted in changes in

TABLE 1

LIFE EXPECTANCY FOR PERSONS WITH SPINAL CORD INJURIES WHO SURVIVE AT LEAST 24 HOURS
POSTINJURY BY AGE AT INJURY AND NEUROLOGICAL CATEGORY

Age at Injury (yrs)	Normal*	C1-4 (Frankel Grade A, B, C)	C5-8 (Frankel Grade A, B, C)	T1-S5 (Frankel Grade A, B, C)	Frankel Grade D
5	70.8	37.3	47.7	55.7	61.4
10	65.9	32.9	43.1	51.0	56.6
15	61.0	28.5	38.4	46.3	51.8
20	56.3	25.3	34.3	42.1	47.5
25	51.6	22.4	30.5	38.1	43.3
30	46.9	19.3	26.5	34.0	39.0
35	42.2	16.5	22.9	30.0	34.6
40	37.6	14.2	19.5	26.2	30.3
45	33.0	12.2	16.4	22.6	26.0
50	28.6	9.7	13.1	18.7	21.9
55	24.4	7.3	10.2	15.0	18.1
60	20.5	5.0	7.8	11.6	14.8
65	16.9	3.5	5.8	8.9	11.8
70	13.6	2.2	4.0	6.7	9.0
75	10.7	1.3	2.7	4.8	6.7
80	8.1	0.3	1.6	3.2	4.6

*Normal values are from 1988 U.S. Life Tables for the general population.

demographics, with needs for the typical older patient with a fall being different from the needs of an inner city minority patient with a gunshot wound.

BACKGROUND

Until the 20th century, SCIs resulted in an early demise, usually due to respiratory failure, urosepsis, massive decubitus ulcers, or renal failure. The often quoted Edwin Smith Egyptian Surgical Papyrus describes SCIs by stating, "Thou shouldst say concerning one having a dislocation of the vertebrae of his neck while he is unconscious of his two legs and two arms and his urine dribbles an ailment not to be treated."[4]

The first large-scale exposure of modern medicine to SCIs occurred during World War I. Although the anatomy, neurology, and complications of SCI were better understood, treatment and patient survival remained at a primitive level. The modern era of SCI began during World War II, during which great advancements were made in the areas of emergency evacuation, the treatment of infection, and social attitudes toward disability. The pioneers delivering service to patients with SCIs used two lessons from WWI: 1) war results in many disabled combatants; and 2) unless social attitudes were changed, another generation of persons with disabilities would exist where nothing would be expected and behaviors such as drug addiction, hopelessness, and dependency would be the norm.[3]

The first SCI units were begun in England soon after the start of World War II. The first facility that combined acute medical care and rehabilitation was Stoke Mandeville Hospital in England under the directorship of Sir Ludwig Guttman in 1944. Guttman promoted the idea that a person with an SCI, although disabled, could be a healthy and productive member of society. Combining this new philosophy with excellence in medical care and rehabilitation was the first real breakthrough in care for patients with SCIs.[2]

The first SCI centers in the U.S. also began during WWII in Veterans Administration hospitals. During this time, the U.S. was experiencing large polio epidemics. The March of Dimes helped fund large programs to provide rehabilitation to people with residual paralysis from polio. The 1940s and 1950s saw medical rehabilitation evolve. "Physiatrists" emerged during WWII as specialists who supervised the medical management of patients with disabilities and rehabilitation programs. Rehabilitation specialists, such as physical therapists, occupational therapists, vocational counselors, and psychologists also developed during this period. Along with rehabilitation professionals, the way in which rehabilitation was delivered also evolved.

Rehabilitation in the U.S. has traditionally used a "team approach." The team is comprised of the patient/family, physiatrists, therapists, nursing, psychologists, and, if needed, other rehabilitation professionals such as vocational counselors. The team meets on a regular basis, discussing and establishing realistic goals, documenting progress, and planning discharge to home. In the past, the overall goals were to regain or maintain health and maximize the independence of the person with the disability. A person's rehabilitation program was individualized by assessing their strengths, needs, abilities, and preferences.

Between the 1960s and the 1980s, there was an explosion in the number of rehabilitation units. This explosion was fueled by: 1) an improvement in trauma and general medical care which has resulted in more patients surviving with significant disabilities, therefore becoming candidates for rehabilitation; 2) having adequate numbers of rehabilitation professionals to staff these facilities; and 3) the fee for a service reimbursement system not only funded rehabilitation but also made it financially beneficial to start rehabilitation programs in acute care hospitals.

Spinal Cord Injury Programs

Under the leadership of Dr. John Young, the first regional SCI system was established in Phoenix in 1970. The National Institute on Disability and Rehabilitation Research helped fund this and subsequent regional SCI systems to determine whether this model would optimize clinical and rehabilitation outcomes. The initial network in 1972 consisted of six centers. By 1990, 19 centers were receiving government funding. These programs were committed to a "system of care" concept that included: 1) modern emergency medical services as an entry point to the system; 2) Level One trauma centers available within the system; 3) comprehensive SCI inpatient rehabilitation; 4) psychosocial and vocation services; and 5) adequate follow-up care after discharge. A research component of the model system was to develop a national database for SCIs.

Concurrent with the establishment of federally funded SCI centers were the development of other SCI rehabilitation programs that met the criteria established by the Commission on the Accreditation of Rehabilitation Facilities (CARF) (4891 East Grant Road, Tucson, Arizona). Other organizations that created program criteria for the care of trauma patients include the Uniform Data System, which tracks rehabilitation outcomes for selected disabilities including SCIs, and the American College of Surgeons, which is in charge of the accreditation of trauma centers (Uniform Data System Management Service, 232 Parker Hall, 3435 Main Street, SUNY South Campus, Buffalo, New York 14214-3007, and the American College of Surgeons, 633 North Saint Clair Street, Chicago, Illinois 60611).

Historically, there were two models for SCI rehabilitation programs: rehabilitation units in acute care hospitals, and free-standing rehabilitation centers. There were many positive reasons why both of these types of programs flourished during the 1970s and early 1980s. Free-standing rehabilitation hospitals, by definition, provide rehabilitation as their principle product. If positioned to have a rehabilitation referral base, these free-standing facilities could have the volume of patients to create a thorough or comprehensive skill level and would not have to compete with other programs or products seen in acute care hospitals.

On the other hand, SCI programs in acute care hospitals have had the historical opportunity to provide continuity of care from emergency medical services to acute care through acute inpatient rehabilitation. Few centers, however, have maximized this opportunity by providing rehabilitation and acute care in adjoining physical locations while utilizing the same nursing and rehabilitation staffs. An example of this is the

Spine Cord Injury Unit operated by Froedtert Memorial Lutheran Hospital and The Medical College of Wisconsin in Milwaukee. In this program, new SCI patients are admitted to an SCI unit, which contains both acute care and rehabilitation beds plus therapy areas, all in the same physical space. The SCI team is consulted on the day of admission and services start on the first day. The same physiatrists, physical therapists, occupational therapists, psychologists, social workers, nurses, and nurse case managers provide care whether the SCI patient is in an acute care or a rehabilitation bed. The goals of early intervention include minimizing complications (e.g., decubitus ulcers and contractures), preparing the patient and family for rehabilitation, minimizing depression by educating the patient regarding the goals of rehabilitation and what is possible (changing the focus from recovery to realistic rehabilitation goals), and providing improved continuity in medical and rehabilitation.

In most SCI programs, the long-term care (medical and rehabilitation services) provided following discharge has centered on outpatient SCI clinics, usually staffed by physiatrists and nurses. Most follow-up care is in the form of yearly clinic evaluations. Few attempts have been made to provide primary care to this population. As expected, post-injury care tends to be fragmented. A holistic exception to this is the Veterans Administration system that has promoted SCI clinics as the principal point of service for veterans with SCI.

BENEFITS OF THE MODEL SYSTEMS (SCI UNITS)

One of the initial rationales for supporting dedicated SCI programs was the expectation that clinical outcomes would improve both due to increased experience by a focal team treating these injuries and the increased volume of patients needed to support the development of clinical guidelines and protocols. Participants in the model system SCI project have published numerous papers and reports on improving clinical outcomes. Highlights include: 1) increasing rates of incomplete injuries, which translates into greater potential for neurological recovery (44.3%

incomplete in 1973-77 vs. 56.7% in 1987-89); 2) decreasing numbers of patients requiring acute hospitalization (.61 per year in 1973-75 vs. .31 in 1986-89); 3) fewer complications (e.g., decubitus ulcers or contractures) for patients admitted to an SCI program within 24 hours of injury; 4) lower medical costs for acute care of patients admitted within 24 hours to an SCI center (a $5,000 savings in 1992); and 5) shorter rehabilitation stays compared to other rehabilitation units (52.7% of what was reported by UDS in 1991).

Improved outcomes in rehabilitation has been harder to prove by model systems SCI programs. Part of this difficulty is due to the fact that model systems programs tend to admit the patients with more severe injuries and with less potential to make gains in typical areas measured by outcome tools, such as the functional independence measurement (FIM).[5] The FIM evaluates independence by measuring 18 items covering mobility, activities of daily living, sphincter control, communication, and social integration. One long-term area in which there has been poor outcomes is employment among the SCI population, which is one of the areas that is poorly assessed by the FIM. Despite a healthy economy, only 20%-30% of the SCI population are working.[8]

A major benefit of the model systems SCI program has been the large number of scientific and educational papers, reports, books, and audiovisual aids produced. More than 1000 peer-reviewed articles have been published on this subject.[8] SCI programs have also had opportunities to interact through several professional organizations, such as the American Spinal Injury Association (ASIA), the National Spinal Injury Association, the International Medical Society of Paraplegia (IMSOP), and the American Paraplegic Society.

Few areas of rehabilitation have kindled the commitment and fervor seen with service delivery for people with SCIs. Part of this is due to the opportunities to work with a younger population over long periods of time and be part of a process where patients gradually regain their sense of individuality and progress to become active, healthy, and productive members of society. An example of this fervor and commitment is a quote from Herbert Talbot: "Man does not live by bread alone, but by faith, by admiration, by sympathy." It is not enough to teach the disabled how to keep alive and earn a living. We must help them to find the joy in living, to regain their faith in themselves, to feel again the glow of being admired, and to know the solace of sympathy. It calls to that combination of compassion and imagination that have ever been the mark of the great physician. In no other activity does the science of medicine need more to be complemented by the art.

Over the past year, we have many times repeated that rehabilitation must be a product of its time and place; it must serve here and now, and it must, by the precepts of Western civilization, acknowledge the primacy of the individual. Parenthetically, it is worth remarking that the individual may attain a high level of self-expression and self-satisfaction when he/she relates personal efforts to those of a group. "However it may be sought, the longing for fulfillment lies in every heart, this urge of every human to be somebody, but above all to be him/herself must never be far from our thoughts. Without it, the processes of rehabilitation become no more than a mechanical tour de force."[3]

TRENDS IN THE 1990S

The decline in "hospitalized days" (acute and rehabilitation) following SCIs has continued. In 1973-77 the mean length of stay in the hospital was 144.8 days, in 1989-92 it was 77.5 days, and in 1998 it was 37 days.[1] Part of this decline can be attributed to better acute care and more efficient rehabilitation. Another factor in declining lengths of hospitalization has been the pressure of health-care reform to decrease costs, third-party payor case managers limiting funding, and the use of clinical pathways that attempt to standardize inpatient goals. Despite the initial concern that shorter lengths of hospitalization would result in decreases in rehabilitation outcomes, FIM outcomes for SCI have had little change.[7] Whether the result of shorter lengths of hospitalization is complications and readmission is still being studied.

The epidemiology of SCI is changing. Specifically, SCI from violence has increased from 13.9% in the 1970s[8] to 29.5% in 1991-94. Violence, specifically gunshot wounds, differs from closed trauma in the neurological outcomes (73% are paraplegic and 57.6% are complete), decreased initial acute hospitalizations (2 days less than motor-vehicle accidents), a disproportionate number of Hispanics and African Americans (African Americans account for 29.9% of SCIs vs. being only 12% of the general population) and this population has poorer outcomes with respect to follow-up statistics, the number of decubitus ulcers, return to work, or the use of vocational and educational resources.[8]

Funding for SCI care is evolving away from a fee-for-service reimbursement to negotiated reimbursement and upcoming a prospective payment system from Medicare.

The 1990s were turbulent times not only for patients with SCIs but for those needing rehabilitation in general. Decreased lengths of hospitalization meant rehabilitation programs needed to increase the number of patients to keep their units full. Prospective payment for skilled nursing facilities for Medicare-funded rehabilitation caused the widespread cancellation of programs and, for the first time, an oversupply of therapists. Several SCI programs have developed other products lines, such as traumatic brain injury rehabilitation, to keep their beds full.

A NEW MODEL FOR SCI PROGRAMS

SCI programs are facing a number of new challenges, including decreased reimbursement for inpatient rehabilitation, decreasing occupancy in rehabilitation units, and identifying innovative approaches to dealing with individuals with SCIs due to violence, and a potential increase in fragmentation due to HMOs. At the same time, the previous model for SCI care (Figure 1) is being questioned. The earlier model with its emphasis on lengthy inpatient rehabilitation is clashing with recent trends to decrease cost, whether reimbursement can fund previous levels of rehabilitation, its lack of committed long-term care, and questions of patient satisfaction with rehabilitation goals in the acute SCI period when the patient has not been able to reside in their community. Another weakness is that, overall, the old model was not responsive to the needs of persons that change over time due to aging,

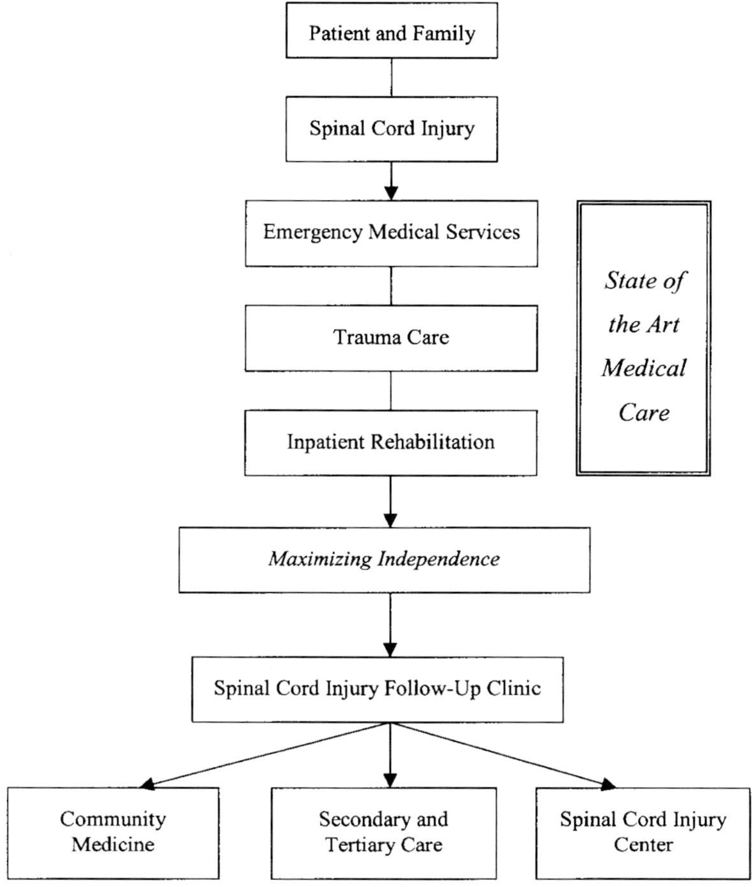

Figure 1: The traditional model of a regional SDI center.

changes in their support system, or changing life goals.[8] As the number of persons surviving with SCIs increase, it is becoming more apparent that the notion that SCI is a stable disability is false.[8] The long-term follow-up care offered by traditional SCI programs without a clear objective to provide primary care has promoted fragmented care and some consumer dissatisfaction.[9]

One positive element of health-care reform is the development of a performance improvement model as advocated by both the Joint Commission for the Accreditation of Hospitals and CARF. Performance improvement fits a research model of studying costs (efficiency) and outcomes (effectiveness) as a routine part of managing medical and rehabilitation services. Within this concept, it will be easier to study alternative models to traditional SCI care. Figure 2 illustrates an

alternative model of SCI care. The initial emphasis remains on state-of-the-art efficient acute care. The rehabilitation component has more of a medical model—patients are discharged to a safe environment when they are medically stable. The focus on rehabilitation can be shifted to the outpatient side. This especially fits in with the increase in SCI due to gunshot wounds, with its population highest in larger urban settings. Providing more organized outpatient rehabilitation facilities will not only be less costly, but will be more effective because persons with an SCI can use their experience in their communities to prioritize their own rehabilitation goals.

It is no secret that HMOs would like to avoid costly patients such as with SCI. By 5 years post-injury, the majority of persons with SCIs will have Medicare or Medicaid as their medical

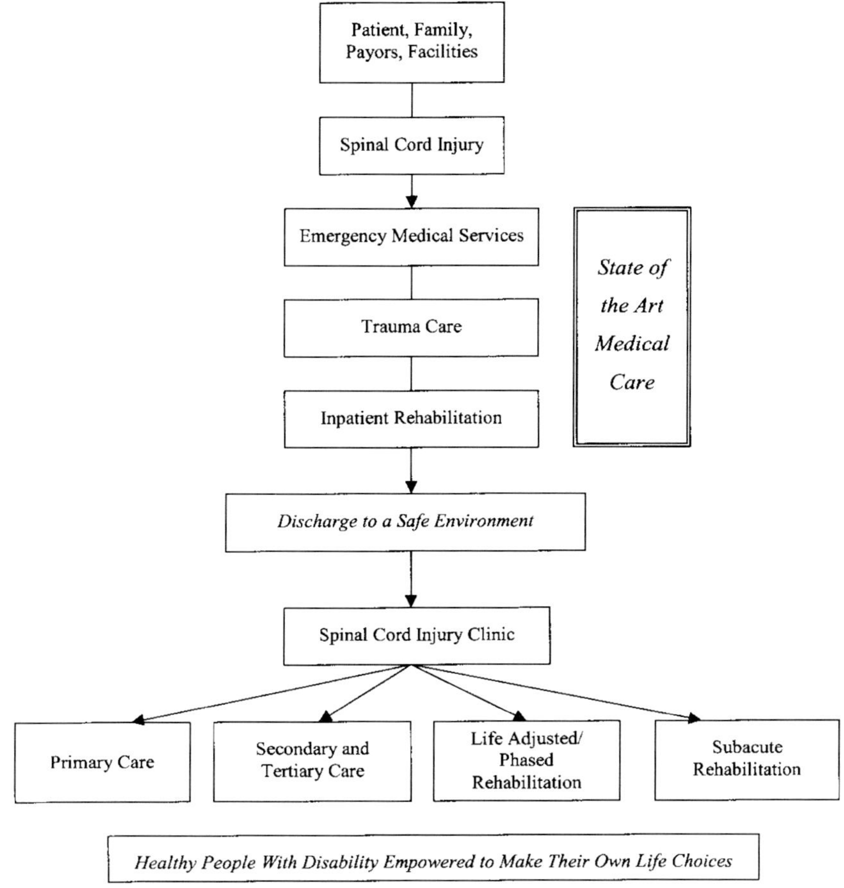

Figure 2: Alternative model of an SCI system of care.

insurance provider. The failure of HMOs to develop programs for senior citizens will permit a window of time when people with SCIs still have a choice regarding their ongoing medical needs. If the future of SCI rehabilitation is in the outpatient arena, the ability to provide primary care will not only provide an access point for initial rehabilitation, but will also be an opportunity to study the long-term health-care needs in a model that will integrate rehabilitation issues.

Although SCI programs and units are facing a seemingly ever-changing health-care environment, these changes also will provide the opportunity to continue the traditions and progress of the past 50 years. Not to evolve has many risks. Sir Ludwig Guttman's prophetic comments 30 years ago still ring true: "The fragmentation of the management of the spinal paraplegic and tetraplegic into immediate, intermediate treatment and the long-term physical, psychological and social rehabilitation including domestic and professional or industrial resettlement, called rehabilitation, has, as a rule, proved unsatisfactory, and from all that I have seen in many countries, often disastrous."[6]

REFERENCES

1. **Annual Report for the Model Spinal Injury Care Systems.** Birmingham, Ala: National Spinal Cord Injury Statistical Center, 1998
2. Cole TM: Spinal cord injury and trauma, in Day SB (ed): **Trauma.** New York, NY: Plenum, 1973, pg 303-327
3. Dick TBS: Traumatic paraplegic pre-Guttmann. **Paraplegia** 7:173-178, 1969
4. Elsberg CA: The Edwin Smith Surgical Papyrus, and the diagnosis and treatment of injuries to the skull

and spine 5,000 years ago. **Ann Med Hist 3:**271-279, 1931

5. Granger CV, Hamilton BB: The uniform data system for medical rehabilitation report of the first admissions for 1992. **Am J Phys Med Rehabil 28:**545-555, 1994

6. Guttman L: **Spinal Cord Injuries Comprehensive Management and Research. 2nd ed.** Oxford: Blackwell Scientific, 1976, p 9

7. Morrison SL, Stanwyck D, Daviou P: The effect of shorter lengths of stay on inpatient and outpatient outcomes of spinal cord injury rehabilitation. **J Spinal Cord Med 20:**151, 1997

8. Stover SL, DeLisa JA, Whiteneck GG (eds): **Spinal Cord Injury. Clinical Outcomes from the Model Systems.** Gaithersburg, Md: Aspen, 1995

9. Waring WP, Ardner M, Hurkett C, et al: Primary health care for people with spinal cord injuries: the consumers' perspective. **J Spinal Cord Med 18:**143, 1995

CHAPTER 25

Prevention of Spinal Cord Injury

Fred H. Geisler, MD, PhD

Traumatic injuries consume a major amount of health care resources. Estimates place the total cost of traumatic injuries at 40% of all health-care expenditures in the United States. Head and spinal cord injury have the highest morbidity, mortality, and cost to society of any disease among the youth of America. The incidence of death for these injuries is estimated at greater than 140,000 per year, with more than 60 million persons seeking medical care.[41,42] An estimated $170 billion was spent in 1988, the last year with published statistics. These figures include between 10,000 and 12,000 spinal cord injuries (SCIs) each year, with the majority of the victims less than 30 years of age.[4,7,23,26,31,34,36,55] The lifetime cost of directly caring for a disabled SCI victim has been estimated to exceed $600,000.[47] Additional costs associated with SCI victims include loss of wages and alterations necessary in their families for aiding in their care. The Oregon State Health Division has determined the following annual estimates for its population: 5% are involved in trauma, 0.825% have a major injury as defined by the Injury Severity Score (score >13), and 0.165% have a major injury to the head or spinal cord.[4]

The majority of the traumatic injuries are preventable; 70% of motor-vehicle accidents (MVAs)[26,31,32,34] are a result of human error[17] and 91% of MVA-associated SCI occurs in unrestrained passengers.[49] Because a time cure for SCI neurological deficits is unavailable, the elimination of these devastating injuries is currently the only means to prevent lifelong disability.[20] Currently, the medical treatments available for the treatment of SCI are: 1) rapid emergency medical technician response, delivery of patient, and protocol-based therapy; 2) the mechanical stabilization of spinal fracture both internally and externally to prevent shifting of the vertebral fragments and resulting spinal cord re-injury; 3) intensive care management to optimize cardiopulmonary function in the acute post-injury period and minimize secondary neurological damage; and 4) drug pharmacotherapy with methylprednisolone[7-14] and Sygen.[24]

Although in an individual case, some or all of these treatments may contribute to a recovery that is greater than expected or partial recovery that occurs earlier than projected, the majority of patients are unfortunately left with a severe neurological deficit.[18,25,27,46,52,53] The programs for the prevention of SCI are not only the first line of defense, but also the only true line of defense. There is currently no medical cure for the vast majority of paralyzed patients accounting for approximately 50% of all SCIs.

MVAs are the most common cause of SCI,

with drugs or alcohol frequently a contributing factor.[15] Falls and diving injuries are the next most common causes;[51] specifically, diving results in about 1000 SCIs per year, with 95% of these injuries resulting in quadriplegia.[50] SCI results from violent assaults or gunshot wounds in many instances, and sports and recreational activity account for 7% to 15%.[33,38] The exact frequency of each mechanism varies considerably in different geographical areas, seasons of the year, and socioeconomic groups.

Adolescents have a higher incidence of neurological injury because of increased risks taken during the developmental stage.[26,31,32,34] Peer pressure, combined with poor judgment, are often the stimuli that result in an injury with potentially lifelong disability. Twelve- to 14-year-old children begin taking dares as a substitute for game playing.[30] During their high school years, adolescents undergo a period of self-centeredness with feelings of invulnerability.[37] Risky behavior is common in this age group because of their disregard for consequences and their limited experience.[28] When compared with adults, adolescents drive more at night on weekends, drive faster, use shorter braking distances, and more frequently pass through an intersection on a yellow light.[5,21,39] In addition to their risky behavior, adolescents wear safety belts less frequently, exposing themselves to greater potential injury.[16] This is also the period in their life in which patterns are set for adult behavior and, hence, a prevention program can have potential long-term benefits.[29]

Within the field of injury prevention, there are three categories of techniques: 1) automatic protection devices; 2) laws or rules that require a behavioral change; and 3) changing the risk-taking behavior.[20] Protection devices include side-impact protection panels, airbags, and automatic restraint systems in cars. The use of these devices does not require the cooperation of the individual for their function. Laws or rules that require a behavioral change include seat-belt laws, motorcycle helmet laws, diving restrictions, and modification of the rules of sports games. Automobile seat belts reduce both injury and death by approximately 50%.[44] Although the most difficult, the most effective method for reducing SCI is persuading individuals to lessen the level of risk that they are willing to take.

Prevention measures have been instituted in other areas when a contributing factor has been identified.[56] Athletic SCIs were studied with a registry system and high-risk activities demonstrated. For football, this was found to be axial loading of the cervical spine.[57] Rule changes by the National Collegiate Athletic Association and the National Federation of State High School Associations were established to eliminate the intentional use of the helmet to ram or strike the opponent.[43] Significant reductions in the SCI rate were noted after these rule changes were instituted.[57] Similarly, the Canadian Committee on Prevention of Spinal Injuries has adopted rule changes to decrease the incidence of injury in ice hockey.[54] SCIs resulting from use of the trampoline were analyzed and found to occur in skilled performers attempting a complex routine. Because adequate safeguards have not been developed for the trampoline, the Academy of Pediatrics has recommended that it be removed from school physical education classes and halted in competitive sports activity.[2,3] Other examples of prevention of SCI include advice on the management of breech presentation during childbirth[6] and the avoidance of SCI during occlusion of the descending thoracic aorta during surgery.[35,40]

THE THINK FIRST FOUNDATION

The Think First program was conceived in 1986 as the National Head and Spinal Cord Injury Prevention Program. The Think First Foundation was established in July 1990. The Foundation's Board of Directors is comprised of 30 members, many of whom are neurosurgeons. The Foundation's programs are implemented by more than 200 state and local chapters throughout the country.

Think First For Kids

Think First for Kids is a comprehensive brain and spinal cord injury-prevention program that targets children in Grades 1-3 and is implemented in the classroom by adults such as teachers and school nurses, within the school system. The program has a separate curriculum for each grade, with visual aids including a "Street Smart: A Think First Adventure" video, a set of five classroom posters, a set of five color comic strips, and a set of five black-and-white comic strips. Each curriculum is divided into six lessons that addresses topics including: anatomy of the brain and spinal cord; vehicle, water, bicycle, sports and recreational safety; safety around weapons; and creative problem solving.

Think First For Teens

This unique community outreach program targets junior-high and high school students. Through a network of more than 200 local programs throughout the United States, Canada, Mexico, and Chile, Think First For Teens has been presented to more than 5.7 million students from 1990 to 1998. Each program includes a sponsoring licensed physician and program coordinator who presents this free-of-charge course to schools, church, and civic groups, as well as community clubs. Follow-up activities are conducted to continually reinforce the accident prevention message in the school and community.

The Think First For Teens program is comprised of four parts: 1) an education program targeted at teens and young adults; 2) activities that reinforce the educational program; 3) raising public awareness of neurological injury and its consequences; and 4) working to establish registries and support public policies that enhance injury prevention measures and research. This program[19,20] reinforces prevention as a medical approach and reminds us that it is an old concept rooted in the foundation of medicine with a quote from Louis Pasteur, "When meditating over a disease, I never think of finding a remedy for it, but instead, a means of preventing it."

The cornerstone of the Think First For Teens program[20] is the educational effort aimed at adolescents. The devastating effects of risk taking and the vulnerability of the potential victim are discussed. Peer pressure, the major reason for risk taking, is dealt with directly. Adolescents are taught that they have the power to control the consequences of their actions. The program is presented in school systems in small classroom settings. First, a 15-minute film "On the Edge" is shown that presents interviews with youths who have sustained a neural injury and discusses the risk-taking behavior responsible for the accident

and the subsequent consequences. A health-care professional then reviews the definitions, types, and causes of neural injuries. The final third of the presentation is held with a youth suffering from a post-traumatic injury in a discussion-and-answer session related to the personal account of the physical, emotional, and social consequences of the injury and subsequent disability. In some presentations of the program, a wheelchair obstacle course is set up in which students can experience wheelchair mobility or paramedics are present to discuss initial management and treatment of injury victims.

The reinforcement activities include the posting of signs in high-risk areas where diving is potentially unsafe, school and community bulletin boards, school health fairs, and substance-free graduation events. These activities are important adjuncts to the primary education, as it is not reasonable to assume that all adolescent behaviors can be changed by a 1-hour classroom presentation.

ASSESSING THE EFFECTIVENESS OF THE PREVENTION PROGRAMS

The effects of the prevention programs can be measured in three ways: 1) assess the information retained after attending a program; 2) monitor changes in risk-taking behavior; and 3) determine whether the injury rate has decreased in populations exposed to the program.[20] Several studies regarding the efficacy of these programs have been published. In 1984, a Florida group noted that the incidence of SCI had decreased in the counties using the Think First For Teens program, relative to the nonparticipating counties.[50] A group from Oregon investigated changes in students' knowledge, attitude, and behavior following an educational assembly program.[45] They found that significant knowledge was retained by the students. However, this additional knowledge did not result in changes in attitude or observed behavior. They noted that a reinforcement program would be needed for an optimum prevention program.[45] A group from Missouri was able to demonstrate an increase in both the awareness and the behavior of the participants.[22] Furthermore, they found that several years after attending the program, the risk-taking attitudes were favorably modified, indicating that the information delivered at the program was retained.[22]

A Detroit group identified an increase in the number of gunshot SCI victims in their local community.[58] They questioned these patients for perceived causes. All the activities involved taking risks that placed them at the wrong place at the wrong time. This information led to a program to inform youths of the consequences of their potential risk-taking activities.

A group from Australia also embarked on an SCI prevention program and concluded that the youths retained the information delivered at the program.[59,60] A global spine and head injury prevention project has been initiated to determine the causes of SCI in the third-world countries.[1]

Two chapters of the Think First Foundation have recently completed evaluation studies (unpublished) to determine the efficacy of a comprehensive brain and spinal cord injury prevention curriculum titled Think First For Kids on first, second, and third grade students in the Portland, Oregon and San Diego, California metropolitan areas. The intervention was school-based and teacher-delivered at large.

The Portland, Oregon study was a pre-post comparative design without randomization. The curriculum was tested in 55 selected classrooms in seven elementary schools during two school years, 1995 and 1997, and compared to 43 classrooms in six control schools. The results showed a statistically significant increase (P<0.01) in knowledge of healthful injury prevention in all three grades at the treatment schools. Additionally, there was a greater increase in treatment school scores associated with the lower socioeconomic rank in Grade 3 (P=0.0066) and a decreased treatment effect with increasing socioeconomic rank in Grade 2 (P=0.0016). For Grade 3, there was a significant increase in scores in the Weapons Safety unit (P=0.0237) among the treatment schools compared to control schools.

The San Diego study was a pre-post comparative randomization design. The intervention measured knowledge and self-reported behaviors among 1977 students in eight action schools in two school districts compared to eight control schools, matched by school district, socioeconomic status, reading level, and race/ethnic composition. Students in the intervention schools had significantly greater improvement in post-test scores and within individual curriculum areas when compared to matched control schools. Both studies provided promise that early intervention school-based injury prevention education may have a public health impact.

Public awareness is important because most people are unaware of the vast magnitude of the current problem and the limited resources applied to combat it. Current estimates indicate that the total federal research budget for all spinal injuries was a relatively meager $160 million, compared to the $1400 million awarded to the National Cancer Institute and the $930 million to the National Heart, Lung, and Blood Institute. Local registries accumulate data relative to the target group of prevention programs and provide the basis for studies on the effectiveness of care and rehabilitation.

CONCLUSION

Current knowledge suggests that a substantial number of SCIs can be eliminated by preventive measures. No cure for a devastating SCI exists either now or in the foreseeable future. It is commonly accepted that prevention is the best cure and should be vigorously pursued by all. Prevention programs are noted to have a beneficial effect on adolescents, the age group at greatest risk of SCI. Despite preventive measures that are available and effective in changing attitudes and lowering the injury rate, they do not enjoy widespread application.[48] Clearly, these prevention programs deserve vigorous, constant support to ensure their continued dissemination and use. It is hoped that the widespread use of prevention programs will reduce the number of patients who require therapy for SCI. The prevention of SCI will always be a better form of medical treatment than any intervention after an injury has occurred.

REFERENCES

1. Alexander E Jr: Global spine and head injury prevention program (SHIP). **Surg Neurol** 38:478-479, 1992 (Editorial)
2. American Academy of Pediatrics: Committee on Accident and Poison Prevention and Committee on

Pediatric Aspects of Physical Fitness, Recreation, and Sports. **Pediatrics 67:**438-439, 1981

3. American Academy of Pediatrics: Committee on Accident and Poison Prevention and Committee on Pediatric Aspects of Physical Fitness, Recreation, and Sports. Policy Statement. Trampolines. **Pediatrics 67:** 438, 1981

4. Baker SP, O'Neill B, Ginsburg MJ, et al: **The Injury Fact Book. 2nd ed.** New York, NY: Oxford University Press, 1992

5. Baker SP, O'Neill B, Karpf RS: **The Injury Fact Book.** Lexington, Mass: DC Heath & Co, 1984, pp 219-249

6. Bhagwanani SG, Price HV, Laurence KM, et al: Risks and prevention of cervical cord injury in the management of breech presentation with hyperextension of the fetal head. **Am J Obstet Gynecol 115:**1159-1161, 1973

7. Bracken MB: Incidence of acute traumatic hospitalized spinal cord injury in the United States, 1970-1977. **Am J Epidemiol 113:**615-622, 1981

8. Bracken MB: Treatment of acute spinal cord injury with methylprednisolone: results of a multicenter, randomized clinical trial. **J Neurotrauma 8 (Suppl):** S47-S52, 1991

9. Bracken MB, Collins WF, Freeman DF, et al: Efficacy of methylprednisolone in acute spinal cord injury. **JAMA 251:**45-52, 1984

10. Bracken MB, Holford TR: Effects of timing of methylprednisolone or naloxone administration on recovery of segmental and long-tract neurological function in NASCIS 2. **J Neurosurg 79:**500-507, 1993

11. Bracken MB, Shepard MJ, Collins WF, et al: Methylprednisolone or naloxone treatment after acute spinal cord injury: 1-year follow-up data. Results of the second National Acute Spinal Cord Injury Study. **J Neurosurg 76:**23-31, 1992

12. Bracken MB, Shepard MJ, Collins WF, et al: A randomized, controlled trial of methylprednisolone or naloxone in the treatment of acute spinal cord injury. Results of the Second National Acute Spinal Cord Injury Study. **N Engl J Med 322:**1405-1411, 1990

13. Bracken MB, Shepard MJ, Hellenbrand KG, et al: Methylprednisolone and neurological function 1 year after spinal cord injury. Results of the National Acute Spinal Cord Injury Study. **J Neurosurg 63:**704-713, 1985

14. Bracken MB, Shepard MJ, Holford TR, et al: Administration of methylprednisolone for 24 or 48 hours or tirilazad mesylate for 48 hours in the treatment of acute spinal cord injury. Results of the third National Acute Spinal Cord Injury Randomized Controlled Trial. National Acute Spinal Cord Injury Study. **JAMA 277:**1597-1604, 1997

15. Carter RE Jr: Traumatic spinal cord injuries due to automobile accidents. **South Med J 70:**709-10,1977

16. Committee on Trauma Research Commission on Life Sciences, National Research Council, Institute of Medicine: **Injury in America: A Continuing Public Health Problem.** Washington, DC: National Academy Press, 1985, p 164

17. Council on Scientific Affairs: Automobile-related injuries, components, trends, and prevention. **JAMA 249:**3216-3222, 1983

18. Dolan EJ, Tator CH: The effect of blood transfusion, dopamine, and gamma hydroxybutyrate on post-traumatic ischemia of the spinal cord. **J Neurosurg 56:** 350-358, 1982

19. Eyster EF, Watts C: The National Head and Spinal Cord Injury Prevention Program. **J Med Assoc Ga 78:** 333-338, 1989

20. Eyster EF, Watts C: An update of the National Head and Spinal Cord Injury Prevention Program of the American Association of Neurological Surgeons and the Congress of Neurological Surgeons. Think First. **Clin Neurosurg 38:**252-260, 1992

21. Finn P, Bragg BWE: Perception of the risk of an accident by young and older drivers. **Accid Anal Prev 18:** 289-298, 1986

22. Frank R, Bouman D, Cain K: A preliminary study of a traumatic injury prevention program. **Psych Health 6:** 129-140, 1992

23. Frankel HL, Hancock DO, Hyslop G, et al: The value of postural reduction in the initial management of closed injuries of the spine with paraplegia and tetraplegia. **Paraplegia 7:**179-192, 1969

24. Geisler F: **Past and Current Human Spinal Cord Injury Drug Trials. 2nd ed.** Park Ridge Ill: American Association of Neurological Surgeons, 1998

25. Geisler FH: Acute management of cervical spinal cord injury. **Md Med J 37:**525-530, 1988

26. Griffin MR, Opita JL, Kurland LT, et al: Traumatic spinal cord injury in Olmsted County, Minnesota, 1935-1981. **Am J Epidemiol 121:**884-895, 1985

27. Guha A, Tator CH, Rochon J: Spinal cord blood flow and systemic blood pressure after experimental spinal cord injury in rats. **Stroke 20:**372-377, 1989

28. Irvin C, Millstein S: Biopsychosocial correlates of risk-taking behavior during adolescence. **J Adolesc Health Care 7 (Suppl):**82S-96S, 1986

29. Jessor R: Adolescent development and behavioral health, in Matarazzo J, Weiss S, Herd J (eds): **Behavioral Health: A Handbook of Health Enhancement and Disease Prevention.** New York, NY: John Wiley & Sons, 1984, pp 69-90

30. Jessor R: Cited by Lewis CE, Lewis MA: Peer pressure and risk-taking behaviors in children. **Am J Publ Health 74:**580-584, 1984

31. Kalsbeek WD, McLaurin RL, Harris BSH III, et al: The National Head and Spinal Cord Injury Survey: major findings. **J Neurosurg 53 (Suppl):**S19-S31, 1980

32. Kraus JF: Epidemiology of head injury, in Cooper PR (ed): **Head Injury.** Baltimore, Md: Williams & Wilkins, 1987, pp 1-14

33. Kraus JF, Conroy C: Mortality and morbidity from injuries in sports and recreation. **Annu Rev Publ Health 5:**163-192, 1984

34. Kraus JF, Franti CE, Riggins RS, et al: Incidence of traumatic spinal cord lesions. **J Chronic Dis 28:** 471-492, 1975

35. Laschinger JC, Izumoto H, Kouchoukos NT: Evolving concepts in prevention of spinal cord injury during operations on the descending thoracic and thoracoabdominal aorta. **Ann Thorac Surg 44:** 667-674, 1987

36. Le CT, Price M: Survival from spinal cord injury. **J Chronic Dis 35:**487-492, 1982

37. Lewis CE, Lewis MA: Peer pressure and risk-taking behaviors in children. **Am J Publ Health 74:**580-584, 1984

38. Maiman D, Kunelius D, Weiss H: Diving associated spinal cord injuries during drought conditions: Wis-

consin, 1988. **Morbid Mortal Weekly Report 37:** 453-464, 1988

39. Matthews ML, Moran AR: Age differences in male drivers' perception of accident risk: the role of perceived driving ability. **Accid Anal Prev 18:**299-313, 1986

40. Molina JE, Cogordan J, Einzig S, et al: Adequacy of ascending aorta-descending aorta shunt during cross-clamping of the thoracic aorta for prevention of spinal cord injury. **J Thorac Cardiovasc Surg 90:** 126-136, 1985

41. National Center for Health Statistics: **Advance Report of Final Mortality Statistics, 1985.** Washington, DC: U.S. Government Printing Office, 1987

42. National Center for Health Statistics: **Current Estimates from the National Health Interview Survey, United States, 1985.** Washington, DC: U.S. Government Printing Office, 1986

43. National Collegiate Athletic Association: **National Collegiate Athletic Association Football Rules, Changes and/or Modifications. January 23, 1976. Rule 2, Section 24; Rule 9, Section 1, Article 2-L; Rule 9, Section 1, Article 2-N,** 1976

44. National Highway Traffic Safety Administration: **Fatal Accident Reporting Systems, 1987.** Washington, DC: US Department of Transportation, 1988

45. Neuwelt EA, Coe MF, Wilkinson AM: Oregon Head and Spinal Cord Injury prevention program and evaluation. **Neurosurgery 24:**453-458, 1989

46. Piepmeier JM, Lehmann KB, Lane JG: Cardiovascular instability following acute cervical spinal cord trauma. **Cent Nerv Syst Trauma 2:**153-160, 1985

47. Public Health Service: **Healthy People 2000. National health Promotion and Disease Prevention Objectives-Full Report and Commentary.** Washington, DC: US Department of Health and Human Services, Public Health Service, No. PHS 91-50212, 1991

48. Rice M: Cost of Injury in the U.S.: A Report to Congress. Institute for Health and Aging, University of California and Injury Prevention Center, The John Hopkins University, 1989

49. Schmidt G, Hawks R, Anston F: **Fact Pack, Prevention of Head and Spinal Cord Injury Facts.** Tallahassee, Fla: Florida Interagency Office of Disability Prevention, 1989

50. Shaw LR, McMahon BT, Bruce JH: The Florida approach to spinal cord injury prevention. **Rehabil Lit 45:**85-89, 1984

51. Stover SL, Fine PR: **Spinal Cord Injury: The Facts and Figures.** Birmingham, Ala: National Spinal Cord Injury Statistical Center, The University of Alabama at Birmingham, 1986

52. Tator CH: Hemodynamic issues and vascular factors in acute experimental spinal cord injury. **J Neurotrauma 9:**139-141, 1992

53. Tator CH: Review of experimental spinal cord injury with emphasis on the local and systemic circulatory effects. **Neurochirurgie 37:**291-302, 1991

54. Tator CH, Edmonds VE: National survey of spinal injuries in hockey players. **Can Med Assoc J 130:** 875-880, 1984

55. Thomas JP: Introduction, in Young JS, Burns PE, Bowen AM, et al (eds): **Spinal Cord Injury Statistics: Experience of the Regional Spinal Cord Injury Systems.** Phoenix, Ariz: Good Samaritan Medical Center, 1982, pp 1-10

56. Torg JS: Epidemiology, pathomechanics, and prevention of athletic injuries to the cervical spine. **Med Sci Sports Exerc 17:**295-303, 1985

57. Torg JS, Vegso JS, Yu A, et al: Cervical quadriplegia resulting from axial loading injuries: cinematographic, radiographic, kinematic, and pathologic analysis. Presented at the American Orthopaedic Society for Sports Medicine Interim Meeting, Atlanta, GA, February 8-9, 1984

58. Weingarden SI, Graham PM: Targeting teenagers in a spinal cord injury prevention program. **Paraplegia 29:** 65-69, 1991

59. Wigglesworth EC: Towards prevention of spinal cord injury: the role of a national register. **Paraplegia 26:** 389-392, 1988

60. Yeo JD, Walsh J: Prevention of spinal cord injuries in Australia. **Paraplegia 25:**221-224, 1987

CHAPTER 26

PAST AND CURRENT HUMAN SPINAL CORD INJURY DRUG TRIALS

FRED H. GEISLER, MD, PHD

There have been eight prospective drug trial studies completed on human acute spinal cord injury (SCI). These can be separated into three categories of investigation: 1) studies with methylprednisolone sodium succinate (MPSS);[5, 8,9,11-13,15,16,64] 2) studies with GM-1 ganglioside;[34,35,37,39,41] and 3) small patient-number pilot studies with TRH[66] and nimodipine.[65] Three studies from the MPSS and GM-1 groups entered patients in the 1980s: the first National Acute Spinal Cord Injury Study (NASCIS 1),[10,14] the second National Acute Spinal Cord Injury Study (NASCIS 2),[5,7,9,11,12] and the Maryland GM-1 Ganglioside Study.[36-40] Two studies entered patients in the 1990s: the third National Acute Spinal Cord Injury Study (NASCIS 3)[15,16] and the Sygen (GM-1) Acute Spinal Cord Injury Study.[33] Preliminary data presented in this chapter are based on a presentation at the Congress of Neurological Surgeons in Seattle, Washington in October 1998 on the Sygen (GM-1) Acute Spinal Cord Injury Study. The topic of reviewing acute human SCI studies has been tabulated and recently commented on by several groups.[6,32,34,77]

THE NASCIS 1 STUDY

The NASCIS 1 study began entering patients in 1979, with the results published in 1984 and 1985.[10,14] This study compared the administration of two dosage regimens of intravenously administered MPSS for 10 days: 100 mg or 1000 mg. During the planning stage, it was decided not to include a placebo group because many investigators believed that, in some cases, the patients would be denied a potentially beneficial therapy. By design, the study was randomized, prospective, double-blinded, and multicentered. Only SCI patients admitted to a participating center within 48 hours of injury were eligible for inclusion. In this study, an SCI was defined as any loss of motor or sensory function below the level of injury. Motor function was assessed by testing 14 muscles on each side of the body on a 0- to 5-point scale. Sensory function (light touch and pinprick sensation) from C2 to S5 was assessed as normal, decreased, or absent. Neurological examinations were performed on admission and at 6 weeks, 6 months, and 1 year after injury. It was concluded that no difference in neurological recovery of motor function or sensation was noted between the two treatment groups at 6 weeks and 6 months after injury. The authors noted that wound infections of both trauma and operative sites were more prevalent in the high-dose regimen. With no placebo group, the results are consistent with either both treatment protocols being good or bad, as the study demonstrated no difference between them.

In a retrospective scrutiny of the study, it was noted that most patients were admitted late in the 48-hour entry window, there was no uniform medical or surgical protocol used by all centers, and there was no detailed description of the medical care. The distribution of the initial severity of SCI between groups was not specified. Radiological description and anatomic location of injury were not noted.

THE NASCIS 2 STUDY

After completion of the NASCIS 1 study, new animal SCI investigations with MPSS revealed that very high doses of MPSS were required for improvement after SCI.[17,49,56] For the greatest effect, treatment with MPSS also needed to begin promptly, within minutes or a few hours. A mechanism of action for the neuroprotective effects of MPSS was believed to be a reduction in lipid peroxidation[2,47,48,50] and increased blood flow.[1,61,84] High doses of naloxone were also noted to improve blood flow and motor ability up to 12 hours after injury.[25,26]

The NASCIS 2 study entered patients from May 1985 to December 1988, and the results were published in 1990.[11-13] This study compared placebo, MPSS (a 30-mg/kg bolus followed by 5.4 mg/kg/hr for 23 hours), and naloxone (a 5.4-mg/kg bolus followed by 4.0 mg/kg/hr for 23 hours). By design, this was a randomized, prospective, double-blinded, multicenter study. Randomization was performed within 12 hours of injury, and patients were separated into two groups based on their entry time: <8 hours or >8 hours from injury. An SCI diagnosed by a physician was necessary for entry into the study; no initial degree of injury severity was required. Motor function was assessed by testing 14 muscles on each side of the body on a 0- to 5-point scale, and sensory function (light touch and pinprick sensation) from C2 to S5 was assessed as normal, decreased, or absent. Neurological examinations were obtained on admission and at 6 weeks, 6 months, and 1 year after injury.

It was concluded that patients treated with MPSS within 8 hours of injury had a significantly increased recovery of neurological function observed at 6 weeks, 6 months, and 1 year after the SCI injury. Patients treated with MPSS after 8 hours were noted to recover less motor function in both the MPSS and the naloxone groups compared with placebo. The medical complications were the same for all three groups.

The history of the release of the NASCIS 2 results was controversial and deserves a review. The results of NASCIS 2 were announced by the National Institutes of Health (NIH) in public press releases[19,20] and in faxes[81] sent to emergency rooms before any scientific publication of the study. The National Institute of Neurological Disorders and Stroke press release[20] of March 30, 1990 claimed, "The study is the first to demonstrate positive results from treatment in acute spinal cord injury, and points out the importance of early treatment. The conclusion is based on a randomized trial of 487 patients with acute spinal cord injury treated in 10 collaborating centers in the United States." *The New York Times*[57] reported, "For the first time, researchers have shown that drug treatment can reduce paralysis and other disability in people with serious spinal cord injury." The NIH press releases about the "significant improvement" in SCI were widely reported in the news media.[3,53,54,56,57,62,83] Other press releases[55,82] have reaffirmed the NIH's enthusiastic support of the reported positive results. After such a dramatic announcement, clinicians expected that conclusive, scientifically presented results would be promptly released, and that an indication for MPSS in acute SCI would be sought from the Food and Drug Administration (FDA). Unfortunately, neither of these expectations has been met.

The total number of patients entered into the study was 487. There was no difference in benefit following the administration of MPSS or naloxone between the treatment groups. However, in a subgroup analysis of patients, a positive drug effect was reported. The number of patients in the two subgroups was analyzed to determine whether the positive drug effect of MPSS was much less. There were only a total of 127 patients treated <8 hours after injury, with 62 in the MPSS group and 65 in the placebo group. There were even fewer in the partial neurological deficit subgroup (17 in the MPSS group and 22 in the placebo group), which contributed heavily to the total changes in their group as a whole. Additionally, the study admitted patients with no motor deficits and minor neurological deficits as well as patients with cauda equina injury. No details of the distribution of initial neurological deficits in these patients have been presented. Furthermore, no analysis of the subgroup of patients with a major neurological injury from a pure SCI has been presented, although this is the claimed positive result of the study. These facts present the clinician's difficulty in accurately interpreting the results of the study, as the population studied has not been completely specified. Additional problems in interpreting the study occurred since the results were presented as a change in motor score and not a functional scale, leaving the possibility that even if the effect is statistically significant, it could be clinically insignificant.

Many critiques of the limitations of NASCIS data reporting and interpretation have appeared in letters to editors,[22,52,68-70,76,78] articles,[23,51,63] and chapters in books.[32,34] Several retrospective studies following the results of NASCIS 2 have attempted to determine the effects of steroids. The results of these studies have been mixed.

- A study in Japan,[64] not yet reported in English, appears to have been modeled on NASCIS 2. However, its methodology was not clearly reported. Among other difficulties, it may not have been a prospective and randomized study.[6] It was not blinded, as the placebo patients received only standard treatment with no placebo medication administered. There were 53 centers and 158 patients were admitted, with a 25.9% dropout rate. Therefore, its statistical properties seem doubtful.
- A study by George et al[42] included 145 acute SCI patients and found MPSS (n=80) to provide a nonsignificant decrease in mortality and a significantly poorer discharge mobility compared to patients who did not receive MPSS (n=65). The authors did not note any difference in the functional independence measurement (FIM) rehabilitation score. This was not a randomized prospective trial and, hence, caution should be utilized in interpreting the authors' conclusions.
- A study by Glandiuk et al[31] included 32 acute SCI patients and was not able to come to a conclusion on efficacy but found MPSS patients to have longer hospital stays (44.4 days vs. 27.7 days, P=.065), at an estimated cost of $51,504 per patient.
- A study by Gerndt et al[43] in which 93 patients who received MPSS and 47 who did not receive MPSS were compared; MPSS patients were found to have early infectious complications and no difference in long-term outcome.
- A study by Prendergast et al[67] compared MPSS therapy (n=54) and no MPSS therapy (n=29) after penetrating wounds causing acute SCI; they concluded

that MPSS might impair recovery of neurological function.
- A study by Levy et al[60] compared patients receiving MPSS (n=55) or no MPSS (n=181) with acute SCI from penetrating wounds and found no benefit in the patients who received MPSS.

Although these studies do not present a uniform opinion, as a whole, they certainly do not confirm a dramatic benefit following the use of MPSS. It is of note that these studies have a similar number of patients (or potential statistical power) as the subgroup reported in NASCIS 2 with beneficial effects of MPSS.

Nesathurai[63] recently published in the *Journal of Trauma* an extensive and negative critique of the NASCIS 2 and 3 studies. In the article, several of the same points made here were made. It was concluded that the meaning of the studies "remains unclear," not only statistically but also clinically. Nesathurai states: "To help resolve this dilemma, an impartial, blue-ribbon panel of clinicians and statisticians should be appointed to reanalyze the NASCIS 2 and 3 primary data." The "blue-ribbon panel" is of course the FDA. An FDA review for drug indication would have clarified these issues. Unfortunately, no FDA review process has been sought yet, although the original announcement of a positive drug effect of MPSS by the NASCIS group and the NIH study was produced in 1990. Coleman, along with 14 spinal surgeons, provides a recent detailed review of the history of reported results along with a statistical and clinical critique. They found major deficiencies in the reporting, questionable statistical methodology, and a lack of any independent review or verification of the authors' claimed beneficial effect of methylprednisolone in acute major SCI (Coleman WP, et al: A critical appraisal of the reporting of the National Acute Spinal Cord Injury Studies (II and III) of methylprednisolone in acute spinal cord injury. *J Spinal Disord* 13:185-199, 2000).

THE NASCIS 3 STUDY

NASCIS 3 randomized 499 patients into three parallel groups within 8 hours of injury: 1) NASCIS 2 MPSS bolus and infusion for 23 hours; 2) NASCIS 2 MPSS bolus and infusion for 48 hours; and 3) NASCIS 2 MPSS bolus and infusion of tirilazad for 24 hours. The results of the 6- and 12-month follow-up have become available.[6,16] The authors recommended, based on trends in the data and analysis of adjusted data analysis, that if the administration of MPSS were initiated within 3 hours of the injury, then prolonging the therapy from 24 to 48 hours provided no benefit and increased the incidence of severe sepsis and pneumonia. However, if the initiation of MPSS were between 3 and 8 hours from the injury, then the neurological recovery was enhanced by the continuation of MPSS from 24 to 48 hours.

The study allowed the entry of patients with a broad definition of SCI as declared by the investigator, without a stated clinical scale criteria. This allowed many patients with questionable SCIs into the study. For instance, in the 24-hour MPSS group, 24.7% (41 of 166 patients) had normal motor scores on admission. It is unclear how the inclusion of patients with normal motor scores at baseline can provide information regarding recovery from a major SCI with a major motor deficit. Furthermore, when the patients with no motor loss are removed from analysis by simple subtraction, two thirds of the difference between the recoveries of the patients entered at 3 to 8 hours who received MPSS at 24 vs. 48 hours is lost (the main recommendation of the paper). Data regarding the patients with a major SCI were not presented. As the study did demonstrate an increase in complications due to infections with the longer administration of MPSS and because any beneficial effect is in doubt, caution should be exercised by the clinician before utilizing MPSS as a 48-hour treatment.

Investigation of Thyrotropin-Releasing Hormone in SCI

Thyrotropin-releasing hormone (TRH) has been shown to provide enhanced outcome in animal models following acute SCI.[27-29] This led to a small-number pilot study by Pitts et al.[66] The prospective placebo-controlled study was double-blinded to TRH or normal saline, with the patients stratified by complete and incomplete SCI. The patients were recruited in a 2-year period starting in July 1986 from a single center. Patients were entered within 12 hours of injury. The TRH was administered as an intravenous bolus of 0.2 mg/kg followed by a 0.2-mg/kg/hr iv infusion for 6 hours (n=11); the normal saline placebo was administered using an identical schedule (n=9). Neurological examination at baseline and 1-year follow-up utilized the NASCIS 2 motor and sensory scales and included the Sunnybrook grade. Of the 20 patients entered, two died and five withdrew, leaving 13 patients to complete the study, with a dropout rate of 35%. The authors reported no significant difference in the neurological outcome between the treatment groups. In a study with this small sample size and high drop-out rate, it is basically impossible to demonstrate a significant effect of TRH even though the enhanced recovery might have been large enough to be clinically important (Type II statistical error). Thus, this study does not provide negative information on the efficacy of TRH, but rather provides the safety information on the administration of TRH (FDA Phase I trial) and provides the basis for a larger clinical trial (FDA Phase II or III trial).

Investigation of Nimodipine in SCI

Nimodipine, a calcium channel blocker, was investigated in a prospective block-randomized single-center study by Petitjean et al.[65] Nimodipine was administered as a 0.015-mg/kg iv bolus over 1 hour followed by 0.03 gm/kg/hr iv for 7 days if the patient's mean arterial blood pressure was lower than 60 mg Hg. MPSS was administered as a 30-mg/kg iv bolus over 1 hour followed by 5.4 mg/kg/hr iv for 23 hours. The four treatment groups comprised the following: 1) MPSS only (n=27); 2) nimodipine only (n=27); 3) both MPSS and nimodipine (n=27); and 4) no pharmacological treatment (n=25). The administration of the study drug treatment was not blinded. Neurological examinations were performed at baseline and at 1-year follow-up. Patients were treated with early surgical decompression and stabilization. The authors reported no difference between the treatment groups on neurological outcome. They did note a higher incidence of infectious complications in patients receiving

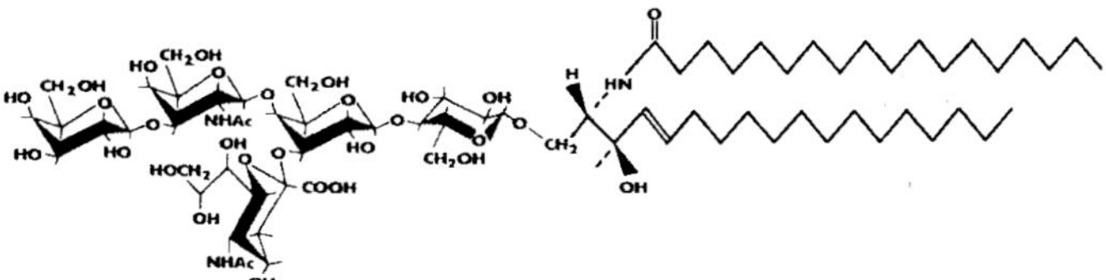

Figure 1: Molecular structure of Sygen.

MPSS treatment. This study, like the TRH study, is a small-number study and subject to Type II statistical errors, meaning that a useful clinical result could exist in either MPSS or nimodipine and not be detectable in a study with this sample size. This study fails to confirm the NASCIS 2-reported enhanced recovery with MPSS, provides information that the MPSS has an increased infectious complication rate, and provides the basis for a larger study on nimodipine in SCI patients.

THE MARYLAND GM-1 GANGLIOSIDE STUDY

Sygen (monosialotetrahexosylganglioside GM-1 sodium salt) (Figure 1) is a naturally occurring compound in cell membranes of mammals and is especially abundant in the membranes of central nervous system cells. Acute neuroprotective and longer-term regenerative effects in multiple experimental models of ischemia and injury have been reported. The proposed mechanisms of action of Sygen include anti-excitotoxic effects, apoptosis prevention, and neuro-reintegration enhancement. Clinical trials using Sygen in stroke, Parkinson's disease, and other entities are ongoing or previously reported.

A single-center Phase I trial of Sygen in acute SCI entered patients between January 1986 and May 1987 at the Maryland Institute for Emergency Medical Services System in Baltimore, Maryland, and was reported in the *New England Journal of Medicine* in 1991.[37,40] This prospective double-blinded clinical trial randomized 37 patients (23 cervical and 11 thoracic) to either placebo or 100 mg of Sygen iv qd for a planned 30-day treatment period, with the first dose administered within 72 hours of injury.

All patients received a course of MPSS therapy with a dose of approximately one tenth that of the NASCIS 2 dose recommendation. The results of the NASCIS 2 trial were not reported until after the completion of patient entry into the Maryland study.

All patients admitted to the Maryland Institute for Emergency Medical Services System with a spinal cord or column injury during the 16-month entrance period were considered for the study. The criteria for inclusion included the following: 1) patient consent was obtained; 2) there was no contraindication to GM-1; 3) female patients were surgically sterile or postmenopausal; 4) the patient was at least 18 years old; and 5) an SCI with a major motor deficit of 3/5 in hands or legs. The criteria for exclusion were: 1) the patient had sustained a premorbid major medical illness (e.g., end-stage diabetes or heart disease); 2) the patient was likely to be lost to follow-up; 3) the patient was involved in other experimental drug protocols; and 4) the patient had significant damage to the cauda equina.

A standard medical protocol was utilized that included: 1) initial assessment and spinal immobilization; 2) medical management to correct neurogenic shock to optimize tissue perfusion and oxygenation; 3) 250 mg of iv-administered MPSS on admission and 125 mg every 6 hours for 72 hours; 4) continuous iv-administered dopamine hydrochloride for most patients to reverse the neurogenic shock and maintain a normal to high-normal blood pressure; 5) prompt anatomic alignment of the spinal bony elements; 6) radiological diagnostics (radiograph, myelogram, computed tomography scan); 7) prompt surgical decompression of neural elements if closed spinal alignment failed to relieve the bony compression; and 8) stabilization of bony instability.[33]

The American Spinal Injury Association (ASIA) motor score and the Frankel classification grade[30] were used to assess the neurological injury at baseline (Table 1) and at follow-up.

TABLE 1

THE FRANKEL CLASSIFICATION[30] GRADING SYSTEM

Grade A	Complete neurological injury—No motor or sensory function clinically detected below the level of the injury.
Grade B	Preserved sensation only—No motor function clinically detected below the level of injury; sensory function remains below the level of injury but may include only partial function (sacral sparing qualifies as preserved sensation).
Grade C	Preserved motor non-functional—Some motor function observed below the level of the injury, but is of no practical use to the patient.
Grade D	Preserved motor function—Useful motor function below the level of the injury; patient can move lower limbs and walk with or without aid, but does not have a normal gait or strength in all motor groups.
Grade E	Normal motor—No clinically detected abnormality in motor or sensory function with normal sphincter function; abnormal reflexes and subjective sensory abnormalities may be present.

Analysis of the Maryland study[41] disclosed the following:[32,34,35,37-40] 1) the baseline ASIA Impairment Severity (AIS) grade greatly affects the recovery pattern; 2) the distribution of the motor recovery scores is highly non-normal; 3) nonparametric statistics are necessary for data analysis; 4) functional improvement (winners in a binomial analysis) could be based on the proportion of patients with a large change in clinically relevant neurological function; and 5) significant drug effect was apparent (P=0.034) as seen in the proportion of marked recoveries. This main statistical test showed an enhancement in the fraction of patients obtaining an improvement of two Frankel grades, clearly a large and clinically relevant enhancement of neurological recovery. This Phase II study provided the rational for the multi-center Sygen Acute Spinal Cord Injury Study.

The proposed mechanism of recovery was hypothesized to be that GM-1 enhances function or potency of the damaged white matter passing through the level of the injury, thus allowing increased function at caudal neurological levels.[4,18,21,24,44-46,58,59,71-75,79,80,85] Animal experiments indicate that motor recovery occurs with only 5% of axons surviving through the injury site.[85] The enhanced motor function recovery of GM-1 treated patients may be related to increased survival of axons at the injury site or, possibly, the GM-1 augmentation of the response of the neurons in the conus to the decreased input from the damaged white matter tracts passing through the injury site. Apoptosis prevention may also be an important mechanism of action of GM-1 in improving the outcome following SCI. This study formed the basis of the larger multicenter study utilizing Sygen (GM-1) in the treatment of patients with acute SCI.

The Sygen Acute Spinal Cord Injury Study was sponsored by the Fidia Pharmaceutical Corp., Washington, DC. It was designed to determine the efficacy and safety of Sygen in the treatment of patients with acute SCI following standard treatment with MPSS. The first public presentation of preliminary data analysis and results occurred at the Congress of Neurological Surgeons in Seattle, Washington on October 8, 1998 (Sygen (GM-1 Ganglioside) Acute Spinal Cord Injury Study, by Fred H. Geisler, M.D., Ph.D., F.C. Dorsey, Ph.D., F. Patarnello, Ph.D., G. Grieco, M.D., D. Poonian, and R. Fiorentini, M.D.). This study was conducted over a 6-year data collection phase at 28 neurotrauma centers (Table 2) in the U.S. and Canada.

Study Design

The Sygen Acute Spinal Cord Injury Study is a prospective double-blinded randomized stratified multi-center trial studying the efficacy and safety of Sygen in the treatment of patients with acute SCI following standard treatment with MPSS. The study was initially stratified by level (cervical and thoracic) and baseline severity (AIS A, B, and C+D), with block randomization into three parallel-treatment groups (placebo, low-dose Sygen, and high-dose Sygen). The patients in all groups received a bolus dose followed by 56

TABLE 2

SYGEN (GM-1) PRINCIPAL INVESTIGATORS AND CENTERS

Principal Investigator	Center
Janet Alteveer, MD	Cooper Hospital, University Medical Center, Camden, NJ
Lee V. Ansell, MD	University of Texas Health Science Center, Houston, TX
Gregory J. Bennett, MD	University of Buffalo, Buffalo, NY
Edward C. Benzel, MD	University of New Mexico, Albuquerque, NM
Charles L. Branch, MD	Bowman Gray School of Medicine, WinstonSalem, NC
Richard Bucholz, MD	St. Louis University Hospital, St. Louis, MO
James E. Burgess, MD	Fairfax Hospital, Falls Church, VA
George R. Cybulski, MD	Northwestern University Medical School, Chicago, IL
Gail Delaney, MD	Victoria Hospital, London, Ontario, Canada
Herbert H. Engelhard, MD, PhD	Northwestern University Medical School, Chicago, IL
Mahmood Fazl, MD	Sunnybrook Health Science Center, North York, Ontario, Canada
Kevin Foley, MD	Semmes-Murphey Clinic, Memphis, TN
Gerard Fulda, MD	Medical Center of Delaware, Newark, DE
M. Sean Grady, MD	University of Washington, Seattle, WA
P. W. Hitchon, MD	University of Iowa Hospitals and Clinics, Iowa City, IA
Katharyn Holloway, MD	Medical College of Virginia, Richmond, VA
Arnie Jackson, MD	University of Alabama Hospital, Birmingham, AL
Nachshon Knoller, MD	Maryland Institute for Emergency Medical Services Systems, Baltimore, MD
Daniel P. Lammertse, MD	Craig Hospital, Englewood, CO
Peter L. Lane, MD	Victoria Hospital, London, Ontario, Canada
Dennis Maiman, MD, PhD	Medical College of Wisconsin, Milwaukee, WI
Lawrence Marshall, MD	University of California at San Diego, Medical Center, San Diego, CA
Duncan McBride, MD	Harbor/University of California at Los Angeles Medical Center, Torrance, CA
Michael Miner, MD, PhD	Ohio State University Hospitals, Columbus, OH
Steven E. Murk, MD	University of Texas Health Science Center, San Antonio, TX
Kristjan T. Ragnarsson, MD	Mt. Sinai Medical Center, New York, NY
Walker Robinson, MD	Maryland Institute for Emergency Medical Services Systems, Baltimore, MD
Michael Rosner, MD	University of Alabama Hospital, Birmingham, AL
Paula Stewart, MD	Charlotte Rehabilitation Hospital, Charlotte, NC
Dan R. Thompson, MD	The Mercy Hospital of Pittsburgh, Pittsburgh, PA
Peter C. Wemer, MD	Santa Clara Valley Medical Center, San Jose, CA
Jack E. Wilberger, Jr., MD	Allegheny General Hospital, Pittsburgh, PA
C. Wilmot, MD	Santa Clara Valley Medical Center, San Jose, CA

days of study treatment. The placebo group had a loading dose of placebo and then 56 days of placebo. The low-dose Sygen group had a 300-mg loading dose followed by 100 mg/day for 56 days. The high-dose Sygen group had a 600-mg loading dose followed by 200 mg/day for 56 days.

Originally, it was planned to have 720 completed patients (240 per each of the three initial treatment groups). For inclusion in the study, patients were required to have a major SCI, defined as a neurological deficit in one lower limb with a total ASIA motor score of <15 (from a possible 25 points). Patients had to have a neurological deficit from an SCI with the potential for recovery. Thus, patients with spinal cord transection or penetration, as well as patients with a significant cauda equina, plexus, or peripheral nerve injury, were excluded from the study. All patients received the NASCIS 2 recommended dose regimen of MPSS <8 hours after the SCI. The study medication was initiated <72 hours after the SCI, but after completion of the MPSS therapy, to avoid a possible drug-drug interaction effect between MPSS and Sygen.

Patients had an emergency room evaluation, received MPSS, and had a baseline evaluation just prior to the first dose of study medication. Thus, the baseline examination to which all subsequent examinations are compared is performed after the 24-hour MPSS was administered and after the initial hemodynamic resuscitation, mechanical decompression, and multiple neurological

TABLE 3

AIS SCALE (PRE-TREATMENT ONLY)

Grade A	Complete: No motor or sensory function is preserved in the sacral segments S4-5
Grade B	Incomplete: Sensory but not motor function is preserved below the neurological level and extends through the sacral segments S4-5
Grade C	Incomplete: Motor function is preserved below the neurological level, and the majority of key muscles below the neurological level have a muscle grade <3/5
Grade D	Incomplete: Motor function is preserved below the neurological level, and the majority of key muscles below the neurological level have a muscle grade ≥3/5
Grade E	Normal: Motor and sensory functions are normal

examinations had been performed by the medical staff. The increased neurological function between the emergency room examination and the baseline examination is thus not included in the study follow-up neurological improvement analysis. Following a loading dose of three times the daily dose, study medication was administered intravenously for 29 days and either intravenously or intramuscularly for 28 subsequent additional days. Follow-up evaluations were performed at 4, 8, 16, 26, and 52 weeks after the initiation of treatment.

The data accuracy and integrity were maintained by a comprehensive protocol. More than 8 million values were included in the efficacy and safety data collected and managed in this study. The data in the case report forms were periodically verified by independent study monitors at each site throughout the study. An adjudication committee reviewed the clinical data for consistency of the medical information. An extramural monitoring committee (Michael D. Walker, M.D., chair) provided guidance throughout the patient entry period. After the planned interim analysis of the first 180 patients was completed at the 26-week follow-up evaluations, the extramural monitoring committee observed an age imbalance among the treatment groups. The committee then recommended: 1) adding additional stratification by age ("younger" <29 years vs. "older" ≥29 years) to correct a baseline imbalance, and 2) dropping the high-dose group.

The pre-treatment neurological assessment included both the AIS (Table 3) and a detailed ASIA motor and sensory examination. The modified Benzel classification (Table 4) and a detailed

TABLE 4

MODIFIED BENZEL CLASSIFICATION (AT 4, 8, 16, 26, AND 52 WEEKS FOLLOW-UP)

Grade	Description	AIS Grade
I	Complete—No motor or sensory function is preserved in the sacral segments S4-5	A
II	Sensory preservation—Sensory but no motor function is preserved in the sacral segments S4-5	B
III	Motor function is preserved below the neurological level, and the majority of key muscles below the neurological level have muscle grades <3/5. Unable to walk	C
IV	Some functional motor control below the level of injury that is significantly useful (i.e., assist in transfers, etc.). Unable to walk independently	D or high C
V	Motor function allows walking with or without assistance, but significant problems secondary to lack of endurance or fear of falling limit patient mobility. Limited walking	
VI	Independent ambulation >25 feet but may have difficulties with micturition and/or dyscoordination	
VII	Neurologically intact with the exception of minimal deficits that cause no functional difficulties	

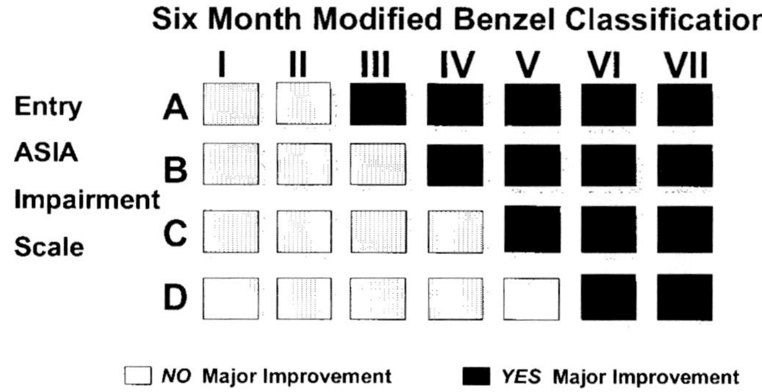

Figure 2: Major improvement criterion: AIS/Benzel neurological improvement.

ASIA motor and sensory examination were performed at 4, 8, 16, 26, and 52 weeks after the SCI. A scale different from the baseline measurement was used because it includes an assessment of the patient's walking ability and expands the "D" classification from that of the AIS. Because most patients have an unstable spinal fracture at baseline, it is not possible to assess walking ability and, hence, the use of different baseline and follow-up scales is necessary.

Note that the definitions of the Benzel I, II, and III categories are essentially the same as the AIS A, B, and C categories, respectively. The categories from IV to VII of the Benzel scale expand the AIS to include degrees of walking and, hence, provide functional information on the patient's clinical status.

A "marked improvement" is defined as at least a two-grade improvement in the Benzel equivalent of the baseline AIS. This is shown graphically in Figure 2. Let us take a baseline AIS "A" as an example. To be considered a major improvement, a Benzel score between III and VII would be needed on follow-up (the dark squares in this figure). This criterion sets a high hurdle for neurological recovery and is, unarguably, a clinically relevant change. This definition of marked recovery allows the use of a single outcome measure for populations of different patient baseline severity.

There were several primary pre-planned outcome measures in this study. The proportion of marked improvement (two grades) vs. no marked improvement in the AIS/Benzel grade change between treatment groups at 26 weeks is a dichotomous comparison. This timeframe was prespecified as the principal endpoint. The ASIA motor, sensory, bowel, and bladder score improvements at Week 26 are investigated using an ANCOVA model with center, stratum, and treatment. An AIS/Benzel 26-week grade change adjusted for baseline AIS will also be analyzed.

Secondary pre-planned outcome measures and analyses are: 1) mortality rate; 2) time course to recovery; 3) sensory function recovery; and 4) subgroup analysis with regard to strata, time to entry, surgery timing, traction timing, and MPSS and study medication timing.

Study Data Description

The Sygen study is the largest prospective SCI drug trial ever conducted—797 patients randomized in a 5-year recruitment period in 28 neurotrauma centers in North America. All 12-month follow-up data collection was completed in February 1998. Figure 3 shows the total number of patients in the study over the enrollment period: 3130 patients were screened in the 28 centers, with 2333 not qualified using the exclusion criteria of the study. The vast majority of the patients considered not qualified had spinal fractures with no or minimal neurological deficits. Of the 797 patients randomized and entered into the study, 37 were considered truly ineligible and are included in the safety analysis only. These patients met one of the prespecified exclusion crite-

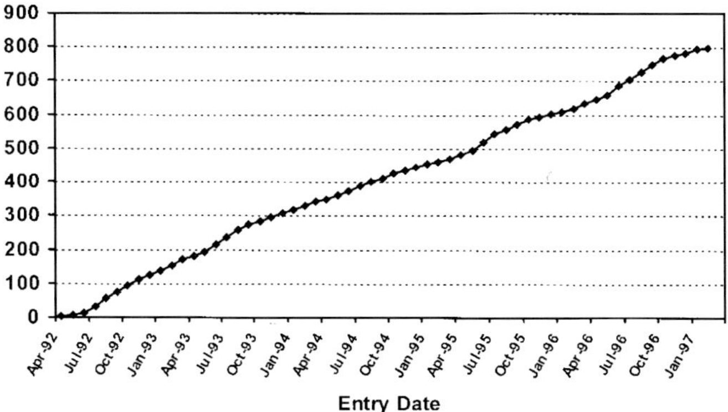

Figure 3: Enrollment in the Sygen (GM-1) Acute Spinal Cord Injury Study.

TABLE 5

PATIENT ENROLLMENT BY BASELINE SEVERITY AND ANATOMIC REGION

Anatomic Region	Baseline AIS Grade			
of Injury	A	B	C+D	Total
Cervical	332	113	134	579
Thoracic	150	18	13	181
Total	482	131	147	760

ria and should not have been enrolled in the study. Thus, 760 patients are included in the efficacy analysis data set. This study is a unique database of acute SCI with 8 million total data values, more detail than in any previous study.

The accounting of the efficacy analysis data set of baseline severity and anatomic region is shown in Table 5. Note that the largest severity group in both the cervical and thoracic region is those rated "A" in the AIS scale. Also note the fewer number of patients categorized in "B" and "C+D" in the thoracic region compared to the cervical region. Cervical traction was used in 395 patients, and 600 patients underwent a spinal operation.

Safety Data

The safety data disclosed that adverse events were consistent with the acute SCI population and that there were no noteworthy differences between the treatment groups in frequency or severity of events. An anticipated dose-associated pattern of modest elevations in cholesterol and triglycerides in the Sygen groups during the treatment phase was noted. This change has been observed in other studies with Sygen and is not clinically relevant. Detailed safety analysis disclosed no noteworthy drug side effects or complications. The only noteworthy difference between the Sygen 100 mg- and the placebo-dose groups was that early termination of either study medication due to death was higher in the placebo-treated patients (12/345=3.5%) than with the Sygen 100 mg-treated group (5/348=1.4%).

The overall death rate was 5.9%. There were no statistically significant differences among the treatment groups. In Figure 4, the death rate is presented as the fraction of patients surviving as a function of log time, separated by treatment groups. A higher percentage of patients died who were treated with 200 mg of Sygen (10/102=9.8%) than with either 100 mg of Sygen (18/348=5.2%) or placebo (19/345=5.5%) (P=0.213, Fisher's exact test). Survival analysis indicated generally longer times from injury to death for both Sygen-treated groups compared to placebo-treated patients, but the differences were not statistically significant (P=0.2905, log rank chi-square test).

The population characteristics of the treatment groups were examined, and there were no unexpected observations of mechanism of in-

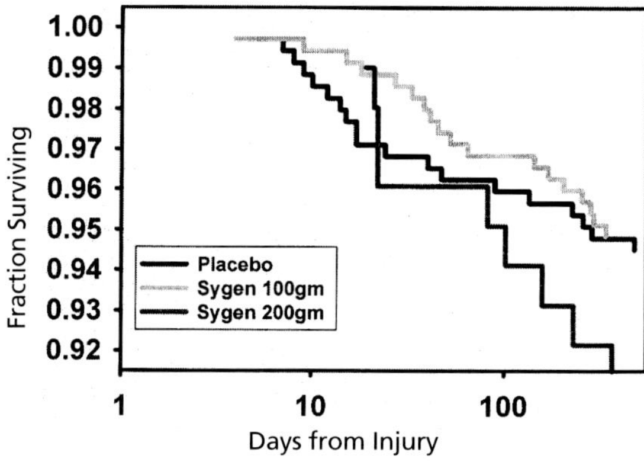

Figure 4: Survival by treatment group (there were 49 deaths among the 797 patients).

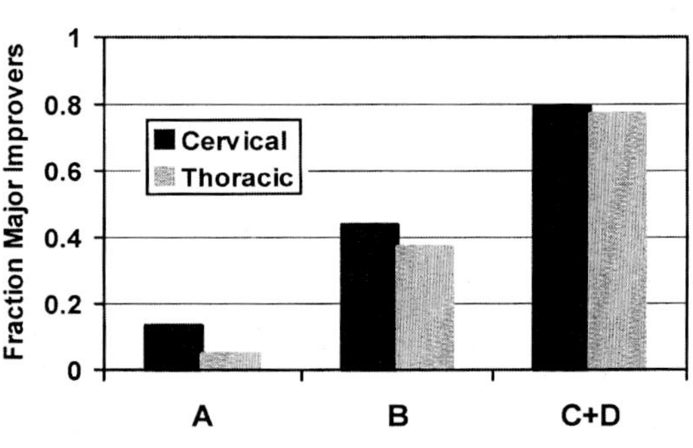

Figure 5: Week 26 AIS/Benzel major improvers by baseline AIS strata and level.

jury, neurological level distribution, or age or sex distribution. These demographics were similar to those reported historically with regard to these parameters. The median timing of the medical events was as follows: SCI to emergency room 20 minutes; SCI to MPSS <2 hours; SCI to cervical traction <6 hours if used, and SCI to surgery <4 days if operated. There were no noteworthy differences between the treatment groups in these timings.

Efficacy Evaluations

Differences in the baseline AIS strata strongly determined the fraction of major improvers at Week 26. This fraction of major improvers at Week 26 is presented in Figure 5 as a function of baseline AIS strata and anatomic region. Note that for all of the baseline severity grades, the thoracic group had a smaller proportion of major improvers than the cervical group. Among all Sygen 100 mg- and placebo-treated patients combined, dramatically different patterns of marked recovery at Week 26 were associated with the three baseline AIS groups: A (11.3%), B (42.4%), and C+D (75.2%). ASIA motor scores also had quite different recovery patterns associated with the baseline AIS groupings, some of which were statistically intractable because the median and mean were both located in the large spike at zero recovery and, thus, prevent meaningful use of these distributions in any form of multivariant analysis. The time course of the marked recovery

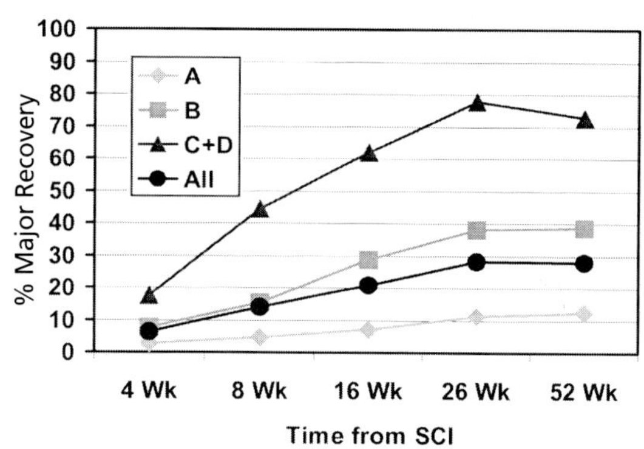

Figure 6: Major recovery pattern of the placebo group by baseline severity (n=330).

in the placebo group is presented in Figure 6. A detailed Benzel outcome grade at Week 26 by baseline AIS strata in the placebo group is presented in Figure 7. This graph presents the percentage Benzel outcome for each baseline AIS. Note that for the A group, more than 75% of the outcomes are 1 or no improvement, for B group, the probability is relatively flat across all outcomes, and for C and D groups, the outcome is heavily weighted to a large change with many improving to near or at normal.

The fraction of major improvers at Week 26 by baseline AIS strata and the start of the bolus dose of MPSS <3 hours compared to >3 hours is

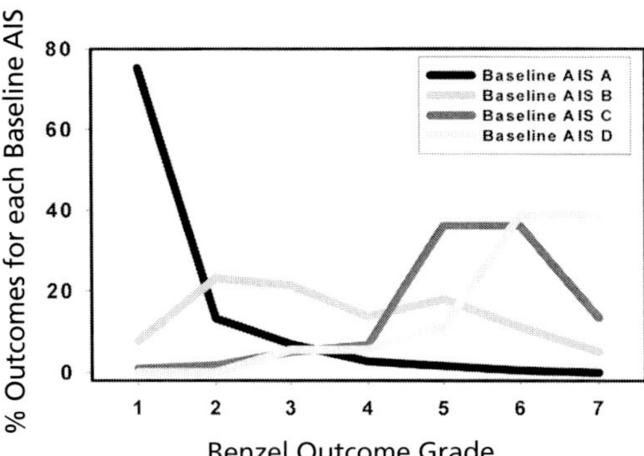

Figure 7: Week 26 Benzel outcome grade by baseline AIS strata.

TABLE 6

PATIENT ENROLLMENT BY TREATMENT GROUP AND STRATA: AGE, INJURY LEVEL, AND BASELINE AIS

	Placebo	Sygen 100 mg
Age <29 years old	163	157
Age ≥29 years old	167	174
Cervical region injury	248	257
Thoracic region injury	82	74
Baseline AIS Grade A	215	206
Baseline AIS Grade B	52	63
Baseline AIS Grade C	55	53
Baseline AIS Grade D	8	9
Total	330	331

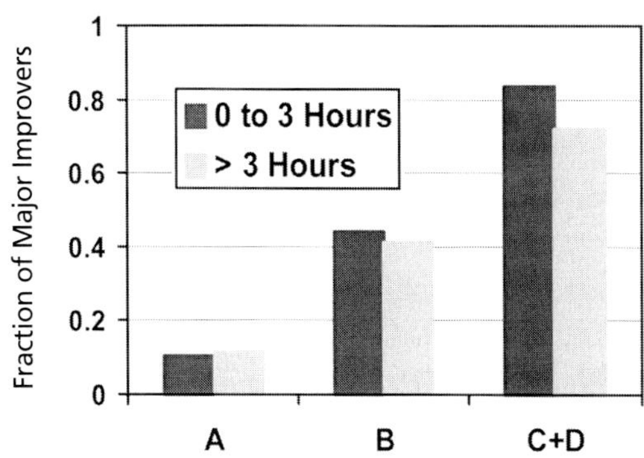

Figure 8: Week 26 AIS/Benzel major improvers by baseline AIS strata and MPSS timing.

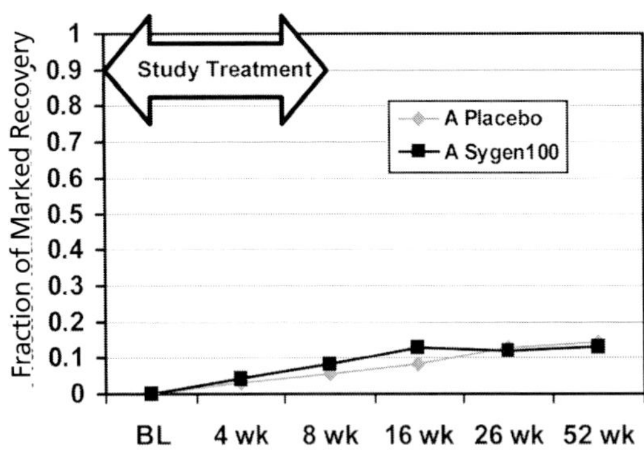

Figure 9: Baseline A: marked recovery (two-grade improvement using the AIS/Benzel classification system) by visit.

shown in Figure 8. Note that the timing of MPSS initiation is not an important prognostic variable, with only a mild nonstatistical difference in the C+D subgroup.

The patient enrollment by treatment group and the strata of age, anatomic region, and baseline AIS are shown in Table 6. This table compares the placebo and the Sygen 100-mg groups, for which subsequent analysis is presented. When the distribution across strata for these groups is performed, no noteworthy differences are noted in the strata of age, anatomic region, or baseline severity. The treatment groups are thus considered equivalent at baseline and, hence, should yield valid statistical conclusions.

Figure 9 represents the fraction of major improvers in baseline A over the follow-up period. Note that among the baseline A patients, the major improvement rate at Week 26 is only 12%. Note also the separation at Weeks 8 and 16 for Sygen and the placebo groups, favoring the drug. A recovery pattern implying a 2-month earlier recovery is noted.

The baseline B patients separated by placebo and Sygen 100 mg are shown in Figure 10. Note the earlier and enhanced recovery of the Sygen group in the baseline B patients. At Week 26, the Sygen group had a 55% major improvement rate. This is a greater than 30% increase over the placebo rate at Week 26.

The data for the baseline C+D patients are presented in Figure 11. At the end of the study treatment period, the Sygen group had a signifi-

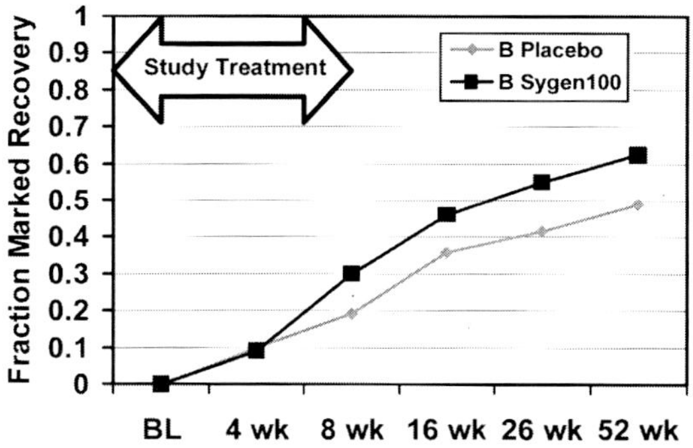

Figure 10: Baseline B: marked recovery (two-grade improvement using the AIS/Benzel classification system) by visit.

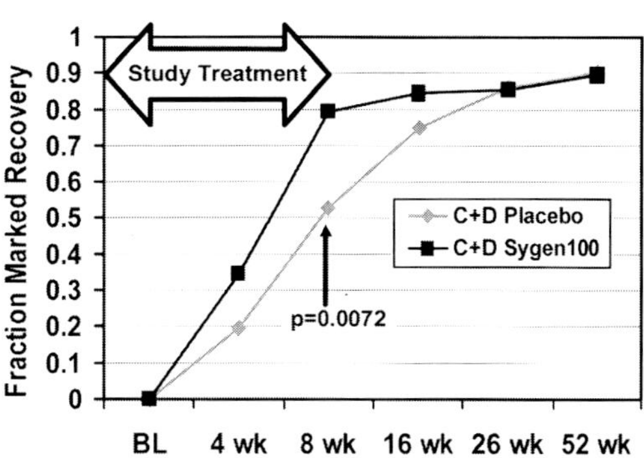

Figure 11: Baseline C+D: marked recovery (two-grade improvement using the AIS/Benzel classification system) by visit.

cantly greater proportion of major improvers than the placebo group (P=0.0072). This significance was lost in later follow-up as a result of a ceiling effect in which both groups had an 86% major improvement rate at Week 26.

The proportion of major improvers by placebo vs. Sygen 100 mg for all groups combined is shown in Figure 12. At the end of the study drug treatment period (Week 8), 21.3% of all randomized Sygen 100 mg-treated patients as opposed to 14.2% of placebo-treated patients had attained a marked recovery (P=0.003). At Week 16, the proportions were 25.9% for Sygen 100 mg vs. 21.5% for placebo-treated patients (P=0.043). The protocol-specified principal endpoint, the Week 26 difference, is not statistically significant. A Fisher's exact test of the 2 by 5 table of the time at which marked recovery was first

obtained (Table 7) yields a P value of 0.026, indicating that Sygen 100 mg-treated patients who attained marked recovery did so earlier than placebo-treated patients.

At the end of the 2-month treatment period, 21.3% of the Sygen patients had attained major improvement. This was not observed in the placebo group until Week 16. This implies that major recovery occurred approximately 2 months earlier in the Sygen group. The result of the sum of the three different baseline groups is highly dependent on the proportion contributed by each of the groups before the outcomes are summed together. Thus, caution should be used in interpreting the results of this composite index of outcomes when considering what can be expected from an individual patient at a particular baseline severity.

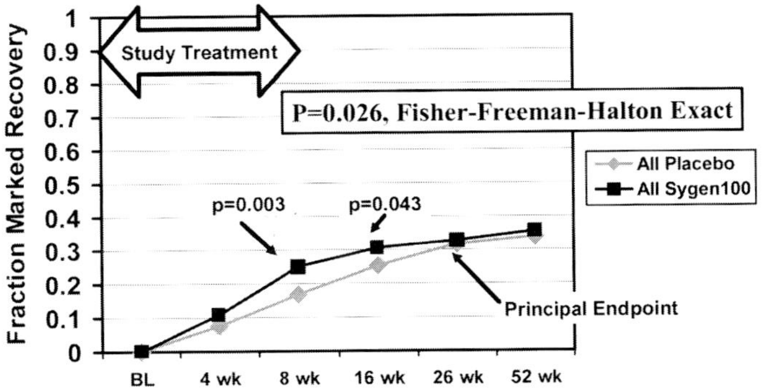

Figure 12: All patients: marked recovery (two-grade improvement using the AIS/Benzel classification system) by visit.

TABLE 7

TIME AT WHICH MARKED RECOVERY WAS OBTAINED

Treatment Group	Marked Recovery				No Marked Recovery	Total
	Week 4	Week 8	Week 16	Week 26		
Sygen 100 mg	33 (9.5%)	41 (11.8%)	16 (4.6%)	12 (3.4%)	246 (70.7%)	348 (100%)
Placebo	21 (6.1%)	28 (8.1%)	25 (7.2%)	24 (7.0%)	247 (71.6%)	345 (100%)

Beneficial drug effect was also observed in analysis of the sensory data. Repeated-measures analyses of variance for total ASIA sensory scores through Week 52 demonstrated the effects of Sygen 100 mg over placebo ($P=0.0776$ and $P=0.0168$ for pinprick and light touch, respectively). Repeated-measures analyses of variance through Week 52 of changes in sensory deficit levels to light touch testing yielded P values of 0.0412 and 0.0621 for the absolute level and relative level, respectively.

There were strong correlations between the recovery of the motor levels and that of the sensory levels. The sensory assessments were continuous from C2 to S5. However, the ASIA motor score consists only of assessments of neurological function in the upper and lower limbs and fails to assess recovery between T2 and Ll. Thus, patients with recovery confined to this portion of the spinal cord had no possibility of observable motor recovery.

Patients who had a spinal operation within the first year of injury vs. patients without any spinal operation were compared in Figure 13. This pre-planned analysis of the non-operated patients vs. the operated patients disclosed a dif-

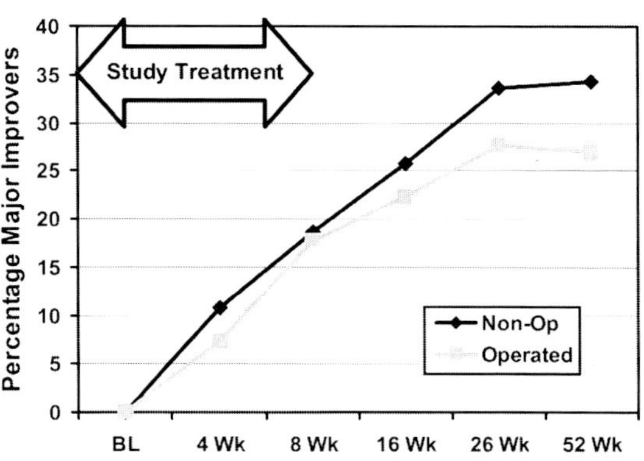

Figure 13: Operated (n=521) vs. non-operated (n=140) patients (placebo and Sygen 100 mg).

ference favoring a better outcome in the non-operated patients. This suggests that the non-operative or "spinal cord contusion" patients had more potential for recovery. When the operated vs. non-operated patients are separated by treatment group (Figure 14), a large difference is noted between the non-operated Sygen and placebo groups. At the end of the study treatment period, the major recovery rate for non-operated placebo was 7% vs. 30% for Sygen. This is a four-

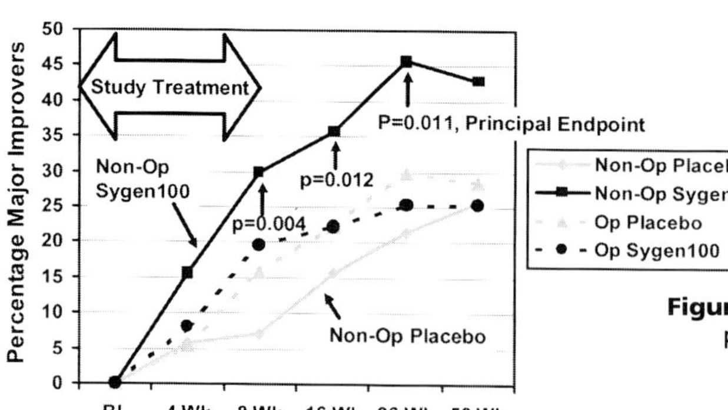

Figure 14: Operated vs. non-operated patients by treatment group.

fold increase in the proportion of major improvers. At Week 26, the major improvement rate in this group for placebo was 22% vs. 46% for Sygen. This is more than a two-fold increase. Note the highly significant P values at Weeks 8, 16, and 26. Furthermore, note that the total proportion of major improvers in the placebo group at Week 26 had already been surpassed by Week 8 in the Sygen group. Non-operated patients comprised those not requiring spinal cord decompression or stabilization of the spinal column. These patients have an inherently greater potential for neurological recovery. There is no compression on the spinal cord to limit drug delivery and impair the natural healing mechanism of the spinal cord, and they are not likely to suffer mechanical re-injury to the spinal cord, as they are not mechanically unstable.

Conclusions of the Sygen Acute SCI Study

An analysis of the data indicates that the Sygen 100 mg and placebo groups are comparable at baseline. No noteworthy differences in medical/surgical management occurred between the groups. No clinically relevant safety issues associated with Sygen were identified. The prespecified primary outcome measure of two grade changes in the AIS/Benzel category for all patients (the arithmetic composite of the three different types of recovery curves) had a statistically significant P<0.05 at 8 and 16 Weeks, with Sygen favored over placebo, and was not statistically significant at Week 26, the principal endpoint. A Fisher's exact test of the 2 by 5 table of the time that marked recovery was first obtained yields a P value of 0.026, indicating that the Sygen 100 mg-treated patients who attained marked recovery did so earlier than the placebo-treated patients. The Sygen 100 mg-treated group had greater and earlier recovery than the placebo-treated group consistently across all baseline severity groups. Patients in A had an earlier modest effect, possibly constrained by the generally small rate of recovery among those in that category. Patients in B had an earlier and greater drug effect observed. Patients in C+D had an earlier effect but exhibited a ceiling effect in late recovery

measurement. An increased improvement in sensory function was noted in the Sygen 100 mg-treated group over the placebo-treated group in both light touch and pinprick sensation. A large drug effect was seen in the non-operated patients. A pattern of positive drug effect response is consistent across primary and secondary efficacy measures, including bowel, bladder, and sensory recovery.

The data analysis conclusions are consistent with known pathophysiology of acute SCI in which recovery and treatment effect potential is largest among patients in the B category and patients with "spinal cord contusions," in which the largest beneficial Sygen treatment differences were observed in these groups also. When all baseline severities are combined, the Sygen-treated patients who had major recovery at Week 26 recovered approximately 2 months earlier than the placebo-treated patients.

Sygen administered as a 300-mg loading dose followed by daily 100-mg doses for 56 days appeared to be safe and to enhance recovery from acute SCI. It is hoped that further analysis of the historical SCI studies reviewed here, along with future drug trials, will provide useful therapy to improve the ultimate neurological function of SCI victims and provide additional information on the nature and recovery patterns in SCI patients.

References

1. Anderson DK, Means ED, Waters TR, et al: Microvascular perfusion and metabolism in injured spinal cord after methylprednisolone treatment. **J Neurosurg 56:**106-113, 1983
2. Anderson DK, Saunders RD, Demediuk P, et al: Lipid hydrolysis and peroxidation in injured spinal cord: partial protection with methylprednisolone or vitamin E and selenium. **Cent Nerv Syst Trauma 2:** 257-267, 1985
3. AP Wire Service: Spine Treatment to Be Publicized. **The New York Times.** New York, NY, 1990, p A21
4. Benzel EC, Larson SJ: Functional recovery after decompressive spine operation for cervical spine fractures. **Neurosurgery 20:**742-746, 1987
5. Bracken MB: Methylprednisolone in the management of acute spinal cord injuries. **Med J Aust 153:** 368, 1990 (Letter)
6. Bracken MB: **Pharmacological Interventions for Acute Spinal Cord Injury, Vol 1999.** The Cochrane Library, Cochrane Reviews, 1999
7. Bracken MB: Pharmacological treatment of acute

spinal cord injury: current status and future projects. **J Emerg Med 11 (Suppl 1)**:43-48, 1993

8. Bracken MB: Steroids after spinal cord injury. **Lancet 336**:279-280, 1990

9. Bracken MB: Treatment of acute spinal cord injury with methylprednisolone: results of a multicenter, randomized clinical trial. **J Neurotrauma 8 (Suppl 1)**: S47-S52, 1991

10. Bracken MB, Collins WF, Freeman DF, et al: Efficacy of methylprednisolone in acute spinal cord injury. **JAMA 251**:45-52, 1984

11. Bracken MB, Holford TR: Effects of timing of methylprednisolone or naloxone administration on recovery of segmental and long-tract neurological function in NASCIS 2. **J Neurosurg 79**:500-507, 1993

12. Bracken MB, Shepard MJ, Collins WF Jr, et al: Methyl prednisolone or naloxone treatment after acute spinal cord injury: 1-year follow-up data. Results of the second National Acute Spinal Cord Injury Study. **J Neurosurg 76**:23-31, 1992

13. Bracken MB, Shepard MJ, Collins WF Jr, et al: A randomized, controlled trial of methylprednisolone or naloxone in the treatment of acute spinal cord injury. Results of the Second National Acute Spinal Cord Injury Study. **N Engl J Med 322**:1405-1411, 1990

14. Bracken MB, Shepard MJ, Hellenbrand KG, et al: Methylprednisolone and neurological function 1 year after spinal cord injury. Results of the National Acute Spinal Cord Injury Study. **J Neurosurg 63**:704-713, 1985

15. Bracken MB, Shepard MJ, Holford TR, et al: Administration of methylprednisolone for 24 or 48 hours or tirilazad mesylate for 48 hours in the treatment of acute spinal cord injury. Results of the third National Acute Spinal Cord Injury randomized controlled trial. National Acute Spinal Cord Injury Study. **JAMA 277**:1597-1604, 1997

16. Bracken MB, Shepard MJ, Holford TR, et al: Methylprednisolone or tirilazad mesylate administration after acute spinal cord injury: 1-year follow up. Results of the third National Acute Spinal Cord Injury randomized controlled trial. **J Neurosurg 89**: 699-706, 1998

17. Braughler JM, Hall ED: Lactate and pyruvate metabolism in injured cat spinal cord before and after a single large intravenous dose of methylprednisolone. **J Neurosurg 59**:256-261, 1983

18. Ceccareli B, Aporti F, Finesso M: Effects of brain gangliosides in functional recovery in experimental regeneration and reinnervation, in Porcellati G, Ceccarelli B, Tettamanti G (eds): **Advances in Experimental Medicine and Biology.** New York, NY: Plenum Press, 1976

19. Cook L, Rowan C: **The Results of a Controlled Multicenter Clinical Trial in the Treatment of Spinal Cord Injury.** Bethesda, Md: National Institute of Neurological Disorders and Stroke (www.ninds.nih.gov), 1990

20. Cook L, Rowan C, Shaffer S: **National Acute Spinal Cord Injury Study.** Bethesda, Md: National Institute of Neurological Disorders and Stroke (www.ninds.nih.gov), 1990

21. Di Gregorio F, Ferrari G, Marini P, et al: The influence of gangliosides on neurite growth and regeneration. **Neuropediatrics 15**:93-96, 1984

22. Ducker TB: Medical treatment in spinal cord injuries. **J Spinal Disord 9**:381, 1996 (Editorial)

23. Ducker TB, Zeidman SM: Spinal cord injury. Role of steroid therapy. **Spine 19**:2281-2287, 1994

24. Epstein N, Hood DC, Ransohoff J: Gastrointestinal bleeding in patients with spinal cord trauma. Effects of steroids, cimetidine, and mini-dose heparin. **J Neurosurg 54**:16-20, 1981

25. Faden AI, Jacobs TP, Holaday JW: Endorphins in experimental spinal injury: therapeutic effect of naloxone. **Ann Neurol 10**:326-332, 1981

26. Faden AI, Jacobs TP, Holaday JW: Opiate antagonist improves neurological recovery after spinal injury. **Science 211**:493-494, 1981

27. Faden AI, Jacobs TP, Smith MT: Thyrotropin-releasing hormone in experimental spinal injury: dose response and late treatment. **Neurology 34:** 1280-1284, 1984

28. Faden AI, Salzman S: Pharmacological strategies in CNS trauma. **Trends Pharmacol Sci 13**:29-35, 1992

29. Faden Al, Yum SW, Lemke M, et al: Effects of TRH-analog treatment on tissue cations, phospholipids and energy metabolism after spinal cord injury. **J Pharmacol Exp Ther 255**:608-614, 1990

30. Frankel HL, Hancock DO, Hyslop G, et al: The value of postural reduction in the initial management of closed injuries of the spine with paraplegia and tetraplegia. **Paraplegia 7**:179-192, 1969

31. Galandiuk S, Raque G, Appel S, et al: The two-edged sword of large-dose steroids for spinal cord trauma. **Ann Surg 218**:419-427, 1993

32. Geisler F: Past and current human spinal cord injury drug trails, in Benzel EC, Tator CH (eds): **Contemporary Management of Spinal Cord Injury.** Park Ridge, Ill: American Association of Neurological Surgeons, 1995, pp 261-268

33. Geisler FH: Acute management of cervical spinal cord injury. **Md Med J 37**:525-530, 1988

34. Geisler FH: Clinical trials of pharmacotherapy for spinal cord injury. **Ann NY Acad Sci 845**:374-381, 1998

35. Geisler FH: GM-1 ganglioside and motor recovery following human spinal cord injury. **J Emerg Med 11 (Suppl 1)**:49-55, 1993

36. Geisler FH: GM-1 ganglioside in human spinal cord injury. **J Neurotrauma 9 (Suppl 2)**:S517-S530, 1992

37. Geisler FH, Dorsey FC, Coleman WP: Correction: recovery of motor function after spinal-cord injury—a randomized, placebo-controlled trial with GM-1 ganglioside. **N Engl J Med:325**:1659-1660, 1991 (Letter)

38. Geisler FH, Dorsey FC, Coleman WP: GM-1 ganglioside in human spinal cord injury. **J Neurotrauma 9 (Suppl 1)**:S407-S416, 1992

39. Geisler FH, Dorsey FC, Coleman WP: Past and current clinical studies with GM-1 ganglioside in acute spinal cord injury. **Ann Emerg Med 22**:1041-1047, 1993

40. Geisler FH, Dorsey FC, Coleman WP: Recovery of motor function after spinal-cord injury—a randomized, placebo-controlled trial with GM-1 ganglioside. **N Engl J Med 324**:1829-1838, 1991

41. Geisler FH, Dorsey FC, Patarnello F, et al: SYGEN Acute Spinal Cord Injury Study. **Neurotrauma 15:** 868, 1998 (Abstract)

42. George ER, Scholten DJ, Buechler CM, et al: Failure of methylprednisolone to improve the outcome of spinal cord injuries. **Am Surg 61**:659-664, 1995

43. Gerndt SJ, Rodriguez JL, Pawlik JW, et al: Conse-

quences of high-dose steroid therapy for acute spinal cord injury. **J Trauma** 42:279-284, 1997

44. Gorio A: Gangliosides as a possible treatment affecting neuronal repair processes. **Adv Neurol 47:** 523-530, 1988

45. Gorio A: Ganglioside enhancement of neuronal differentiation, plasticity, and repair. **CRC Crit Rev Clin Neurobiol 2:**241-296, 1986

46. Gorio A, Ferrari G, Fusco M, et al: Gangliosides and their effects on rearranging peripheral and central neural pathways. **Cent Nerv Syst Trauma 1:**29-37, 1984

47. Hall ED: Inhibition of lipid peroxidation in CNS trauma. **J Neurotrauma 8 (Suppl 1):**S31-S41, 1991

48. Hall ED: The neuroprotective pharmacology of methylprednisolone. **J Neurosurg 76:**13-22, 1992

49. Hall ED, Braughler JM: Glucocorticoid mechanisms in acute spinal cord injury: a review and therapeutic rationale. **Surg Neurol 18:**320-327, 1982

50. Hall ED, Wolf DIL, Braughler JM: Effects of a single large dose of methylprednisolone sodium succinate on experimental posttraumatic spinal cord ischemia. Dose-response and time-action analysis. **J Neurosurg 61:** 124-130, 1984

51. Hanigan WC, Anderson RJ: Commentary on NASCIS-2. **J Spinal Disord 5:**125-133, 1992

52. Hardy R: Commentary on spinal cord injury: role of steroid therapy. **Neurosurgery Q 6:**71-72, 1996

53. Helms D: New Hope for Spinal Injuries. **Newsweek.** Chicago, 1990, p 50

54. Kotulak R: Drug Reduces Paralysis from Spinal Injuries. **Chicago Tribune.** Chicago, 1990, p 1

55. Larsen N, Clipper S: **Prolonged Treatment with Methylprednisolone Improves Recovery in Spinal Cord Injured Patients.** Bethesda, Md: National Institute of Neurological Disorders and Stroke, National Institutes of Health (www.ninds.nih.gov), 1997

56. Leary W: Delay Seen In Publicizing Spinal Drug. **The New York Times.** New York, NY, 1990, p C5

57. Leary W: Treatment Is Said to Reduce Disability From Spinal Injury. **The New York Times.** New York, NY, 1990, pp 1 and 26

58. Ledeen RW: Biology of gangliosides: neurotigenic and neuronotrophic properties. **J Neurosci Res 12:** 147-159, 1984

59. Ledeen RW: Ganglioside structures and distribution: Are they localized at the nerve ending? **J Supramol Struct 8:**1-17, 1978

60. Levy ML, Gans W, Wijesinghe HS, et al: Use of methylprednisolone as an adjunct in the management of patients with penetrating spinal cord injury: outcome analysis. **Neurosurgery 39:**1141-1149, 1996

61. Means ED, Anderson DK, Waters TR, et al: Effect of methylprednisolone in compression trauma to the feline spinal cord. **J Neurosurg 55:**200-208, 1981

62. National New York Times: Spine Treatment to Be Publicized. **The New York Times National.** Washington, DC, 1990, p A21

63. Nesathurai S: Steroids and spinal cord injury: revisiting the NASCIS 2 and NASCIS 3 trials. **J Trauma 45:** 1088-1093, 1998

64. Otani K, AH, Kadoya S, et al: Beneficial effect of methylprednisolone sodium succinate in the treatment of acute spinal cord injury. **Sekitsui Sekizui J 7:** 633-647, 1994

65. Petitjean ME, Pointillart V, Dixmerias F, et al: [Medical treatment of spinal cord injury in the acute stage]. **Ann Fr Anesth Reanim 17:**114-122, 1998 (Fr)

66. Pitts LH, Ross A, Chase GA, et al: Treatment with thyrotropin-releasing hormone (TRH) in patients with traumatic spinal cord injuries. **J Neurotrauma 12:** 235-243, 1995

67. Prendergast MR, Saxe JM, Ledgerwood AM, et al: Massive steroids do not reduce the zone of injury after penetrating spinal cord injury. **J Trauma 37:** 576-580, 1994

68. Rosner MJ: Methylprednisolone for spinal cord injury. **J Neurosurg 77:**324-327, 1992 (Letter)

69. Rosner MJ: National acute spinal cord injury study of methylprednisolone or naloxone. **Neurosurgery 28:** 628-629, 1991 (Letter)

70. Rosner MJ: Treatment of spinal cord injury. **J Neurosurg 80:**954-955, 1994 (Letter)

71. Sabel B: Anatomic mechanisms whereby gangliosides induce brain repair: what do we really know, in Stein D, Sabel B (eds): **Pharmacological Approaches to the Treatment of Brain & Spinal Cord Injury.** New York, NY: Plenum Press, 1988

72. Sabel BA, DelMastro R, Dunbar GL: Reduction of anterograde degeneration in brain damaged rats by GM1-gangliosides. **Neurosci Lett 77:**360-366, 1987

73. Sabel BA, Dunbar GL, Stein DG: Gangliosides minimize behavioral deficits and enhance structural repair after brain injury. **J Neurosci Res 12:**429-443, 1984

74. Sabel BA, Slavin MD, Stein DG: GM1 ganglioside treatment facilitates behavioral recovery from bilateral brain damage. **Science 225:**340-342, 1984

75. Sabel BA, Stein DG: Pharmacological treatment of central nervous system injury. **Nature 323:**493, 1986

76. Shapiro SA: Methylprednisolone for spinal cord injury. **J Neurosurg 77:**324-327, 1992 (Letter)

77. Tator C, Fehlings M: Review of clinical trials of neuroprotection in acute spinal cord injury, **Neurosurg Focus 6(1),** American Association of Neurological Surgeons, 1999

78. Taylor TK, Ryan MD: Methylprednisolone in the management of acute spinal cord injuries. **Med J Aust 153:**307-308, 1990 (Letter)

79. Toffano G, Savoini G, Aldinio C, et al: Effects of gangliosides on the functional recovery of damaged brain. **Adv Exp Med Biol 174:**475-488, 1984

80. Walker MD: Acute spinal-cord injury. **N Engl J Med 324:** 1885-1887, 1991

81. Walker MD: New Treatment for Acute Spinal Cord Injury Bethesda, Md: National Institute of Neurological Disorders and Stroke (www.ninds.nih.gov), 1990

82. Warren M, Oliver N, Thomas A: Curing Paralysis: A Total NIH Research Effort. Bethesda, Md: National Institutes of Health (www.ninds.nih.gov), 1996

83. Weiss R: Drug reduces paralysis after spinal injury, **Science News of the Week137:**212, 1990

84. Young W: Blood flow, metabolic and neurophysiological mechanisms in spinal cord injury, in Becker D, Povlishock J (eds): **Central Nervous System Trauma Status Report.** Rockville, Md: National Institutes of Health, 1985, pp 463-573

85. Young W: Recovery mechanisms in spinal cord injury; implications for regenerative therapy, in Seil FJ (ed): **Neural Regeneration and Transplantation.** New York, NY: Alan R Liss, 1989, pp 157-169

HOME STUDY EXAMINATION FOR

*Contemporary Management of Spinal Cord Injury: From Impact to Rehabilitation**

CHAPTER 1

THE CONTRIBUTIONS OF ALLEN, RIDDOCH, AND GUTTMAN TO THE HISTORY OF SPINAL CORD INJURY:

Match each of items 1 through 10 to a related item in A through J.

1. Described spinal cord injury (SCI) as an illness not to be treated.
2. Demonstrated spinal reflexes in humans.
3. Described first operative laminectomy.
4. A neurosurgeon famous for noninvasive treatment of SCI.
5. Developed an SCI center at Stoke Mandeville Hospital.
6. Devised a reproducible SCI animal model.
7. The first to markedly decrease the early mortality of traumatic paraplegia.
8. Hypothesized that a secondary injury was caused by the retraction of the spinal cord to injury.
9. Demonstrated that myelotomy could improve function in an animal model.
10. Performed myelotomy in a patient with SCI.

  (A) George Riddoch
  (B) Ludwig Guttmann
  (C) Edwin Smith Papyrus.
  (D) Reginald Alfred Allen
  (E) Hippocrates
  (F) Vidus Vidius
  (G) Paulus of Aegena
  (H) William J. Mixter
  (I) Head and Riddoch
  (J) Charles Frazier

CHAPTER 3

EPIDEMIOLOGY AND GENERAL CHARACTERISTICS OF THE SPINAL CORD INJURED-PATIENT

1. The incidence of complete SCI is declining. This may be attributed to all of the following *except:*
(A) the increasing use of seat belts.
(B) the increasing use of air bags.
(C) the increasing use of child restraint systems.
(D) the use of gangliosides to manage SCI.

2. Regarding the type of spinal column injury and its affect on severity of SCI, which of the following is *false?*
(A) Thoracic injuries have a higher incidence of complete myelopathy than cervical injuries.
(B) Anterior dislocations and fracture dislocations have a higher percentage of complete myelopathy than compression fractures or burst fractures.
(C) With complete injuries, neurological recovery is greater with thoracic and lumbar fractures than with cervical injuries.
(D) In patients with complete myelopathy, the likelihood of neurological recovery is approximately the same as in cervical and thoracic injuries.

---

* Answers to questions are on page 365. To apply for Category 1 Continuing Medical Education credits, see instructions in the front of this book or on the evaluation card enclosed with this book.

3. Which of the following is *false?*
   (A) There is high morbidity associated with non-neurological associated injuries.
   (B) Motor-vehicle accidents are the most common cause of isolated SCI associated with multiple trauma.
   (C) There is no alteration of mortality in patients with SCI who also have incurred multiple trauma.
   (D) SCIs in multiple trauma patients are more severe than in those with isolated SCI.

CHAPTER 4

CLINICAL MANIFESTATION OF ACUTE SPINAL CORD INJURY

1. Which of the following is a combined spinal cord and cauda equina injury?
   (A) central cord syndrome
   (B) anterior cord syndrome
   (C) cauda equina syndrome
   (D) conus medullaris syndrome

2. SCIWORA:
   (A) is most common in young adulthood.
   (B) produces the clinical findings of the anterior spinal artery syndrome.
   (C) is commonly associated with penetrating injuries.
   (D) is a very common syndrome.

3. In patients with impaired consciousness and a high level of suspicion for SCIs, which of the following is not a diagnostic clue for the presence of an SCI?
   (A) hypotension
   (B) paradoxical respiration
   (C) the absence of priapism
   (D) Horner's syndrome

CHAPTER 5

CELLULAR, IONIC, AND BIOMOLECULAR MECHANISMS OF THE INJURY PROCESS

1. A free radical is:
   (A) an antioxidant.
   (B) a wild one from a past generation.
   (C) a form of superoxide dismutase.
   (D) a molecule with a free electron in an outer orbital.
   (E) none of the above

2. Superoxide dismutase converts:
   (A) hydrogen peroxide to water and oxygen.
   (B) oxygen to superoxide.
   (C) superoxide to hydrogen peroxide.
   (D) superoxide to water.
   (E) hydrogen peroxide to hydroxyl radicals.
   (F) none of the above

3. Intracellular calcium ionic activity is normally closest to:
   (A) 0.0005 mM.
   (B) 0.005 mM.
   (C) 0.05 mM.
   (D) 0.5 mM.
   (E) 5.0 mM.
   (F) 50.0 mM.

4. Cyclo-oxygenase converts arachidonate to:
   (A) glutathione.
   (B) prostaglandin.
   (C) leukotriene.
   (D) nitric oxide.
   (E) xanthine.
   (F) none of the above

5. Opiate receptor blockers include:
   (A) naloxone.
   (B) nalmefene.
   (C) nor-binaltorphimine.
   (D) dynorphin.
   (E) naltrexone.
   (F) none of the above

6. Excessive calcium entry into axons:
   (A) closes membrane potassium channels.
   (B) blocks phospholipase activity.
   (C) inhibits lipid peroxidation.
   (D) reduces protease activity.
   (E) decreases phosphatase activity.
   (F) none of the above

7. The recommended dose of methylpred-
   nisolone for a 65-kg person with acute SCI
   (<8 hours) is approximately:
   (A) 10 mg per day.
   (B) 100 mg per day.
   (C) 1,000 mg per day.
   (D) 10,000 mg per day.
   (E) 100,000 mg per day.
   (F) none of the above

8. High-dose methylprednisolone should be
   considered for acute SCI if the patient is
   within:
   (A) 1 hour after injury.
   (B) 2 hours after injury.
   (C) 4 hours after injury.
   (D) 8 hours after injury.
   (E) 16 hours after injury.
   (F) none of the above

9. NMDA receptors are activated by:
   (A) glutamate.
   (B) norepinephrine.
   (C) serotonin.
   (D) acetylcholine.
   (E) GABA.
   (F) none of the above

10. The following has not been or is not being
    tested in clinical trials of SCI:
    (A) methylprednisolone sodium succinate.
    (B) naloxone.
    (C) GM-1 (monosialic ganglioside).
    (D) tirilazad mesylate.
    (E) superoxide dismutase.
    (F) none of the above

CHAPTER 7

RESUSCITATION AND EARLY MEDICAL MANAGEMENT OF THE SPINAL CORD INJURY PATIENT

1. The optimal position in which a victim
   with a suspected cervical spine injury is
   kept at the scene of the accident in prepara-
   tion for transport to a health care facility is:
   (A) the prone position.
   (B) supine with the head turned to the side.
   (C) supine with "eyes forward" position.
   (D) the lateral decubitus position.

2. The preferred method for maintaining an
   airway in a patient with suspected cervical
   spine injury and upper airway obstruction is:
   (A) needle cricothyroidectomy.
   (B) surgical cricothyroidectomy.
   (C) tracheostomy.
   (D) nasotracheal intubation with manual
       in-line immobilization of the neck.

3. Ventilation in a spine-injured patient may
   be compromised by associated:
   (A) open pneumothorax.
   (B) flail chest.
   (C) tension pneumothorax.
   (D) paralysis of the diaphragm.
   (E) all of the above

4. The most common cause of cardiorespira-
   tory failure in an SCI patient is:
   (A) severe systemic sepsis.
   (B) air embolism.
   (C) fat embolism.
   (D) hypovolemic shock.

5. The hallmarks of neurogenic shock are
   hypotension with:
   (A) tachycardia.
   (B) bradycardia.
   (C) tachypnea.
   (D) hyperpyrexia.

6. Initial management of a patient in neurogenic shock should include:
    (A) Trendelenburg position.
    (B) dopamine.
    (C) fluids.
    (D) elastic stockings.
    (E) all of the above

7. The return of bulbocavernosus reflex in a completely paraplegic individual implies that:
    (A) the patient has a functional disorder.
    (B) the patient is not longer in spinal shock and the spinal cord is probably transected.
    (C) there is good potential for recovery of all neurological function.
    (D) there is selective impairment of the autonomic nervous system.

8. Major classes of pharmacological agents that may offer potential neural protection in SCI patients are:
    (A) antioxidants.
    (B) opiate receptor antagonists.
    (C) neurotransmitter receptor blockers.
    (D) anti-inflammatory agents.
    (E) all of the above

9. The inspiratory mode on a ventilator that delivers a preset volume in synchrony with the patient's respiratory effort of waiting for preset negative inspiratory force before delivering the volume is designated:
    (A) control mode.
    (B) assist/control mode.
    (C) intermittent mandatory ventilation.
    (D) synchronized intermittent mandatory ventilation.

CHAPTER 8

IMAGING OF SPINAL CORD INJURY

1. What is the initial investigation of choice in acute spinal injuries?
    (A) plain films
    (B) CT scan
    (C) tomography
    (D) MRI

2. What type of injury is CT best at identifying?
    (A) ligamentous injury
    (B) horizontally oriented fractures
    (C) vertically oriented fractures
    (D) spinal cord parenchymal injuries

3. Which of the following is correct regarding MRI?
    (A) It is the only imaging modality capable of directly imaging the spinal cord parenchyma
    (B) It is relatively insensitive in detecting cortical fractures
    (C) It is poor at identifying ligamentous injuries
    (D) only A and B
    (E) all of the above

4. Which of the following is correct concerning T1-weighted MRIs?
    (A) CSF appears bright on these images.
    (B) They generally give the best anatomic detail.
    (C) Edema is acute spinal injuries is best seen on these images.
    (D) only A and B
    (E) all of the above

5. Disadvantages of MRI in trauma include:
    (A) substances with ferromagnetic properties (such as some bullets).
    (B) the patient must remain still for at least several minutes during MRI.
    (C) MRI may underestimate ossification of the posterior longitudinal ligament.
    (D) only A and B
    (E) all of the above

6. The normal distance between the air column in the trachea and the anterior margin of the vertebral body at C2 in the adult is:
   (A) less than 7 mm.
   (B) greater than 7 mm.
   (C) less than 22 mm.
   (D) greater than 22 mm.

7. Jefferson's fractures:
   (A) involve the ring of the atlas.
   (B) are best visualized on lateral plain films.
   (C) are caused by hyperextension.
   (D) only A and B
   (E) all of the above

8. Bilateral facet dislocations:
   (A) are rarely associated with SCI.
   (B) are visualized by the classic appearance of the "bow tie" sign on plain films associated with this injury.
   (C) are associated with 50% or greater subluxation at the involved level.
   (D) are rarely associated with disc herniation.

9. Cervical lamina fractures:
   (A) usually occur in the lower cervical spine.
   (B) are often seen in older patients.
   (C) are best seen on anteroposterior plain film radiographs.
   (D) only A and B
   (E) all of the above

10. Radiological signs that correlate with potential spinal injury include all of the following *except:*
    (A) focal widening of the facet joints.
    (B) focal widening of the interspinous distances.
    (C) vertebral displacement greater than 1.5 mm.

(D) disruption of the posterior vertebral line.

CHAPTER 9

IMMOBILIZATION AND TRACTION

1. Regarding halo ring placement, which of the following is *not true?*
   (A) The ring should be fitted to allow approximately 1 inch of skull clearance.
   (B) Pin tightening may require intravenous sedation.
   (C) The frontal pins should be placed in line with or medial to the supraorbital notch.
   (D) The frontal pin torque in an adult should be 6 to 8 pounds.

2. The most frequent problem associated with the halo is:
   (A) loss of spinal alignment.
   (B) pin injection.
   (C) cerebrospinal fluid leakage.
   (D) pin breakage.

3. Regarding spinal traction, all of the following are true *except:*
   (A) The timing for spinal realignment is controversial.
   (B) Rapid spinal realignment by traction may be associated with improved neurological outcome.
   (C) More weight may be applied when using a halo ring for traction than when using Gardner-Wells tongs.
   (D) Five pounds of traction per injured spinal level is the generally applied clinical guideline.

4. Traction is contraindicated with: I) hangman's fractures; II) atlanto-occipital dislocation; III) facet dislocations; or IV) ankylosing spondylitis complicated by fracture.
   (A) I and III only.

(B) II and IV only.
(C) I, II, and III only.
(D) IV only.

5. Adjunctive measures to traction in achieving alignment include all of the following *except:*
   (A) muscle relaxants.
   (B) altering the angle of traction.
   (C) reverse Trendelenburg position.
   (D) weight in excess of 80 lb.

6. Contraindications for the use of a Stryker frame include:
   (A) midcervical fracture dislocation.
   (B) associated head and spinal cord injury.
   (C) significant pre-existing pulmonary problems.
   (D) lumbar fracture.

7. Documented neurological deterioration after SCI has occurred in all of the following situation *except:*
   (A) Roto bed rotation.
   (B) halo placement.
   (C) surgical intervention.
   (D) CT scanning.

8. Cervical manipulation is:
   (A) preferred to traction as the means of realignment of facet dislocations.
   (B) best undertaken with fluoroscopic monitoring.
   (C) indicated prior to attempting traction for fracture/dislocation.
   (D) not associated with any significant risk of neurological deterioration.

CHAPTER 10

ANESTHESIA AND CRITICAL CARE MANAGEMENT OF SPINAL CORD INJURY

1. Which one of the following muscle relaxants act by depolarization of the neuromuscular junction?
   (A) curare
   (B) atracurium

(C) succinylcholine
(D) mivacurium
(E) all of the above

2. Which of the following statements is *true* concerning succinylcholine?
   (A) It may be safely used at about 1 week following SCI.
   (B) The principal risk of its use in the SCI patient is sudden hypokalemia.
   (C) The use of this agent infrequently results in apnea.
   (D) This agent has a rapid onset and short half life.

3. The intubation method of choice in the SCI patient requiring emergency intubation is:
   (A) oral intubation with manual in-line traction.
   (B) blind nasotracheal intubation.
   (C) fiberoptic nasotracheal intubation.
   (D) tracheotomy.

4. The agent with the greatest alpha 1 adrenergic activity is:
   (A) phenylephrine.
   (B) ephedrine.
   (C) dobutamine.
   (D) isoproterenol.

5. Regarding the laryngeal mask airway, which one of the following statements is *true?*
   (A) It may be used in the awake patient.
   (B) It protects against the aspiration of gastric contents.
   (C) It must be inserted under direct vision.
   (D) It is possible to deliver 25 cm of water positive pressure with this device.

6. Regarding ventilation in the quadriplegic patient, which one of the following statements is *true?*
   (A) Vital capacity is greater in the supine than in the upright position.
   (B) The use of an abdominal binder can increase the vital capacity in the upright position.
   (C) The large percentage of patients with an injury level at C4 or below should be able to be weaned from ventilatory sup-

port.
(D) Vital capacity eventually returns to 60% of the baseline predicted value.
(E) all of the above

7. To calculate the systemic vascular resistance, all of the following are needed *except:*
(A) mean arterial pressure.
(B) central venous pressure.
(C) pulmonary artery wedge pressure.
(D) cardiac output.

CHAPTER 11

PATIENT SELECTION AND TIMING OF SURGICAL INTERVENTION

1. Regarding the management of acute spinal cord injury, which of the following is *true?*
(A) Traction reduction is rarely associated with increased neurological deficit.
(B) There is no evidence that pharmacological support of mean arterial pressure in the presence of spinal shock affects outcome after spinal cord injury.
(C) Patients with intramedullary hemorrhage have a poor prognosis for neurological recovery.
(D) Early surgery is associated with an increased incidence of complications.

2. Which is the following is *true?*
(A) The small incidence of acute disc herniation associated with acute spinal cord injury does not justify magnetic resonance imaging or computed tomography myelography in all patients.
(B) There is no meaningful difference among "primary" injuries that appear clinically complete.
(C) Methylprednisolone influences the recovery of nerve roots but not long tracts.

(D) Surgical studies have shown that the time limit for effective decompression after spinal cord injury is 8 hours.
(E) none of the above

3. Which is the following is *true?*
(A) Central cord injury is a contraindication to surgical intervention.
(B) There is no evidence that surgical decompression can influence the incidence of chronic deterioration after central cord injury.
(C) Hand-held myometry is less sensitive to changes in motor function than American Spinal Injury Association (ASIA) grading.
(D) Small prospective studies are particularly vulnerable to type II errors.
(E) Neurological recovery cannot be expected if decompression is delayed for more than 1 month.

CHAPTER 12

SURGICAL TECHNIQUES: CRANIOCERVICAL JUNCTION

1. Which of the following are suitable fixation techniques when the posterior arch of the atlas is disrupted?
(A) Gallie fusion.
(B) C1-2 lateral mass screw fixation.
(C) Brooks fusion.
(D) Halifax clamp fixation.

2. Concerning MRI, which one of the following is *true?*
(A) Imaging is contraindicated with titanium implants.
(B) Only views in the anatomical position are obtained.
(C) Bony injury is better defined than with CT.
(D) MRI is useful in demonstrating contusion of the neuraxis.

3. Concerning craniocervical junction trauma, which of the following is *true?*
(A) Atlanto-occipital injuries often require 20 kg of skull traction for reduction.

    (B) Internal fixation is always required.

    (C) Soft-tissue injury is seldom significant.

    (D) Methods of internal fixation may immobilize uninjured segments.

4. Concerning C1-2 lateral mass screw fixation, which of the following is *true?*
   - (A) Brooks fusion has been shown to be more mechanically stable.
   - (B) Atlantoaxial subluxation must be reduced preoperatively.
   - (C) Integrity of the lateral masses is unnecessary.
   - (D) Fixation may be used in conjunction with Gallie fusion.

5. In transoral surgery:
   - (A) the base of C2 is inaccessible.
   - (B) implants are contraindicated because of the risk of infection.
   - (C) the transverse ligament may be removed in cases of odontoid fracture.
   - (D) a posterior fixation will require a second-stage procedure.

6. Regarding nonunion of craniocervical fractures, which of the following is *false?*
   - (A) May involve soft-tissue elements.
   - (B) May lead to late instability.
   - (C) Will usually correct with prolonged halo jacket immobilization.
   - (D) Is less common in the subaxial cervical spine.

7. Occipitocervical fixation using the Ransford loop:
   - (A) requires fixation down to C7.
   - (B) has shown that distraction between the occiput and C2 can be achieved.
   - (C) requires an intact C1.
   - (D) should be applied with the patient's head extended.

8. In atlantoaxial rotatory dislocation:
   - (A) closed reduction may be performed up to 1 year after injury.
   - (B) the anterior approach allows bilateral access to the lateral mass joints.
   - (C) the injury is relatively more common in adults than in children.

    (D) only one lateral mass joint may be dislocated.

CHAPTER 13

SURGICAL TECHNIQUES: CERVICAL SPINE STABILIZATION

1. Transodontoid screw fixation:
   - (A) preserves motion at C1-2.
   - (B) may best be suited for acute Type II odontoid fractures.
   - (C) may be difficult in the barrel-chested, bull neck patient.
   - (D) should be avoided in the presence of transverse ligament rupture.
   - (E) all of the above

2. Posterior spinal fixation techniques for atlantoaxial instability include:
   - (A) C1-2 transarticular screw fixation.
   - (B) a combination of wiring and bone grafting of C1 and C2.
   - (C) occiput-to-C2 fusion using plates and screws.
   - (D) Halifax clamp fixation of C1-2 lamina in the presence of intact posterior elements.
   - (E) all of the above

3. Posterior C1-2 transarticular screw fixation:
   - (A) is biomechanically superior to other fixation methods.
   - (B) avoids the need for halo bracing postoperatively.
   - (C) should be performed only after preoperative CT and/or MRI document the absence of an anomalous vertebral artery and intact C1 lateral mass and C2 pars interarticularis.
   - (D) in experienced hands, may be the optimal method for atlantoaxial fixation.
   - (E) all of the above

4. The mechanism of injury that produces unilateral and bilateral interfacetal dislocation is:
   - (A) compression-fixation.
   - (B) vertical compression.

(C) distraction-flexion.
(D) compression-extension.
(E) distraction-extension.

5. Regarding Halifax clamps, all of the following are *true* except:
    (A) it is an accepted technique for C1-2 fixation.
    (B) it has been used to achieve fixation of the mid and lower cervical spine.
    (C) it provides greater rotational stability than transarticular screw fixation.
    (D) its application requires intact posterior elements.

6. The Caspar anterior cervical plating system:
    (A) relies on bicortical screw purchase.
    (B) is a locking screw system.
    (C) is available only in stainless steel.
    (D) never requires plate bending.

7. The Morscher-Synthes anterior cervical plating system:
    (A) uses an expansile head anchor screw that locks to the plate.
    (B) uses a smaller diameter screw inserted through the plate into the expansile head, coupling the plate and anchor screw.
    (C) requires an assistant to help secure the plate during both preparation and screw placement.
    (D) cephalad screw holes are angled 12°, thereby placement in the upper cervical spine (or at the cervicothoracic junction if the plate is reversed) may be facilitated because drilling does not have to be perpendicular to the plate.
    (E) all of the above

8. The Manny-Stillerman anterior cervical device:
    (A) avoids the need to prepare and place the screw through the plate.
    (B) consists of shorter, larger diameter screws.
    (C) includes an insert screw that engages the anchor screws.
    (D) uses a drill guide that is secured to the

spine and helps maintain coronal plane orientation.
    (E) all of the above

9. The surgical management of traumatic atlantoaxial instability and unstable Type II fractures includes all of the following *except:*
    (A) occiput-to-C2 fusion.
    (B) posterior C1-2 transarticular screw fixation.
    (C) anterior transodontoid screw fixation.
    (D) wiring constructs of the posterior elements of C1 and C2.

10. C1-2 rotational stability is best provided by:
    (A) the Brooks wiring procedure.
    (B) posterior transarticular screw fixation.
    (C) Halifax interlaminar clamp fixation.
    (D) the Gallie fusion technique.

CHAPTER 14

SURGICAL TECHNIQUES: THORACIC AND LUMBAR

1. Regarding the use of the internal spinal fixation to obtain indirect spinal canal decompression, which of the following is *true?*
    (A) The patient should have less than 30% canal compromise.
    (B) The patient should have *complete* neurological injury.
    (C) The posterior longitudinal ligament should be intact.
    (D) Correction of kyphotic deformity is not necessary for satisfactory decompression.
    (E) none of the above

2. Regarding the use of laminectomy in traumatic injuries, which of the following is *not true?*
    (A) Laminectomy can further compromise spinal instability.
    (B) Neural arch fracture with posterior impingement is an accepted indication for laminectomy.
    (C) Detection of a dural tear on a CT scan frequently necessitates laminectomy for

repair.

(D) Laminectomy is rarely needed in the surgical treatment of thoracolumbar fractures.

3. Fill in the blanks with the most appropriate approach choice from below:

(A) low profile anterior fixation device

_______________.

(B) high profile anterior fixation device

_______________.

(C) T4 flexion-compression injury with a centrally located retropulsed fragment

_______________.

(D) L5 flexion-compression fracture with left L5 root dysfunction

_______________.

Choices:

(X) left-sided approach
(Y) right-sided approach
(Z) neither

CHAPTER 15

SURGICAL TECHNIQUES: LUMBOSACRAL AND SACROPELVIC FIXATION

1. Where do the common and internal iliac veins lie in relation to their corresponding arteries?
(A) lateral and anterior
(B) lateral and posterior
(C) medial and anterior
(D) medial and posterior

2. The lumbosacral junction is unique in that it has:
(A) the largest amount of flexion and extension motion in the lumbar spine.
(B) the largest amount of lateral bending in the lumbar spine.
(C) the least amount of axial rotation in the lumbar spine.
(D) all of the above

3. Regarding sacral screw placement and fixation, which of the following is *true*?
(A) Directing sacral screws medically or laterally (away from the sagittal plane) increases pull-out resistance.
(B) Bone density and quality are not related to pedicle screw pull-out strength.
(C) Sacral screws cannot be placed in the alae.
(D) There are no known risks of overpenetrating the anterior sacral cortex with a screw.

4. The location of the lumbosacral pivot point is:
(A) the anterior-most aspect of the L5-S1 intervertebral disc space.
(B) the anterior-most aspect of the L5 inferior end plate.
(C) the posterior-most aspect of the S1 superior end plate.
(D) the posterior-most aspect of the L5-S1 intervertebral disc space.

5. The medial safe zone for S1 pedicle screw placement is from the sacral promontory medially to the:
(A) internal iliac artery laterally.
(B) internal iliac vein laterally.
(C) lumbosacral trunk laterally.
(D) sacroiliac joint laterally.

6. Stress shielding can:
(A) occur when spinal instrumentation is extremely rigid.
(B) reduce the load-bearing capacity of the spine to a less than normal physiological level.
(C) lead to progressive loss of bone mineral content.
(D) lead to failure of a bony arthrodesis.
(E) all of the above

7. Pseudarthrosis rates increase in patients with:
(A) tobacco use.
(B) advantaged age.

(C) non-instrumented fusion operations.
(D) a multilevel fusion operation.
(E) all of the above

8. The unit rod:
    (A) is most often used for patients with neuromuscular scoliosis and pelvic obliquity.
    (B) has more tendency to migrate or shift than two L rods.
    (C) is ideally inserted between the cortical bone tables of the ilium and its inferior-most aspect should lie posterior to the sciatic notch.
    (D) all of the above

9. Which of the following is/are *true* regarding pelvic vascular anatomy?
    (A) The common iliac veins converse on the right side of the fourth lumbar vertebra.
    (B) The internal iliac veins lie lateral to the sacroiliac joints.
    (C) The internal iliac arteries do not have contact with the bony sacrum.
    (D) all of the above

10. Biomechanical testing has demonstrated which of the following?
    (A) Flexion constitutes the largest directional force borne by the lumbar spine under physiological conditions.
    (B) Constructs utilizing sacral pedicle screws or iliac screws usually fail at the most caudal bone-metal interface.
    (C) Constructs which utilize the ilium for fixation increase the rigidity of sacro-pelvic fixation if they project anterior to the lumbosacral pivot point.
    (D) all of the above

CHAPTER 16

PENETRATING INJURIES

1. After a spinal gunshot wound, which clinical problem is least likely?
    (A) myelopathy
    (B) nerve root injury
    (C) spinal instability

2. In which clinical situation is there most consensus on operative intervention?
    (A) complete spinal cord deficit
    (B) nerve root injury
    (C) progressive neurological deficit

3. Progress in survival after penetrating spinal cord injury is due to:
    (A) an improvement in surgical technique.
    (B) the use of steroids.
    (C) improved systemic care.

4. Complications after penetrating spinal cord injury may include:
    (A) cerebrospinal fluid fistula.
    (B) meningitis.
    (C) intraspinal hemorrhage.
    (D) all of the above

5. Stab wounds of the spine:
    (A) are more frequent than gunshot wounds.
    (B) classically result in Brown-Séquard syndrome.
    (C) have been reported most frequently in the United States.

CHAPTER 17

PEDIATRIC SPINAL CORD INJURY

1. Regarding the biomechanics and anatomy of the pediatric spine, which of the following statements is *false?*
    (A) Incomplete development of the uncinate processes allows reduces the ability of the spine to withstand extreme flexion and rotational forces.
    (B) The fulcrum of motion occurs at approximately C5-6 in young children.
    (C) Excessive sagittal motion can occur due to the geometric configuration of the vertebral bodies.
    (D) The orientation of the facets joints in young children is more horizontal which permits excessive motion.

(E) Ligaments and paraspinous muscles do not become fully supportive until puberty.

2. Regarding the pathological findings in pediatric spinal trauma, which of the following statements is *true?*
   (A) Vertebral body fractures are the most commonly seen injury in children under 8 years of age.
   (B) Epidural hematoma is rarely found.
   (C) Ligamentous injuries are not commonly seen in young children.
   (D) Fractures in young children frequently involve the growth zone of the vertebral endplates.

3. Regarding the injury patterns seen in the pediatric age group, which one of the following statements is *false?*
   (A) Injury patterns vary depending on the age of the patient
   (B) Overall, bony fractures comprise the largest single group of injuries
   (C) The syndrome of SCIWORA is more often seen in adolescent children.
   (D) Age-related differences in injury patterns are related to variations in anatomy and biomechanics of the spine.

4. Regarding neonatal spinal cord injury, which of the following statements is *true?*
   (A) Birth injuries often result in severe unrecoverable neurological dysfunction.
   (B) Neonatal spinal cord injuries are usually associated with breech presentation.
   (C) The mechanism of injury usually involves longitudinal traction coupled with hyperextension.
   (D) The cervicothoracic junction is especially vulnerable to this type of injury.
   (E) all of the above

5. All of the following are *true* statements regarding occipitoatlantal (OA) dislocation *except:*
   (A) A retropharyngeal hematoma seen on a plain lateral cervical spine radiograph may provide a clue to the diagnosis.
   (B) The true incidence of OA dislocation is higher than that recognized clinically.
   (C) Once recognized, OA dislocation should be immediately reduced with skeletal traction.
   (D) Optimum management of OA dislocation involves surgical fixation and immobilization in a halo vest as soon as possible.
   (E) OA dislocation is primarily a ligamentous rather than bony injury.

6. All of the following are *false* statements regarding atlantoaxial (AA) rotary luxation atlantoaxial *except:*
   (A) The most common cause of atlantoaxial rotary luxation is inflammatory conditions involving the upper respiratory tract and pharynx.
   (B) All cases of atlantoaxial rotary luxation require surgical fixation and stabilization.
   (C) Treatment of this condition depends on the integrity of the transverse ligament.
   (D) Neurological symptoms never occur with AA luxation.

7. Regarding axis fractures in children, which one of the following statements is *true?*
   (A) Odontoid fractures occur more commonly in young children than teenagers and adults.
   (B) Most odontoid fractures in children require surgical stabilization and fusion.
   (C) Failure to recognize and treat an odontoid fracture in a young child may lead to late atlanto-axial instability and/or os odontoideum.
   (D) In young children, odontoid fractures usually extend into the axis body (type III fracture).

8. Regarding SCIWORA, which of the following statements is *true?*
   (A) Most cases of SCIWORA involve the thoracic spine.
   (B) All children with SCIWORA present with severe neurological injury from the outset.
   (C) SCIWORA is invariably associated with

significant spinal trauma.
(D) The cervical spine is most commonly affected in cases of SCIWORA.

9. All of the following radiographic studies would be appropriate in the evaluation of a child with SCIWORA *except:*
(A) magnetic resonance imaging.
(B) polytomography.
(C) dynamic flexion and extension films.
(D) computed tomography.
(E) all of the above

10. Regarding prognosis of children with spinal cord injury, which of the following statements is *most accurate?*
(A) Children unequivocally have a better prognosis for neurological recovery than do adults with similar injuries.
(B) There is significant evidence that the spinal cord in children exhibits greater plasticity than in adults.
(C) Functional recovery is primarily related to the severity of the initial neurological injury.
(D) Prognosis is mostly related to the location and type of injury sustained.

CHAPTER 20

PREVENTION AND TREATMENT OF MEDICAL COMPLICATIONS

1. Regularly encountered problems in SCI patients during initial assessment include all of the following *except:*
(A) hypovolemia.
(B) hypoventilation.
(C) autonomic dysreflexia.
(D) bradycardia.

2. All of the following are true *except:*
(A) plethysmography is a good diagnostic test for calf deep vein thrombosis (DVT).
(B) venography is a good diagnostic test for calf DVT.
(C) Doppler ultrasound is a good diagnostic

test for proximal DVT.
(D) symptoms and signs are nonspecific in DVT.

3. Hypoxia in an SCI patient with a lesion at C6 cannot be explained by:
(A) increased bronchial secretion.
(B) loss of abdominal tone.
(C) paralysis of the external intercostal muscles.
(D) paralysis of the diaphragm.
(E) paralytic ileus.

4. Successful extubation of SCI patients is most likely:
(A) in lesions above C4.
(B) if at the time of extubation, respiration rate (RR) <40/min, $PaO_2 = 70$ mm Hg, $PaCO_2$ <50 mm Hg.
(C) if at the time of extubation, RR <40/min, $PaO_2 = 80$ mm Hg, $PaCO_2$ <50 mm Hg.
(D) if at the time of extubation, RR <30/min, $PaO_2 = 70$ mm Hg, $PaCO_2$ <50 mm Hg.

5. Recognized methods to prevent atelectasis and pneumonia are:
(A) assisted coughing whenever necessary.
(B) incentive spirometry whenever necessary.
(C) changing the patient's position every 8 hours.
(D) A and B
(E) A, B, and C

6. A diagnosis of neurogenic pulmonary edema is most often accompanied by:
(A) raised central venous pressure.
(B) raised blood pressure.
(C) raised pulmonary capillary wedge pressure.
(D) normal pulmonary capillary wedge pressure.

7. Gastrointestinal trauma in an SCI patient with a lesion at T4 can present with all of the following *except:*
(A) anorexia and nausea.
(B) hypovolemia.
(C) abdominal guarding.

(D) abdominal distention with air-fluid levels on x-ray.

(E) a negative peritoneal lavage.

8. The following agent(s) are used as a first line therapy in bowel management in SCI patients:
(A) high-fiber diet and bran.
(B) senna and bisacodyl.
(C) lactulose.
(D) enemas.

9. Nutritional requirements of SCI are complicated by:
(A) fever and sepsis.
(B) altered gastrointestinal mortality.
(C) pressure ulcers.
(D) paralysis of the respiratory muscles.
(E) all of the above

CHAPTER 21

UROLOGICAL MANAGEMENT OF THE SPINAL CORD INJURY PATIENT

1. The innervation of the detrusor muscle is:
(A) somatic via the pudendal nerves.
(B) sympathetic via the hypogastric nerves.
(C) parasympathetic via the pelvic nerves.
(D) dual, autonomic, and somatic.

2. The urethral sphincter mechanism consists of:
(A) proximal autonomic and distal somatic components.
(B) three distinct musculofascial elements.
(C) parasympathetic longitudinal and circulatory arranged slow-twitch fibers.
(D) purinergic nerve supplied fast-twitch muscle.

3. The initial urological management of the SCI patient includes:
(A) cystography for gross hematuria.
(B) a CT scan for suspected renal injury.

(C) suprapubic catheter or urethral stenting for urethral rupture.
(D) all of the above

4. During a prolonged spinal shock phase:
(A) bladder management is optimized by an indwelling catheter.
(B) intermittent characterization is associated with fewer infectious complications.
(C) bladder emptying is best achieved by the Credé method and Valsalva maneuver.
(D) bladder areflexia portends absence of long-term recovery.

5. Intermittent catheterization in the acute hospital setting:
(A) should be undertaken only by nursing.
(B) cannot be taught to patients.
(C) leads to the development of resistant uropathogens.
(D) should be a sterile procedure.

6. Recovery of bladder function after injury:
(A) never occurs within the first 6 months.
(B) should be treated with parasympathetic agonists and the Credé method.
(C) may be monitored with urodynamics and postvoid residuals.
(D) may be hastened with pharmacological manipulation.

7. Urodynamic studies:
(A) are not indicated when a balanced bladder is achieved.
(B) are always predicted by the level of injury.
(C) have largely been replaced by ultrasound for functional evaluation.
(D) provide a measurement of the relationship between the bladder and urethra.

8. Renal deterioration may be a result of :
(A) high-pressure bladder storage.
(B) high-pressure voiding.
(C) upper urinary tract infection.

(D) combinations of internal and external sphincter dyssynergia.
(E) all of the above

9. Autonomic dysreflexia is characterized by:
(A) hypertension, bradycardia, and bladder distention.
(B) hypotension, tachycardia, and bladder collapse.
(C) failure of response to prophylactic.
(D) failure of response to prophylactic calcium channel blockers.

10. Urethral obstruction in the SCI patient may be:
(A) distal sphincter dyssynergia.
(B) proximal sphincter dyssynergia.
(C) combined proximal and distal sphincter dyssynergia.
(D) treated with sphinctcrotomy.
(E) all of the above

CHAPTER 22

SPINAL ORTHOTICS

1. The goals of spine bracing include all of the following *except:*
(A) restriction of movement.
(B) spinal realignment.
(C) the elimination of segmental motion.
(D) trunk support.

2. The parallelogram-like bracing effect and snaking are most commonly observed following bracing of the:
(A) cervical spine.
(B) thoracic spine.
(C) lumbar spine.
(D) thoracolumbar junction.

3. Limited cervical bracing techniques:
(A) are more effective than cervical shoulder bracing techniques.
(B) do not substantially restrict movement in any direction.

(C) enhance the parallelogram-like bracing effect.
(D) are usually extremely uncomfortable.

4. Cervical-thoracic bracing techniques are most effective at:
(A) the occipital-C1 joint.
(B) the C1-2 joint.
(C) the C3-4 joint.
(D) the mid-to-low cervical region.

5. Which of the following is most often associated with the snaking phenomenon?
(A) the Minerva jacket
(B) soft cervical collars
(C) thoracic and thoracolumbar braces
(D) the halo vest

6. The halo apparatus can apply which of the following forces to the spine?
(A) distraction
(B) compression
(C) segmental complex forces
(D) all of the above

7. Complications of orthotics include all *except* which one of the following?
(A) pain
(B) pressure
(C) psychological dependence
(D) osteoporosis
(E) axial muscle weakness

8. The halo:
(A) provides restriction of capital flexion and extension movements.
(B) provides restriction of all segmental movement of the spine, particularly in the mid-cervical region.
(C) is least effective in the cervical-thoracic region.
(D) is associated with no significant risks.

9. The conformation of the orthosis to the torso:
(A) is of minimal importance.
(B) is important in reducing focal pressure points.
(C) is seldom associated with augmentation

of stability.
(D) does little to promote the maintenance of the cylindrical body shell.

10. The conformation and close fit between the anterior and posterior halves of the spinal brace:
(A) are unimportant.
(B) are critical for the brace to stabilize the spine.
(C) decrease the efficacy of bracing.
(D) always augment patient comfort.

CHAPTER 23

FUNDAMENTALS, TECHNIQUES, AND EXPECTATIONS OF THE REHABILITATION PROCESS

1. The most common cause of traumatic spinal cord injury in the United States is:
(A) fall.
(B) diving accident.
(C) motor vehicle crash.
(D) bullet wound.
(E) football injury.

2. The highest spinal level allowing independence in all self-care and mobility at a wheelchair level is:
(A) C2.
(B) C4.
(C) C7.
(D) T6.
(E) L3.

3. Of the following, which is the most common cause of death after spinal cord injury?
(A) pneumonia
(B) heart attack
(C) pulmonary embolus
(D) pressure ulcer
(E) renal failure

4. Spasticity unresponsive to all other measures usually responds to:
(A) dantrolene.
(B) intrathecal baclofen.
(C) botulinum toxin.
(D) diazepam.
(E) gabapentin.

5. A person admitted with spinal cord injury and an ASIA Impairment Scale grade of B has what chance of improving to an ASIA grade of D?
(A) 5%-10%
(B) 15%-20%
(C) 25%-30%
(D) 55%-60%
(E) 80%-85%

CHAPTER 24

THE SPINAL CORD INJURY UNIT IN THE NEW MILLENNIUM: A PARADIGM SHIFT

1. Which of the following is/are responsible for the increased survival rates of individuals with SCIs?
(A) advent of antibiotics
(B) development of emergency medical system
(C) advent of specialized SCI centers
(D) all of the above

2. The interdisciplinary approach to rehabilitation:
(A) is synonymous with the multidisciplinary approach.
(B) involves minimal communication between team members.
(C) requires communication, collaboration, and input from all team members.
(D) requires a strict team hierarchy.

3. The therapist responsible for evaluating and upgrading swallowing disorders is the:
(A) physical therapist.
(B) occupational therapist.
(C) speech therapist.
(D) recreation therapist.

4. The therapist primarily responsible for evaluating and upgrading feeding, dressing, bathing, and oral facial hygiene is the:
   (A) physical therapist.
   (B) occupational therapist.
   (C) speech therapist.
   (D) recreation therapist.

5. The recreation therapist:
   (A) assists the patient in developing alternative leisure activities.
   (B) educates the patient about the availability of specialized equipment and adaptive sports.
   (C) helps to integrate the patient into the community with recreational trips to shopping centers, grocery stores, and restaurants.
   (D) all of the above

6. How many hours of therapy each day must a patient must be able to participate in to be admitted to an acute rehabilitation program?
   (A) 1 hour
   (B) 2 hours
   (C) 3 hours
   (D) 4 hours

7. The average cost of acute and rehabilitation care for an individual with high-level quadriplegia is:
   (A) $200,000.
   (B) $150,000.
   (C) $100,000.
   (D) $50,000.

8. The average annual follow-up expense for an individual with high-level quadriplegia is:
   (A) $60,000.
   (B) $40,000.
   (C) $30,000.
   (D) $20,000.

9. The long-term provider of primary care for a patient with an SCI is the:
   (A) primary care physician.
   (B) neurosurgeon.
   (C) physiatrist.
   (D) A and C

10. Which category of SCI statistically has the shortest life span?
    (A) incomplete paraplegia.
    (B) complete paraplegia.
    (C) incomplete quadriplegia.
    (D) complete quadriplegia.

CHAPTER 25

PREVENTION OF SCI

1. Approximately how many SCIs occur in the United State per year?
   (A) 1,000
   (B) 10,000
   (C) 100,000
   (D) 1,000,000

2. The majority of SCI are preventable.
   (A) True
   (B) False

3. Adolescents have a higher incidence of neurological injury than other age groups because of:
   (A) increased risk-taking behavior.
   (B) poor judgment.
   (C) peer pressure.
   (D) all of the above

4. Neurological injury has been shown to be decreased by the techniques of:
   (A) automatic protection devices.
   (B) laws or rules that require a behavioral change.
   (C) changing risk-taking behavior.
   (D) all of the above

5. The major effort of the Think First program is:
   (A) to lobby the U.S. Congress for neurosurgical funding.
   (B) to research funding.
   (C) an educational program aimed at adolescents.
   (D) finding a cure for SCI.

CHAPTER 26

PAST AND CURRENT HUMAN SPINAL CORD INJURY DRUG TRIALS

1. In retrospect, the major study design deficiency of the NASCIS 1 study for interpreting the results was:
   (A) the doses of study medication.
   (B) the time of administration of the study medication.
   (C) no placebo group with which to compare the study drug group.
   (D) controlling wound infections.

2. The NASCIS 2 study:
   (A) reported improvement of neurological function between methylprednisolone and placebo with hundreds of patients in both groups.
   (B) reported a statistically significant improvement in functional outcome between the methylprednisolone and placebo treatment groups.
   (C) reported a clear definition of the degree of SCI necessary to enter the study.
   (D) was universally accepted without criticism.
   (E) none of the above

3. The GM-1 Maryland Acute Spinal Cord Injury Study:
   (A) was a small study in terms of number of patients that reported a statistically significant beneficial drug effect.
   (B) was a multicenter study design.
   (C) demonstrated that surgical intervention was beneficial to the ultimate outcome of the patients.
   (D) reported an increased complication rate in the GM-1 study group.

4. The NASCIS 3 and the Sygen Acute Spinal Cord Injury studies *both:*
   (A) have a multicenter, placebo controlled, randomized, prospective study design.
   (B) require years to collect the necessary patient numbers.
   (C) rely on statistical analysis to interpret the results of the study to determine if the recovery of the study drug group is significant larger than the expected recovery in the reference group.
   (D) all of the above

INDEX

Figures and tables are indicated by an f or t following the page.

C

Contemporary Management of Spinal Cord Injury: Impact to Rehabilitation

ANSWERS TO HOME STUDY EXAMINATION

Chapter 1
1. C   2. A   3. G   4. B   5. B
6. D   7. I   8. D   9. D   10. J

Chapter 3
1. D   2. C   3. C

Chapter 4
1. D   2. B   3. C

Chapter 5
1. D   2. C   3. A   4. B   5. D
6. F   7. D   8. D   9. A   10. E

Chapter 7
1. C   2. D   3. E   4. A   5. B
6. E   7. B   8. E   9. D

Chapter 8
1. A   2. C   3. D   4. B   5. E
6. A   7. A   8. C   9. D   10. C

Chapter 9
1. C   2. B   3. C   4. B   5. D
6. C   7. D   8. B

Chapter 10
1. C   2. D   3. A   4. A   5. D
6. E   7. C

Chapter 11
1. C   2. E   3. D

Chapter 12
1. B   2. D   3. D   4. D   5. C
6. D   7. B   8. D

Chapter 13
1. E   2. E   3. E   4. C   5. C
6. A   7. E   8. E   9. C   10. B

Chapter 14
1. C   2. C
3. A = X, B = Y, C = X, D = Z

Chapter 15
1. B   2. D   3. A   4. D   5. B
6. E   7. E   8. A   9. C   10. D

Chapter 17
1. B   2. D   3. C   4. E   5. C
6. C   7. C   8. D   9. E   10. C

Chapter 20
1. C   2. A   3. D   4. D   5. D
6. C   7. C   8. A   9. E

Chapter 21
1. C   2. A   3. E   4. B   5. D
6. C   7. D   8. E   9. A   10. E

Chapter 22
1. C   2. A   3. B   4. D   5. D
6. D   7. D   8. A   9. B   10. B

Chapter 23
1. C   2. C   3. A   4. B   5. C

Chapter 24
1. D   2. C   3. C   4. D   5. D
6. C   7. B   8. D   9. D   10. D

Chapter 25
1. B   2. A   3. D   4. D   5. C

Chapter 26
1. C   2. E   3. A   4. D

PREVIOUSLY PUBLISHED BOOKS IN THE
Neurosurgical Topics SERIES

Charles H. Tator, CM, MD, MA, PhD, FRCSC, FACS, graduated from the Faculty of Medicine, University of Toronto in 1961. After an internship at the Toronto General Hospital, he entered the School of Graduate Studies at the University of Toronto in the Division of Neuropathology and received an M.A. and a Ph.D. He then trained in neurosurgery at the University of Toronto and became a Fellow of the Royal College of Physicians and Surgeons of Canada in Neurosurgery. Dr. Tator's research career began in 1969 as Assistant Professor at the University of Toronto. In 1974 he was appointed Associate Professor, and in 1980 he was promoted to Full Professor. Dr. Tator was the Director of the Toronto Hospital Neurosciences Centre (1993-1998) and Associate Director of the Playfair Neuroscience Unit at the Toronto Hospital (1990-1999); he recently completed a 10-year term as Dan Family Professor and Chairman of Neurosurgery at the University of Toronto (1989-1999).

Since l969, Dr. Tator's principal area of research has been in spinal cord injury, with additional research in brain tumors. He is currently President of Think First Canada Penser d'Abord, an injury prevention Foundation. His research achievements include the development of experimental laboratory models of acute spinal cord injury which closely stimulate spinal cord injury in humans and new methods of injury evaluation. Using these models and outcome measures, he characterized several fundamental mechanisms of injury in the traumatized spinal cord, both experimentally and in humans. In particular, he showed with a variety of techniques that spinal cord injury causes major damage to the vessels including vasospasm and reduction in flow. At the cellular level, he has shown that injury causes profound biochemical effects in spinal cord neurons such as increased intracellular calcium. He has also demonstrated that a variety of therapeutic strategies can ameliorate some of these vascular and biochemical changes.

Currently, Dr. Tator's major research program is in regeneration of the spinal cord after trauma. His clinical research has included the development of a multidisciplinary acute spinal cord injury unit, and he showed that these units can reduce mortality, morbidity, and costs of care of patients with spinal cord injury. His research into the epidemiology and prevention of spinal cord injury has revealed a rising incidence of spinal cord injury due to sports and recreation, and the effectiveness of prevention programs.

Edward C. Benzel, MD, is Director of Spinal Disorders at the Cleveland Clinic Foundation in Cleveland, Ohio. He was previously Professor and Chief of Neurosurgery at the University of New Mexico School of Medicine. Prior to that, he was Assistant Professor and Chief of Neurosurgery at Louisiana State University at Shreveport. Dr. Benzel received a BS in Chemical Engineering at Washington State University and an MD from the Medical College of Wisconsin. He completed his residency training in neurosurgery and a fellowship in spine surgery at the Medical College of Wisconsin.

Dr. Benzel is a member of the AANS Publications Committee. He is a past president of the AANS/CNS Joint Section on Disorders of the Spine and Peripheral Nerves. His membership in professional organizations includes the National Rehabilitation Association, the American Medical Association, the Congress of Neurological Surgeons, the American Association of Neurological Surgeons, the Society of Critical Care Medicine, and the Neurotrauma Society. In addition to authoring and editing multiple books, Dr. Benzel has authored more than 40 chapters and 90 refereed manuscripts. He is a member of the editorial review board for the *Journal of Neurosurgery* and *Neurosurgery* and is an ad hoc reviewer for several other journals.

His specialty and expertise are in the areas of spinal trauma, complicated spinal disorders, peripheral nerve, trauma, and critical care.

AANS Publications Office
Lebanon, New Hampshire

Editors
Gay Palazzo
Joanne B. Needham

Compositor
Barbara Jones

Indexer
Gay Palazzo

Reference Editor
Kim DeVillers